LIFE IS MOVEMENT

THE PHYSICAL RECONSTRUCTION AND REGENERATION OF THE PEOPLE

(A DISEASELESS WORLD)

By

EUGEN SANDOW

PROFESSOR OF NATURAL THERAPEUTICS.
INSTRUCTOR IN PHYSICAL CULTURE TO H.M. THE KING.
AND AUTHOR OF "CONSTRUCTION AND RECONSTRUCTION OF THE HUMAN BODY."

Originally Published in 1920

PUBLISHED BY O'Faolain Patriot L L C, Copyright 2012

info@physicalculturebooks.com

ISBN-13: 978-1475277913

ISBN-10: 1475277911

Published in the United States of America

To Order More Copies Visit: PhysicalCultureBooks.com

The information contained in this publication is for historical and educational purposes only and is not designed to and does not provide medical, nutritional, or health advice, diagnosis, or opinion for any health or individual problem. The material presented is not a substitute for medical or other professional health services from a qualified health care provider who is familiar with the unique facts of the individual, and should not be used in place of a visit, call, consultation, or advice of a physician or other healthcare provider. Individuals should always consult a qualified health care provider about any health concern and prior to undertaking any new treatment. The publisher assumes no responsibility and specifically disclaims all liability for any consequence relating directly or indirectly to any action or inaction that a reader takes based on any information contained herein.

Be advised that no one should undertake exercises in the nature of those addressed in this book without prior consultation with a physician. Nor does the publisher make any representations concerning whether any of the exercises or suggestions provided by the trainers or physical fitness specialists featured in this book would be effective or appropriate for the reader's needs or expectations. The publisher expressly disclaims any and all responsibility and/or liabilities that might result from the uninformed or misinformed application of the techniques identified herein as well as for any unsupervised physical fitness training.

Finally, the publisher disclaims any and all liabilities arising from the use of any equipment featured in this book and makes no representations as to the utility, safety, or adequacy of the equipment generally or with respect to any specific purpose.

FOREWORD.
BY SIR ARTHUR CONAN DOYLE.

IN the course of a fairly busy literary life, in which I have essayed most things within the scope of a writer, I have never once had the experience of getting between an author and his audience by saying a few words in advance. There is an obvious impertinence in the intrusion. And yet here I find myself not only doing this very thing, but even going out of my way to volunteer for it. I can only excuse myself by my conviction of good work, the national work, which Mr Eugen Sandow has done in this country, which makes it a duty to say a word, when one can, on its behalf.

If there were any antagonism between matter and spirit the case would be very different. If it could be shown that the body developed at the expense either of the mind or of the character, then physical degeneration might be accepted as the price which the human race must pay for its mental and spiritual advance. But the facts are the very opposite. Vice and ignorance are the companions of ugliness. That which is physically beautiful stands in the main for that which is mentally sane, and spiritually sound. The classic ages of Greece, which showed the highest intellectual average seen in this world in a single population, produced also the finest physical types which the sculptor has ever committed to marble. The man who can raise the standard of physique in any country has done something to raise all other standards as well.

The strength of a nation is measured by the sum total of the strength of all the units which form it. It is a truism that anything which raises any portion of a man, his body, his character, his intelligence, increases to that extent the strength of the country to which he belongs. Therefore, since the State is so interested in these matters, it has every reason to examine into them and to regulate them. The truth is an obvious one, but it is only within our lifetime that it has been practically applied. " Parents may do what they like with their children. A man may do what he likes with himself." So ran the old heresy, which ignored the fact that the State must look after the health of its own component parts. Then came the Education Act of 1870. It was a great new departure. What it said was: " No, your mind is not your own. It belongs to the State. Therefore we must force you to keep yourself in better order." That is as far as we have got yet in State ownership of the individual. But it is evident that the same principle may be applied to the body as well as the mind.

Meanwhile Mr Eugen Sandow and his schools are doing something—as much as a great expert can do—to fill this national want. He has first arrested the attention of our public, shown it the pristine perfection of the human body, and systematised the methods by which it may be preserved. It is my appreciation of the national quality of his services, and the really vital aim towards which they have been directed, which must be my excuse if for a moment I have intruded upon the patience of his readers. It is my firm conviction that few men have done more for this country during our generation than he, and that his schools have appreciably improved our physique. Every word which he writes upon the subject deserves the most careful consideration, not only of the general public, but also of the medical faculty with whom he has always loyally worked.

ARTHUR CONAN DOYLE.

IMPORTANT NOTICE TO THE READER.
FROM THE AUTHOR.

I HAVE written this book with pleasure but not for pleasure. It is, on the other hand, a serious attempt to grapple with one of the greatest problems that has ever confronted the civilised to meet a crisis beside which the terrible blood-bath from which the world has just emerged is but a bagatelle. For it deals with the serious menace of physical deterioration and the prevention and eradication of disease, the most devastating enemy that humanity has ever had to face. Where war has killed its millions, disease has killed and is killing its tens of millions.

HUNTING DOWN DISEASE.

This book, I hope, will help to elucidate many mysteries not only to the average man and woman but even to the medical profession itself, mysteries that should not be mysterious, and which must no longer remain mysteries. It is an attempt to unravel the tangling and tangled threads of Health and Disease, to trace to its fount and origin the one true cause of disease, to reveal the one and only method of preventing or overcoming it radically and permanently, and to point out the only and natural way to attain and maintain perfect health in a disease-proof body.

It will be observed that I am, for obvious reasons, dealing with the whole question of health from the national point of view, and that, for this reason, I am advocating the methods I describe principally as a preventive of disease, because I am naturally anxious that the children should have the benefits of these methods from early childhood to fortify them against that very large percentage of disease which we now know is preventable and avoidable. "If," said the late King Edward, " disease is preventable, why not prevent it." Well, here is the way and the only way, always provided the children receive good nourishment, fresh air and other essentials of healthy growth as well.

But—and I wish those who are actually in a state of disease at present to make special note of this—although my book is mainly directed to the physical upbuilding of the children and the prevention of disease, the principle involved in preventing disease, especially in the children, applies with equal force to adults and for the cure of existing disease. My ultimate aim being the total eradication of disease, as far as that is humanly possible, it stands to reason that the methods I advocate must eliminate the mass of existent disease as the very first step towards that goal.

What I suggest should be done in the case of children for the future will be found by adults to be quite as effective in overcoming and banishing already existent disease, so that I hope every adult suffering from disease, as well as all who wish to take the best protective measures against disease, will read and ponder over the advice here given, and consider it as applying directly to themselves. This applies to disease in all its myriad and protean forms, for I contend that all disease has a common cause, and that if we can cure one disease we can cure all disease—as I am about to prove in this book we can—by the logical process of removing the common cause. So, too, we can make a normal body so strongly resistant to disease as to be intolerant of it, or, in other words, prevent all disease.

Circumstances have compelled medical men at last to realise that the prevention of disease is a far more important matter even than its cure. I have asserted that for more than a quarter of a century. Years ago I recognised, as Sir George Newman, Chief Medical Officer of the Board of

Education, now admits, that "the first line of defence is a healthy, well-nourished and resistant body," but I also discovered what even yet the doctors do not seem to fully realise that physical movements, simple and natural in themselves but scientifically applied, are the only methods we possess to build up such a body, and that this method of conquering, preventing and eliminating disease is one within the personal control of each individual to make or mar his or her body and life at will.

HEALTH FROM NATURE ONLY.

This is a solemn thought, and I make the statement with all solemnity. There is, I affirm, only one preventive against disease, viz., to make the body so strong in each of its cells, and to develop all in such equal and harmonious strength, as to make disease impossible either within the body itself or through microbic attacks from without. Just how this can be done I fully explain in these pages.

So far as I can see, the physicians are only groping blindly for some puerile and inefficient substitute because they have not yet wrested the real secret of Health from Nature. They have much, apparently, yet to learn in this direction—and, indeed, I myself, after thirty years' study of the subject, am still but a pupil—and more to unlearn before they can hope to prevent disease, while many age-long traditions must be cast aside before they succeed.

Metchnikoff was right when he called disease a " disharmony." Health, on the other hand, is harmony. A body in which every system, organ, function, and even every cell, are in harmonious balance in every part, can only be secured and maintained as a pianist obtains harmony from the keys of the piano, by the skilful and scientific use and harmonious combination of the voluntary muscles which were given us by the Creator for the express purpose of that physical movement which is the prime factor of life and health.

PATIENT AND HEALER IN PARTNERSHIP.

It is useless to condemn a people who have been, kept so long in ignorance of the most vital subject that affects their whole life and well-being, viz., a knowledge of their own body and how to maintain it in health, but when this elementary lesson is learned and a better system of health education follows, there will be much to be said in favour of the partnership, which Dr Sir George Newman advocates for the future, between the physician, the Public Health Officer and the people. Before the public can become an active partner in such a trinity, however, it must be taught something of the business of the body, or it can be nothing but a sleeping partner in a business of which it is utterly ignorant.

But before even that, medical men themselves will have discovered, as I have done, that the greatest ignorance of all is ignorance of the first law of life, the law of movement and the neglect or transgression of which means weakness or disease. The best health knowledge is the knowledge that leads to health, its attainment and maintenance, and which the people themselves must acquire to be worthy of such a partnership, and that knowledge I have attempted to supply in part, at least, in these pages in the simplest possible language, unburdened by medical camouflage, or foreign terms and phrases.

It has been my object here to clarify such health knowledge as is necessary for the possession and maintenance of a healthy and disease-free body, and to avoid the mystifying language of the regular text-book which too often affrights the sufferer, aggravates his condition by morbid fears, and sets up in his mind an attitude antagonistic to health instead of an outlook of hope.

NAMES MORE DANGEROUS THAN DISEASES.

Medical men too often employ a language descriptive of disease with which they themselves are familiar, but which is alarming and even dangerous to unsophisticated minds. The nomenclature of disease should be simplified for the sake of suffering humanity, and in this book I have studiously avoided, as far as possible, ominous words and foreign or technical expressions for more homely English words and simple illustrations, while my further object has been to create hope rather than despair in the minds of those who have wandered from the somewhat narrow and straight path of Health and Happiness.

The individual examination of school children and of recruits for our citizen army has emphasized the necessity for a system of health culture and natural physical reconstruction by really scientific methods, which, if carried out as I suggest, will check national physical deterioration and make the cure of disease unnecessary by leading to its prevention and complete eradication. If we can, in conjunction with the natural law of life, the law of movement, literally reconstruct a new body or any part of a body out of a feeble and diseased one, as I contend we can, there is no reason whatever why we should not be able to produce men and women with bodies so perfectly balanced in health and strength as to be really immune from disease in any form.

It is essential for the people to know and understand the underlying facts of health before they can hope to conquer disease and prevent it in the future. Without this knowledge it is useless for them to seek health in any other direction, and I hope the medical profession will also begin to recognize this and to apply this knowledge in what is admittedly the noblest of all human professions.

A HEALTH BOOK FOR THE PEOPLE.

For these reasons I want everyone who is in search of health to read these pages carefully and thoughtfully, as they contain health information of priceless value, which, if it will not actually be sufficient to free them from disease or prevent that condition, will at last prove a most helpful signpost to every wanderer on the highway that leads to Health. Those who are actually weak, ailing, or diseased, will find much helpful information in the later chapters of this book, especially that on "Neurasthenia," and the chapter on "How and Why Scientific Physical Movement Cures Disease."

A great world-crusade against physical decadence and disease is going to take place, and we have in our own hands the weapon to destroy these enemies altogether. "All for Health" should be the motto of us all from now forward, and I feel certain that after reading this work many will be eager to render service in this great movement for the uplifting of humanity. As I explain later, I have decided, with the assistance of distinguished patrons and workers, to form an " All-for-Health League "—what, I hope, will be a real League of Nations against Disease—to spread the gospel of physical movement as an agent—I might, indeed, call it | the agent in advance "—of Health.

The objects of the All-for-Health League are more fully set out at the close of this book, but its chief value will be that the men and women who represent it will set up a new ideal and standard in the minds of the people, and especially to the children who will be the men and women of the future and whose health and fitness will be the prime and determining factor in the nation's future. Above all, we must aim at inspiring in them a very different ideal from that which has been so sedulously instilled in the past, the desire and tendency to win a position rich in monetary rewards before the material body is physically secured to support such strenuous mental efforts and to guarantee it against disease. None of us can afford to despise money as a lubricant of the wheels of life, but we must not so lose our sense of proportion as to idolise it or let it become a Moloch to devour our children. The sound body must be a precedent to the sane and receptive mind, and the brain, which is a physical thing of tissue and blood, like the rest of the body, cannot thrive and prosper unless its physical demands are met and satisfied.

There is a great future before such a League if everyone will contribute his mite of service, however small or humble, and with the powerful support of the press which, I am glad to see, realizes the gravity of our present health position and the necessity for new and more comprehensive strategy and tactics in the war against disease and physical deterioration. I want this All-for-Health League to be the equivalent of a great international brotherhood of Free-masonry of Health, with its " lodges " or clubs everywhere throughout the world, in which men and women will rise by degrees or stages to their highest possible standard of physical and organic fitness. Such an institution and organisation will give to the world a higher and loftier ideal of humanity than ever it possessed before, and lead us away from the darkness of the past towards an ideal world in which the sun of perfect health shall rise every day, a translation, indeed, from a pain-fraught existence to something closely approximating to an earthly Paradise, in which no foul thing such as disease can longer exist.

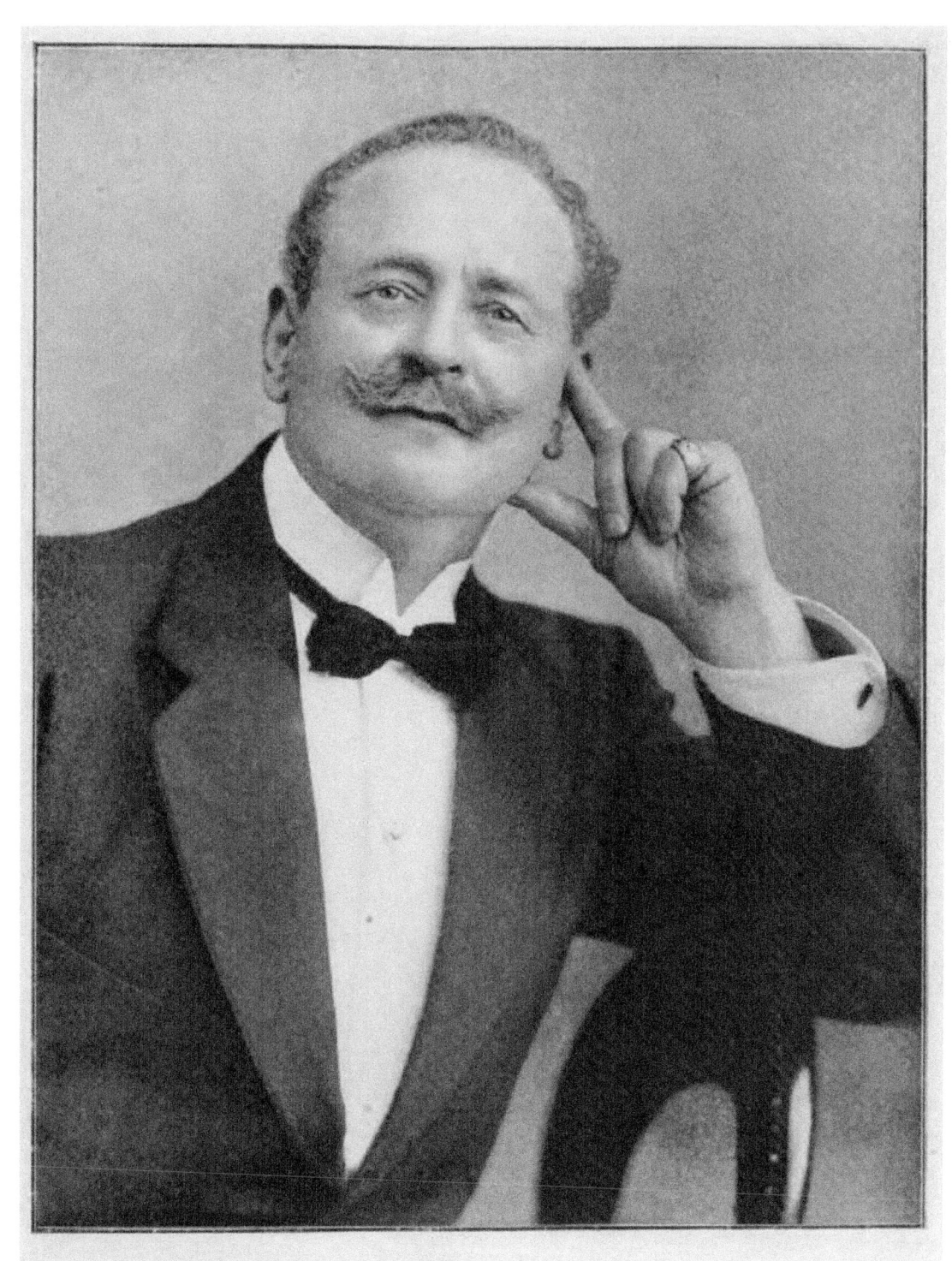

Photo by Warwick Brookes, Manchester

THE AUTHOR AS HE IS TO-DAY.

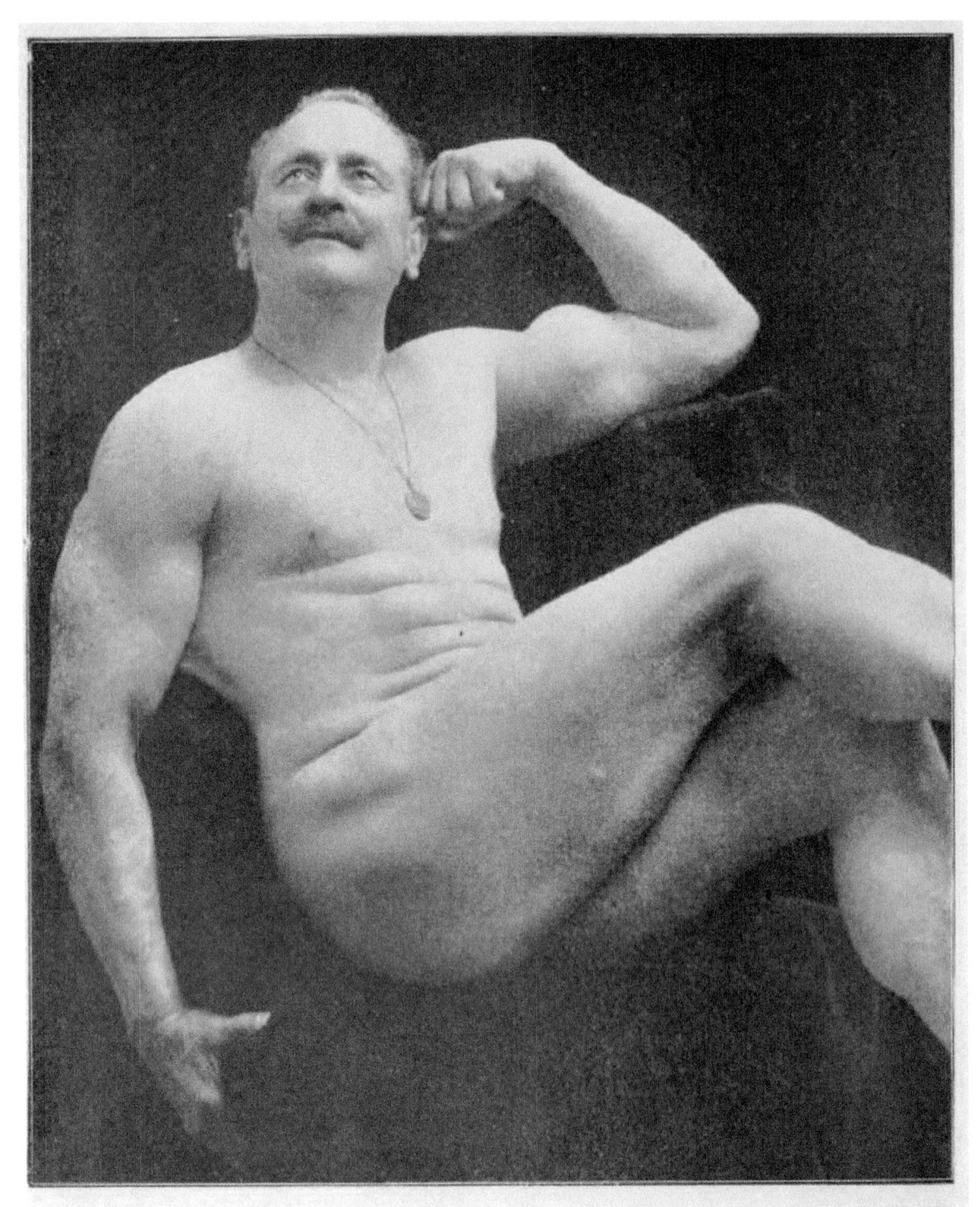

Photo by Warwick Brookes, Manchester.

POWER IN REPOSE.

Photo of the Author, showing excellence of physique at 52.

CONTENTS.

I.	Lessons the War have Taught Us	12
II.	My Grave Warning	42
III.	My World-Startling Claim—A Diseaseless World	77
IV.	The State and the Child	86
V.	The Physical Basis of all Reform	108
VI.	Life is Movement	122
VII.	The Movement that Resists and Defeats Disease	134
VIII.	What is Scientific Physical Movement?	151
IX.	The Physiology of Bodily Reconstruction.	171
X.	The Heart the Root of Remedial or Preventive Physical Culture	184
XI.	The Machinery of National Physical Training	192
XII.	A Well-Nourished Body the First Step in Education	208
XIII.	The Marvels of the Muscular System	215
XIV.	Mind, Muscle and Nerve	226
XV.	Perfect Physical and Mental Balance	236
XVI.	Man's Most Deadly Foe	244
XVII.	Medical Facts for Medical Men	255
XVIII.	The No-Medicine Medical Man of the Future	267
XIX.	The Joy of a Healthy Life	280
XX.	Temporary Aids and Auxiliaries	288
XXI.	The True Position of Sports and Pastimes	301
XXII.	A Word to Parents and Guardians	311
XXIII.	Neurasthenia—A New Conception	322
XXIV.	How and Why Scientific Physical Movement etc.	346
XXV.	Hints for the Prevention of Disease, etc.	397
XXVI.	The All-For-Health League	408

CHAPTER I.

Lessons the War have Taught Us.

In a speech at Manchester in September, 1918, that will become historical, Mr Lloyd George made it quite clear that a new world would emerge from the womb of war, and that its birth or re-birth would be the signal for the active commencement of that great work of re-education and national physical reconstruction in which, as he well said, " all classes must be invited to assist, to co-operate, to devise, and to work out problems and in anticipation of which he said, " minds—expert minds—are already engaged in solving problems

This book is an honest attempt to grapple with the first and greatest of these problems, and is the product of life-long experience, study and research. It will, I trust, be accepted in the spirit in which it is proffered, as my small contribution to this great national endeavour movement. Realising, in the words of the Premier, that the war demanded every ounce of the national energy at home as well as at the Front, publication of this book was purposely postponed until peace had been declared, although most of its contents were written in the days of the nation's travail, and much of what Mr Lloyd George said at Manchester in 1918 had been anticipated in its pages.

It is very gratifying, indeed, to know that with such a driving power behind the State, the most vital and elementary work of reconstruction—viz., the re-building of the 'physique and health of the people, is never again likely to be treated with placid and frigid indifference by a Levite State, but that, more than ever in the history of the nation, the State can be relied upon to play the part of the Good Samaritan in the nation's hour of need. Never was the call for healthy and vigorous men and women more insistent than it is now. I show and prove in these pages that the State may secure and maintain them, and at a price out of all proportion to the immense benefits that will accrue in every department, sphere and phase of the national life. The national house must not only be set in order—it must be built upon a rock.

The following chapter deals with some of the most important features of the Premier's famous speech, a lengthy extract from which is given at the finish.

There have been speeches before that have made history. Sheridan's impeachment of Hastings, Bright's speech on the Crimean War Pitt's speech on the American War of Independence at least moulded if they did not make history. Recently, Mr Lloyd George's epoch-making speech on the future of the British Empire, at Manchester, is probably the most historic public utterance of modern times, and its influence upon the health and physical condition of the people in the future will be great, especially when we remember that the speaker did not merely string together a beautiful series of oratorical pearls, but submitted practical suggestions characteristic of one who won both before and during the war a high reputation for constructive statesmanship. The speech should be printed and circulated in millions, and read by everybody, for in it are to be found the germinal seeds of a new, greater, and better Britain.

The keystone of the Premier's speech is to be found in the following pregnant sentence: " If Britain has to be thoroughly equipped to meet any emergencies of either peace or war, the State must take a more constant and a more intelligent interest in the health and fitness of the people." This confession was wrung from the Premier when it was brought home to him that the physical deterioration of the nation had robbed the State and the Army of quite 1,000,000 citizen soldiers through physical unfitness and disease.

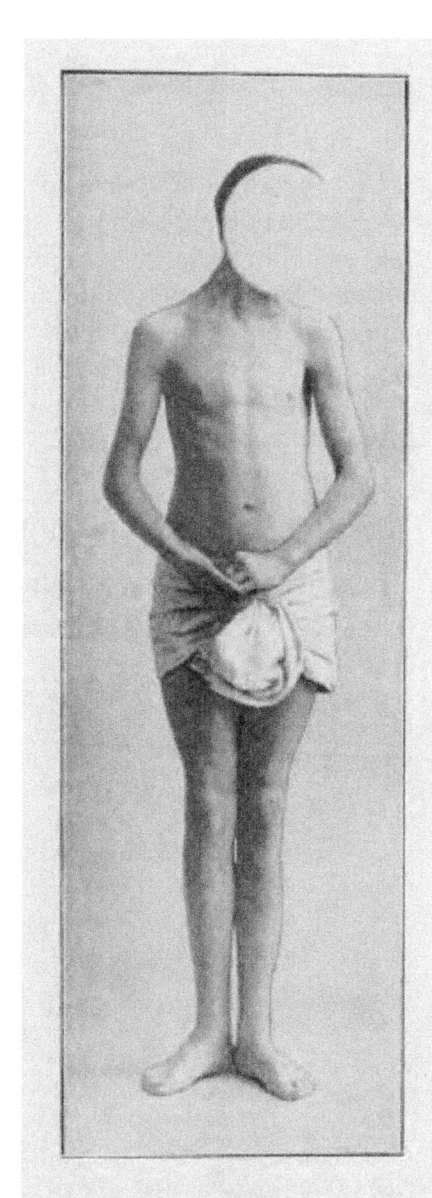

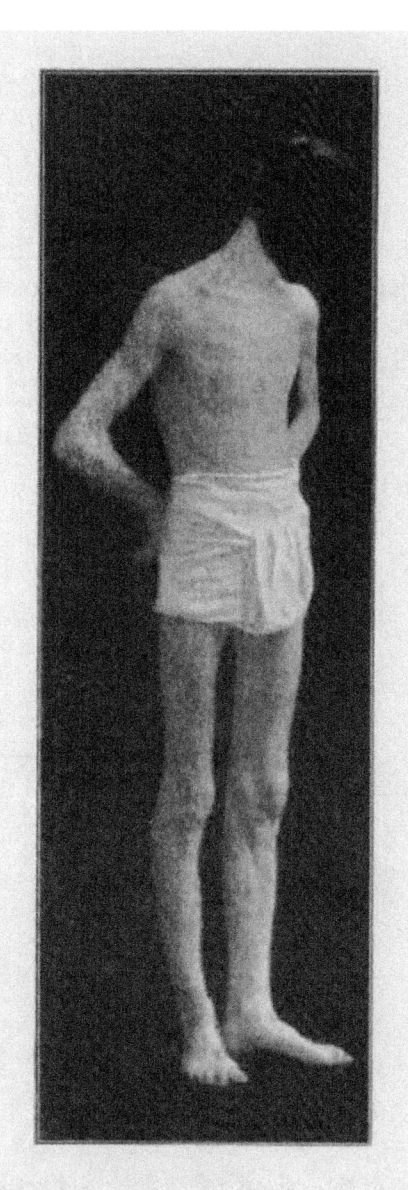

Physical types of the Lost Army of The Rejected mentioned by Mr. Lloyd George in his great speech.

How this physical unfitness and disease handicapped us when suddenly confronted by a crisis that made the threat of the Spanish Armada seem trifling in comparison, came as a revelation to this great leader of the State, and how it almost cost us the victory was subsequently described in the Premier's speech which, in conjunction with Dr Sir George Newman's famous report to Parliament on Medical Education (referred to more fully later), may be said to constitute a veritable Magna Charta for the weak, the ailing, and the diseased in our midst. The keen Celtic brain of Mr Lloyd George realised the gravity of the revelations, and the necessity for reform and reconstruction at the earliest opportunity. Hence the above utterance made with characteristic candour and in defiance of all the traditions of statecraft.

" We have had," said the Premier, " a Ministry of National Service, and carefully compiled statistics as to the health of the people between the ages of eighteen and forty-two. Now that is the age of fitness, the age of strength. You have three grades, Al, B2, and C3, and all I can tell you is this, that the results of these examinations are startling, and I do not mind using the word appalling. I hardly dare tell you the results of same.

" The number of B2 and C3 men throughout the country is prodigious. So much so, that we half suspected the doctors. But there were re-examinations which did not make very much difference, and I apologise to the doctors here for the first time. Now what does it mean? Let us look at it. It means this, that we have used our human material in this country prodigally, foolishly, cruelly. I asked the Minister of National Service how many more men could we have put into the fighting ranks if the health of the country had been properly looked after. I was staggered at the reply. It was a considered reply. It was, £ at least one million.' If we had only had that million the war would have been ended triumphantly before now."

Then followed this solemn warning which should be emblazoned for ever in letters of enduring gold:

" I solemnly warn my fellow-countrymen that you cannot maintain an Al Empire with a C3 population. Unless this lesson is learned the war is in vain."

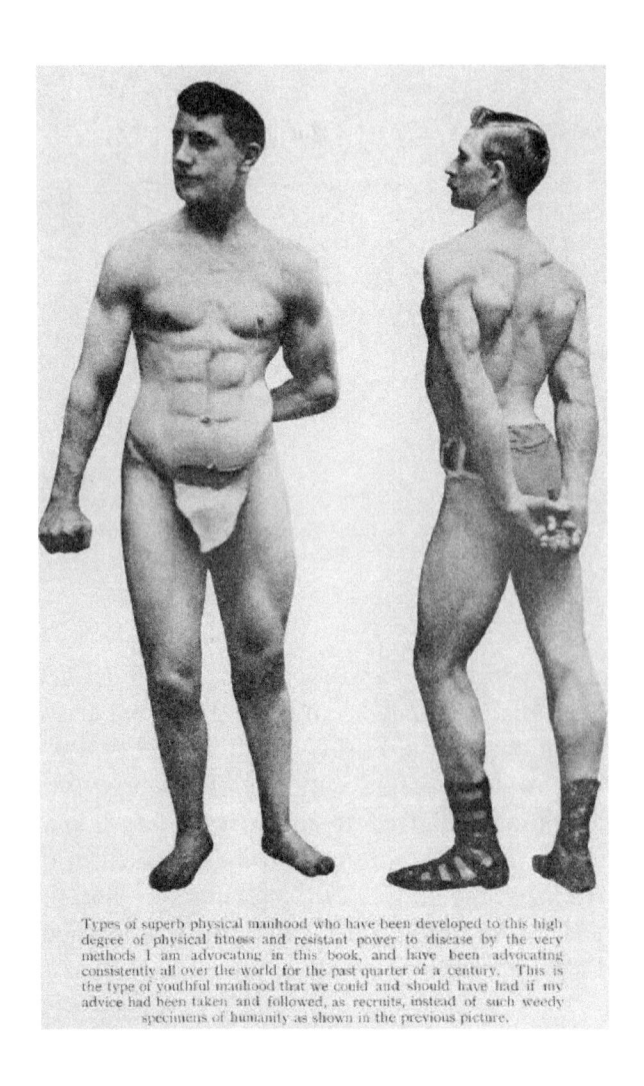

Types of superb physical manhood who have been developed to this high degree of physical fitness and resistant power to disease by the very methods I am advocating in this book, and have been advocating consistently all over the world for the past quarter of a century. This is the type of youthful manhood that we could and should have had if my advice had been taken and followed, as recruits, instead of such weedy specimens of humanity as shown in the previous picture.

AN ALMOST FORGOTTEN WARNING.

The "C3" men largely represented the human physical metal of the nation that had deteriorated through lack of constructive statesmanship in times of peace. It nearly rang the death-knell of the British Empire. For the future we must, in the language of our own unequalled bard, have "metal more attractive."

Over twenty years ago, I myself warned the nation of the danger of physical deterioration, and pleaded the same cause most strenuously, not altogether in vain. So effective was my warning then, and so powerful was my pleading, that a wave of public enthusiasm swept over the country, and after years of continued working, many prominent public men, and distinguished military and naval officers, came to my support. As a result, a Committee was appointed to investigate the facts and take evidence upon every aspect of the serious physical deterioration of the nation. It deliberated long and seriously the question, it called many witnesses, including myself, from all parts of the country, and it issued the customary Report with many excellent recommendations. Unfortunately, with the exception of some slight alterations and improvements of a casual character, the matter ended there so far, at least, as the State was concerned.

Lethargy slowly but surely supplanted enthusiasm, for the driving force of a Lloyd George was lacking. I only wish that the man who uttered the words I have just quoted had been at the helm of State then, for, if so, I firmly believe that steps would at once have been taken by the Government to put the national house in order, and with how much happier results in the great war crisis through which we have passed. I look forward with great hope, therefore, to Mr Lloyd George in this new awakening, and trust that he will remain in office until his already splendid life-work has been crowned with the great achievement of giving the people every opportunity for health and physical fitness.

Not only did I warn the State and the people of this danger over twenty years ago and of many things that have since come to pass, but I pioneered the first great physical regeneration movement in this country. It is not for the sake of idle boasting that I recall these things, but as an object-lesson of great value at the present time. I sounded the first alarm throughout the country as to the national physical deterioration, the increasingly lowered physical standard of our men, women and children, and the gravity of such things from a national and Imperial view-point.

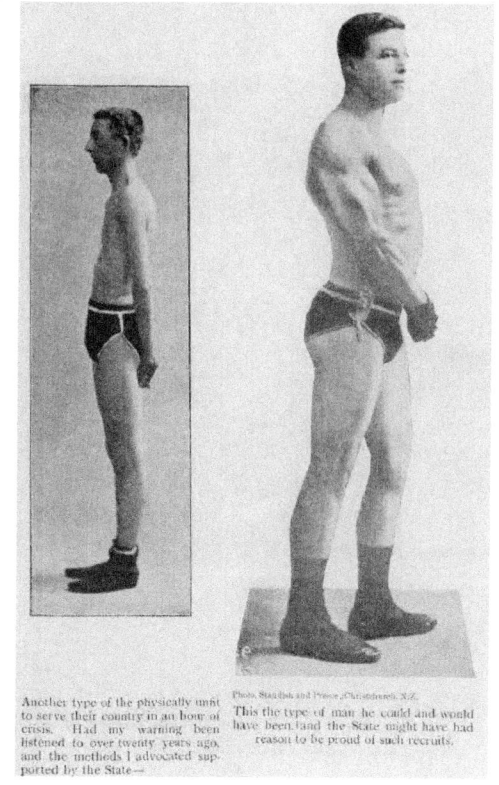

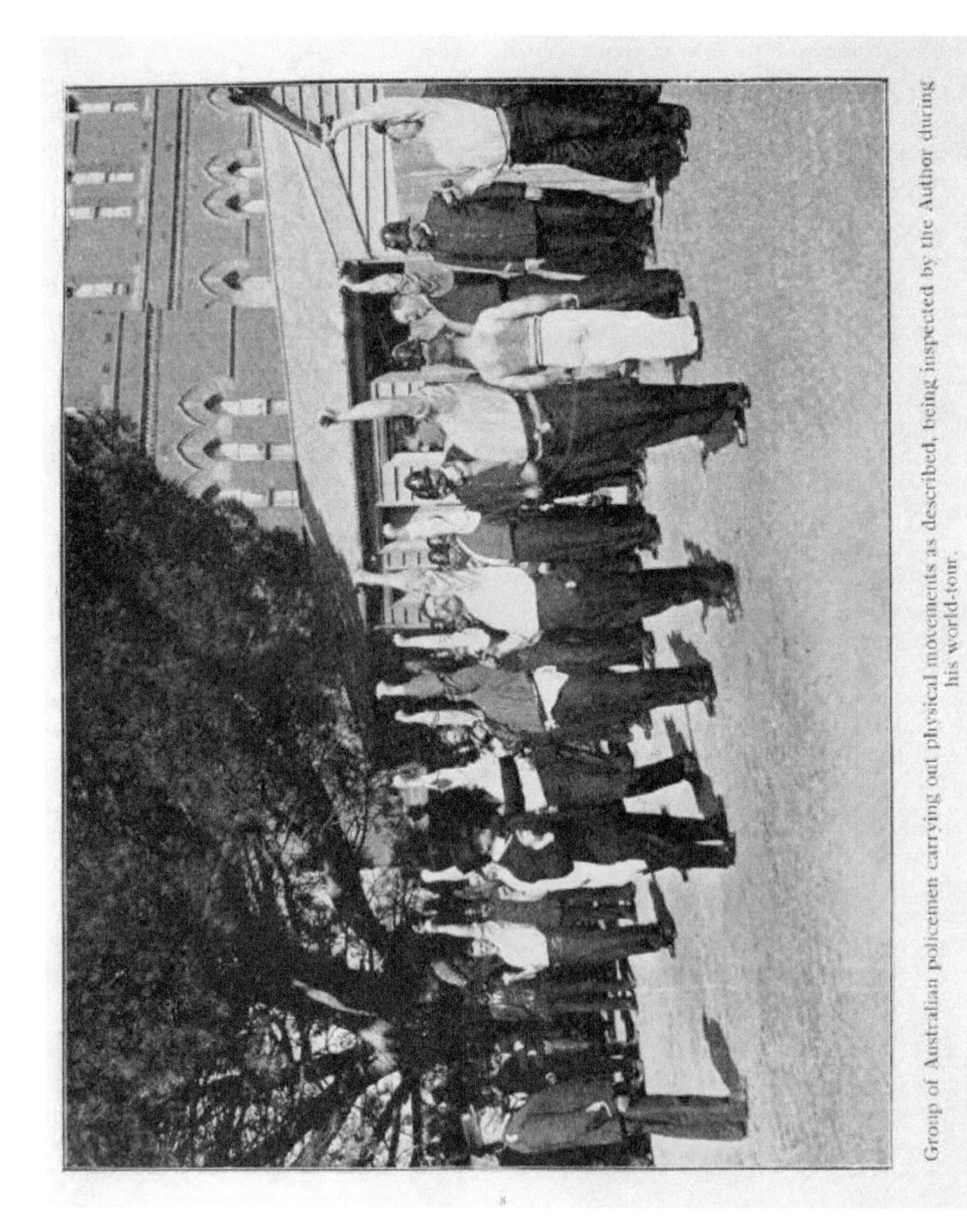

Group of Australian policemen carrying out physical movements as described, being inspected by the Author during his world-tour.

NATION IN A PHYSICAL DECLINE.

I preached the gospel of health and physical culture as essential even then for the salvation of the nation and the Empire, for I saw— and I had unique opportunities for observation—all too plainly that the country was in a serious physical decline, and that a great crisis would at any time threaten it even with the fate of Rome, Greece, and Carthage.

" The glory that was Greece, and the grandeur that was Rome " began to decay from the very moment that those nations began to neglect the physical culture of the body for which they were once so famous. So long as Rome had its amphitheatres thronged with gladiators or Greece its gymnasia full of young athletes, these nations flourished not only in a physical sense but also in every art and science. In time, however, physical neglect led to physical deterioration, as with ourselves, and inevitably also to intellectual weakness of many kinds. Thus the sun went down for ever on Rome and Athens as on Alexandria and Byzantium.

The British Empire was even at the time of my warning threatened with a similar fate, and at the time I pointed out the danger of the national physical deterioration through similar neglect of the body physical. As Sir Robert Hadfield had said, " life had been too easy for us." Civilisation, a faulty education, and luxurious living had set up a softening of the national marrow, muscle and brain. The fabric was poor in quality. The steel of the body—and muscle is to the body what steel is to an engine or a machine, the material of materials—required hardening and tempering. Here, surely, was a splendid work for a Government with a high ideal and the courage to lead the nation towards that ideal, and it is a pity that the opportunity was not then embraced by those in the high seats of authority.

Without any State encouragement or support, but with the patronage of a handful of high-minded public men, I began my own humble crusade against physical deterioration in 1897. I had developed my own body to the highest degree of physical perfection and was generally regarded as " the strongest man in the world," and to-day, even at 52, as the photos of myself will show, that fitness still persists, while I feel as healthy and robust to-day as in the very heyday of my youth. I gave displays of my own strength throughout the country, not for personal vanity or aggrandisement, but because I knew such visible evidence of what could be done by physical self-culture, must have a more inspiring effect on others than hours of talk or volumes of printed matter, must, indeed, make a great and inspiring appeal, especially to the youth of the nation.

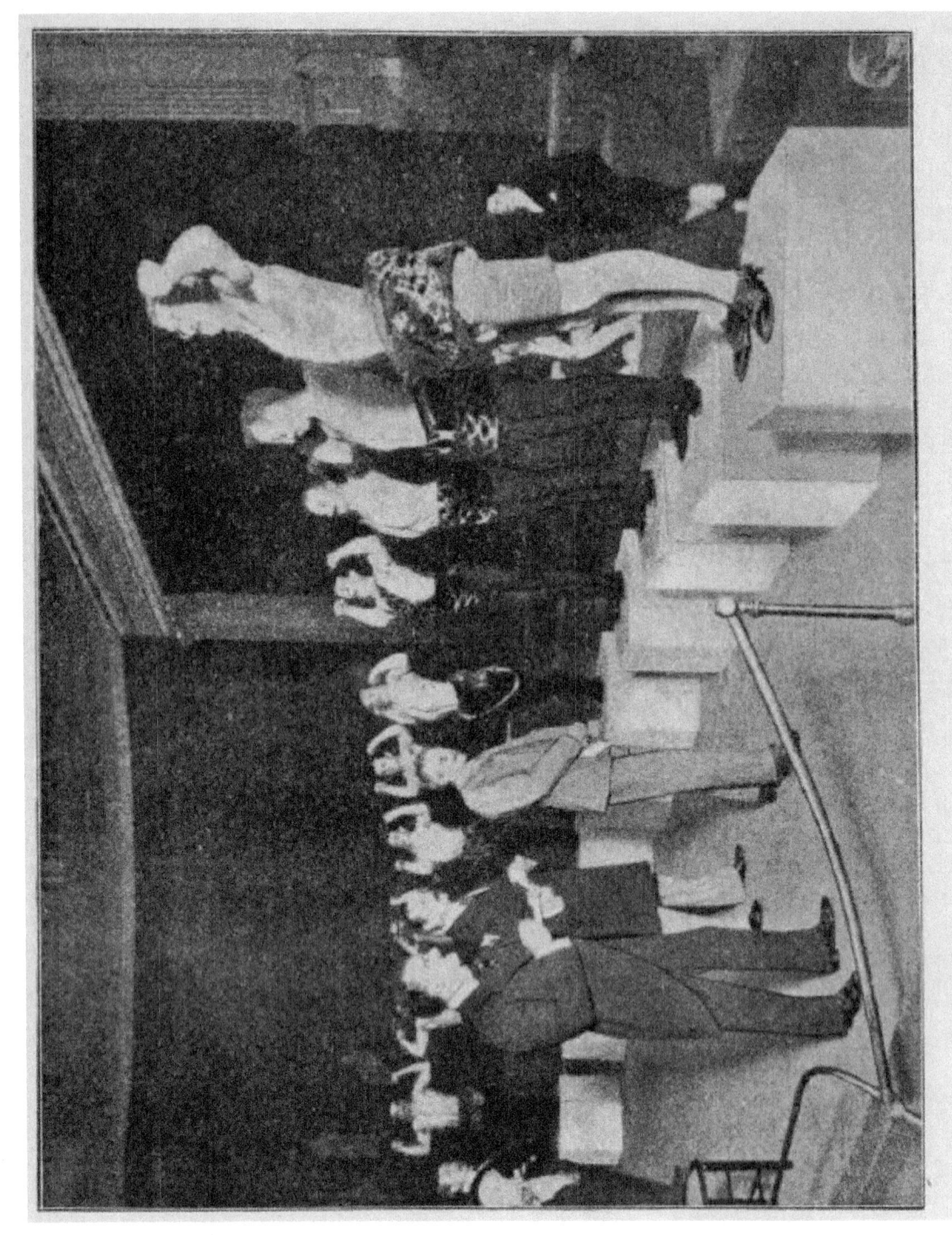

Dr. Sir Arthur Conan Doyle, Sir Charles Lawes, Bart., and the Author judging Gold, Silver, and Bronze Medal Winners from every part of the United Kingdom in the competition at the Royal Albert Hall, for Gold, Silver, and Bronze Statuettes of the Author.

One of hundreds of Clubs for the study and practice of physical culture which sprang up in all parts of the United Kingdom as a result of the Author's grave warning against physical deterioration.

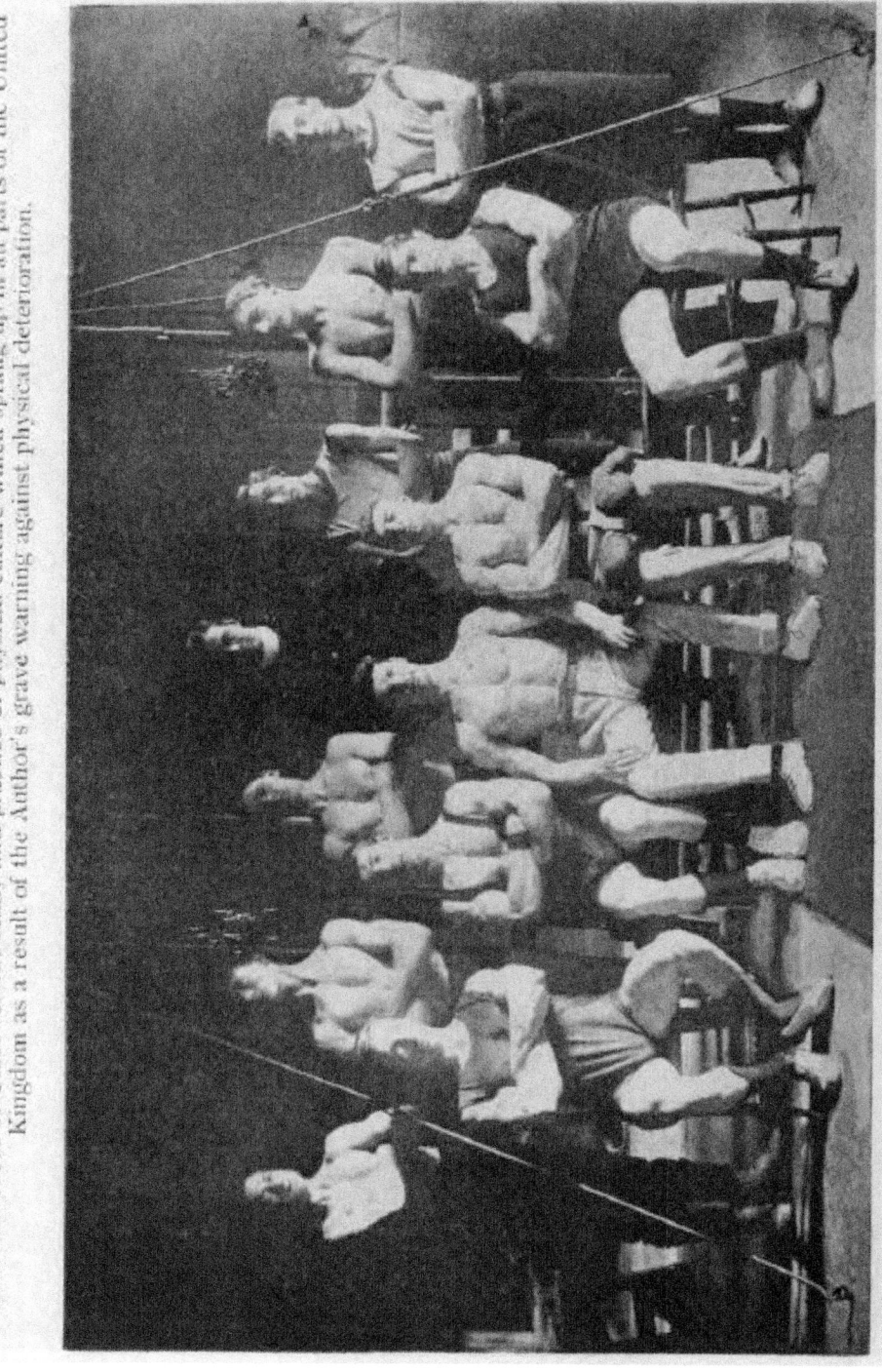

A. CHARL.   A. MOORE.   H. BEST.   REV. P. BROWNING.   J. GRIST.   P. COLLIER.   R. FAULKNER.
R. BERESFORD.   T. HOWE.   A. DANT (Inst.).   A. GOOCH.   T. WADE.

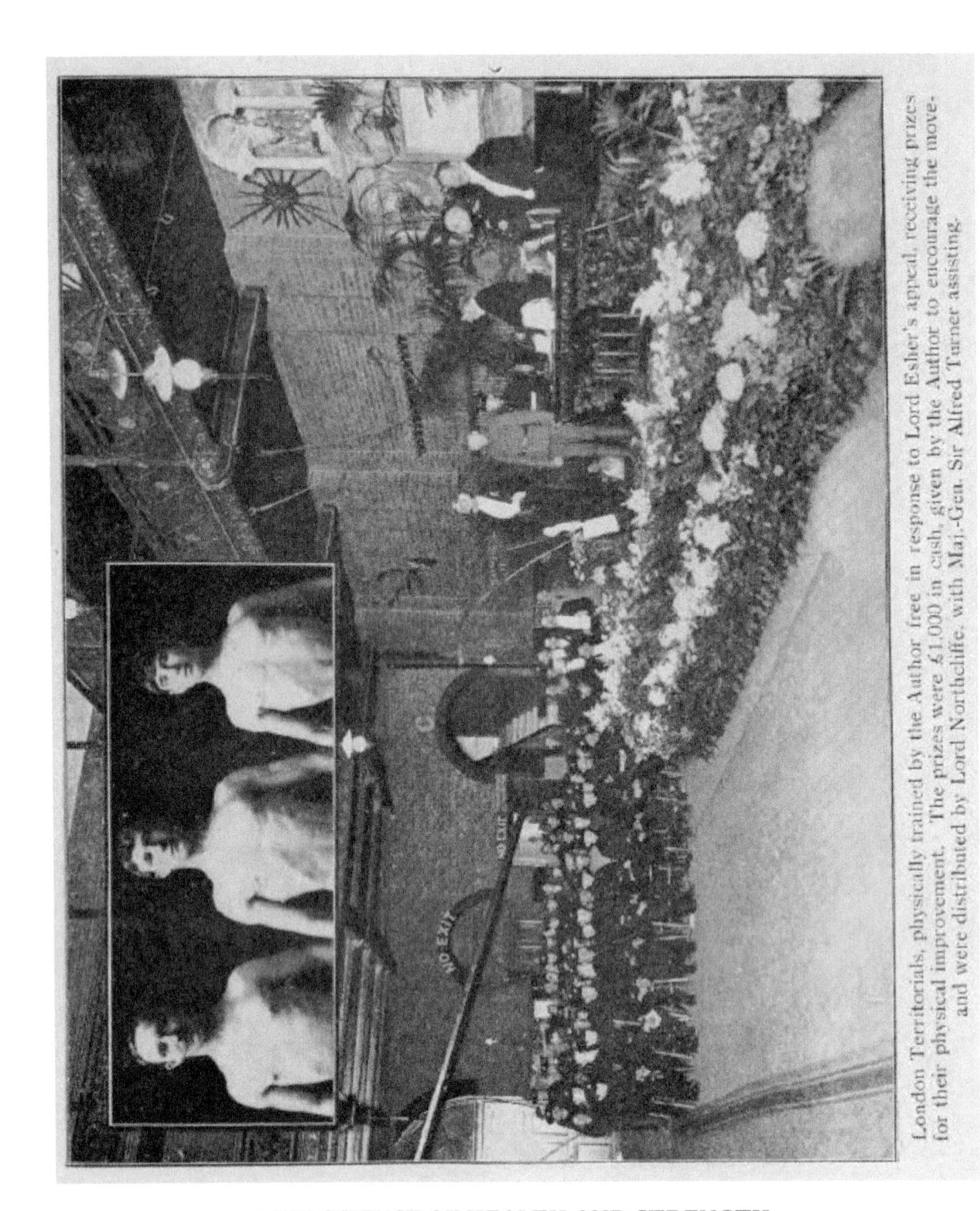

London Territorials, physically trained by the Author free in response to Lord Esher's appeal, receiving prizes for their physical improvement. The prizes were £1,000 in cash, given by the Author to encourage the movement and were distributed by Lord Northcliffe, with Maj.-Gen. Sir Alfred Turner assisting.

THE SCIENCE OF HEALTH AND STRENGTH.

I had not obtained my own health and strength by accident. I was, indeed, on the other hand, a delicate child. But I had proved in my own body that if the attainment and maintenance of health was not an exact science, it was governed by natural, and therefore, exact laws, and was, consequently, obtainable by all. In that, alone, I think I may say with all modesty I have done the

State some service, for tens on tens of thousands immediately flocked to my standard, proving that there was no slackness at least on the part of the people themselves.

For the furtherance of the cause I organised contests throughout the country, offering prizes at great personal expense, while I personally visited the fifty-two counties of England and Wales to adjudicate and award the prizes. A veritable furore in favour of physical culture followed, and the keenest enthusiasm was awakened throughout the length and breadth of the kingdom. Many men, women and children began, for the first time, to take pride in their physical bodies, and to appreciate the value and happiness of physical fitness and health. To still further encourage this splendid spirit of self-culture I spent large sums in prize-money, and gave special gold, silver and bronze medals to those who became the best developed men and the healthiest in each county, among the many thousands who competed.

After the adjudication in this great national contest, I later received the 156 winners (three from each of the 52 counties) at the Albert Hall, London, upon which occasion the best physically developed and physically proportioned man was presented with a gold statuette of myself, eighteen inches high, while the second and third were awarded silver and bronze statuettes. There was an immense gathering—the largest ever seen in that capacious building —to witness the final competition among these 156 splendid physical specimens of the nation for the statuettes, and the takings were handed over to a fund for the widows and orphans who fell in the South African War. The outcome of this was that physical culture clubs were inaugurated in hundreds of cities, towns and villages in the United Kingdom to the great benefit of the national physique. Unfortunately, enthusiasm was subsequently allowed to wane through lack of that State support, which the Premier tells us truly is most essential to-day.

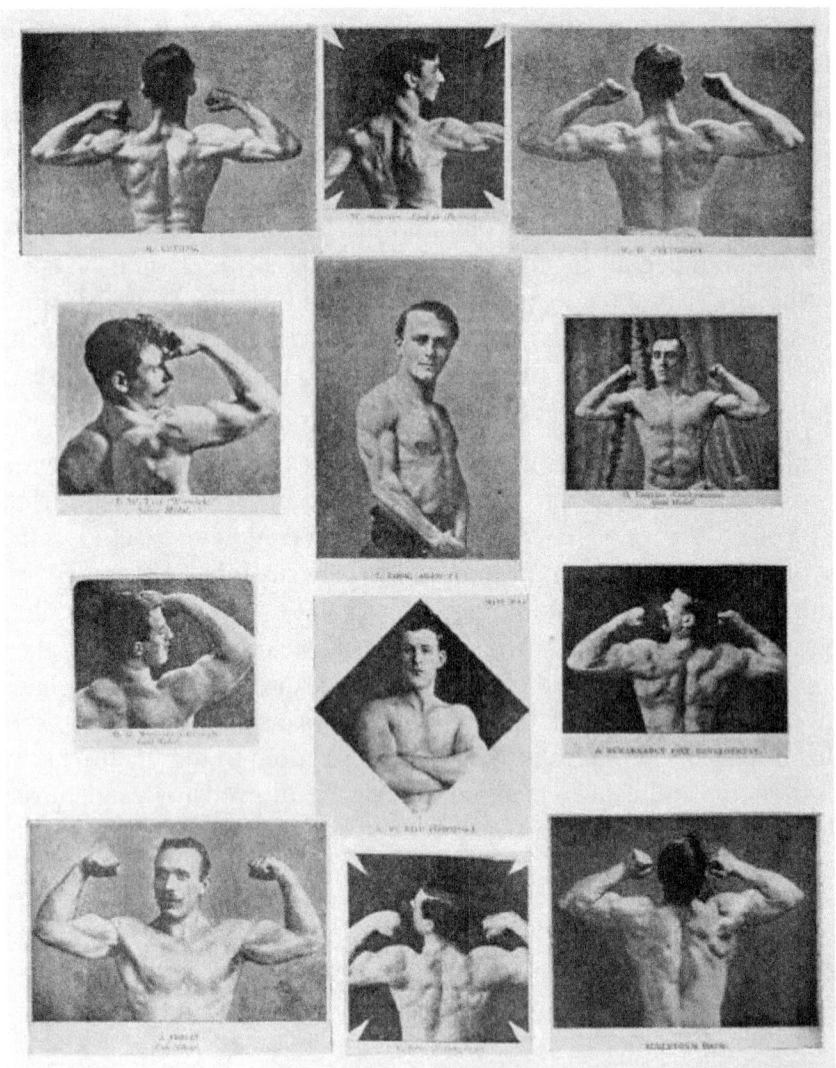

Twelve of the 156 Competitors in the Final Competition at the Royal Albert Hall for the Gold, Silver, and Bronze Statuettes, given by the Author for the best proportioned and developed men in the United Kingdom whose fine physique was obtained by these methods. These prizes were given by the Author to encourage physical education and culture in this country, and the photos show what might have been achieved with State support.

BUILDING A BETTER BRITAIN.

Since then, my own efforts—and it is only with reluctance that I refer to them here not for the purpose of advertisement but because they " point a moral " and, in some degree, help to adorn the Premier's tale of woe—are fairly well known. I travelled personally through nearly all over our Overseas Dominions, through India, Australia, Canada, New Zealand, South Africa, and the Straits Settlements, giving lectures, demonstrations and free training to soldiers, police and fire-fighting forces. Many of those who heard, saw, and were advised by me then, were amongst the best soldiers Great Britain ever put in the field. When Lord Esher made his famous appeal for 11,000 recruits to bring up the London County Regiments of the Territorials to full strength, I volunteered to make myself personally responsible for the physical training necessary to enable them to fulfil the physical requirements. I presented £1,000 in cash prizes as an added inducement to those who accepted my offer and made the greatest development during training, and the result was an improvement of many of the men's physique, averaging three inches upon the chest measurement of every man, and of all other parts in proportion.

In addition to all this, I offered free individual physical training to the lads belonging to the Church Brigade, of which many took advantage, and I have no doubt that many of those were since able to pass the military tests when called up, and so did not help to swell the missing million whom Mr Lloyd George mourned in his Manchester speech.

Hundreds of young men were so improved physically under my tuition as to be able to qualify for commissions, so far, at least, as the physical tests were concerned, and thousands of soldiers of all ranks in the Army have expressed their gratitude to me for the improvement wrought both in their physical condition and their health. When I look back on all this, in the light of recent events, I can quite appreciate the humour of a public man's remark when he complimented me on being the greatest " recruiting sergeant " the Army has ever had.

I think I am, indeed, entitled to say without egotism that but for this great physical culture crusade and revival, and the work subsequently carried on by me as described, the number of rejections for physical unfitness, to which the Premier refers, would have been greater still, and the physical standard of our new Army lower even than it proved to be.

WHAT A PHYSICAL CENSUS WOULD HAVE REVEALED.

If my own modest efforts could achieve such results as these, what might we not expect if the State were to inculcate and foster the desire for physical fitness in the mind of every individual in every village, town, city and county of the British Isles, and, indeed, of the British Empire from childhood, if, indeed, the training of the body were made, as it should be, an essential part of education, and if such a national and scientific system of physical reconstruction as I advocate in these pages were endowed and supported by the State. Indeed, had such State encouragement been offered to the people twenty-one years ago, when I myself fought for such a physical awakening, most of the 1,000,000 men, if not all, whom, according to the Premier, we had most reluctantly to reject as unfit for military service, would no doubt have been available as desirable recruits when so badly needed.

But I would remind the Premier that the danger of our culpable State neglect in the past of " a more constant and a more intelligent interest in the health and fitness of the people " does not end there, for it is not too much to say that yet another 1,000,000 passed into the Army who were not nearly so fit as they should be, while an enormous number of men had to be discharged because physically unfitted to bear the heavy strains of military service. If the male remnant of the nation, ineligible for military service or exempted for skilled service in war work, had also been medically examined, the results would have been still more staggering, while a similar medical examination of all the people, including men, women and children, would have been truly appalling.

It behoves the State, therefore, to awaken itself in the present grave crisis. Such a state of things must not—need not—occur again if we intelligently grapple with the problem, and if the State does its part in encouraging health and fitness among the people.

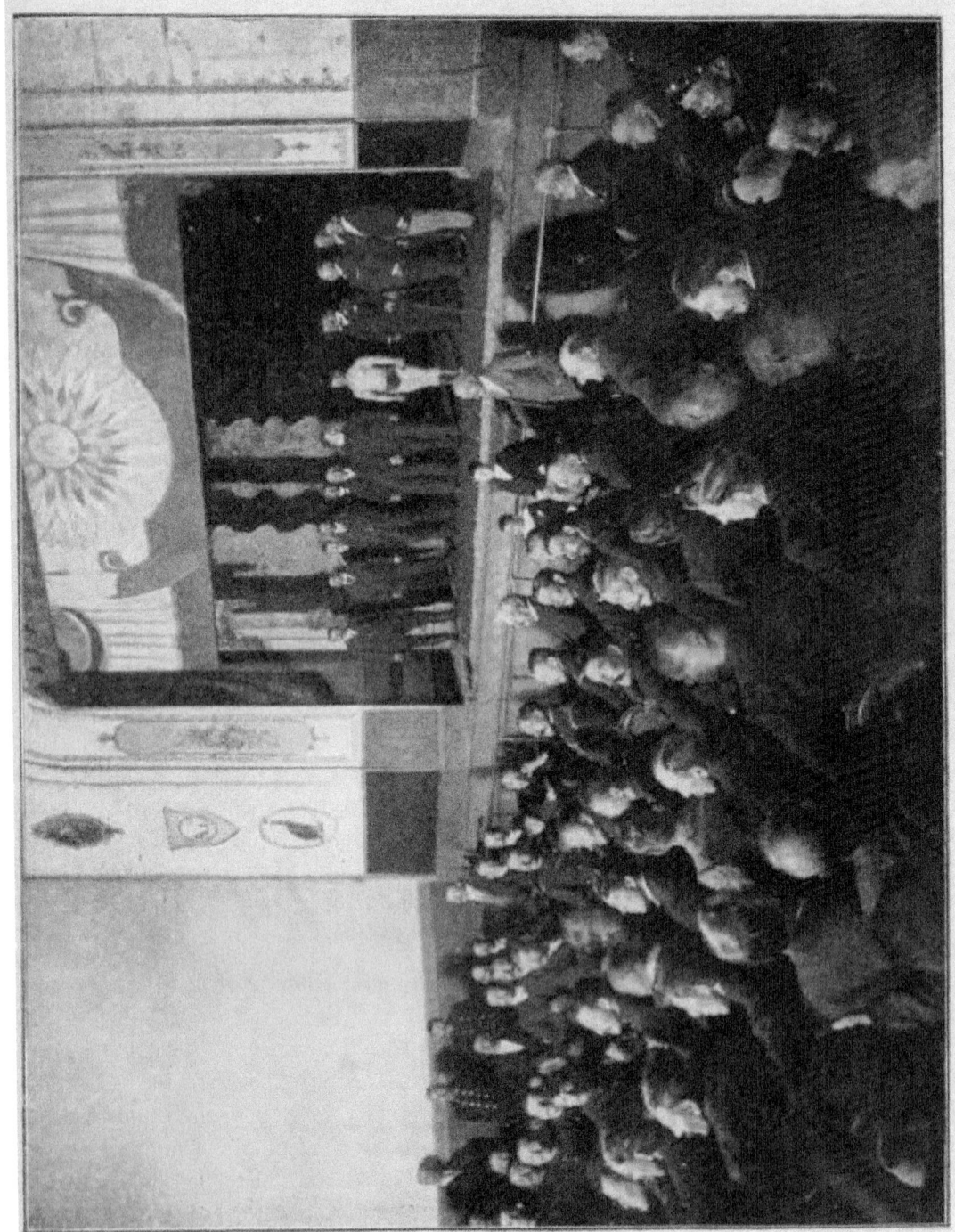

Author giving lecture on anatomy and demonstration in the methods he describes in this book before a body of Australian firemen. The Colonials were a most enthusiastic body of students.

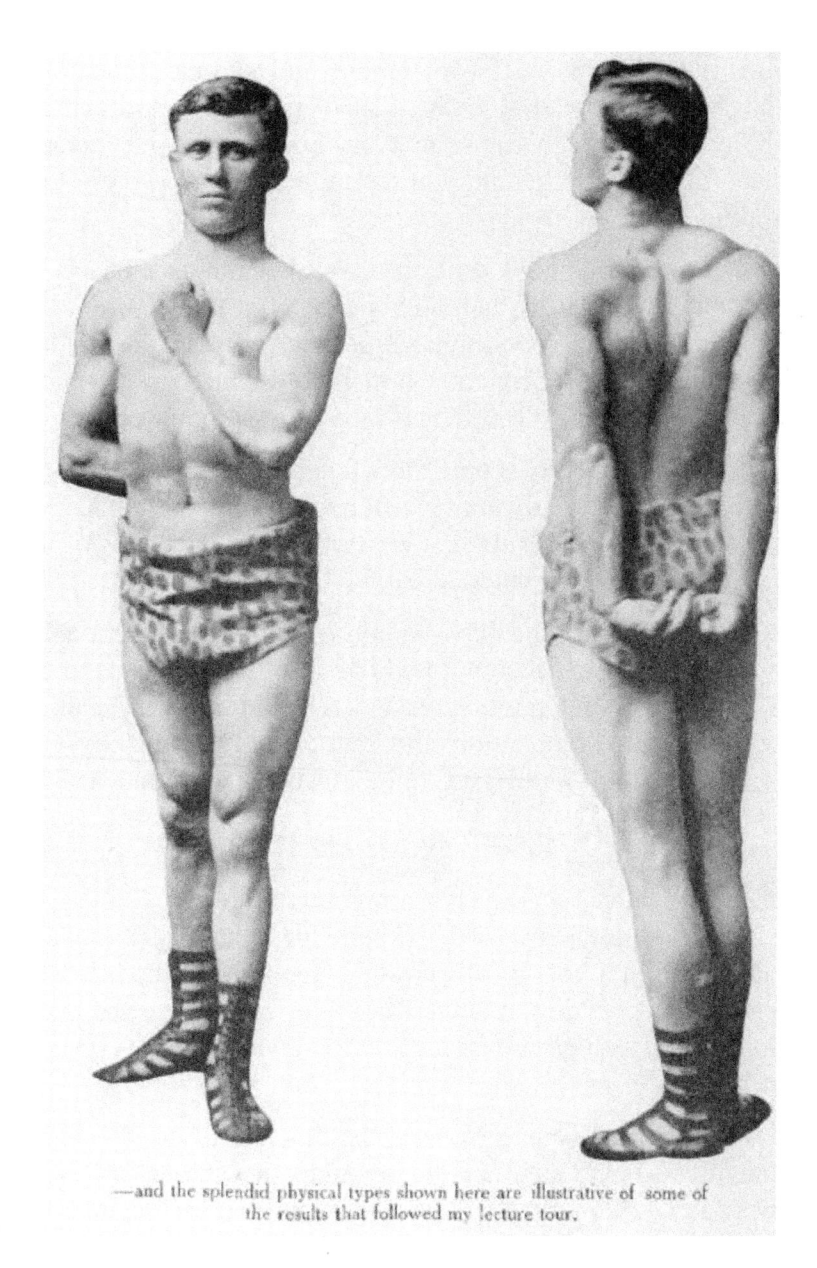

—and the splendid physical types shown here are illustrative of some of the results that followed my lecture tour.

TAKING THE FLOOD TIDE.

Already, even at the time of writing (1917-18), I am pleased to note that there are evidences in many directions that, with Celtic vim and vision, the Premier has set many wheels whirring to discover and provide the necessary " munitions," the best machinery, and the most perfect organisation to ensure the best results in this most vital campaign against our greatest enemy, physical weakness and disease. Perhaps, indeed, it may not be too much to say that the great work of national reconstruction has already begun, although the really critical operations are just about to begin.

THE SKELETON AT THE FEAST.

As the Premier has neatly phrased it, " you must have reconstruction while we have the lessons of the war fresh in our minds. You must reconstruct when the national limbs are supple with endeavour, and before they become stiff with repose and slumber, and you must reconstruct when you see you have behind you that great spirit of patriotism and self-sacrifice which has been raised from the depths of human nature in every house and every breast in this land. You must reconstruct when you have got behind you the momentum of victory to carry you through to an even greater triumph."

It is at just such a moment that this book will make its appearance. I desire to catch the tide of public enthusiasm at its highest, in order that the State may not be allowed to drift with an ebbing tide of public opinion into the shallows or become becalmed in the doldrums of peace and comfort once more. Even at the feast of victory it may not be inadvisable to drag the skeleton of our physical past among the guests and revellers if only as a warning for future conduct.

For if we do not enlist and permanently secure the wholehearted support of the State in this great enterprise, if the State should be negligent, indifferent or parsimonious, if it should leave to private or public enterprise what I say is its first and paramount duty, it is of little use celebrating a victory that will merely postpone a greater defeat.

How can we make each individual a healthy, happy, contented, efficient and intelligent citizen either for peace or war? That is the question to which all other questions of State must be made subsidiary, if we are to have an A1 population and A1 Empire. The health and fitness of the people constitute the corner-stone of a nation, and its foundation is the physique and constitution of the individual. How are we to re-build the Empire on such a deep and sure foundation?

FIT CHILDREN AND FIT ADULTS.

Well-meaning people are already at work. They are going to do it by building us better and more hygienic homes, by banishing slums, by more mental education, by better wages, by sending the people back to the land, and in a host of other ways. Good and desirable as are all these, these methods will never succeed if we do not attend first and foremost to the physical demands and necessities of the individual. Healthy, robust men and women, however few the number, will set an ideal to the whole nation.

" You cannot," as a writer in the Evening News at the time well said, " make a man or a woman A1 by Act of Parliament. Whatever the State, the municipality, the enlightened employer may do, in the end it all comes back to the individual. The State and the town council and the doctor and the teacher can provide the railroad, so to speak, but you have to get up your own steam." The question is how. The individual must first be shown how to get up steam, must possess the knowledge necessary, and must be fitted for the work in every way. Otherwise he could never get up steam at all, produce it in insufficient quantity, or perhaps, attempt to generate it beyond the factor of safety.

It is best, therefore, as in all forms of education, to begin with the child, and to teach and train it from its earliest school days to know, understand and direct the wonderful human engine given to its charge. This may seem a somewhat startling idea to the conservative mind. But, remember, that a few hundred years ago if it had been suggested that every child should be taught to read and write the proposition would have been greeted with ridicule. Not so many years ago, indeed, it was the exception to be able to read and write; to-day there are few, very few, who cannot read and write. So, I contend, that what seems as startling a proposal to-day as was the first Education

Bill will be just as effective in freeing the world from disease as the Education Bill was in banishing illiteracy.

NATIONAL PHYSICAL EDUCATION AND RECONSTRUCTION.

The average individual may be said to live three lives: (1) at school; (2) in the home; (3) in the great world of business. At school, at home, and in the workshop, fair conditions of hygiene must be secured and maintained. In this part of the work the medical profession can, and undoubtedly will, play a prominent and distinguished part. Mr Lloyd George recognises this, but I think, like many others, he is still inclined to overlook the fact that it is the individual rather than his or her environment that first needs consideration and attention. The body, after all, is only the home of the soul, and if the physical home of the soul is first prepared to be a suitable and hygienic dwelling-place for the spiritual tenant of it, that tenant will see to it that the home of the body also fulfils all the requirements and necessities of both for their physical, mental and spiritual well-being.

The child is the kernel of the Empire, and the crux of the whole problem. As the Premier said truly, " it is bad business not to look after the man, the woman, but above all, the child." There are still savage countries where the children are taught from infancy to steal, and to regard theft as the goal to which they have to strive. Needless to say, to be the most successful thief is the aim and ambition of the children. "As the twig is bent the tree grows," and so national physical education must begin by instilling the higher ideal of perfect physical fitness and health in the mind of the child.

ARCHITECTS OF THE NATION.

The teacher and the doctor should be the architects of the new physical structure of the nation, and a building is not begun with the laying of the first brick or even the digging of the foundation, but in the mind of the architect. Education should teach each and every child individually to know and respect itself, to seek to develop its body and mind to the highest possible standard, and if we are to do this with success there should be rewards and honours for health and for freedom from weakness or disease, as well as for the mere accumulation of wealth, which is too often achieved at a cost which no nation can support—viz., that of physical degeneration. The child, too, must be given a new ideal and a new ambition, as I fully deal with in my chapter on the State and the Child.

In this country, mental education has been and is imposed too often on bodies that are unfit physically to support the mental strain, which is undoubtedly one of the causes of our physical decadence as so lamentably revealed in the early days of the war. This is the real reason why our educational methods have proved inferior to Germany's, as Mr Lloyd George admits. But, while military training and conscription such as are employed in Germany may ensure, to some extent, a trained, developed and strong body, in those already sound organically, to support the mental super-structures, such a system would be most injurious to children and the weak, and could never provide that perfect balance which makes the body disease-proof.

Perfect mental and physical balance is, of course, the ideal, and that, I believe, can only be assured to each child under constant medical supervision and direction, by the intelligent use of the discoveries I have made, and by methods which are based on Nature's law, as I show and prove in this book. It is essential, at the very outset, that the child should be taught the beauty, the grandeur and the wonder of the human body which it possesses, and given a high physical ideal and goal. The spirit of imitation, of rivalry, and of emulation latent in every child should be diverted in a right direction.

When I showed, in my own body, the possibilities of physical culture in securing and maintaining health and strength, the cult and culture of the physical body became almost a craze even with adults and the middle-aged. How much more effectively can we stimulate the thoughts and desires of the child towards health-culture by bestowing honours and rewards on the healthiest and fittest of the children in our schools. The head of the school in every form or class should be the healthiest and most physically perfect boy or girl. The boy or girl with the finest physique and constitution would then become the idol and envy of the school, and so the youthful mind would thus early be bent in the proper direction.

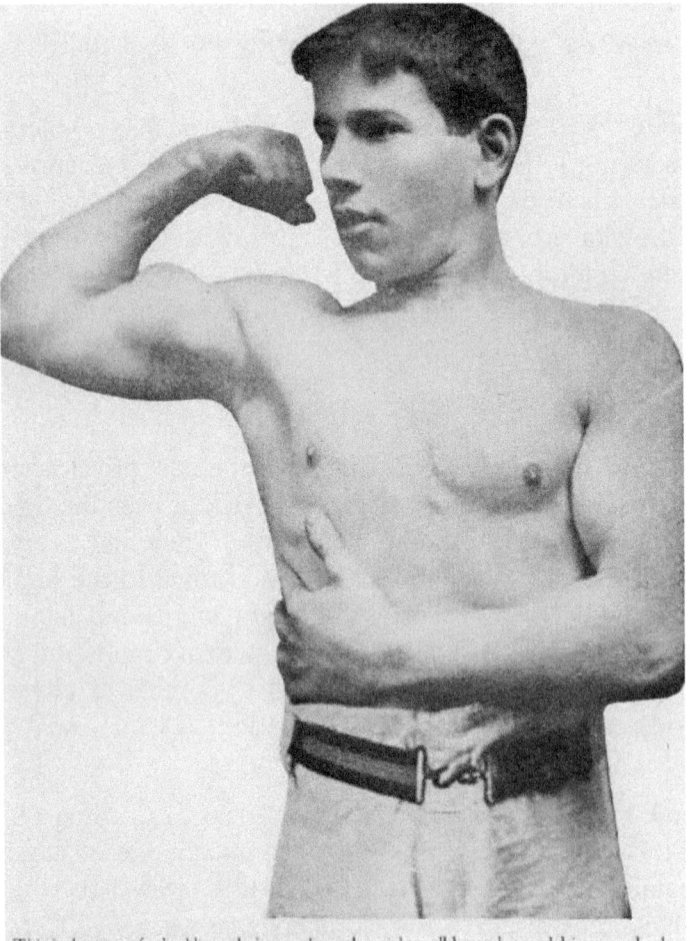

This is the type of a healthy and vigorous boy who might well be such a model in any school, as I suggest here, and whose fine physique and development was the result of careful schooling and practise in these methods of health education and physical reconstruction.

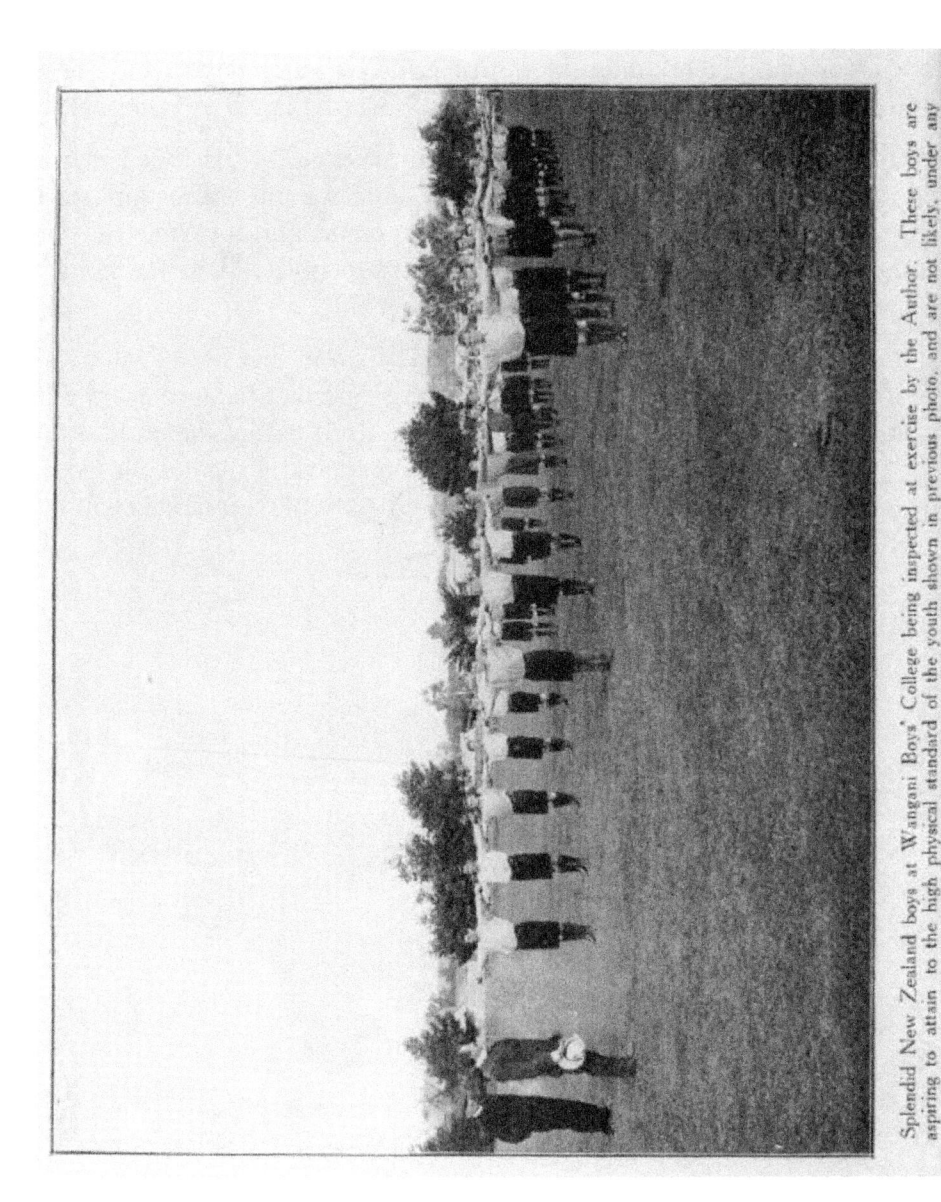

Splendid New Zealand boys at Wangani Boys' College being inspected at exercise by the Author. These boys are aspiring to attain to the high physical standard of the youth shown in previous photo, and are not likely, under any circumstances, to become weaklings, if they continue as they have begun.

DEPRECIATION OF NATIONAL STOCK.

All those, however, of any age who woo health for health's sake, and whose bodies are made and kept in the best physical condition, will find in its ultimate possession a reward far greater than any honours, titles, or distinctions others may bestow on them. They will possess with it a happiness, a sense of joyousness, a capacity for work and play, an exhilaration that the unfit and the unhealthy can never find in all the artificial allurements of a decadent civilisation. They will drink daily from the cup of life a perennial draught more refreshing and more stimulating than the nectar of the gods.

For the State itself, the subject is one of extreme urgency and of the utmost importance, for a depreciated national physique is far more serious and of greater import than the depreciation of the national coinage. The health of the people is the wealth of a State, and yet, as Mr Lloyd George truly said, " we had used our human material in this country profligately, foolishly, cruelly." To prevent further wastage and to make good the cost of war in human life, we will, indeed, require " a more intelligent organisation of the forces which have charge of the health of the nation, national, municipal and medical."

" We have," as the Premier said, "enormous losses to make up —the fallen, the crippled, the mutilated; their case must be particularly thought out—but we must also think of the children who are to fill up the gaps in the generations that are to come, and the State must see that they are built up into a fine, healthy, strong and vigorous people. There is no surer way of strengthening this country than that! I

There is, indeed, no other way, and this, as I show and prove in this book, can only be done by building the bodies of these people so strong and in such perfect balance from childhood that they cannot succumb to disease. The State must prostrate itself before the child. It must stoop if it is to conquer and go on conquering, and a little child must lead it. As Dr Sir George Newman puts it, " a State cannot effectually insure itself against disease unless it begins with its children."

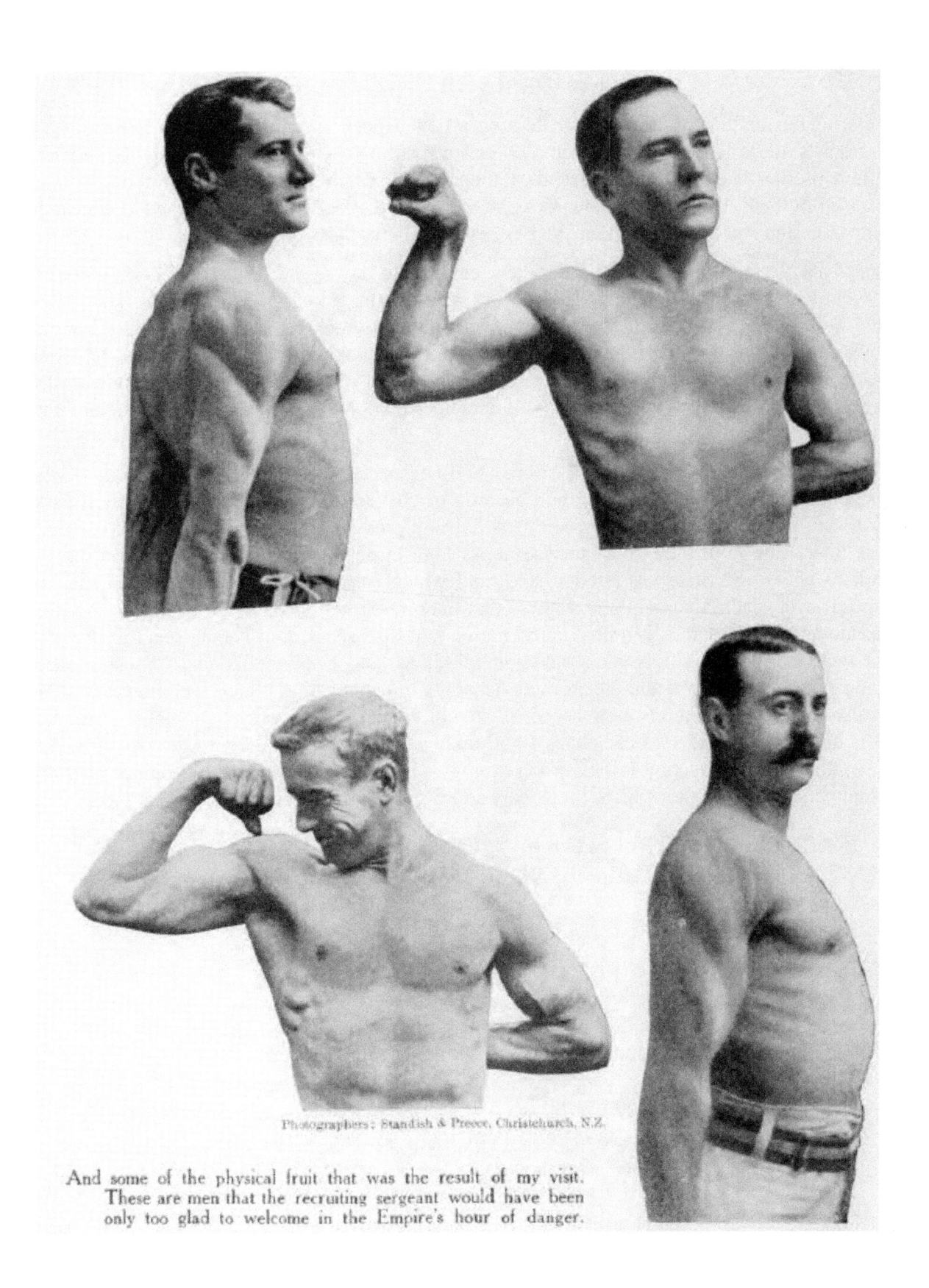

Photographers: Standish & Preece, Christchurch, N.Z.

And some of the physical fruit that was the result of my visit. These are men that the recruiting sergeant would have been only too glad to welcome in the Empire's hour of danger.

NEW IDEALS OF CHILDHOOD.

The struggle for the child must now take on a new aspect. At present the educationalists, the religionists, the reactionists and the employers are rivalling each other over the bodies and brains of the children. The State must assert its authority, and snatch the children from those who seek to traffic in them. Old educational codes and systems must be destroyed, all the old educational compasses and steering gear replenished by new, and new charts prepared.

The physically and often mentally deficient adult of to-day is the product of his teaching and environment. We have worshipped false gods and they have nearly destroyed us. The children must no longer be sacrificed to Mammon, but must be taught to respect a healthy body and robust constitution far more than a fat purse and a big banking account. The child, remember, does not create its own gods. They are created for it. Let us, then, substitute better gods for those that have so basely betrayed us, and give the children a new ideal, a new inspiration, and a new ambition.

If it should seem to the reader that the personal note has obtruded itself somewhat persistently in this chapter, I claim their consideration because of the fact that I have devoted the best part of my life to this subject exclusively, and it is only by proving what is possible and what can be done that I can be of the utmost service in assisting those in authority to accomplish the great work to which the State has put its hand, and which can only be achieved by placing at its disposal every fact, argument and witness that may possibly be of service in the great national crusade against weakness, physical deterioration and disease. If, too, it may seem to the reader that there is an almost irksome reiteration of salient and even vital facts, I must plead the seriousness of my subject and the absolute necessity of driving all the facts well home. Besides, I am dealing with an entirely new aspect of a subject that has never yet previously been fully understood, and which in these pages I am anxious to make clear even to the person with no knowledge of anatomy, physiology or psychology. For these reasons only I introduce only those casual personal references which, I feel, may add weight to my evidence.

EXTRACT REPORTED Verbatim FROM MR LLOYD GEORGE'S GREAT SPEECH AT MANCHESTER, SEPT. 12TH, 1918.

" THE NEW WORLD."

"WE MUST TAKE HEED IN TIME."

Speaking with deep feeling and great force, the Premier said:

" When peace was secured we could then proceed with a clear conscience and a steady nerve to build up the new world in which those who have sacrificed so much might dwell in peace, security and contentment.

" Now, in order to establish the new world, we must take heed in time, lest we fall back into the welter of the old. We must be ready as soon as the unseen hand throws the rainbow of peace on the slide, and be ready—as summarised in one council——to profit by the lesson of the war.

" It has been a most costly schoolmaster in its way. He was not sure it had not been the best in many ways, and the first lesson it had taught us was this—the importance of maintaining the solidity of the British Empire. It had rendered a service to humanity, and the magnitude would appear greater and greater as this generation receded in the past. It had helped to stop the barbarism that was sweeping through Europe.

" To allow such an organisation to fall to pieces after the war would be a crime against civilisation. The British Empire would count more next time than it did in the past, for they knew now what they had to deal with.

Health and Fitness.

" What is the next great lesson of the war? The next great lesson of the war is this—that if the State is to be fairly equipped to face another emergency either of peace or war, the State must take a more constant and more intelligent interest in the health and fitness of the people. If the Empire was to be equal to its task, the men and women who made up the Empire must be equal to theirs.

" How did we stand in the light of that task? We had done great things in the war; we could have accomplished greater if this country had been in condition. War, like sickness, laid bare the weakness of the constitution. What had been ours? Let us talk quite frankly. We had had a Ministry of National Service set up in this country, and since then we had had the most careful compiled statistics of the people—certainly between the ages of 18 and 42.

The Age of Fitness.

" That was the age of fitness, that was the age of strength. What did it reveal? The results of this examination were sufficiently startling, and he did not mind using the word appalling. He hardly dared tell them the results in some parts of Manchester.

" What did this mean? It means this—that we had used our human material in this country profligately, foolishly, cruelly. He asked the Ministry of National Service how many we could have put into the fighting ranks if the health of the country had been properly looked after. He was staggered by the reply. It was a considered reply. They said at least one million men——at least one million men.

If we had only had them, this War would have ended triumphantly ere this.

" There were questions as to whether you ought to put miners back or keep them in the Army—a few tens of thousands—whether you ought to put a few thousand men in munition works—and yet they had a million men who, if the State had taken proper care of the fitness of the people, would have been available for the war.

" The results in agriculture had been almost as disappointing as in almost any other industry. A virile, healthy occupation of that kind ! Everywhere a virile race had been neglected by waste and want of thought—a danger to the State and the Empire.

" I solemnly warn my fellow-countrymen, you cannot maintain an A1 Empire in a C3 population, and unless this lesson is learned the war will have been in vain. Our schooling has cost us dear, but if we make the best use of it I believe it will be worth all in the end, even in the saving of human life.

Health at Home.

" Care for the health of the people was the secret of national efficiency. It was the secret of the national recuperation.

" If the steel is defective through badly ventilated or ill-constructed furnaces or insufficient fuel, if the machinery is inadequately oiled or looked after, or over-worked, if repairs are not done in time or faulty, the machinery is no use. And man is the most delicately constructed of all machines.

" It is bad business not to look after the men, women, and, if I may say so, above all, the children.

" Now the most important workshop in this line is the home. There is a lady over there in the audience accepts my proposition readily. The quality of the steel in the fabric depends upon the home.

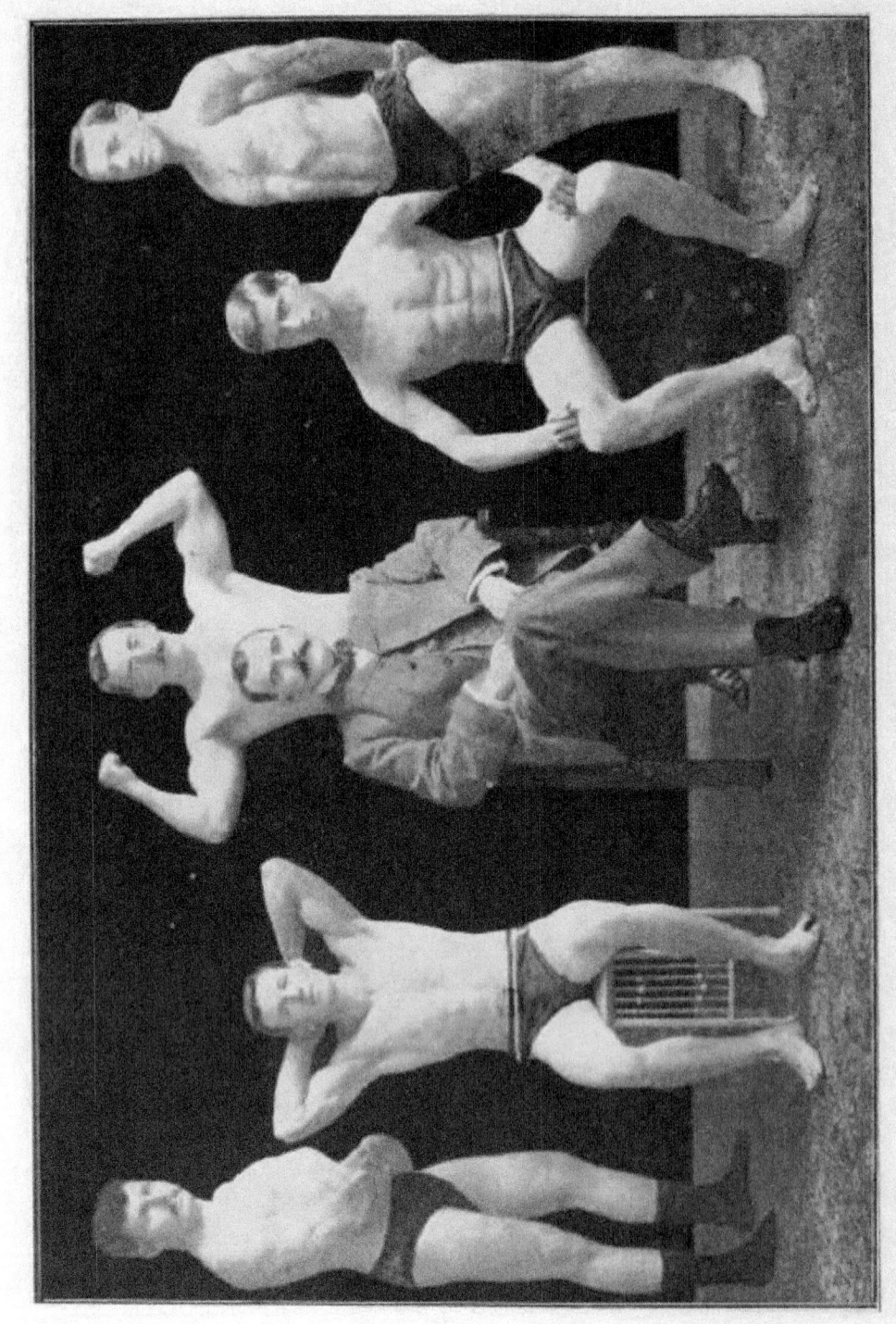

Another group, this time of New Zealand Colonials, who owe their splendid physical development to the methods advocated by me in that country. The figure standing in the centre at back is Mr. Hornibrook, my local representative, whose own magnificent physique was gained in the same way.

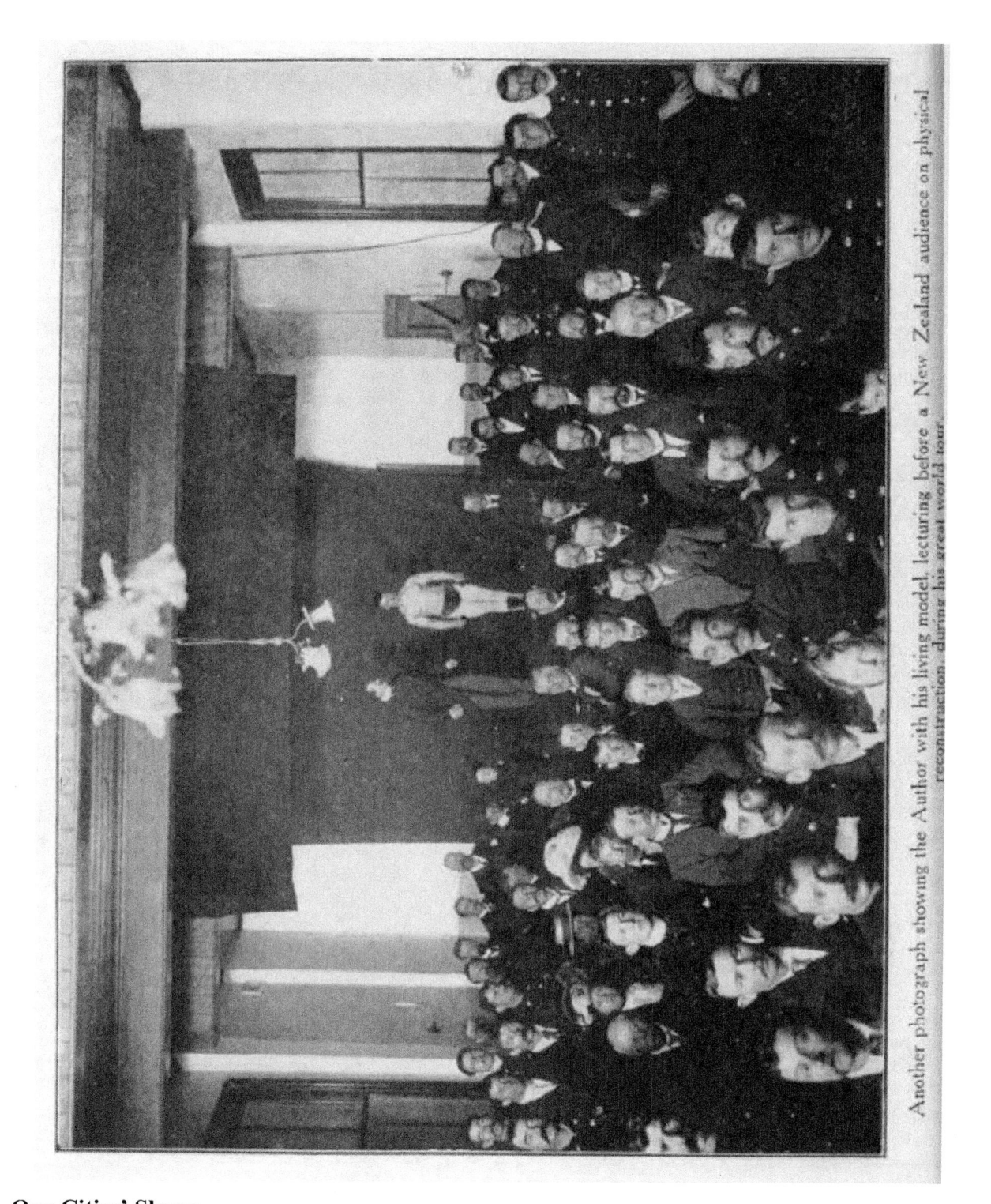

Another photograph showing the Author with his living model, lecturing before a New Zealand audience on physical reconstruction during his great world tour.

Our Cities' Slums.

"If it is unhealthy, ill-equipped, ill-supplied, ill-managed, the quality becomes defective, and it cannot bear the strain. Now, what are the influences which make for the health of the people? The first is the houses in which the people dwell. The problem of housing in this country is the most urgent that awaits treatment.

" We have talked about it, played with it for forty or fifty years, but it has never been really taken in hand. It has only been taken in hand in the way an untidy or slovenly housewife takes up cleaning work. It is that part of the house where the visitor comes and sees which she cleans.

" There has been too much of this thing in our cities—slums, bad houses; they're out of sight. That is not the way to deal with a problem which affects the strength of the nation. It is hopelessly in arrears. No Government, no party has had the courage to grapple in the way a good business man would grapple with some sort of rottenness which he discovered in his business and wasting his capital.

Libraries of Regulations.

" It is equally true of the whole of the public health. We have had Acts of Parliament running into hundreds and hundreds. We have had regulations which would have filled a library. We have had most attractive pictures of model dwellings and endless authorities. But you cannot plough the waste land with writing. You cannot sweep away the slums in Manchester or bind the gaping wounds of the people with red tape.

Wages and Workshops.

" What more have we to do to improve life? We see wages during the war have been raised, and we must see in the future that labour is requited with wages which will sustain life.

" It would be a mistake—in fact, it would be impossible—to attempt a statement of detailed plans in this hour, crowded with other and more important concerns. That is quite true at any moment of the war, but there are minds considering all these points— expert minds—so that when the war is over the nation shall not lose time in setting its house in order. It is idle to pretend that the best method of dealing with all these intricate, delicate, complex problems, far reaching and immense, is in the power of any Government who are necessarily absorbed in the prosecution of this war to a victorious end; but the moment that struggle is over the work of reconstruction must begin.

"You must reconstruct when you have got behind you the momentum of victory to carry you through to an even greater triumph. That is why the whole field of national enterprise, of national endeavour, and national resource, and of material well-being is being examined carefully and prospected with a view to immediate action, before that great spirit grows cold in the frigid atmosphere of self-interest. Let us have it when the nation is riding the chariot of a high purpose, ere it comes down to the dusty road. That is the time to reconstruct, that is the time to build.

The Menace from Within.

" When there is the spirit of fraternity throughout the land, when there is no longer rich and poor, men of one party or other, but one people, one spirit, one purpose, one soul to lift our native land not merely, above the menace of a foreign foe, but above the wretchedness, the squalor, the horror, the misery which so many of the men, women and children who live on the hearthstones of this old land have been enduring. I have been amongst the people, and I know it, and I want to see this thing righted.

" The next thing is we must face these problems with courage. When you come to the war, millions of people are full of courage. But when faced with the problems of peace somehow or other it vanishes. You will never successfully tackle a job of which you are afraid. The next thing is, the effort must be equal to the task."

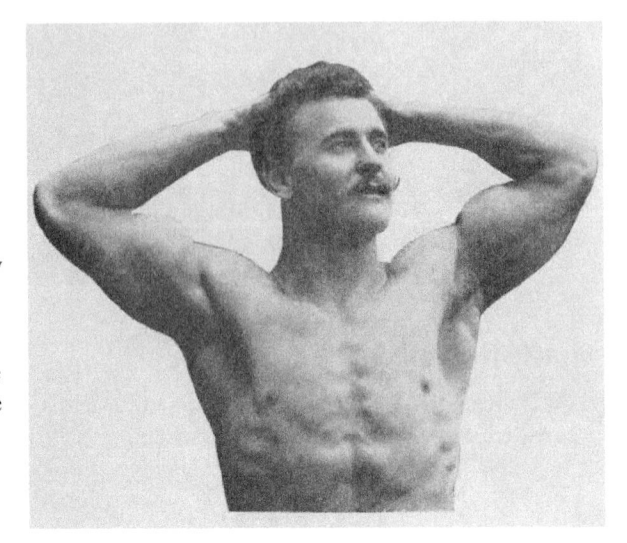

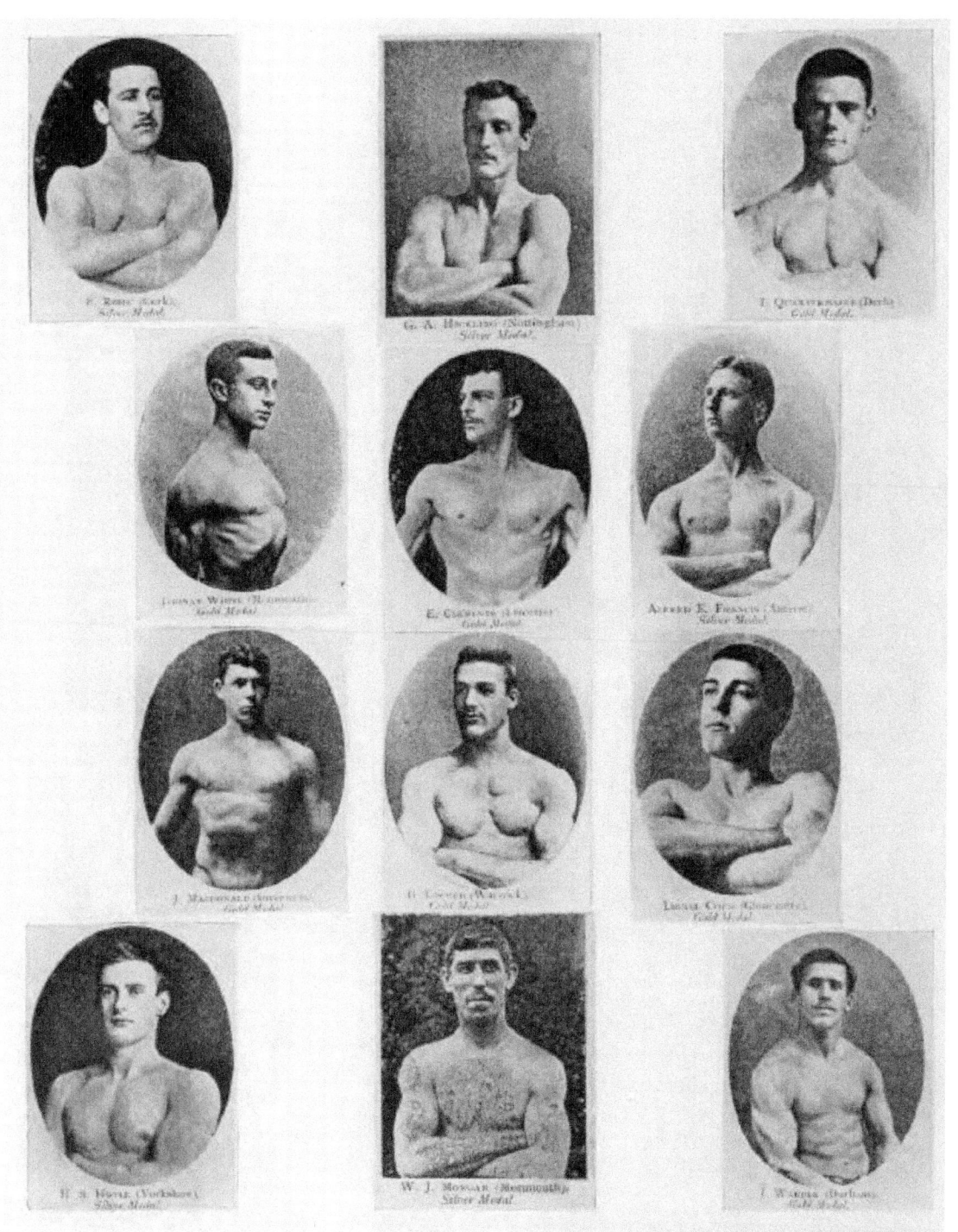

Winners of Gold, Silver and Bronze Medals in various parts of the United Kingdom, who were trained and developed by these methods, and who were among the competitors in the great final contest at the Royal Albert Hall, described in the previous chapter. This gives a slight idea of what could be accomplished if State physical education, as recommended and described here, were made compulsory in all schools from childhood. These were the types so urgently needed, and so often missing, when Britain went to war.

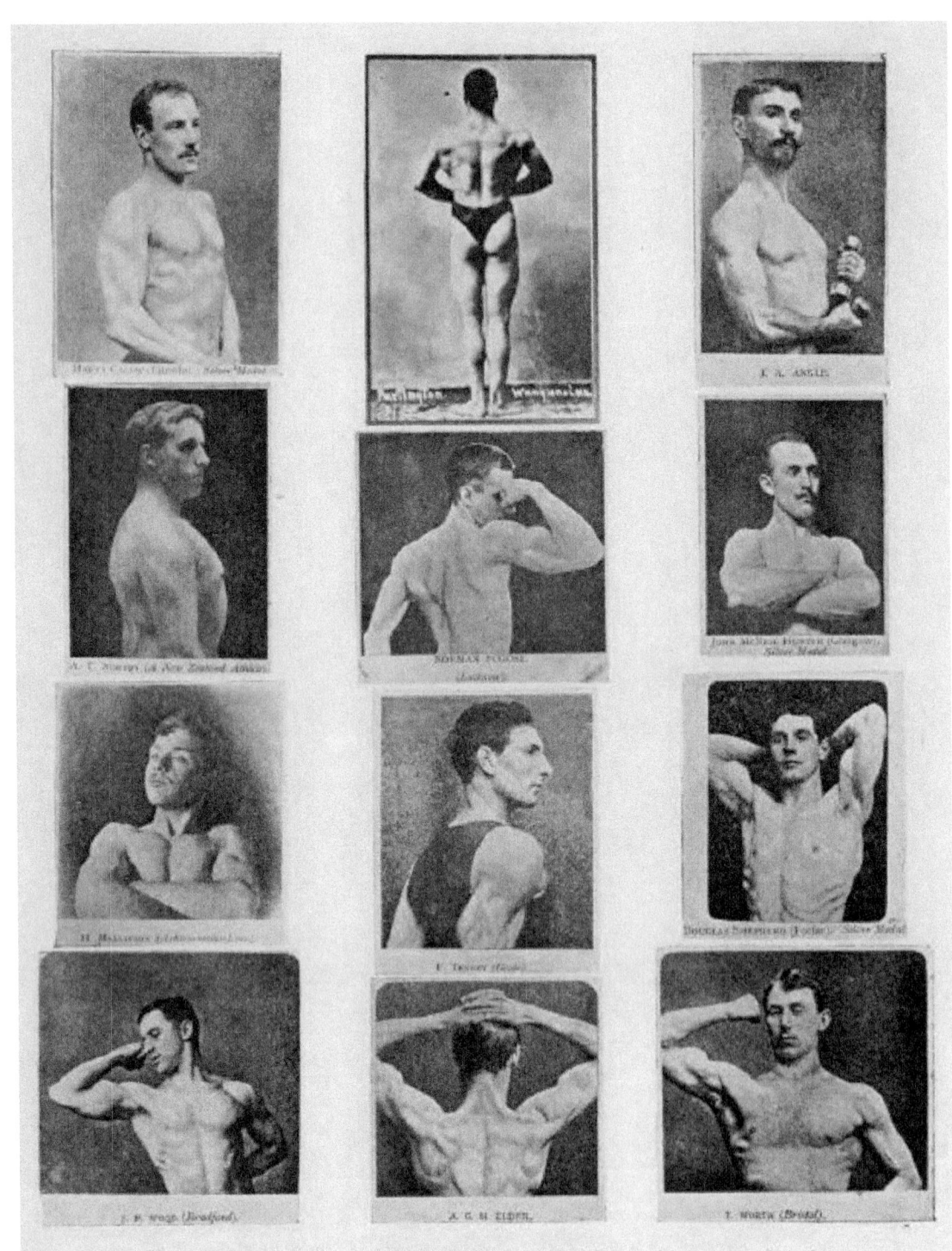

More types of the Gold, Silver and Bronze Medallists who competed at the Royal Albert Hall.

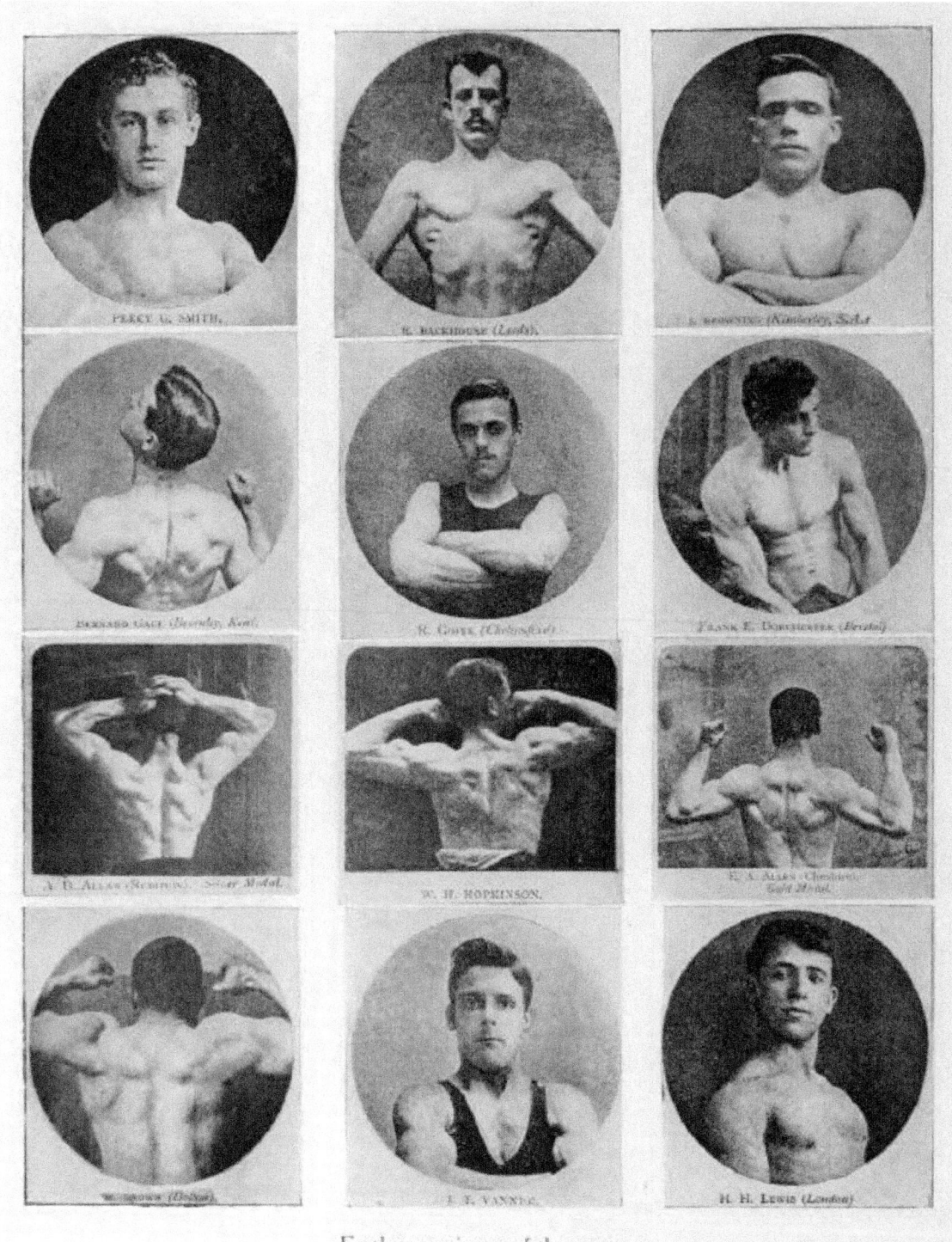

Further specimens of the same.

Another Group of Prize Winners.

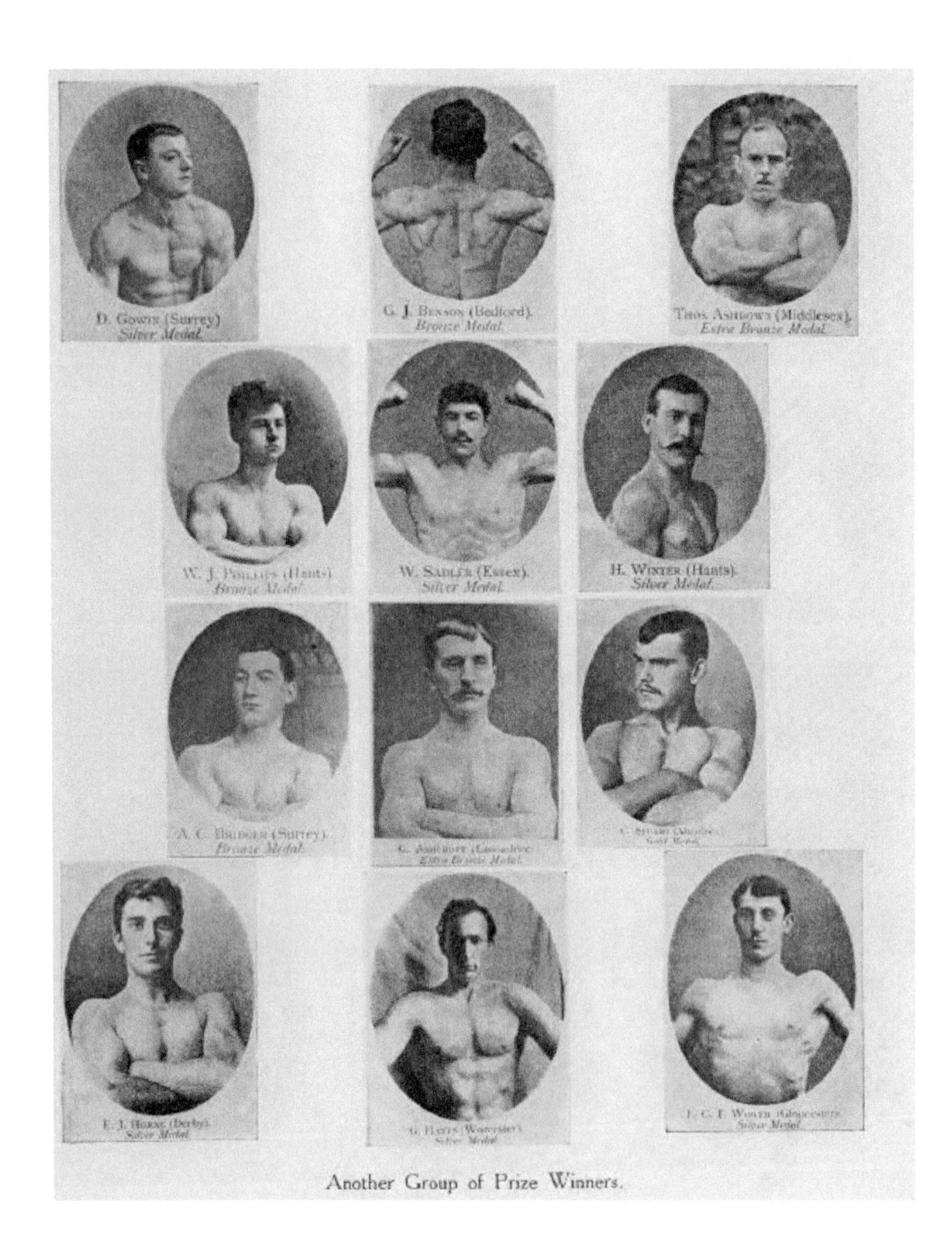

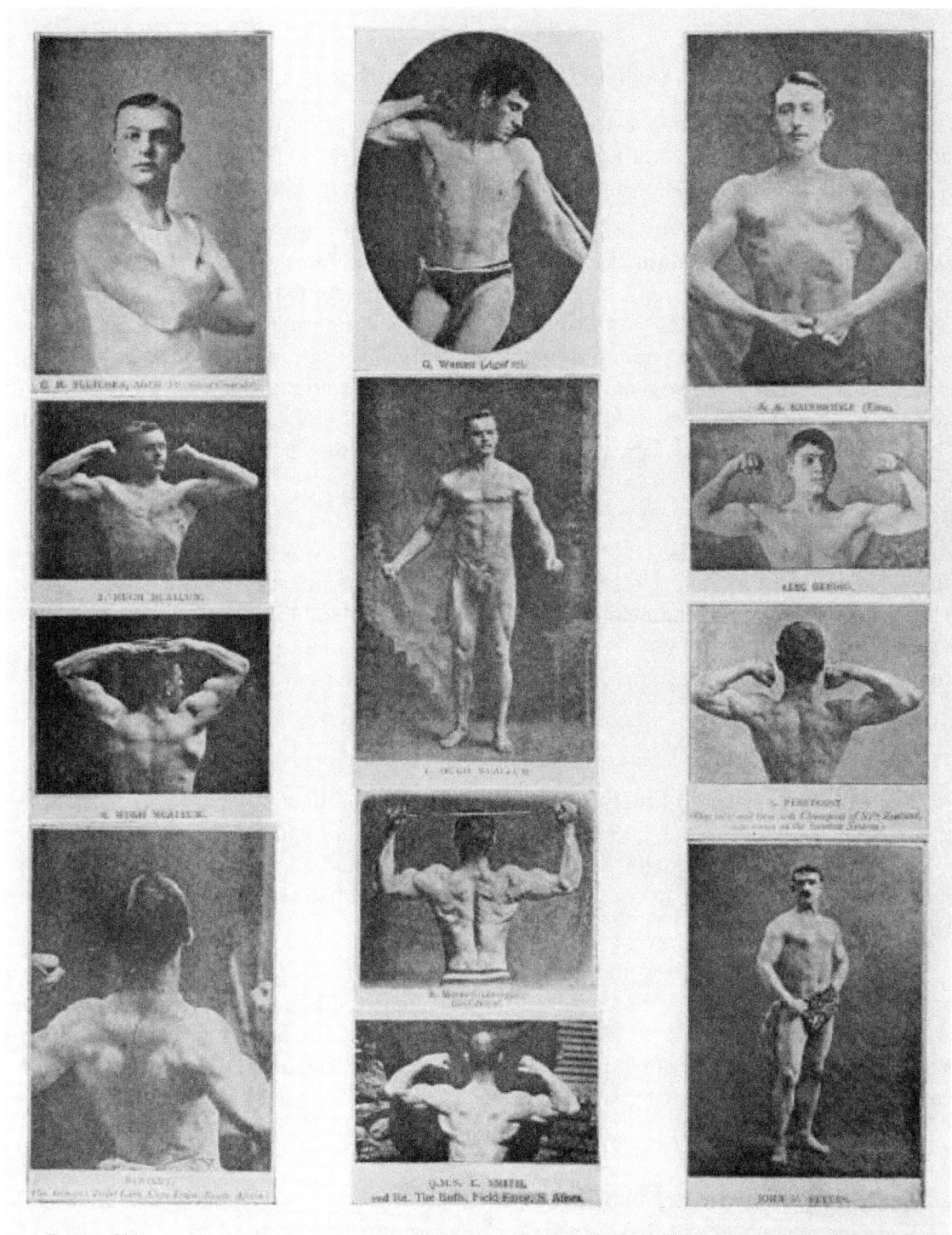

Some of the results of these methods of physical reconstruction which will build the weakest up in strength and resistant power to disease.

CHAPTER II.

My Grave Warning to the Nation.

GREAT and grave as has been the crisis through which we have just passed, a still greater and graver yet confronts us. We were unprepared for war. Let us, at least, be prepared for peace, which will make demands upon each individual little less severe than those of war.

War, " which like the toad, ugly and venomous, wears yet a precious jewel in its head," has at least the uses as it has the discomforts of adversity. It has taught us much, and will, I hope, teach us still more. It has X-rayed deep into every fibre of the modern social system, and has located many blemishes. It has revealed, not a single skeleton, but a veritable army of skeletons, in the cupboard of civilisation. It has pulled down many jerry-built social structures, and torn up still more ramshackle schemes of social construction and reconstruction. It has safely exploded many floating social mines, and cleared the social sea of much drifting and dangerous flotsam and jetsam. It has opened the eyes of the wise and closed the mouths of fools.

THE UNIT OF NATIONAL POWER.

It has shown the world that the real unit of power is MAN—even the humblest human being—and that everything in a country's life depends finally and conclusively upon its man-power—upon the health, happiness, character and efficiency of each and every individual human being, no matter what his social or financial status. We must take mankind more seriously for the future; for, to-day more than ever, we appreciate the deep-biting truth of Goldsmith's words:

> " Ill fares the land to hastening hills a prey,
>
> Where wealth accumulates and men decay."

" War," as the Premier said in his great awakening and illuminating speech at Manchester, to which I have already referred, " had been the most costly schoolmaster any nation had ever had. It had rendered a service to humanity, and the magnitude would appear greater and greater as this generation receded in the past. We have used our human material in this country prodigally, foolishly, cruelly."

Even in the acute crisis of war, indeed, an almost criminally flippant attitude was too often adopted in high places towards the question of individual health and efficiency—an attitude that will be fatal towards a sane outlook for peace times. Here, for instance, is an extract from a report of a London Military Tribunal presided over by a Mr Brinsley Harper during the war. It is indicative of the mental attitude to which I refer:—

HUMOUR IN THE WRONG PLACE.

" I never thought I was so bad until I saw the doctor's certificate," said an appellant to a Mr Brinsley Harper, the chairman. " Ah, there are lots," replied that individual, I who get a terrible shock when medically examined." Such was the happy-go-lucky way of regarding so serious a matter as our individual man-power, debased as it was shown to be to a most dangerous degree, even in such a crisis as that through which the British Empire, and, indeed, the civilised world, has just passed. Yet those very medical examinations revealed facts that were positively of an alarming nature, and were not matters to be regarded lightly.

They led, as a result of the medical examination of many young and middle-aged men for the first time since they had reached adulthood, to surprising and painful revelations as to the physique and health of the nation as a whole. Many, again, who were medically examined by the military doctors, and who had not been medically examined for some years previously in civil life, were surprised to find that they had become unexpectedly unfit physically or were even the victims of some unsuspected form of disease.

Thousands more, having passed the medical tests safely, proved quite unfit, after a very brief military service, for the severe military duties at home or war operations abroad. The taint of tuberculosis, heart trouble, venereal and other microbic diseases, was painfully evident everywhere. What a revelation; but what a harvest of previous information if only it be garnered and stored and profitably used in the future.

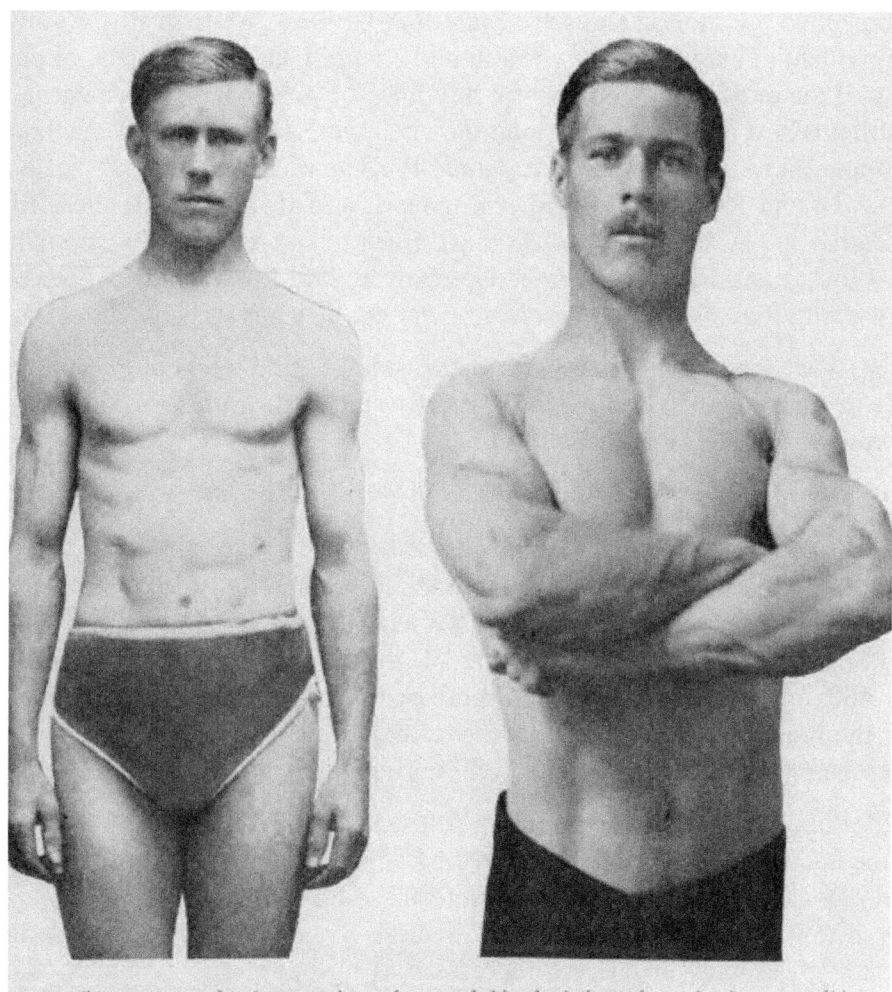

A striking contrast, showing at a glance the remarkable physical transformation from a condition of physical unfitness to an almost perfectly balanced physique, the result of a very short course of physical development and reconstruction by the methods I am now advocating. Had such methods been in vogue before the war, the "terrible shock" so many had on medical examination would have been avoided.

UNFIT AT TWENTY.

Professor Keith, the distinguished physiologist, writing in The Observer, has given some startling evidence as to the physical condition and health of the male population as revealed by these military examinations.

" What," he asks, | are we to regard as an ideal standard of fitness among the young men of a nation? From theoretical reasoning, as well as from practical experience, we expect that if 1,000 young men are collected at random from a population of good health and physique and graded according to their physical fitness the result will be approximately as follows:—

Grade I., 700.   Grade III., 75.

Grade II., 200.   Grade IV., 25.

" What may be called the index grades are I. and IV. Grade I. are men fit for general service—men in the enjoyment of at least average health and strength. Grade IV. men are physically unfit, unequal to any of the duties of a soldier—for any form of physical employment in civil life. We are dealing with a robust and healthy population when we find its youthful manhood yielding us 70 per cent. Grade I. and only 2.5 per cent. Grade IV. The critical line in the scale of fitness lies between Grades II. and III.; the 900 men in Grades I. and II. are more or less fit, but the 100 forming Grades III. and IV. are more or less unfit. Even in an ideal healthy population we expect 10 per cent, of unfit men. In pre-war times Germany is said to have had 16 per cent, of young men who were unfit for active military service; every country has its problem of the unfit.

" I have given what I regard as a satisfactory result of grading young men from a healthy population. To contrast with it I will give a result typical of grading 1.000 men drawn at the present time from one of our large industrial towns:—

Grade I., 190   Grade III., 410

Grade II., 270   Grade IV., 130

" Let us look at the index Grades I. and IV. In Grade I. there are only 190 men in place of 700; in Grade IV. there are 130 in place of 25. When we look for the missing men of Grade I. we find them mostly in the partially unfit group, Grade III. In place of having 900 men more or less fit, we have only 460; and in place of 100 men more or less unfit, 540. The objection might rightly be raised that the present population of our towns and cities is merely a residue left after the fit and young men had gone on active service in the earlier years of the war.

" Only the older and less fit younger men are left, and age has a definite influence on a man's grade. After the age of thirty, men tend to become degraded—to pass from Grades ft. and II. to Grades III. and IV. This tendency proceeds uniformly until about the age of forty-six, and then there is a slump towards the lower grades. Now these objections are perfectly valid; we obtain from such examples a totally erroneous impression as to the relative numbers of the unfit—but they leave us under no illusion as to the total number of our citizens who are physically unfit. Mr Lloyd George is right; their number is appalling."

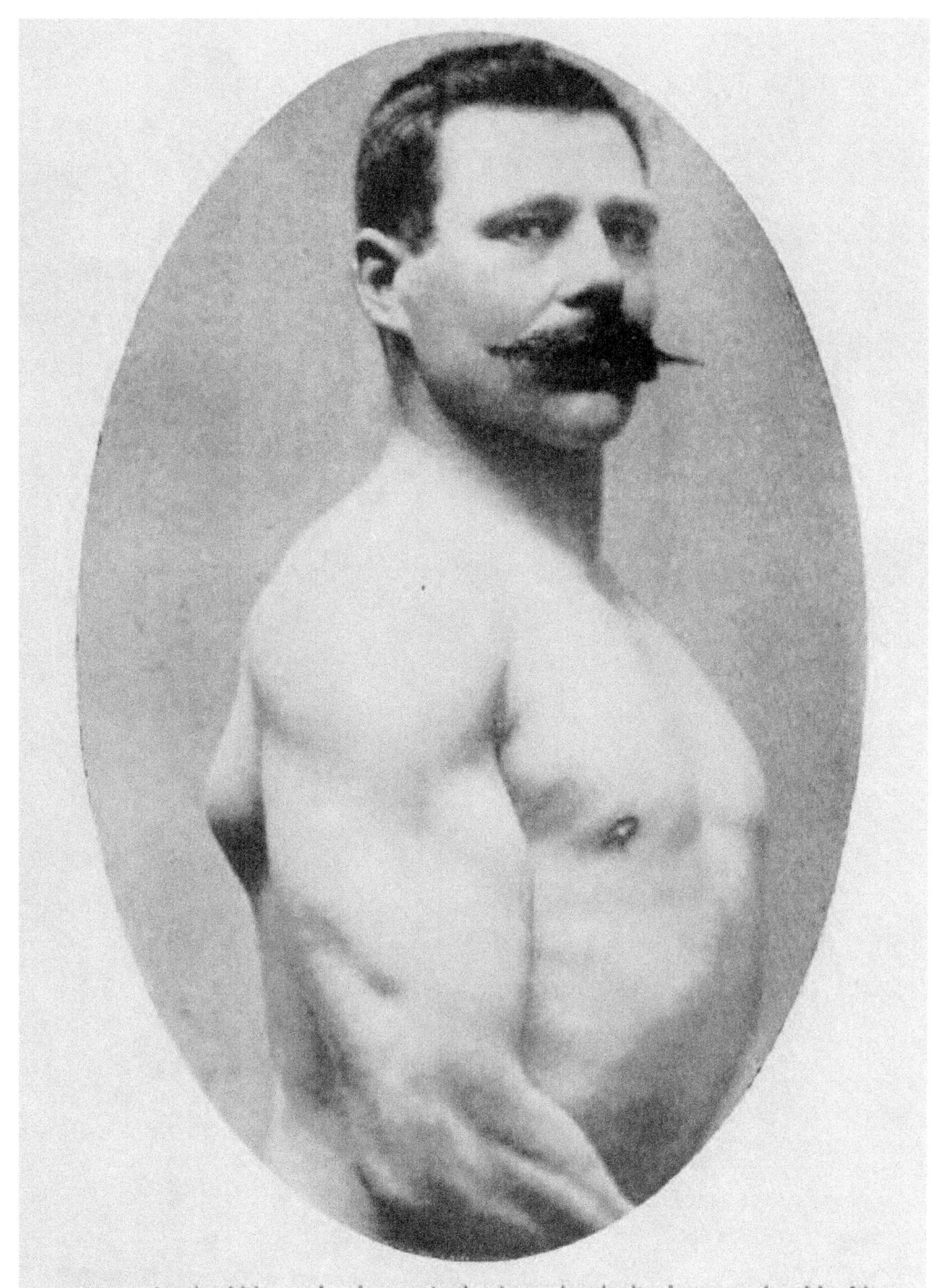

Man as he should be, and as he was in the days when he lived a natural and healthy physically active life. A fine specimen of New Zealander, W. Jarratt, who has done much to spread the gospel of physical and mental efficiency by these methods, to which he owes his own fine development.

Photo by Stannish & Preece, New Zealand.

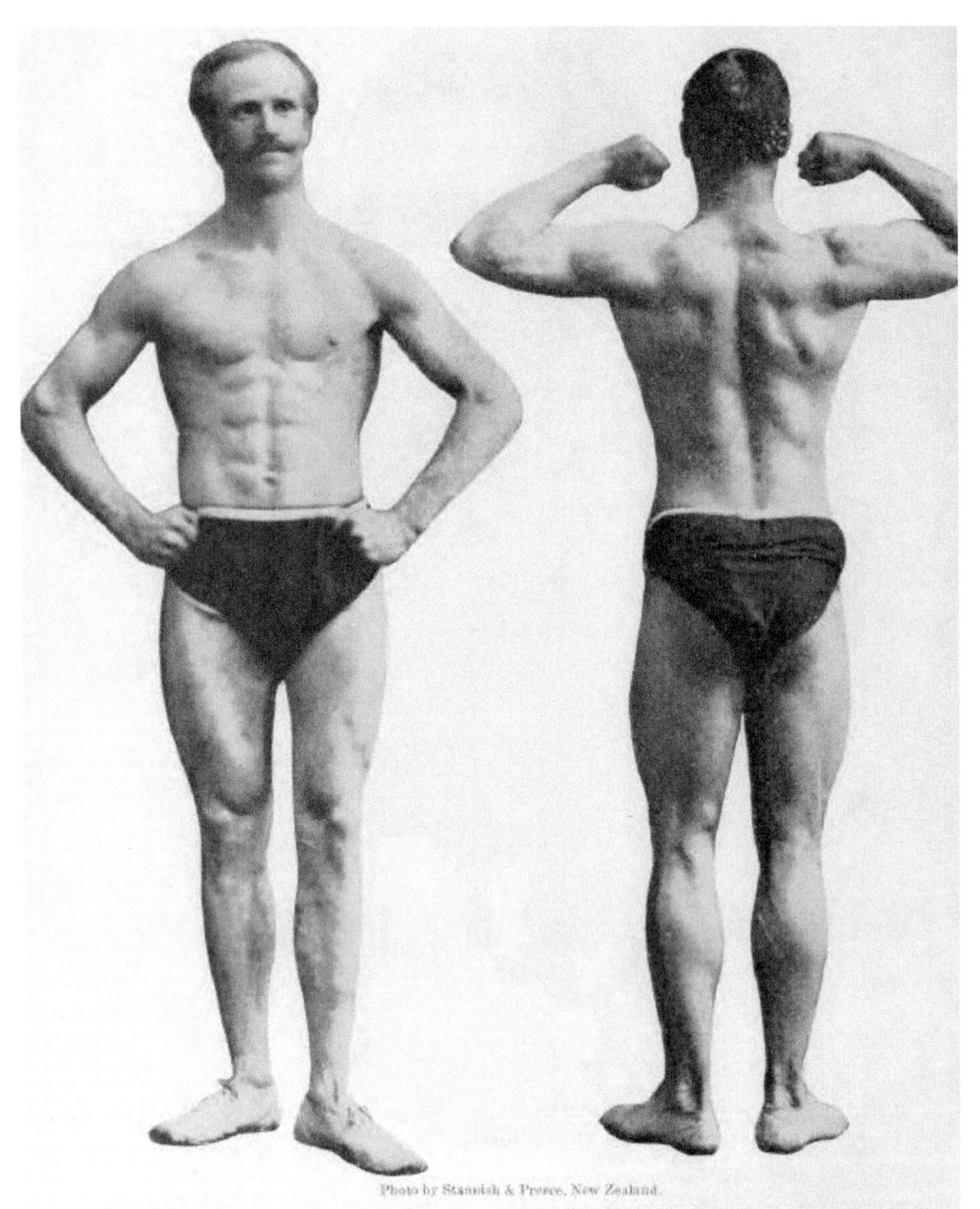

Two splendid physical examples, showing back and front development, whose physique is entirely attributable to scientific methods of natural physical movement as described in these pages.

A BLOW TO A NATION'S PRIDE.

Nor were these revelations after medical examination confined to England. Equally, and in some cases even more alarming, returns were made among the peoples of all the countries affected by the war. The diarist of the Evening Standard said that in America no less than 66 out of every 100 men who volunteered for the American Army had to be rejected as physically unfit. This means roughly that something like 5,000,000 young Americans between the ages of 21 and 31 failed to come up to the A1 standard. Perhaps, after all, this is not to be wondered at, however, in that land of hustle, where health is too often forgotten in the mad race for wealth.

In England, with an out-of-doors and a sport-loving people, the results of the medical examinations shocked us too terribly, and hurt our pride.

Thousands of patriotic men anxious to serve their King and Country were rightly horrified and ashamed at this revelation of their unconscious physical degeneracy. They had believed themselves, as so many mistakenly do, sound and fit until medical tests opened their eyes. Did they expect to have bodies really healthy, fit and strong without that knowledge of their own bodies, and how to keep them in health, which everyone should acquire from childhood, or without that daily and all-round physical movement and consequent development, which the body was meant to have for its own well-being and preservation against disease, and which it naturally received in man's earlier stages of existence?

For years the majority of them had been content to go on earning money with their brains while their bodies wasted and weakened through lack of balanced and natural physical movement. Stripped to a state of nature and medically tested, they suddenly found that, like Macaulay's despised Bengalee, they had grown weak even to effeminacy." They could not stand forth " naked and unashamed." Yet how many more of non-military age are in a similar or worse physical plight to-day, to say nothing of the still more neglected women and children in our midst.

THE RISING VALUE OF MAN.

The fact is that man-power and physical efficiency have too long been despised or neglected in our search after mechanical power and mechanical efficiency or brain-power alone for the wealth it brings, and we were forgetting that, after all, the only wealth is health. Millions have been spent on the invention and perfecting of machinery, while the most wonderful machine in the world— the human body—has been allowed to deteriorate and rust. Hyperdeveloped brains and under-developed bodies have wrought infinite harm.

To-day, man is coming into his own again, and we may with hope look forward to a saner exploitation of human flesh and blood and brain in the future than the gruesome spectacle the world has just witnessed. Let our men of money never forget that money invested in man is as well and as profitably invested as money sunk in land or mines, in inventions or machinery, in horses or dogs or motor-cars, and that it is the deepest interest and duty of the State to cultivate the human soil, to sow it with good seed, to dig it and till it and care for it in every way, to bring it into healthy touch with the air, the sun, the moisture, and all it demands and needs to sustain it and make the human plant grow, just as the agriculturist improves the productive quality of the land by continuous and ordered movement.

The war revealed a people degenerate, diseased, and weak physically, owing to conditions of modern life, in which the physically fittest, by a grim irony, too often survived in the struggle for wealth and position, to leave still weaker and more physically unfit children after them. It has made the physical education and culture of the people imperative, and it is my object in this book to show that this can only be successfully accomplished if the whole subject is taken up seriously and carried out by really scientific methods, and with the support of an efficient and intelligent State organisation, the medical profession, and a qualified and capable executive in every department.

But behind the State we must, as a leader writer in the Evening Standard has well pointed out, have also " the driving power of a resistless public opinion," and what the Daily Mail has pointed out as even more important still, " team work between the doctor and the statesmen "

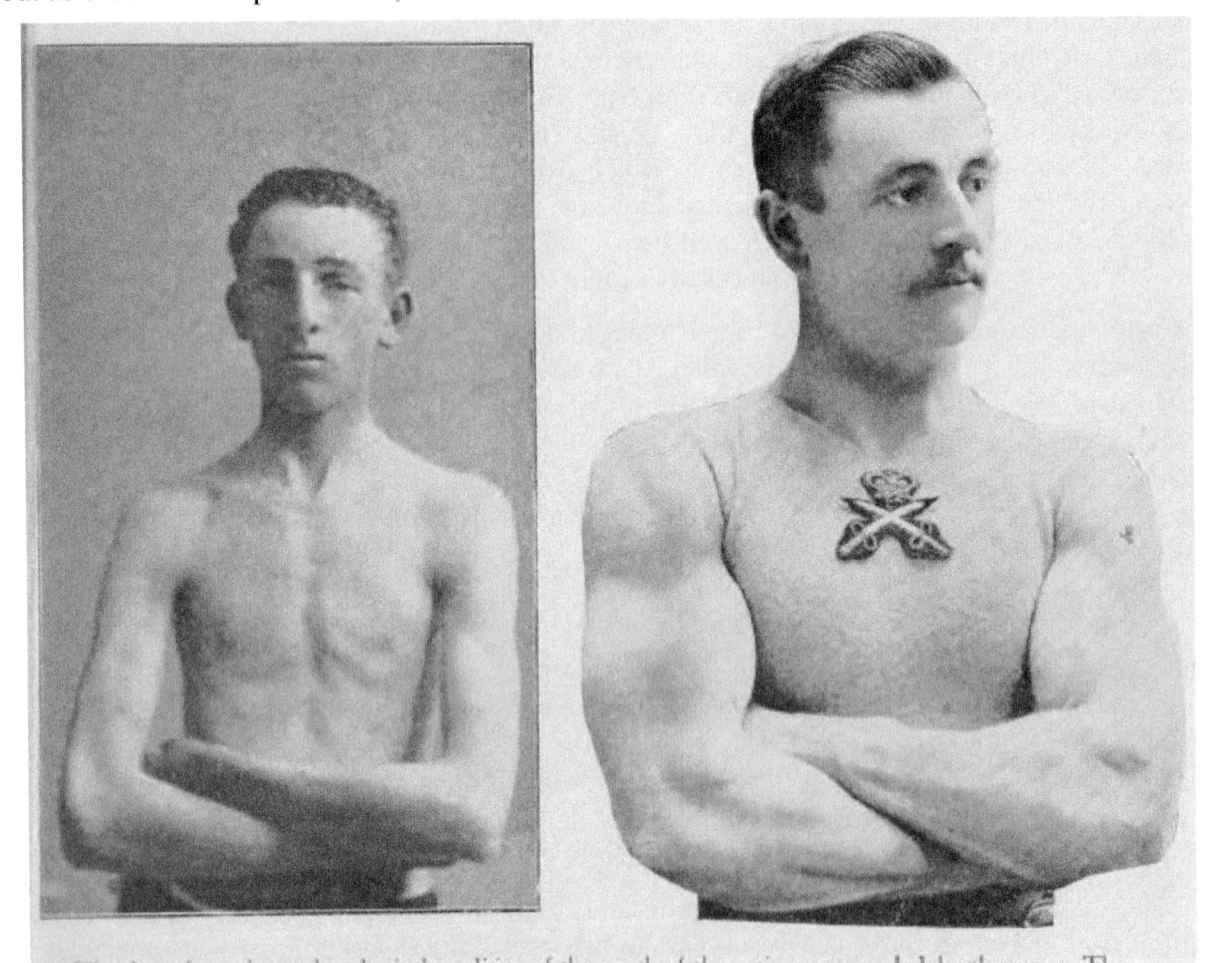

The first photo shows the physical condition of the youth of the nation as revealed by the war. The second shows what can be achieved by scientific methods of physical education and culture, and how imperative such methods are to safeguard us against physical deterioration and disease in the future.

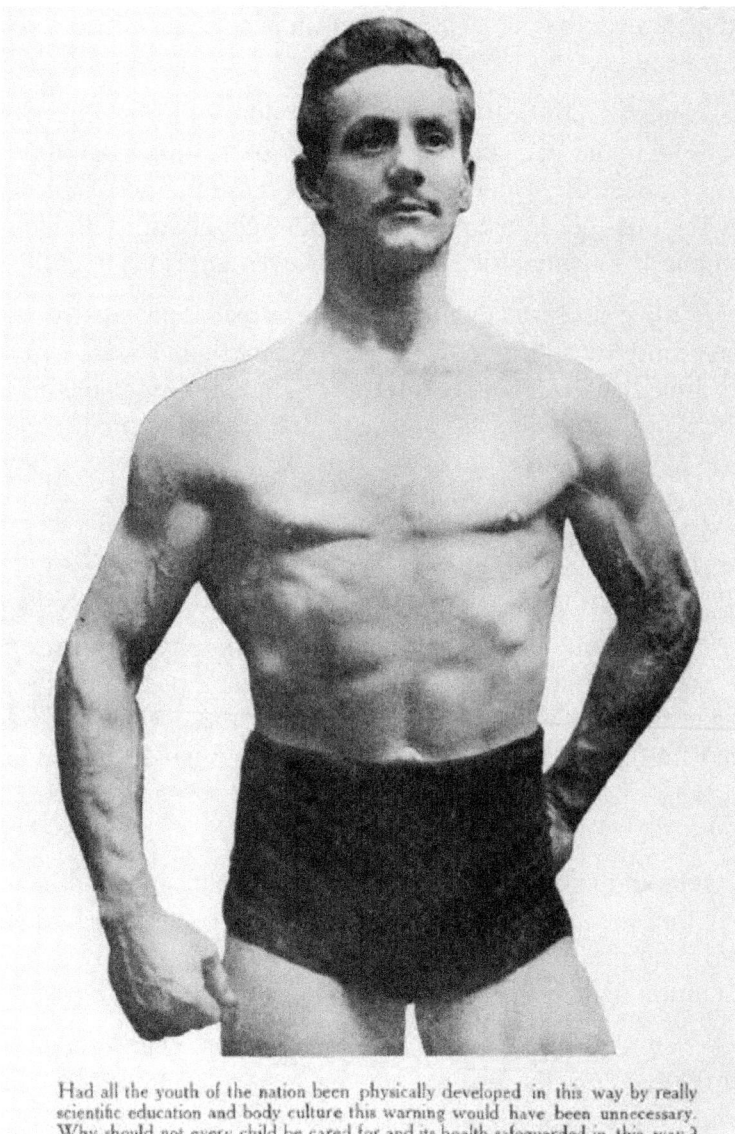

Had all the youth of the nation been physically developed in this way by really scientific education and body culture this warning would have been unnecessary. Why should not every child be cared for and its health safeguarded in this way?

MAKING C3 ADULTS.

Our lack of a scientific system of physical education and health culture in the past has brought us a harvest of physical weakness and ill-health, for, to quote Dr Addison, " we cannot expect to get an A1 population out of C3 homes, habits, work-places or conditions of life," while, unfortunately, he added, the army of C3 men referred to is but " the expression only in adult life of other C3 armies now coming onwards from their cradles." Only such methods as indicated in this book will prevent even A1 babies being perverted into C3 adults.

These changes need not, however, mean efficiency at the price of individual rational enjoyment, but such early education and training will give us a real " merry England " once more, for while, to again quote the Evening Standard, " every child should also be taught that it is a duty to the State to keep himself or herself fit, every child should also be encouraged to enjoy its own life." In this way we can succeed where militarism and materialism have failed in other countries. For no military training can ever be as effective as this civilian education and training from childhood.

When some people suggested physical training for children on the lines followed in our new civilian army there was an immediate outcry, not, however, so much against this military method of physical training as against the danger that this was the thin end of the wedge of militarism. The real danger was the possible introduction into our schools of methods of physical training that would have been totally unsuited for and possibly even injurious to children.

Military physical training is only adapted for those already physically strong and sound in constitution, who have only to be trained specially for particular feats of endurance which are necessary in military life. Such methods would never be successful in the case of children, or even of adults, where the real aim is physical and constitutional reconstruction and the upbuilding of a bod/ strong enough in every part to resist disease. They do not, in short, constitute what I call scientific physical education.

DANGER OF MILITARY METHODS.

In the first place, those who were selected for military service at the beginning of the war represented the very crème de la crème of the nation in the physical sense at least. They were only selected after a most searching medical examination, and passed by the doctor as free from all physical defects and disease. Yet tens of thousands of these young and fit men broke down under the severity and strenuousness of military training, and have been done incalculable injury for life, many collapsing in fits, faints and exhaustion after long marches and heavy military drills.

While of those who endured the training many benefited in physique and health, it is evident that such extemporised and unscientific methods of training were utterly unsuited even for many of those who were passed by the military doctors as Al, but who, in my standardising, would be lower in physical condition than the lowest of all military categories or grades.

Now, what of the others who were rejected altogether, or who were graded in lower categories? In the nation's most critical hour the majority of these were of no military value, and could not even by military drilling or military methods of training be transformed into valuable fighting assets. If we had had such a system of scientific physical education and training as I am now describing, I contend that the majority of these men would never have had to be rejected at all.

If such a system had even been adopted at the beginning of the war, most of these rejects through physical defects and disease could have been gradually made fit to qualify physically as Al men, and so not lost entirely to the nation in so critical a time. Some could have been made fit to pass the severest military examination in a year or less, some might have taken two years, but instead of that all had to be cast into the " scrap-heap " and practically lost to the nation.

To show the value of such methods as these when adapted by military commanders in an emergency, as I am glad to say they were in quite a number of cases, and carried out even in a somewhat hurried and improvised way to meet the exigencies of the moment, some wonderful results were achieved, and officers in high command were amazed at the physical improvement wrought in the men in a very short time. Here is only one instance out of many similar. A Colonel who took especial interest in his men, and who had personally proved the efficacy of these methods, was so delighted with the result that he decided to bring it to the knowledge of those under his command. What was the result? Well, here is an exact copy of a letter I received later on from the Captain and Adjutant of his regiment:—

From Capt. and Adjt. M.V.O.	Liberty Hall,
2/8th Bn.	Kingsthorpe,
Worcestershire Regiment.	Northampton.
	14/1/1915.

To The Director,

Sandow's Curative Institute,

32a St. James' Street, London.

DEAR SIR,

The Commanding Officer has asked me to write to you and tell you that the physique of the men of this Bn. has been enormously improved since they have been carrying out Mr Sandow's exercises, not only in their chest measurements, but in their general health and fitness. I may also add that the C.O. has been complimented three or four times by different Generals on the apparent hardiness and fitness of his men.

(Signed) P. N. Vigors,

Capt. and Adjt., M.V.O.,

2/8th Bn.,

Worcestershire Regiment.

This was accomplished in the case of adults, and under circumstances that considerably modified the value of the methods I am advocating for the upbuilding of the present and coming generations, but it is easy to see what magnificent results we might naturally expect if such methods were made part of the education and upbuilding of every adult from childhood. They would certainly make such revelations as the military tests for recruits have made public impossible in the future, and would have greatly re-enforced our national physical capacity for the stern trial of a war for our very existence as a nation.

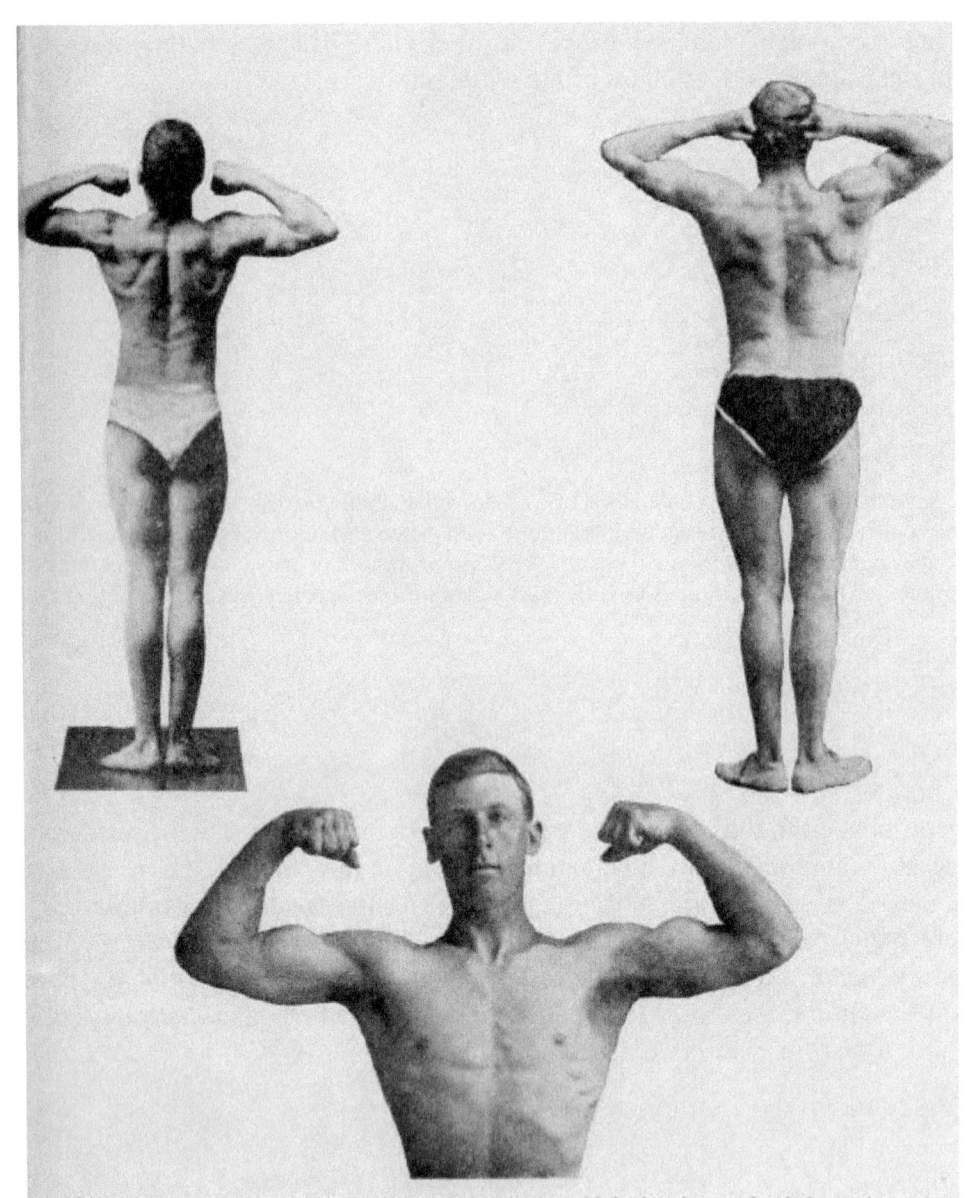

This is what physical education and bodily reconstruction would do for the youth of the nation as it has done for these youths.

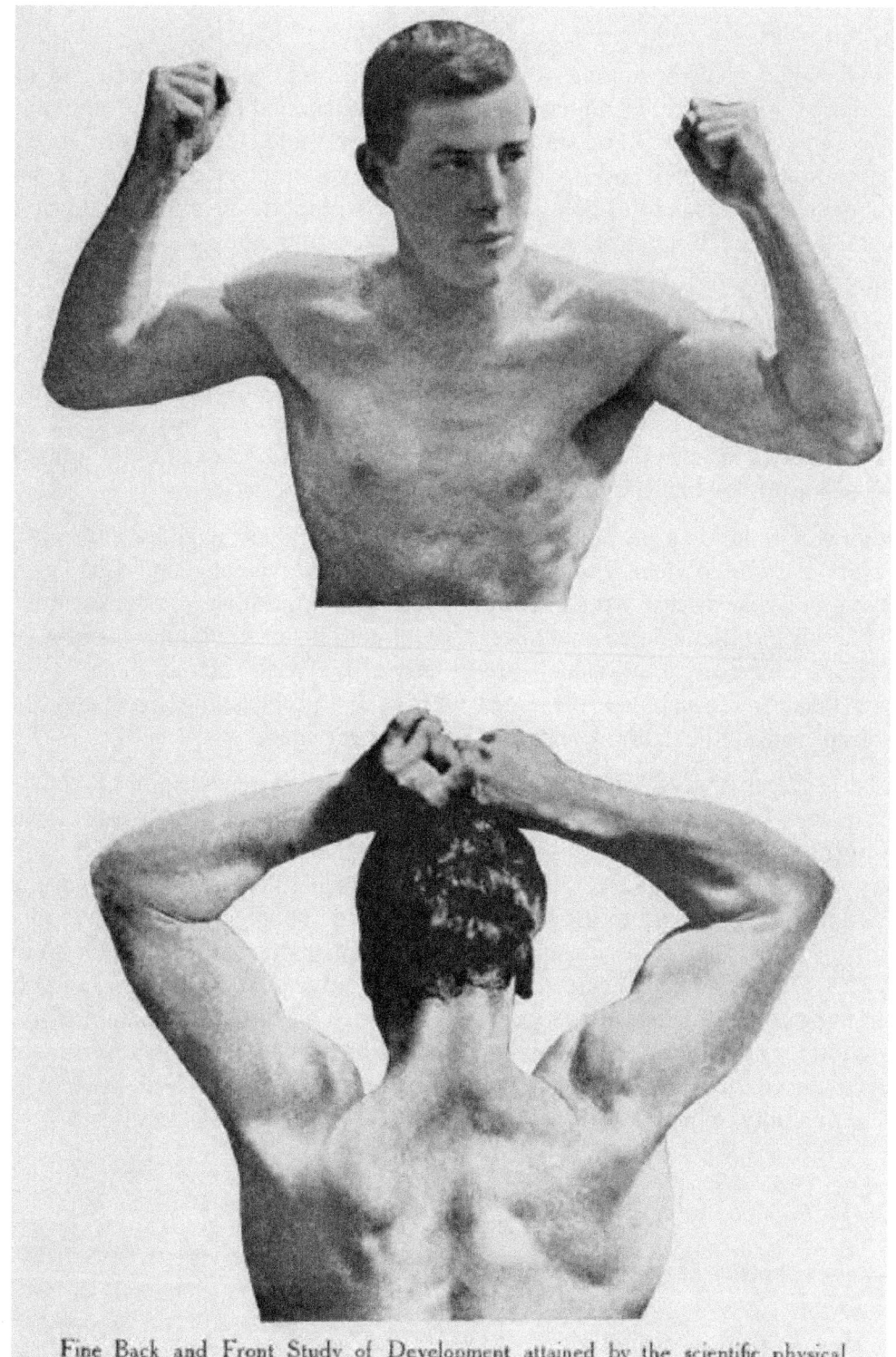

Fine Back and Front Study of Development attained by the scientific physical culture of the body as described in this book.

SCIENTIFIC v. UNSCIENTIFIC METHODS.

When we realise that, at the beginning of the war, only the youngest, healthiest and strongest of the nation came up for medical examination, it will be understood how truly " appalling," to use Mr Lloyd George's word, were these statistics. Indeed, it revealed us almost, as one expressed it to me, as a nation of cripples and invalids. Of those over military age, and the women and children who were left, it is not difficult to imagine how still more appalling would have been the statistics had they also been subjected to a severe medical examination.

One also can imagine the danger of placing these people under a system of physical training of a military type, which wrought so much harm even among the youngest and strongest of the nation and has left many of them infirm and invalid for life. The military system in every country is quite unscientific, and is only fitted for those of the soundest physique and constitution. What the nation requires is a really scientific system of physical education and reconstruction, preferably from the moment a child enters school, so that every one would be taught and trained to health and strength just as to-day they are taught and trained to read and write.

Such a system would build up the body from youth step by step and stage by stage until it was so strong in every part, so perfect in balance and strength everywhere, and with such resistant power in every cell that disease would always attack it in vain. Such a system would deal with each individual on specific and personal lines, according to his or her family history, constitution, temperament, etc., for no two individuals are exactly alike. With such a system it would never again be possible for the nation to be faced with such truly startling figures as the military medical examinations of the nation's manhood have just revealed.

Though the discoveries that followed military medical tests in Great Britain must have alarmed all concerned, they had the one great virtue that they at least put the British Government in possession of a vast store of knowledge and reliable statistics which must prove of the utmost value to any future Ministry of Health, to the medical profession, and to everyone who looks with wise and anxious foresight to the future welfare of the people. Will the State (and, indeed, the States of the world) learn the lesson, and do its or their duty to make such a condition of things impossible in the future? I sincerely hope so, for much can be done to breed better men and women, not only in this, but in every civilised country, if, like the Roman mother, the State regards its children as its jewels. To encourage child-birth, to save and preserve child-life, to reduce preventable disease and mortality, and to make healthy and happy those who survive, should be the first duty of the State. "

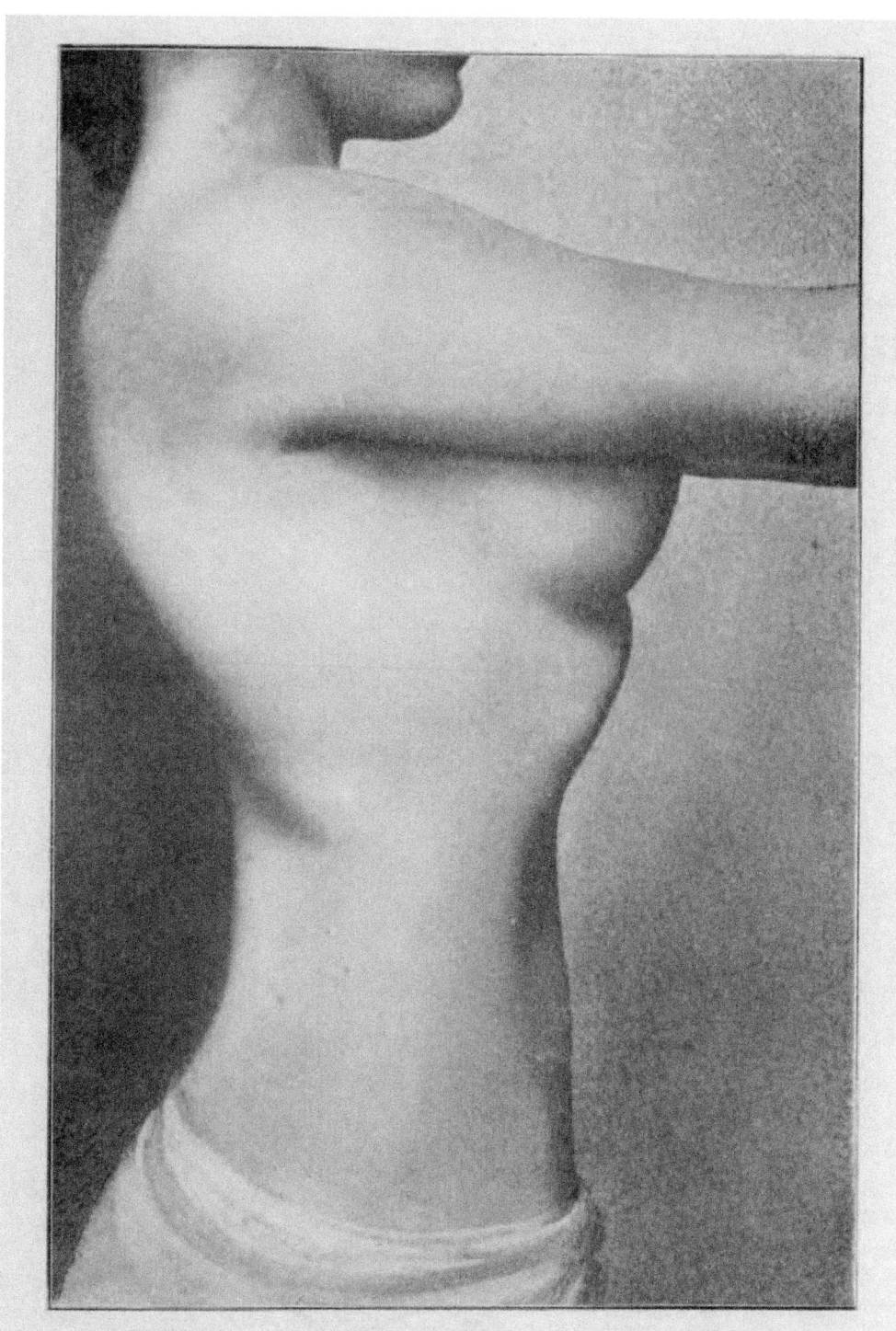

Torso of a beautiful figure, beautifully developed, and as strong as it is beautiful, produced by the methods of body culture herein described. This is the type of woman that the State can have for the mothers of its children if it supports and encourages these methods of body-building from childhood.

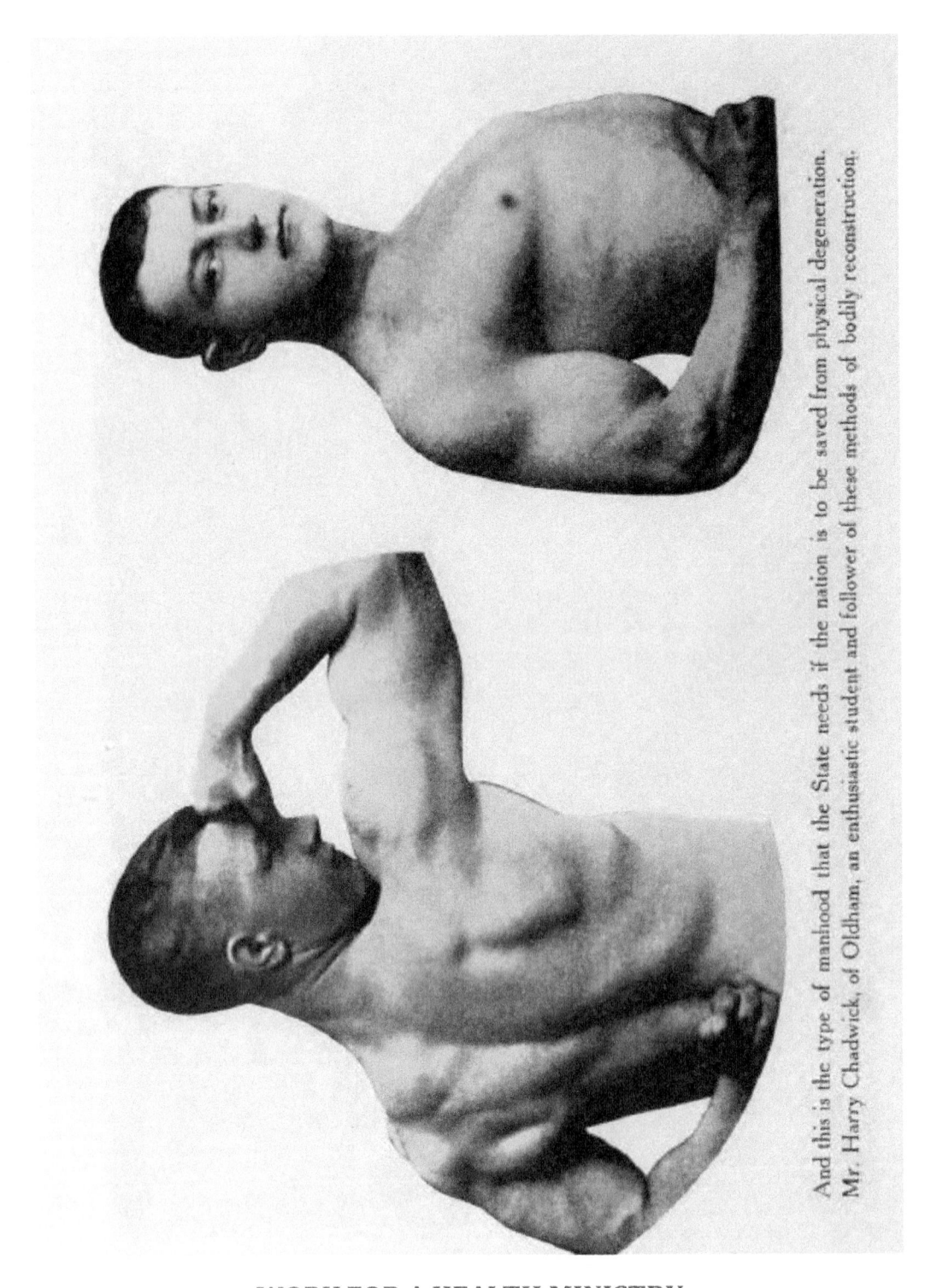

And this is the type of manhood that the State needs if the nation is to be saved from physical degeneration. Mr. Harry Chadwick, of Oldham, an enthusiastic student and follower of these methods of bodily reconstruction.

WORK FOR A HEALTH MINISTRY.

In an editorial on this subject at the time of the revelations, the Daily Mail very rightly pointed out that " the amount of physical unfitness brought to light by the medical examinations has surprised even the doctors. They know that people living in insanitary houses, boys put to hard work before their bones are solid or their muscles strong, men and women working in badly ventilated factories, shop-women and shop-men who stand on their feet for ten hours at a stretch, must almost necessarily suffer from weak lungs, weak hearts, flat foot, curved spine, and other defects, but the amount of ill-health in the country was scarcely suspected.

" Now that the state of matters is made clear," continued the writer, " by statistical records, there should be no delay in taking measures for removing the causes. We have successfully fought the epidemic diseases, small-pox, cholera, and the like, which were destructive so long as their causes remained unknown and unremoved. It will be quite as practicable to remove most of the sources of physical incompetence which not only lessen the pleasure in life of the sufferers, but reduce their value, and often make them a burden to the community. It is said that Dr Addison plans a revolution in the upbringing of children. What we want is a vigorous Ministry of Health to take care of the health of people of all ages, but particularly the young."

This is what I have so long advocated, and I am glad that this distinguished journal, along with the leading periodicals of the day, and medical press, now support me, late in the day as it is. The future of any nation is in the cradles of its children. The physique and health of the child and all children demand attention and care, irrespective of birth or social station, and all should have equal opportunities of health.

All social reform, in fact, must begin in the physical body of the child rather than in its environment. That can be attended to later. But such a revolution in any country's life is not to be lightly begun. It must be begun and carried out on scientific lines.

It must be perfectly organised, and conducted from first to last under strict medical direction and supervision, under the aegis of the State. It must teach men and women and children to understand and care for their own bodies, and to know and obey the laws of health, as does, say, a conscientious and well-schooled athlete. To so educate a child is to put down a good health foundation for life.

PHYSICAL NEGLECT OF THE CHILDREN.

The report of Dr Sir George Newman, K.C.B., F.R.C.P., Chief Medical Officer and Assistant Secretary of the Board of Education, on the physical condition of school children revealed an even more alarming state of things than the military medical examinations, and naturally was widely noted and commented upon by the Press at the time, The Times declaring that " it is now at last realised by the public that something like 1,000,000 children of school age are physically unfit for their school work; more than 2,000,000 children between the ages of 12 and 18 are doing work that is useless as a training for adult life; only a minute proportion of all adolescents in the country are securing an outfit for life in health and in mental and spiritual training.

" The very bad condition of child-life in this country have to some extent been kept stationary during the war by the better food that better wages have secured, but the conclusion of peace, unless the case is specially provided against, will prove a serious set-back, and social deterioration will be accelerated at the very time when it is essential, in view of the losses of the war, to build up a strong and indomitable generation." Steps to prevent degeneration and disease in any and every form, such as I am here advocating, can alone save us from disaster.

In nothing can a State prove more criminal than its neglect of any and every means to ensure and preserve the health of the people. With the passionate appeal of Lord Rhondda still fresh in the memory, it seems utterly incredible that there should be any procrastination in organising the machinery of national health. As his daughter, Viscountess Rhondda, has truly said in a very outspoken article in the Sunday Times, "if the bulk of the disease from which we suffer can be prevented, for Heaven's sake let us prevent it."

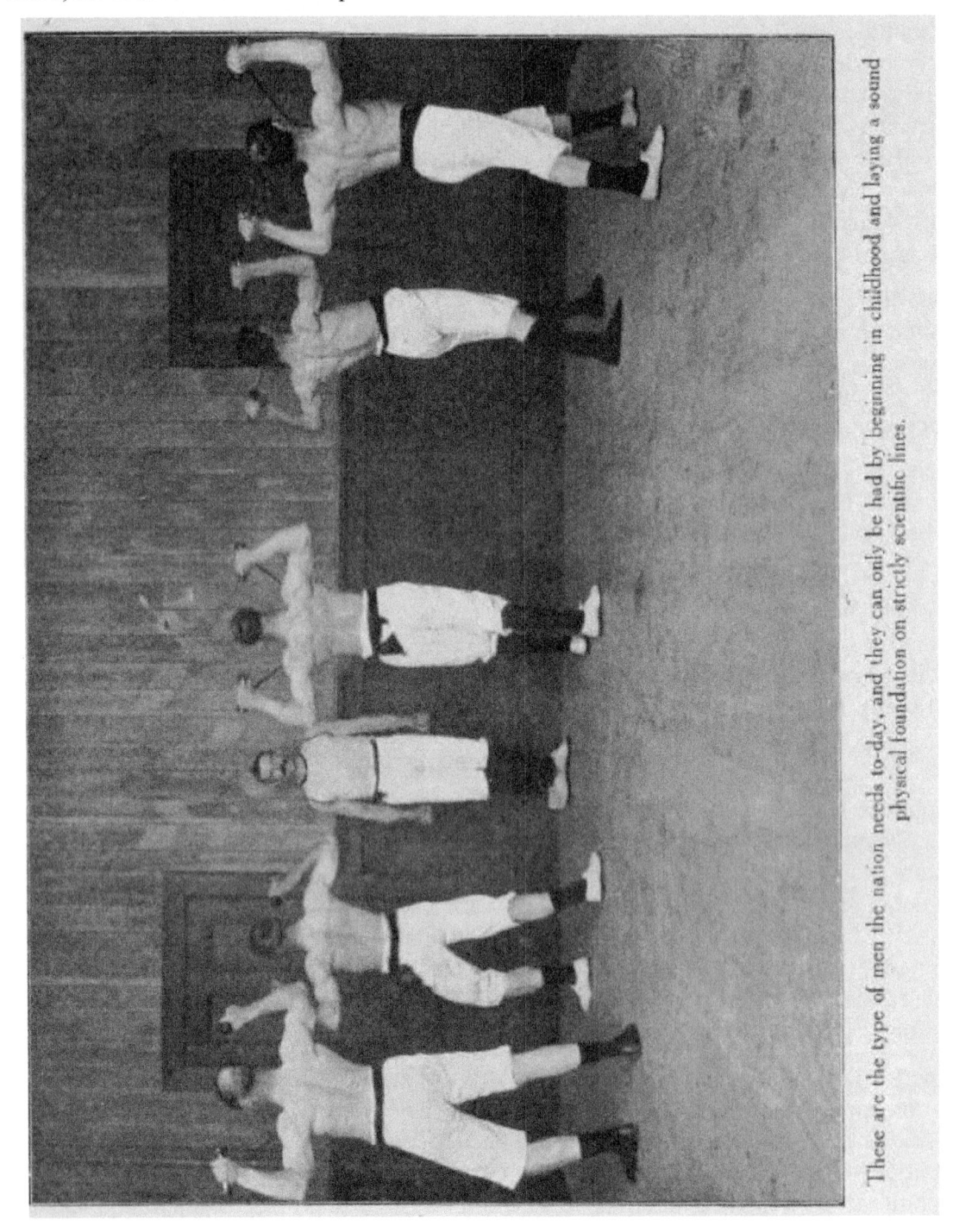

These are the type of men the nation needs to-day, and they can only be had by beginning in childhood and laying a sound physical foundation on strictly scientific lines.

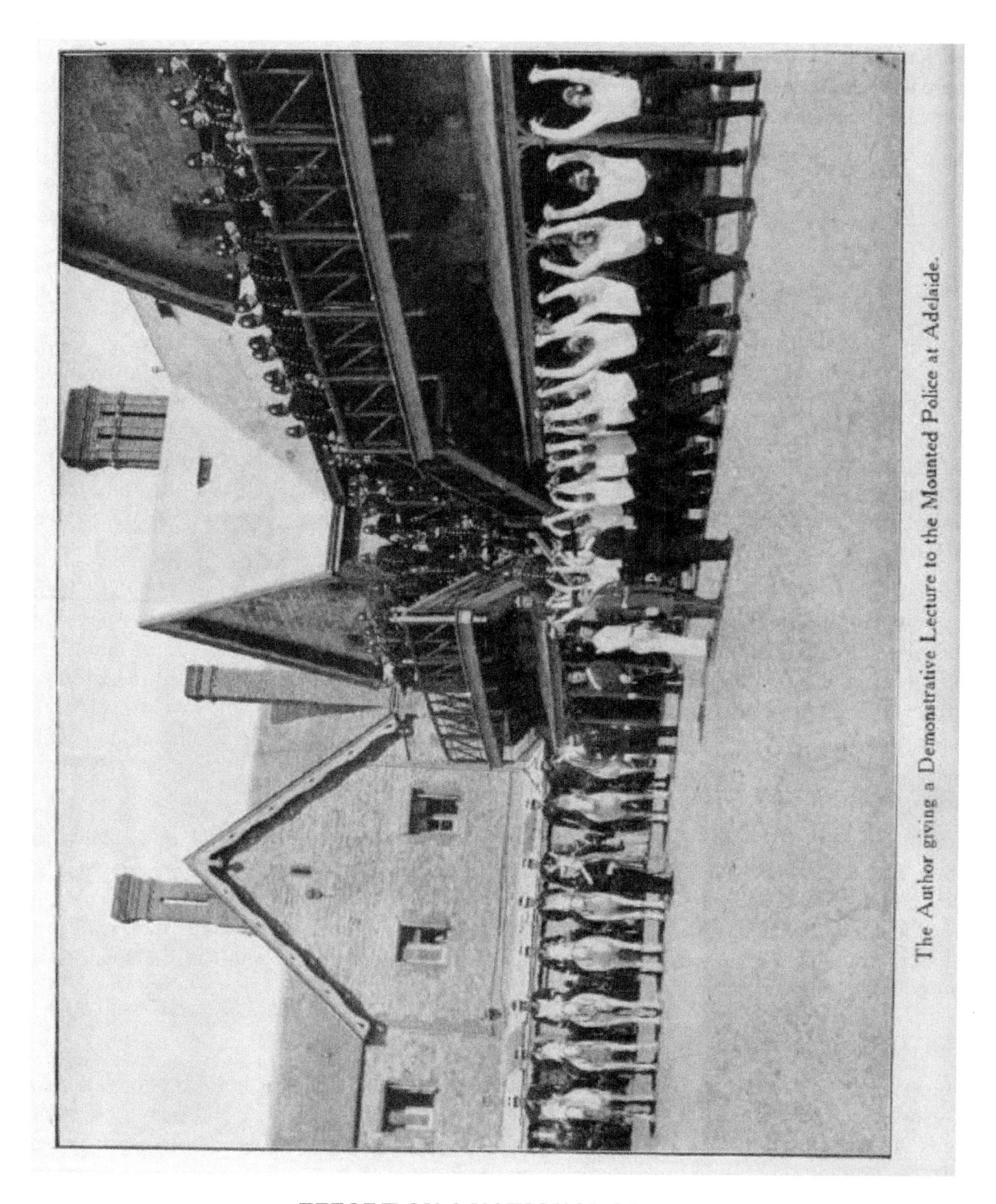

The Author giving a Demonstrative Lecture to the Mounted Police at Adelaide.

EFFORT ON A NATIONAL SCALE.

" It seems, when one stops to consider it, almost unbelievable that in all these years we have never really, as a nation, thought this problem out; never made any serious attempt, on a national scale, to provide ourselves with health. Yet we know that it can be done, for experts tell us that the vast majority of the unfit owe their condition to preventable causes.

"We have fought for liberty, we have insisted upon education, but the one thing that would enable us to enjoy these blessings, to make full use of them, we have left to ignorance, to chance, at best to voluntary effort."

When I first sounded my alarm against the danger of physical deterioration many years ago, I did my very utmost to stimulate such a national movement as Lady Rhondda describes, and it seems a pity that now, after all those years,' my warning must be reiterated with greater emphasis than ever.

PREVENTING PHYSICAL WEAKNESS AND DISEASE.

Medical officers in every part of the country to-day confirm this, and endorse Sir George Newman's observations, while the appalling revelations resulting from the medical examination and treatment of children even on a limited scale—Mr Hayes Fisher, M.P., Minister of Education, himself admitted in the House of Commons that only 39 authorities out of 318 had availed themselves of the power to demand and have medical treatment in public elementary schools—have changed the whole attitude of the medical profession, and compelled them to admit that the work of the medical men in the future must be preventive rather than curative if we are to avert a grave national danger.

Everything, of course, will depend on the nature of the preventive measures adopted whether they achieve success or fail. My contention is that so long as humanity is allowed to physically deteriorate through insufficient movement of the body physical, as it inevitably must through the advance of civilisation and mistaken educational methods, disease can never be prevented, and that, on the contrary, more and more disease and in many new forms will reveal itself as the people grow increasingly weaker. To take the physical body, especially in youth, and to develop it to its highest possible resistant power is the only real preventive of disease, as I show and prove later in this book.

Even in times of peace, life itself is a battle from the cradle to the grave, a battle against foes within and without the body, and, in a physiological sense, at least, it is perfectly true that " peace hath her victories no less renowned than war." Indeed, as a distinguished writer recently said, " it should be the business of those who have the youth of the nation under their care to see that they are educated in accordance with the old ideal of the sane mind in the sound body. Fitness is as necessary for civilian as for military service."

EMPIRES BUILT ON HUMAN FOUNDATION.

Here is a great country—an Empire, indeed, almost too great for human conception—that was only awakened by the stern reveille of war to the fact that its very fibre and being, the human atoms of which it was composed, was in danger. We discovered, in the words of Lord Rosebery, that " an Empire is but little use without an Imperial race." By an effort almost super-human it rallied. Then and then only it was dimly realised that the Empire had been built and was being built upon an insecure foundation. The human material of which it was built and being built had deteriorated to a most alarming degree.

The whole of our far-flung Empire was affected, though less, perhaps, in the Colonies than at home because, I am pleased to say, my own efforts to preach the gospel of physical culture in Canada,. Australia, New Zealand, and South Africa had been well received, and the physical deterioration already checked to some degree. In India, however, a very high percentage of the people have become so physically weak as to be quite unable to withstand the unhealthy climate and pestilential conditions so often associated, and here scientific physical education is even more necessary to combat, prevent and conquer disease than at home. For similar circumstances in India as at home are producing and increasing disease especially just now when there is a great movement afoot to foster education and for the advancement of another stage of civilisation with all its defects and drawbacks as well as its admitted advantages.

The debilitating effect of civilised life and an imperfect or one-sided educational system are the chief causes of this deterioration everywhere. We have forgotten the first principle of education, the stern fact that you cannot develop in a weak, stunted, unhealthy or diseased body a strong, stable and enduring mind. For centuries mind has been cultivated and developed at the expense of body, simply because mental work is deemed to be easier and more profitable than manual.

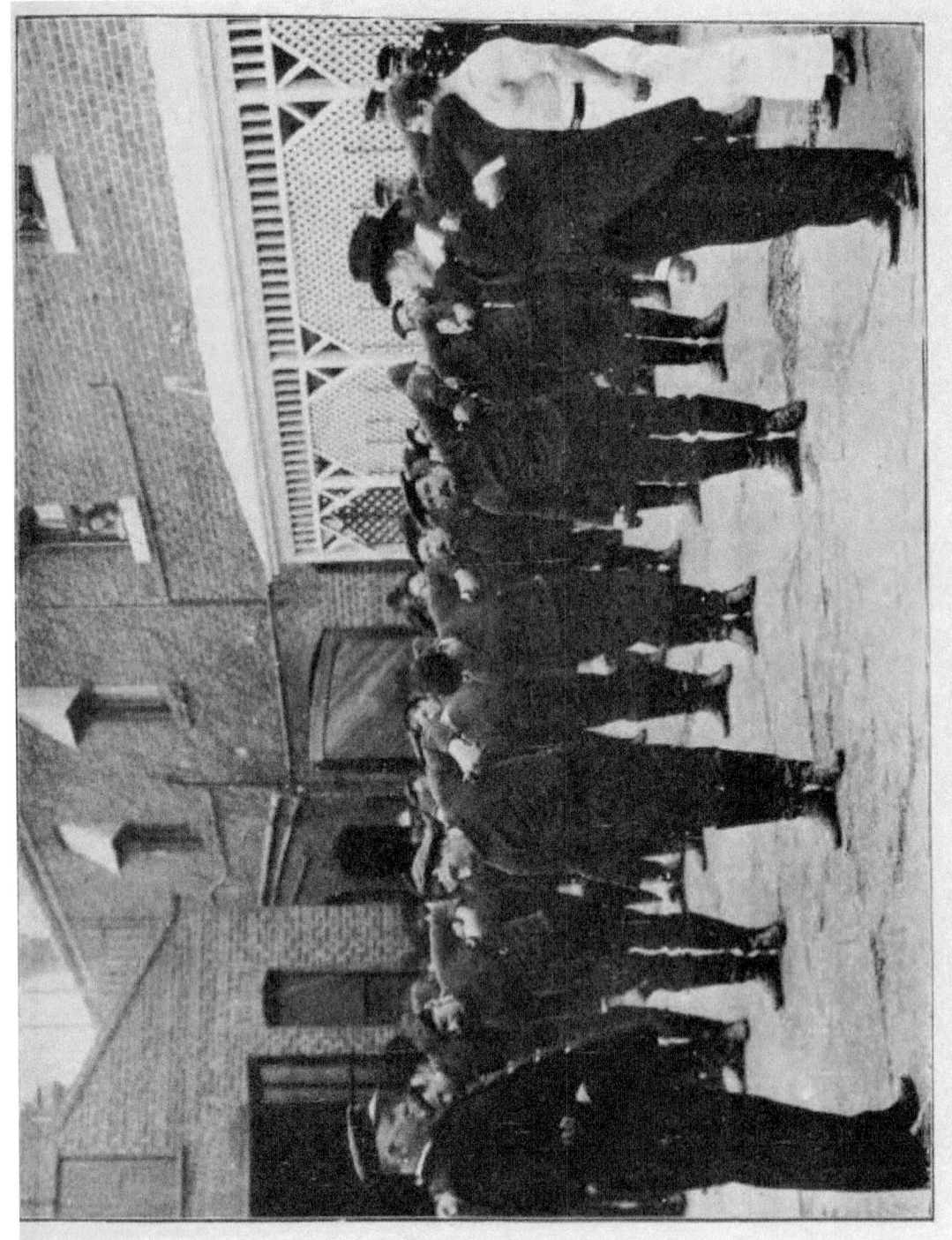

The Author giving personal instruction in these methods of health culture to a squad of Australian firemen, at Adelaide, in his great tour round the world to encourage the people to study and promote physical fitness and health.

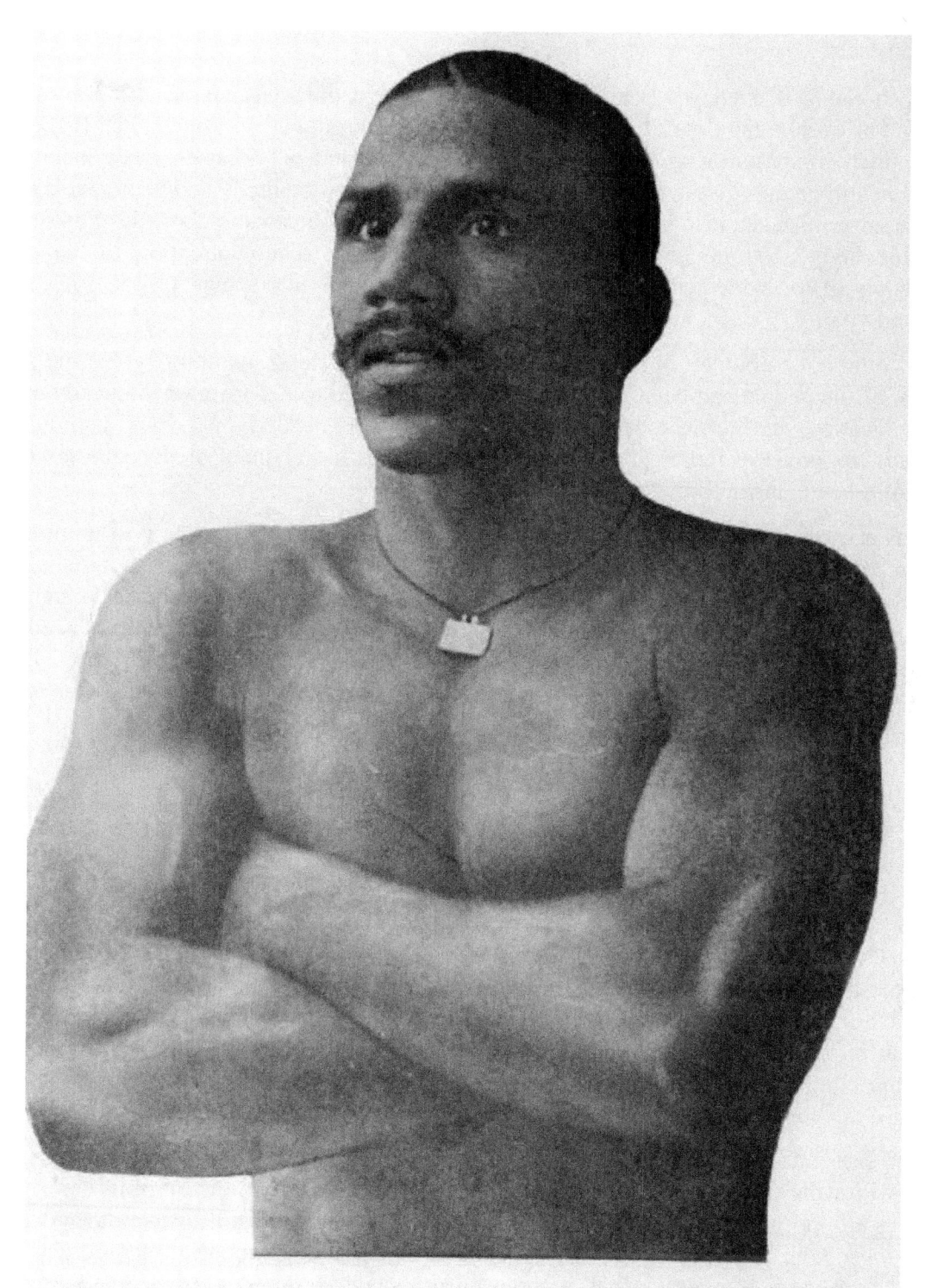

India's reply. Notwithstanding its unhealthy climate, thousands of young Indians, like the above, are now enthusiasts in these methods of developing the body by the methods described here, as a result of the Author's visit to that country.

ARE WE AWAKE YET?

It is questionable if even yet British statesmen and educationalists realise the gravity of the situation. For even at the time of writing, there has been introduced an Educational Bill which is causing much cogitation of grey matter, and which, if carried out as at present conceived, can only end in still greater disaster, so that our last condition shall be really and truly worse than the first. The same mistaken idea seems to exist and persist that you can somehow develop in a weak and feeble body a strong and supple mind, or that some scanty attention to the physical requirements of the body will atone for the deficiency in a child's own physical reservoir of energy and vitality.

When it could not be hidden from the people themselves and those in authority that the physical condition of the people had been, to a great extent, sacrificed to a system of illogically enforced mental education, and it was evident that some reform was needed, one would naturally think that it was the physical rather than the mental condition that claimed precedence in any such scheme of reform, under all the circumstances.

What was my amazement, therefore, on reading even in the light of all these now admitted facts that what was called, or miss-called, an Education Bill had been introduced into Parliament which so completely overlooked the 'probability and danger of still further physical deterioration as to seek to enforce mental pressure on the children, while still treating their physical education and training as of merely secondary consideration. This, too, at the most critical moment in the whole history of the British Empire when it so badly required and still requires physical re-construction.

TRUST THE SCHOOL DOCTOR.

The mere fact that the Bill was introduced as an almost exclusively mental Educational Act shows conclusively that the physical education of the children—who are to be the nation of the future—is not even yet treated as seriously as it ought to be by those in authority. This whole question, indeed, is a medical rather than an educational one, and, unless those in high places realise that real danger arises from any scheme of education that does not make this question first and primarily a medical one, and hand it over to medical rather than educational authorities, it must and will end in signal failure. To quote again from Sir George Newman, " it seems futile to attempt to reform education apart from the physical condition of the child. Physical defect was one of the chief causes of backwardness in schools; there was an accumulation of defective children of the higher ages in the lower standards."

A doctor sees the child when it first crosses the threshold of life. Only a doctor knows the dangers with which its little life is encompassed even from the very moment of its conception. If it survives all pre-natal and post-natal dangers until it enters school, still further dangers threaten it. Only those who know, understand and realise these dangers, as medical men do, can protect the child from them. Any child, that, without proper medical protection, is left at the mercy of educational authorities, who themselves are insufficiently educated in this direction at least, can never be expected to bring forth the best that is in it.

The physical education and training of the children is a matter of the utmost importance apart altogether from the educational aspect. Indeed, to a great degree it is a thing entirely apart from education as the word is used to-day. It is not a matter to be dealt with in an Educational Bill at all, where it receives but the scantiest notice and attention, but which ought to have been itself the object of a special Act of Parliament. In fact, such a vital matter both to the individual and the State should come not so much within the purview of a Minister of Education as of a Minister of Health, and if for this very reason alone the nation ought to have the Ministry of Health which, at the moment of writing is being advocated and which, by the time this book appears, will, I hope, be firmly established.

The whole question ought to be seriously and separately treated by a Ministry or Department of Health, with its own fully equipped medical service, and a really national and scientific system of physical education and bodily upbuilding should be organised and established for every school and institute of learning, on lines such as I suggest in a later chapter of this book.

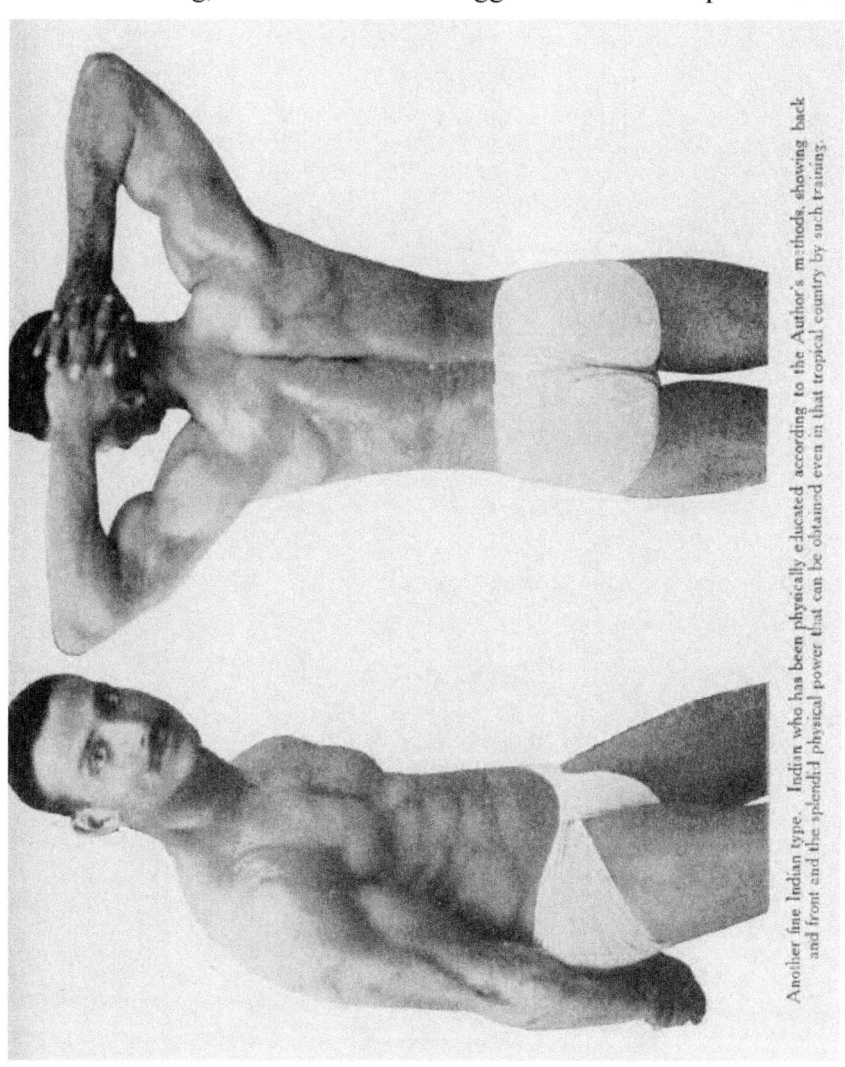

Another fine Indian type. Indian who has been physically educated according to the Author's methods, showing back and front and the splendid physical power that can be obtained even in that tropical country by such training.

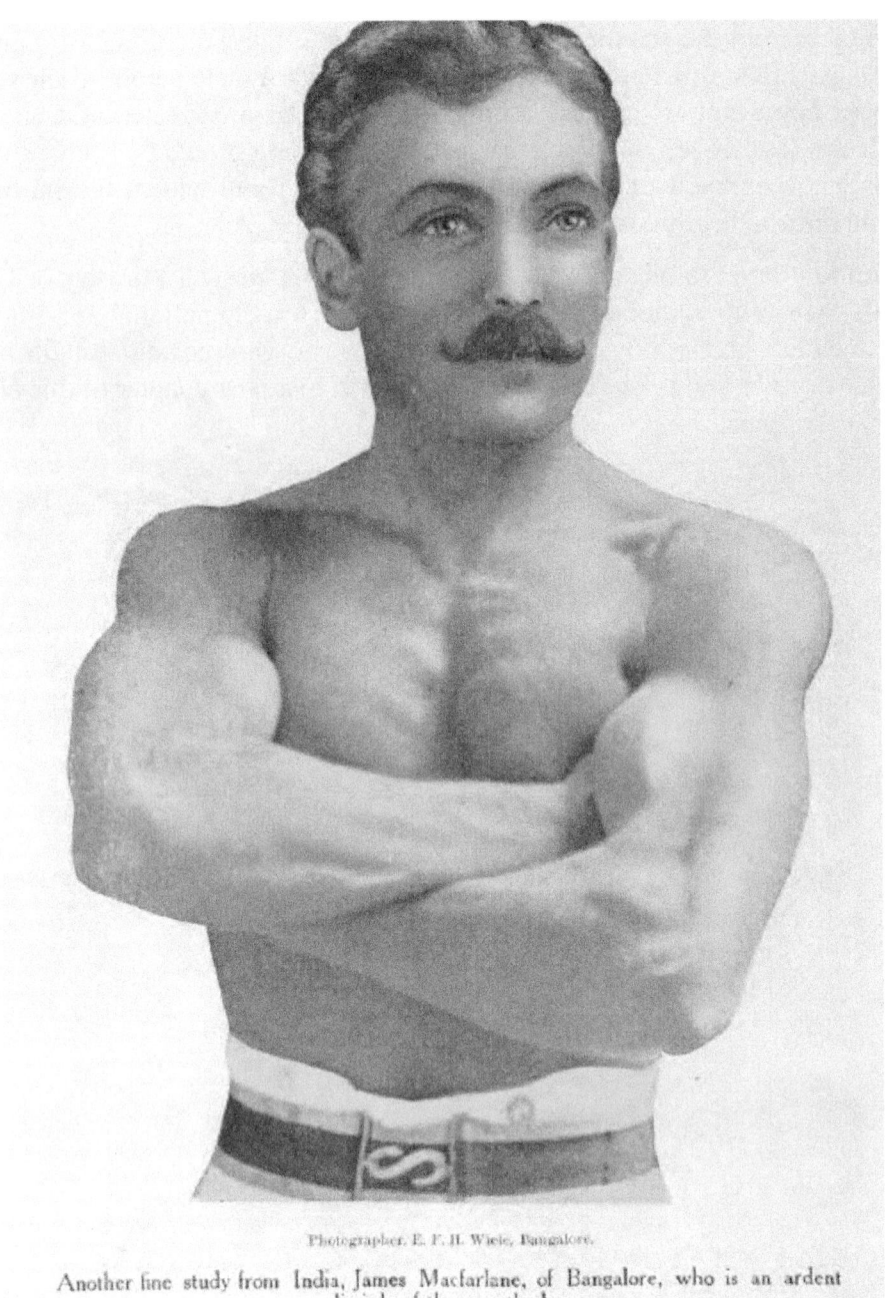

Another fine study from India, James Macfarlane, of Bangalore, who is an ardent disciple of these methods.

HEALTH BEFORE EDUCATION.

Never has the vitality of the people reached a lower ebb than to-day, and it will be still lower for years following the war. Yet at such time it is seriously proposed to add a more severe mental strain than ever upon children who must, of necessity, be poorer in physique and vitality than even the children of our pre-war period. Little wonder that doctors are crying out for more clinics, hospitals, and similar institutions. It is not these we want, but less and less necessity for them.

I am in thorough accord with the views enunciated by Major-General Sir Bertrand Dawson, G.C.V.O., who is no dreamer of dreams but a physician with a sane and clearly defined vision and perception, when he says that " health is a more fundamental need than education, and without doubt the two together form the foundation stone of a State. The changes that have long been germinating and which are soon to see the light (he is referring in a Cavendish lecture to the proposed Ministry of Health) are, as I conceive, the result of the following causes: A growing appreciation of the fact by the profession that much disease is preventable; a growing sense that health is of supreme interest alike to the State and the individual, and that the best means for preserving health and curing disease should be available for (I do not say given to) every citizen, irrespective of his position, and by right and not by favour."

That is, I think, the right medical view, but Sir Bertrand might be a little more explicit and state what he considers to be " the best means " of so going. Personally, I contend that this best method, and indeed, the only one, is by physical education, bodily culture and development, along the lines I have laid down, which would give every child a good physical foundation for the increasing strenuousness of adult life.

The Hon. P. Russell says in his work on " Strength and Diet": "Let the child by all means be taught its letters, its numbers and its maps, but on no account let it leave school and grow up to manhood or womanhood without an adequate and concise course of instruction on the means by which its own strength and value, and the life and value of its children, may best be maintained. The efficiency of the 'physical constitution, the rearing of the children hardy, robust, unaffected, humane, really means the better ability to attain every' sort of learning." But to force mental education on a weak or diseased body is like offering a juicy beefsteak to a man without teeth or giving strong wine to a delicate child. Teachers themselves know that physical incapacity is almost invariably the real cause of mental inefficiency, and that children improve mentally in proportion as they improve physically.

THE RECRUIT OF THE NATION.

The child is the recruit of the nation. It is the unit of the whole national army, whether of defence or offence, the army of workers as well as the army that fights. Why not, then, treat the child from the very beginning at least as well as we do the adult recruit for military purposes. No man is permitted to join or remain in the army unless he is medically fit. Why should a child not first be certified fit before it enters the greatest army of all—the army of the people that determines the fate of a nation. A nation must finally and unalterably stand by the physique of its individual constituents, and the higher the individual physical type the higher will be the mental and moral standard.

Low as was the physical standard of the people at the beginning of the world's greatest struggle, lower as it is to-day than then, it must be still lower in the future when we remember the awful strain through which everyone, civilian and soldier alike, will have passed. The medical opinions which I have quoted here, it must be remembered, are based mainly on pre-war conditions and statistics, or on figures gathered during the earlier stages of the war. If such an Education Bill as that under consideration was destined to put so crushing a burden on those physically unfit children born before and during the war, how are we to expect it to be shouldered by the still more physically unfit children who will come after the war, and born of parents who themselves cannot possibly have escaped physically unscathed or unscarred through such a destructive and testing world struggle.

These children will need infinitely more vigilance .and care physically than even their predecessors, and educational authorities who do not realise this will be guilty of criminal negligence and culpable want of foresight. The public voice must penetrate to the inmost chambers of State, and compel recognition of the vital fact that these children must be given and ensured a sound physical foundation before having their little brains crammed with a mass of indigestible and inassimilable knowledge.

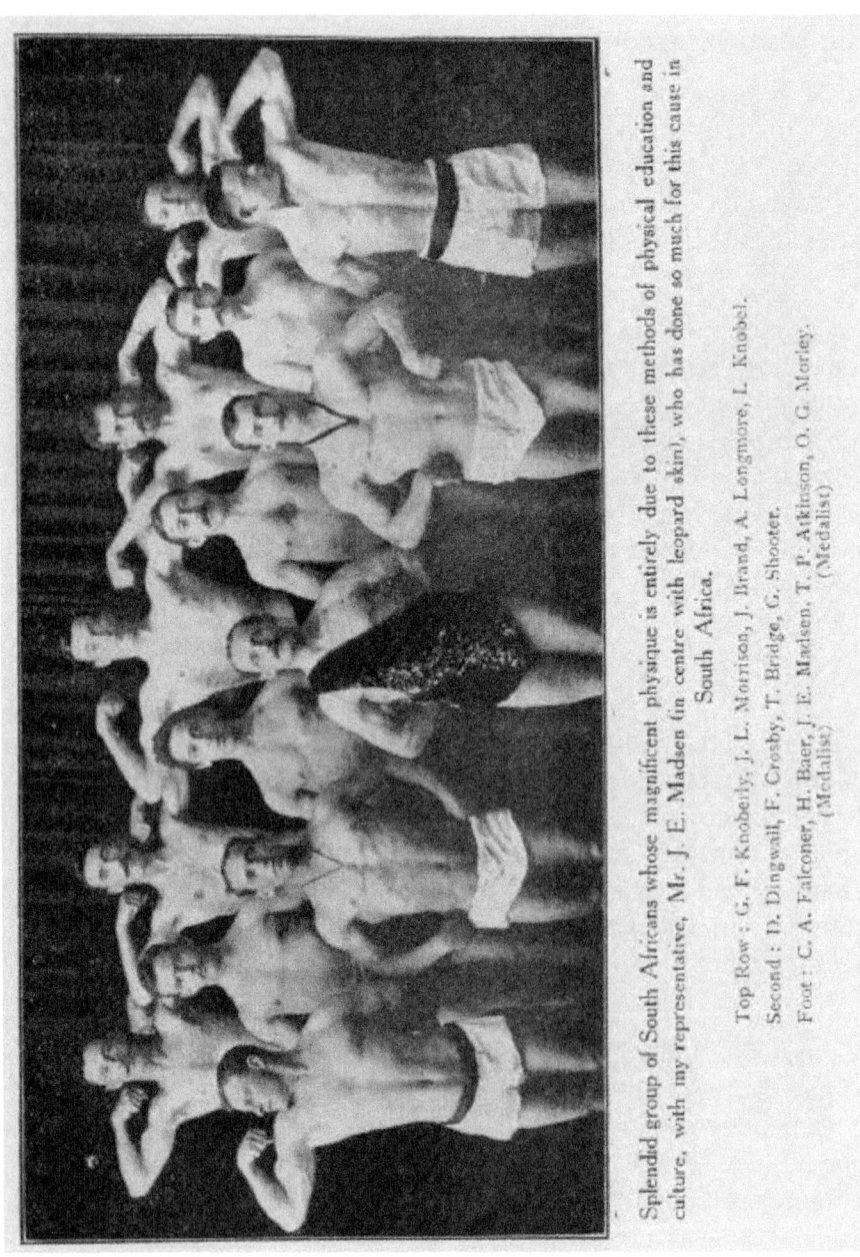

Splendid group of South Africans whose magnificent physique is entirely due to these methods of physical education and culture, with my representative, Mr. J. E. Madsen (in centre with leopard skin), who has done so much for this cause in South Africa.

Top Row: G. F. Knoberly, J. L. Morrison, J. Brand, A. Longmore, L. Knobel.
Second: D. Dingwall, F. Crosby, T. Bridge, G. Shooter.
Foot: C. A. Falconer, H. Baer, J. E. Madsen, T. P. Atkinson, O. G. Morley. (Medalist)

THE AFTERMATH OF WAR.

Scarcely a home in England will remain that has not felt the sting of war just as keenly as if those at home had been actually in the trenches. Thousands and thousands of soldiers can never forget the horrors they have endured or the wounds from which they have suffered. During the war, neurasthenia and nervous disorders have raged to a degree that have never been equalled before. Fathers, mothers, sisters, and daughters have lost their nearest and dearest, and are themselves prostrated with grief and nervous shock. Many have lost friends, businesses, homes, and even the means of subsistence.

Thousands, perhaps millions, who have been patriotically engaged on war work, and who have been, as it were, supported for the time being by a " scaffolding " of their own loyal enthusiasm, will find, when this patriotic " scaffolding " has been removed, that they are the victims of a thousand and one ailments that were overlooked whilst busily engaged. There will be a certain reaction in the case of many who have been overworked during the war pressure, and neurasthenia and other nervous disorders will undoubtedly be more prevalent than ever for a considerable period yet.

THE PEOPLE OF THE FUTURE.

Yet these are the people to whom we must look for the children of the future. What can we expect of the little ones if they are not more than ever cared for instead of adding further burdens to them by a still severer mental strain?

We have no figures to go by as to the exact influence of such a terrible war upon health, but we know that neurasthenia was raging in our midst even before the war, due to modern civilisation, education, and lack of organic or mental and physical balance. We may estimate, therefore, somewhat approximately what will be the nervous condition of the children of the next generation. They can scarcely be otherwise than nervous weaklings, whose bodies will require the most patient nurture and care if their little minds are not to be tortured and strained even to the verge of mental breakdown, and their bodies enfeebled for the ready reception of disease. Higher types cannot be evolved from such material unless we go into the whole subject of physical degeneration and regeneration seriously and in the most thorough and the most scientific manner.

Each child is to the nation just what the cell is to the body, the unit of its life We must evolve better children before we can evolve better men and women, and that can only be done by restoring physical and constitutional health in the really scientific way I describe in this book, which will literally give them better, healthier, stronger and more disease-resistant bodies. Into such a body it will be easy to project all the mental additions and adornments that are necessary to complete what is called its education, and it will be equally difficult for such a body to become receptive to disease.

A STUDY IN BLACK AND WHITE.

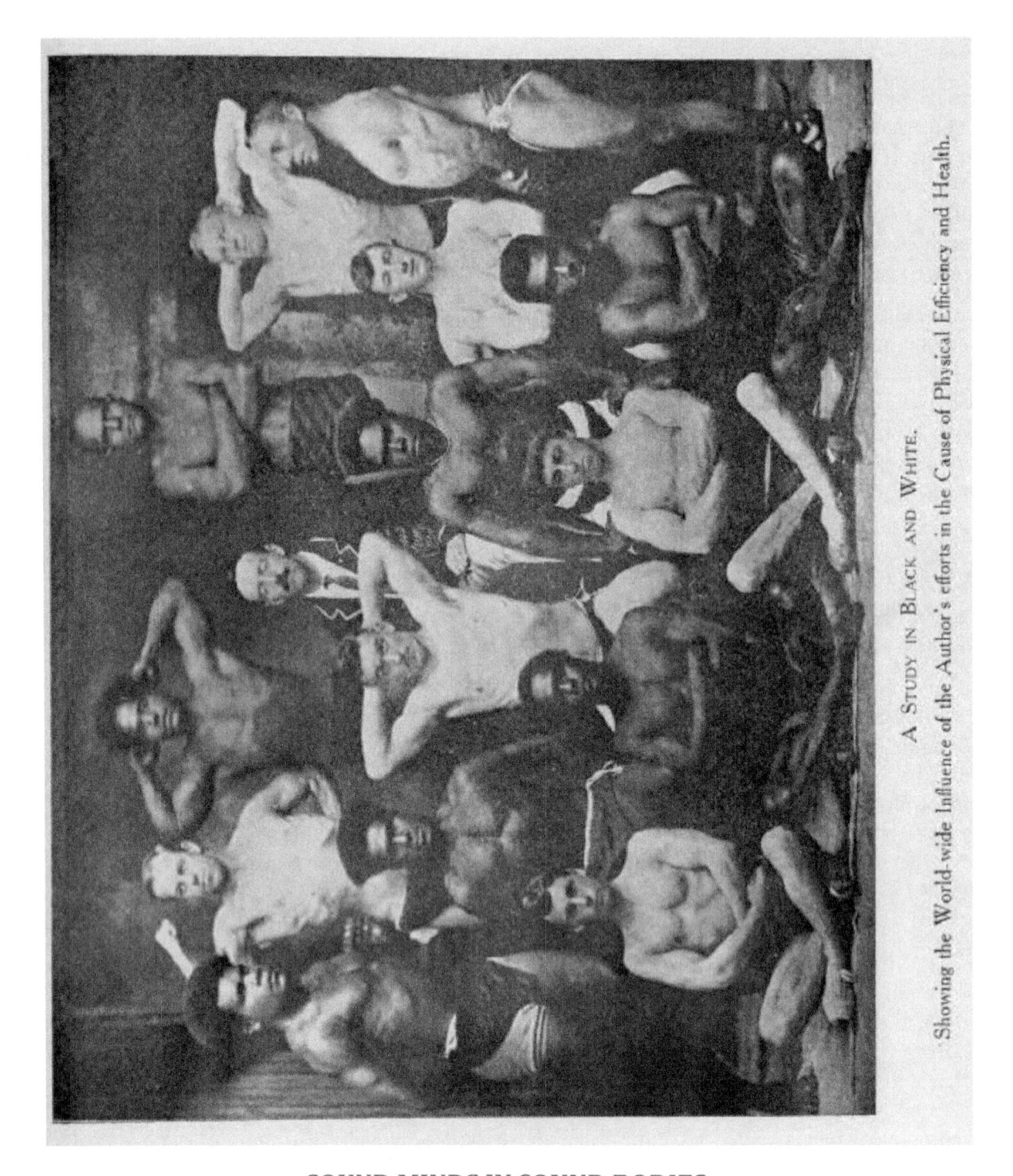

Showing the World-wide Influence of the Author's efforts in the Cause of Physical Efficiency and Health.

SOUND MINDS IN SOUND BODIES.

In face of this crisis, the question then arises, How is it possible for us to reconstruct a nation of better and fitter men and women from the children who have come or will come to us in post-war days, handicapped, as they must be, from birth by their war-affected parentage? How are we to have a mental plan and system of education that will not only enable even a child born physically weak or sickly to bring forth' its best and choicest mental fruit, but will help it to grow up to adolescence and adulthood of robust constitution and free from disease?

For this should be the purpose and end of all education—the attainment of the ancient and classical ideal of a mind and body in perfect health and harmony. Only by placing the supreme power of deciding the child's physical capacity to absorb and assimilate learning in the hands of a medical profession responsible directly and only to the State, generously paid for its services, and having with it the intelligent and willing support of the public, can we have such a system.

All brain work, as medical men know, is a great consumer of vitality, and no child should be allowed by the school medical officer to take up mental work beyond its physical capacity, and without medical permission. Indeed, I would go even further, and would attach the same condition to every student seeking to pursue studies of a very exacting nature, and especially to students wishing to enter the learned professions. The medical officer of any University, college or school, too, should also have the power not only to order a scholar to abstain from continuation mental training as proposed by this immature Education Bill, and to have continuous physical training instead up till 18 years of age if and when desirable.

Personally, I believe that even the mental training already given will have to be most carefully and strictly regulated, at least for the next generation, in our present post-war and seriously depleted state of health and physique, and, if the addition of extra mental training be added, it can, I am afraid, only help to fill hospitals, asylums and infirmaries to overflowing in the near future through mental as well as physical breakdown.

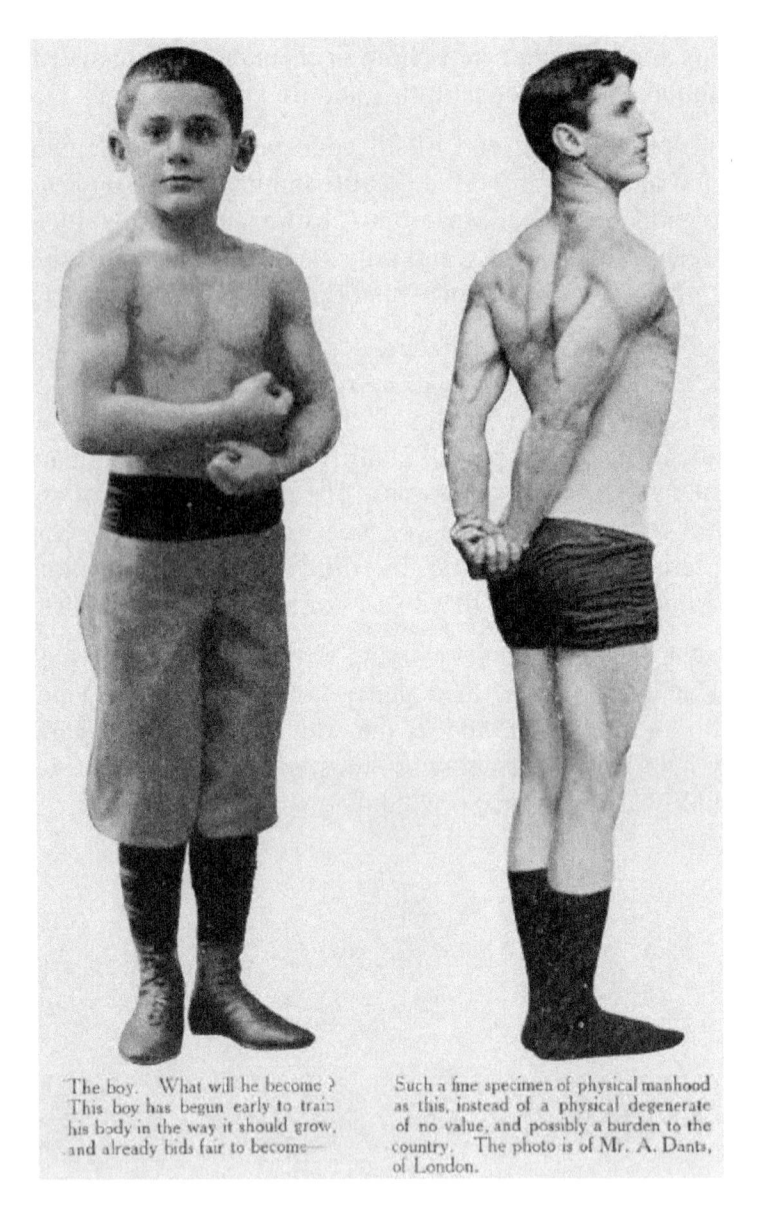

The boy. What will he become? This boy has begun early to train his body in the way it should grow, and already bids fair to become—

Such a fine specimen of physical manhood as this, instead of a physical degenerate of no value, and possibly a burden to the country. The photo is of Mr. A. Dants, of London.

CHILD'S FIRST DUTY TO GROW STRONG.

Any system of miss-called education which provides overfed minds and starved and stunted bodies must finally end in both physical and mental decay. The first duty of the child is to grow and grow stronger, and its natural 'processes of physical growth and development must be encouraged and promoted in every way. After that a mental super-structure can easily be effected. In other words, we must secure for each and every child a sound physical basis by really scientific physical education and training. By that I mean in a nutshell:—

(1) Each child must be considered according to its age, sex, and individual needs before any mental strain is placed upon it. Its physical education and condition must determine its mental education.

{'2) The child must, from its first introduction to school, be kept under the observation and, direction of the school medical officer. so that no child shall be coerced into mental efforts that are prejudicial to its basic physical establishment of health, and it must be medically re-examined periodically.

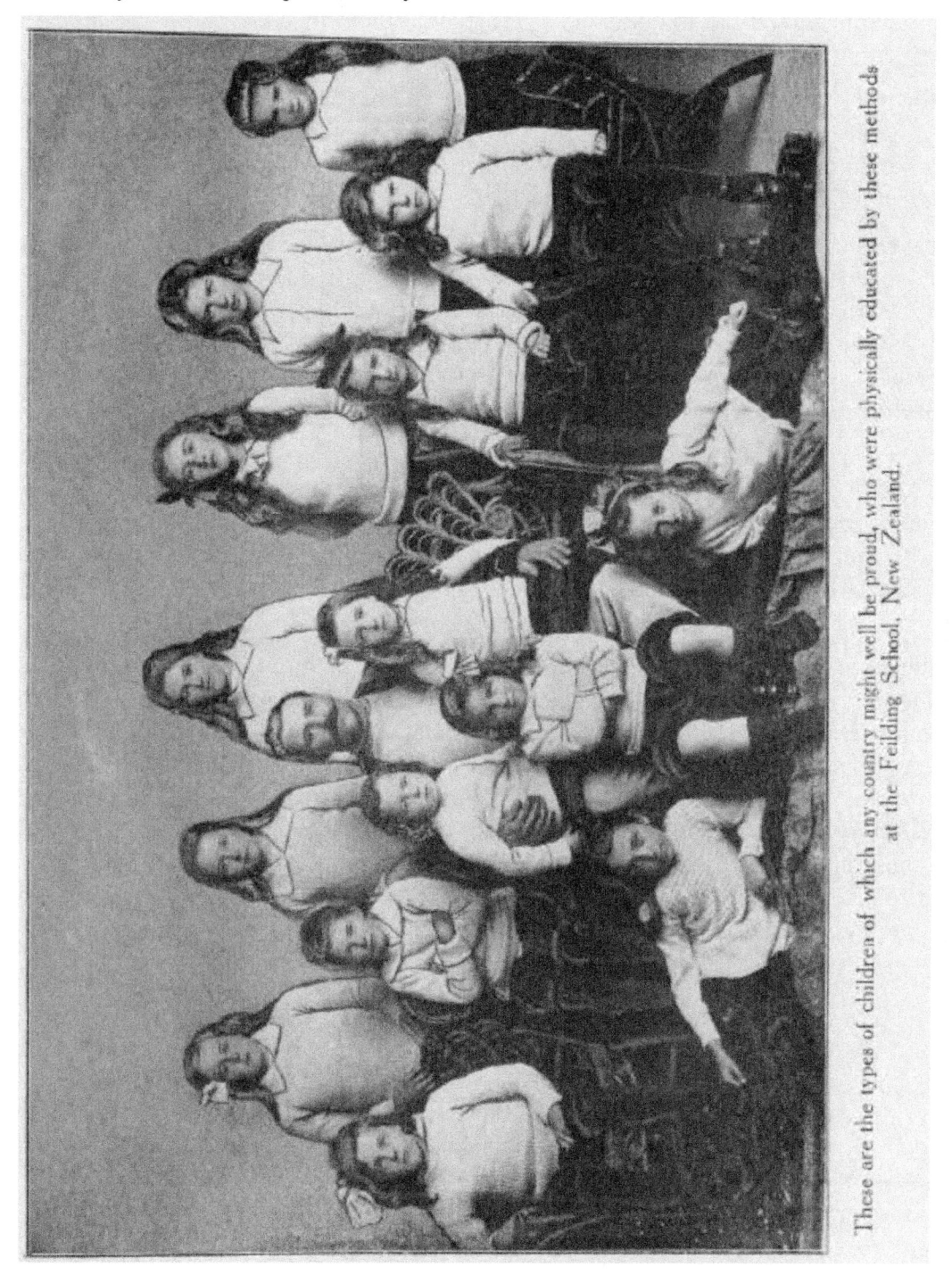

These are the types of children of which any country might well be proud, who were physically educated by these methods at the Feilding School, New Zealand.

MORE CHILDREN AND BETTER.

Before, however, we can either physically or mentally educate the children, we must have the children to educate. As things are, much must be done to encourage child-birth and foster child-life, or we shall soon be without the children to educate. Out of every 1,000,000 babies registered, declares The Observer, 100,000 are stillborn, another 100,000 die before they are a year old, and yet another 100,000 before they are fifteen. One-third of the fewer babies being born die before fifteen. Is comment or criticism necessary in the light of these figures?

Further, as the leader writer of that prominent organ of public opinion points out, " of the rest many grow up stunted, defective and unfit." If we can only save and improve the lives of these survivals by careful and scientific physical education and training, as I know from experience we can, that would be in itself a great work and worthy of our mightiest endeavour. But we need both a higher birth-rate and a higher survival rate.

A medical census of the children of this country would horrify the nation. In America, where the children are even more carefully watched over from birth than in England, such a census revealed the most alarming facts. There are about 20,000,000 pupils in the schools of the United States to-day. It is estimated that 250,000 of these have organic heart disease, a million at least are tubercular, another million have defective hearing, five million suffer from bad sight, six million from tonsils, adenoids, or enlarged glands, while ten million need a visit to the dentist.

If this be so in the United States, we may safely assume that the children in the schools of England to-day are in no better condition. Indeed, from medical reports which I myself have seen from time to time the condition of the school children in England are much worse. These children have existed and survived, but their chances of life and health have been jeopardised and almost destroyed by neglect in infancy.

To quote from the " Daily Mirror," " those who are born should have the best chance of strength and health. But what is the use of trying to eliminate the mentioned mass, ever-increasing, of physical unfitness if we continue adding to it? What is the good of asking the martyred mother of a huge family in a slum to remedy the sickliness of that family by making it a bigger family still? The question has only to be asked for the absurdity of this cruel mania to be revealed to all humane people. We have our 1 surplus 5 population already—all unfit. Let us remedy its unfitness." If we do this and prevent disease in the future, as we undoubtedly can, we will have a people robust and free from disease, and I claim and contend that it is to-day within the power of man now to reach the great ideal of a diseaseless world and a disease-immune people only by the methods of physical reconstruction hereafter described.

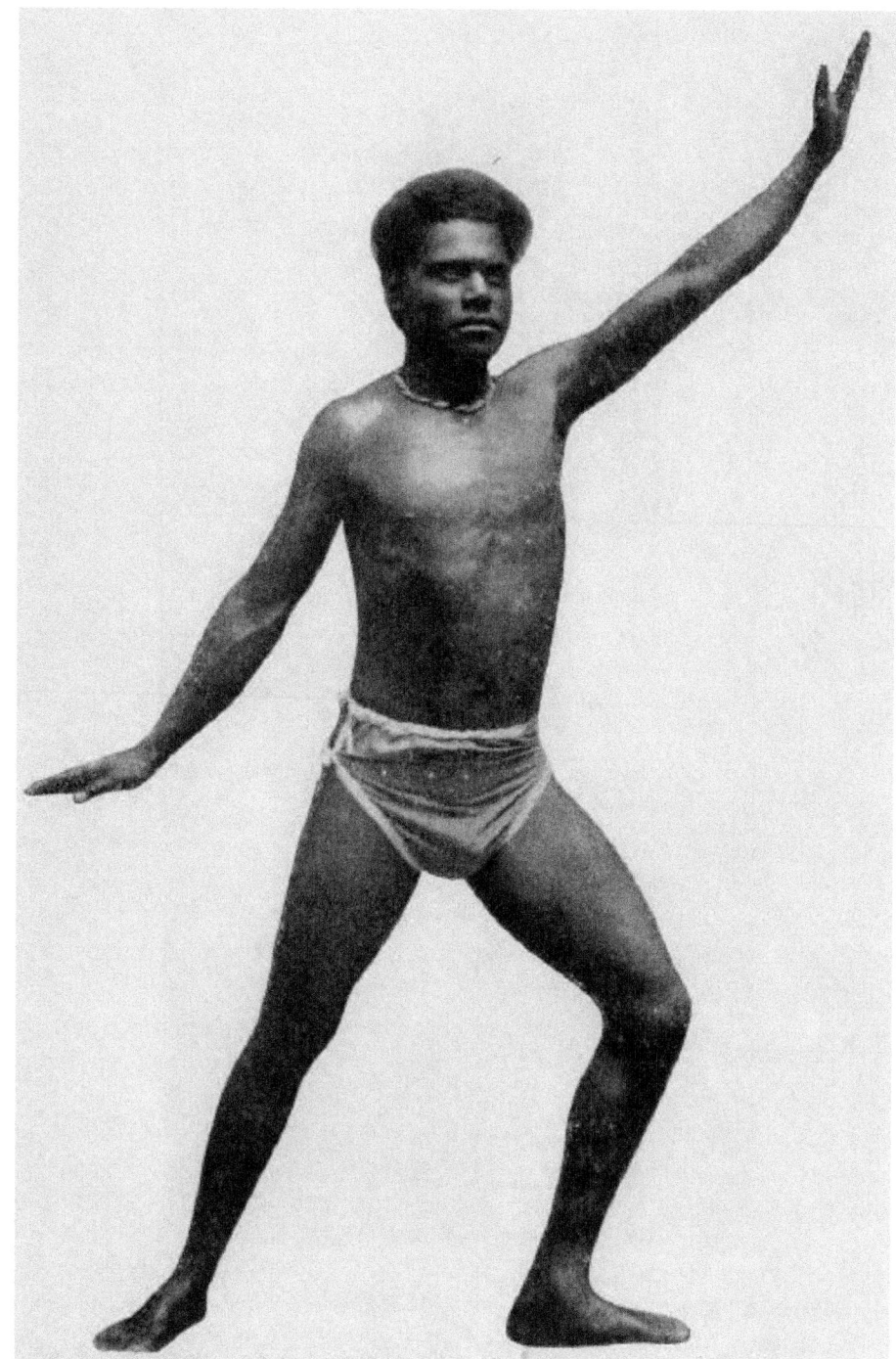

A youthful, and well-formed Fijian, whose body has been developed in grace, strength and suppleness by these methods.

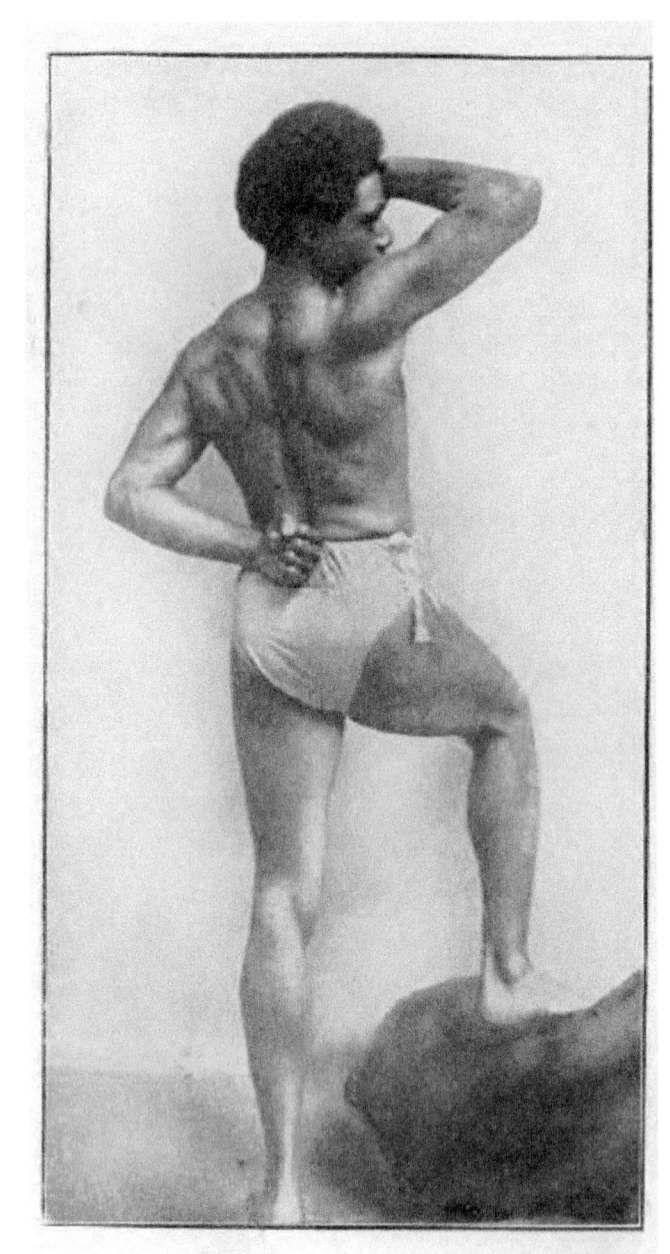

Back view of the same youth.

CHAPTER III.

" My World-Startling Claim "—A Diseaseless World!

IF a man stood on the steps of St. Paul's and proclaimed it possible to prevent disease—even to eradicate it altogether, and give us a diseaseless world—his reception, I know, would be undoubtedly chilling. If he said further that it was possible to replace in a living body a weak or diseased limb with a new and real flesh and blood article, or, what is more remarkable, replace a new and better stomach in place of an old and diseased one, or even to completely rebuild a new and better body out of a feeble and diseased one, most people would smile at him in pity and contempt. In days gone by, he would probably have been crucified, burned at the stake or stoned to death. For, such talk smacks of magic or witchcraft.

Yet all this I say is possible, and possible by easy and accessible methods in consonance with natural physical activities and the ever-changing processes going on unceasingly within the body itself, as I will show and, I think, prove conclusively to the reader's satisfaction.

MAKING A DISEASE-PROOF BODY.

At all times, the man who challenges tradition is liable to be suspected of a personal object in attacking heavily entrenched interests, and has, consequently, received more buffets than rewards. The history of every great invention or discovery has been a history of one long-continued and persistent fight against popular opinion or professional jealousy, usually with tardy and belated honour to the inventor or discoverer, that too often, alas, only came after death. Men like Harvey, Jenner, and Pasteur—Pasteur himself who revolutionised medical science was not even a member of the medical profession—were persons not particularly acceptable for a time to the majority of the medical profession, upon whose traditional corns they trod, until their theories and discoveries were demonstrated and proved in actual practice beyond the shadow of doubt.

So when I boldly put forth the claim that health can be assured to all, and disease eliminated from the human race, I do not, for a single instant, expect so startling a claim to go forth unchallenged, nor do I expect to escape censure, criticism, and even ridicule. There are many searchers after truth, and it is too much to expect that they should be in agreement, especially on a subject which in the past has been so largely Empiric as the prevention or cure of disease and the attainment and maintenance of perfect health.

I hope, however, before the conclusion of this book, to prove beyond the shadow of a doubt that movement is the law of life, that physical movement carried out in a perfectly balanced and scientific way, is essential for the healthy life and working capacity of every cell of the body, that physical movement alone and on scientific lines will make and keep each and every cell of the body so strongly resistant as to be immune from disease or the weakness that makes it liable to disease, that health is proportionate to and determined by the nature and effect of such physical movements, selected, applied and administered as I describe, that, in short, what I call scientific physical movement means health, and that it is because of imperfect or unscientifically ordered movement and, consequently, lack of general bodily balance within, that disease reveals itself in man.

IMPORTANCE OF HEALTH KNOWLEDCE.

I hope to prove conclusively that natural physical movements, so selected and administered, are Dr Nature's sovereign remedy and preventive for all disease, and I hope to show with mathematical exactitude why this must be so, and also to fully establish the truth of my tremendous claim, viz., that such physical movement, adapted to suit our present-day circumstances and environment, can not only prevent and cure disease, but entirely eliminate it in time from the species and give us a world without disease.

To achieve this radically, we must, as I have said, begin with the child—the scientific physical education and physical reconstruction, under medical direction and supervision, of the young.

How much, may I ask, does the average man of to-day—even the man of more than average education—know of his own body, its structure and constitution, and the nature of those wonderful operations that constitute what I may call the mechanics of life and living. He puts food in his mouth and knows little or nothing of how it is transmuted into flesh, blood, bone, nail, hair, sinews and nerve because never taught. How can such a man preserve his body in health against the many enemies ever ready to attack it?

NECESSITY OF PHYSICAL MOVEMENT.

Even the most ancient writers on philosophy and medicine recognised and admitted the value—the necessity, indeed—of physical movement of some kind, in securing bodily, mental, moral and spiritual well-being, although they could not explain or demonstrate the exact and true causes of its power and influence over weakness and disease, and even indeed, over what Shakespeare clearly regarded as incurable, " a mind diseased." Centuries on centuries ago, Pliny wrote:—1It is wonderful how much the mind is enlivened by the motion of the body;" and Democritus declared that " the force of the understanding increased with the health of the body, yet when the body labours under disease, the mind is incapacitated for thinking." " It is exercise alone," said Cicero, " that supports the spirits and keeps the mind in vigour."

Since then, all schools of medical, scientific and educational thought have more and more recognised the necessity and value of rational and natural physical movement in a general way, though they could not explain the how and the why of it. This is just what I propose to do in this book and to do for the first time.

Dr Maudsley, in a lecture before the British Medical Association in 1906 truly said: "In the work of fortifying the body to resist the encroachments of disease, the most simple means are the best, and, it is in the use of simple means that great physicians especially differ from others. Pure air, clean and proper food, regular and adapted exercise, these sum up the measures prescribed as proper to give it inward strength, and to keep it in a sound and supple activity," and also, I may add, to give it mental and moral stability and strength. Dr M'Gregor Robertson put the case even stronger when he declared that " all agree that physical exercise has a potent influence for good, is indeed, as necessary as food and air for the body, both in health and disease."

SCIENCE OF PHYSICAL MOVEMENT.

While this is now almost universally admitted as true, these remarks only apply in a general and indefinite way to any kind of exercise no matter how carelessly or indifferently carried out. It is my object, however, to show there is an actual and exact science of physical movement and this scientific method of applying physical movement is absolutely essential in modern conditions of life to the securing and keeping of health, and for the conquest, prevention and eradication of disease, especially as civilisation and education increasingly diminish the necessity for physical movement in everyday life.

The experience that I have had personally in seeing the miracles that can be and have been achieved by the really scientific selection and application of natural physical movements to a weak, ailing, deformed or diseased body, has convinced me of the influence of natural and simple physical movements, when scientifically employed and carried out, upon junction, and even in changing the constitution and character of an organ. The results of this experience and observation I am embodying in this book, because I firmly believe that they will lead to a revolution in the prevention, treatment and cure of disease.

Only because I honestly believe my own experience in this subject to be unique and of the utmost value of suffering humanity, do I venture to intrude the following personal reference as first hand, definite and credible evidence to help in the establishment of the case I am presenting in this book, and which I am anxious to support by every legitimate evidence and proof at my command.

NO HEALTH WITHOUT STRENGTH.

Practically my whole life-time, as most people know, has been devoted to the study of this subject, from that moment when, as a boy of delicate constitution, with narrow cramped chest and an inborn consumptive tendency, I determined to work out my own physical salvation by building up a body so perfect in every part that, like those of the splendid and ancient heroes whose forms in the early ages were as God intended the human body should be, and who became, therefore, the models of the world's greatest sculptors, it would be so thoroughly and symmetrically developed and balanced in every part and so innately strong as to absolutely defy, resist and conquer disease. For, I contend that only through such physical or, rather constitutional strength can come both physical health and moral courage, because a body can never be made physically strong if it is organically or functionally disordered or ill-regulated, while courage, self-control and other moral attributes are mostly but the expression and evidence of this conscious physical health and strength of constitution.

A weakly man may have a momentary and frenzied strength as in delirium, a coward may conjure up a false and fleeting courage in a situation that endangers himself, but the courage that endures is the true courage, the courage that springs only from the consciousness of a heart organically sound, nerves of steel, firm muscles, a deep, broad chest, and a healthy functioned body in every part.

It was the passion of my own boyhood to become healthy, strong and well developed, and the world knows to-day how well I succeeded in that laudable endeavour. Laudable I say advisedly, for I believe that physical education and bodily culture must teach everyone to respect the body as a Divine gift, to guard it with the most zealous care through life, and to make it the foundation and support of a sound mental and moral structure.

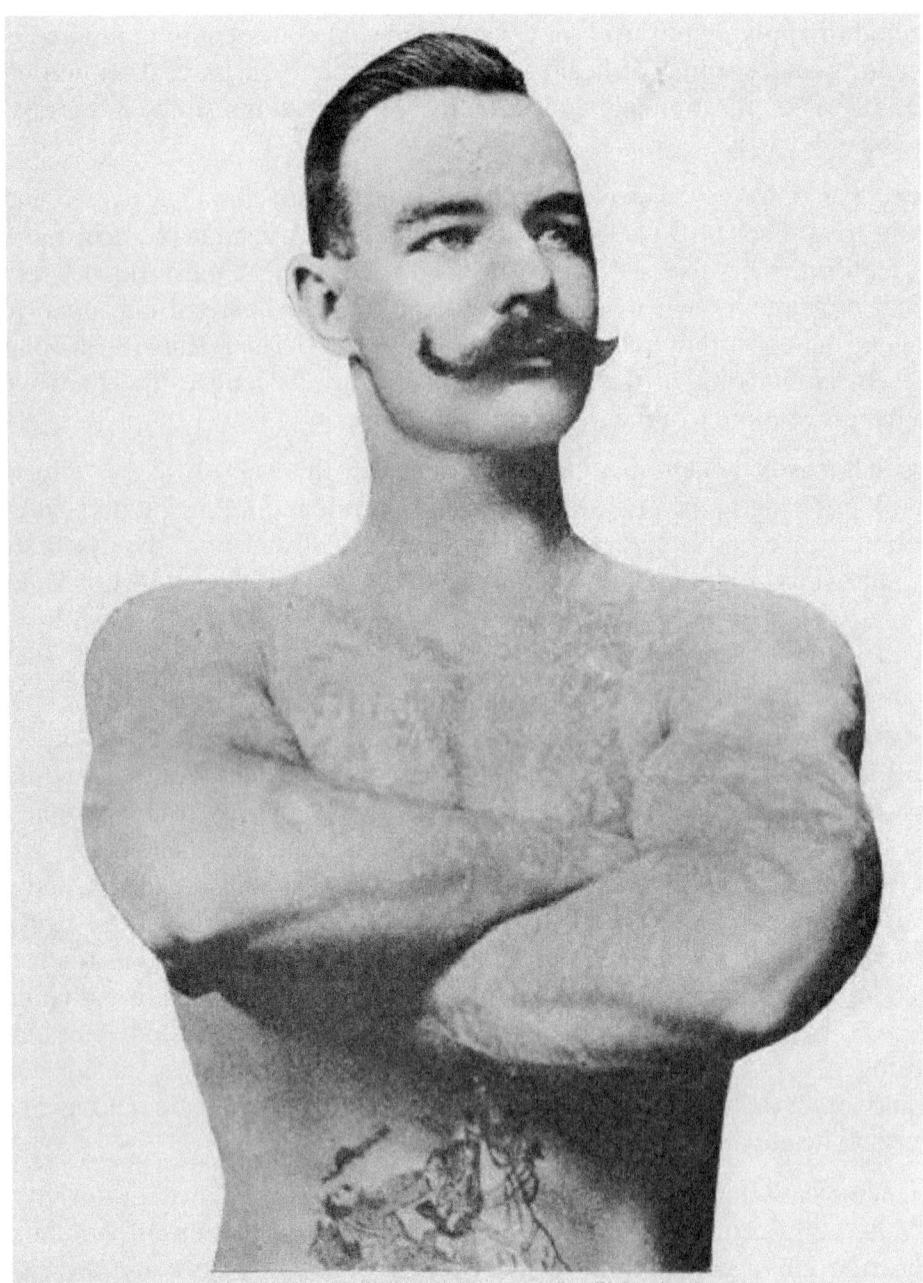

Photographer, The Photographic Studios, Arthur W. Lee, London.

A fine photographic study of the disease-resisting body built up by the absolutely scientific methods recommended by the Author.

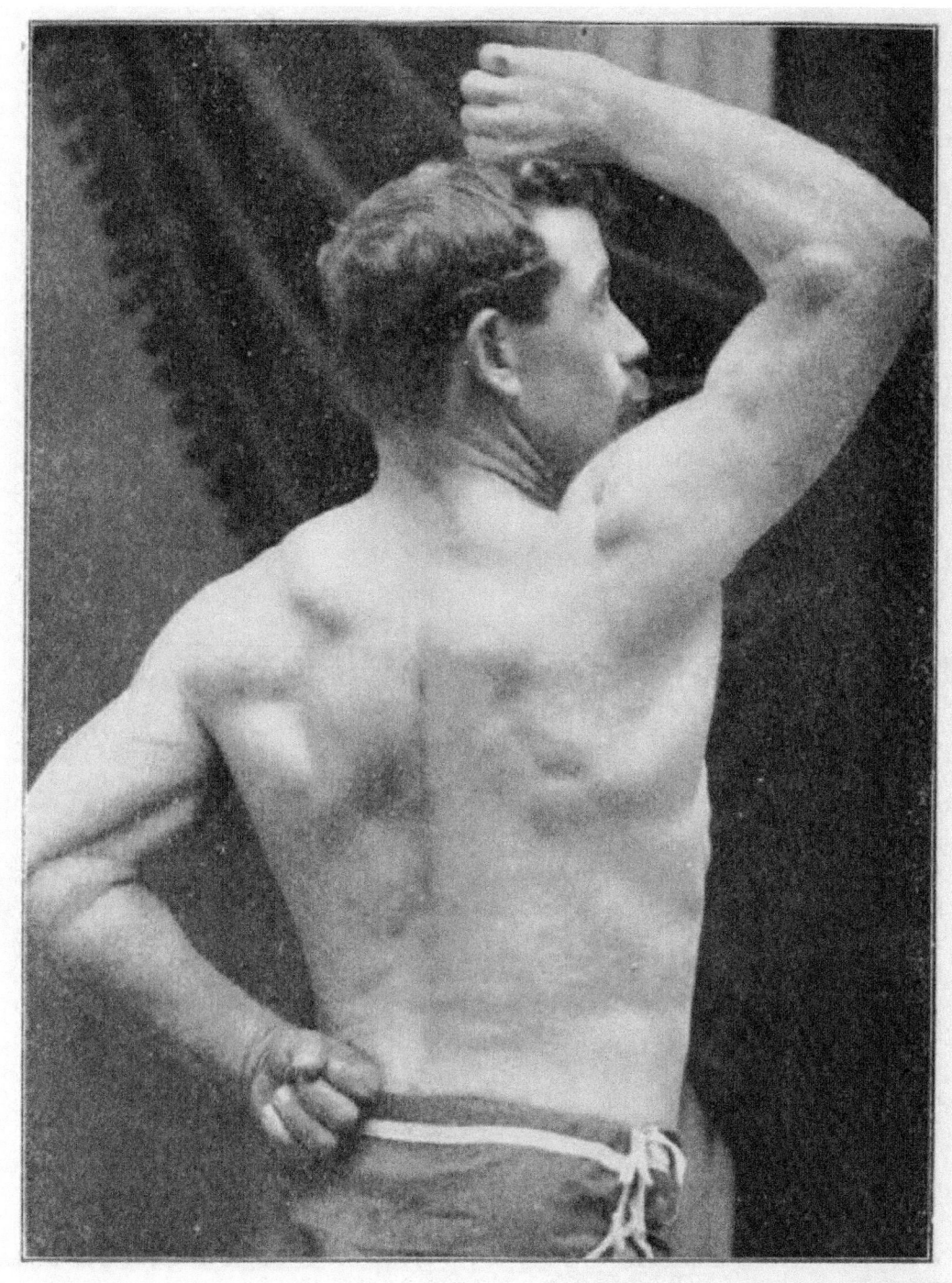

Another enthusiastic follower of these methods.

WORLD CAMPAIGN AGAINST DISEASE.

Since then my chief, almost my sole enthusiasm, has been to achieve similar or approximate results in others who were delicate, diseased, or weak, to give to many thousands the knowledge and experience I had personally acquired, and in this I am glad to say that I have been and continue to be equally successful, often, indeed, to the surprise and amazement of the many medical men who have failed so far to discover or learn how to make and keep the human body so perfectly balanced in strength that it will be able to successfully defy and overcome disease.

I am now convinced, as the result of my long and varied experience, a life-time of study and much experimentation, that disease can be totally eliminated from the human race, when once the States of the civilised world, the doctors, the educationalists, the sociologist, the clergymen, the teachers, and the parents, jointly responsible for the upbringing of the youth of the nation, learn the wonderful therapeutic value of natural and balanced physical movements when harnessed by Science in the manner I am advocating in this book.

The claim that I now advance, despite our enormous and largely avoidable sacrifice of child and patent life, the increasing death toll annually through what I contend is avoidable and preventable disease, may seem a startling claim for any man to make. When the principles I have laid down, however, in the previous chapter are recognised in the education and upbringing of the young, and children are educated as thoroughly and as scientifically in a physical sense as they are mentally to-day, under competent and qualified medical supervision, we can and will attain to the ideal of a diseaseless world, so far at least as gross and deadly disease is concerned. To hasten this it is, as I have said, a prime essential of all elementary education to have every child taught from an early age to know and understand its own body, with all its myriad and marvellous activities, as well as they are at present taught, say, to know and employ the letters of the alphabet or the first principles of arithmetic, for self-knowledge is the beginning of all educational wisdom.

PROCESS OF CONSCIOUS EVOLUTION.

This, then, is the first step in the great work of reconstruction that lies before those responsible for the future of the nation, and, indeed, of the people of the civilised world, for disease knows no frontiers. It is a system of Higher Eugenics that will lead us inevitably to a healthier, more vigorous and more beautiful humanity, help us to breed better men and women without the necessity of statutory measures that insult human intelligence and infringe the liberty of the individual, for it will gradually eliminate the weak, the unfit and the diseased by methods more scientific and beneficent than putting them to death, making them, on the other hand, even in the present generation, and still more in the next, men and women perfect and sound in every physical sense. It is, too, the Higher Ethics, for I am convinced that health and strength foster and ensure morality and virtue, as health and strength cannot long live and flourish in the same human body as immorality and vice.

It is, I believe, too, the real and true gospel of efficiency, for physical fitness is the essential prelude to mental efficiency. It will help us to breed a Spartan race without the cruelties of the Spartan system, or without reversion to the savage principle of killing off the weak, for there will be no weak or diseased left to be killed off until the hour of their natural physical dissolution.

Health and physical strength are the heritage and birth-right of all. That birth-right, of which civilisation has bereft us, we can and must reclaim by a rational return to the great law of life, which is the Law of Movement, a law as exact, as true and as immutable as the Law of Gravitation itself.

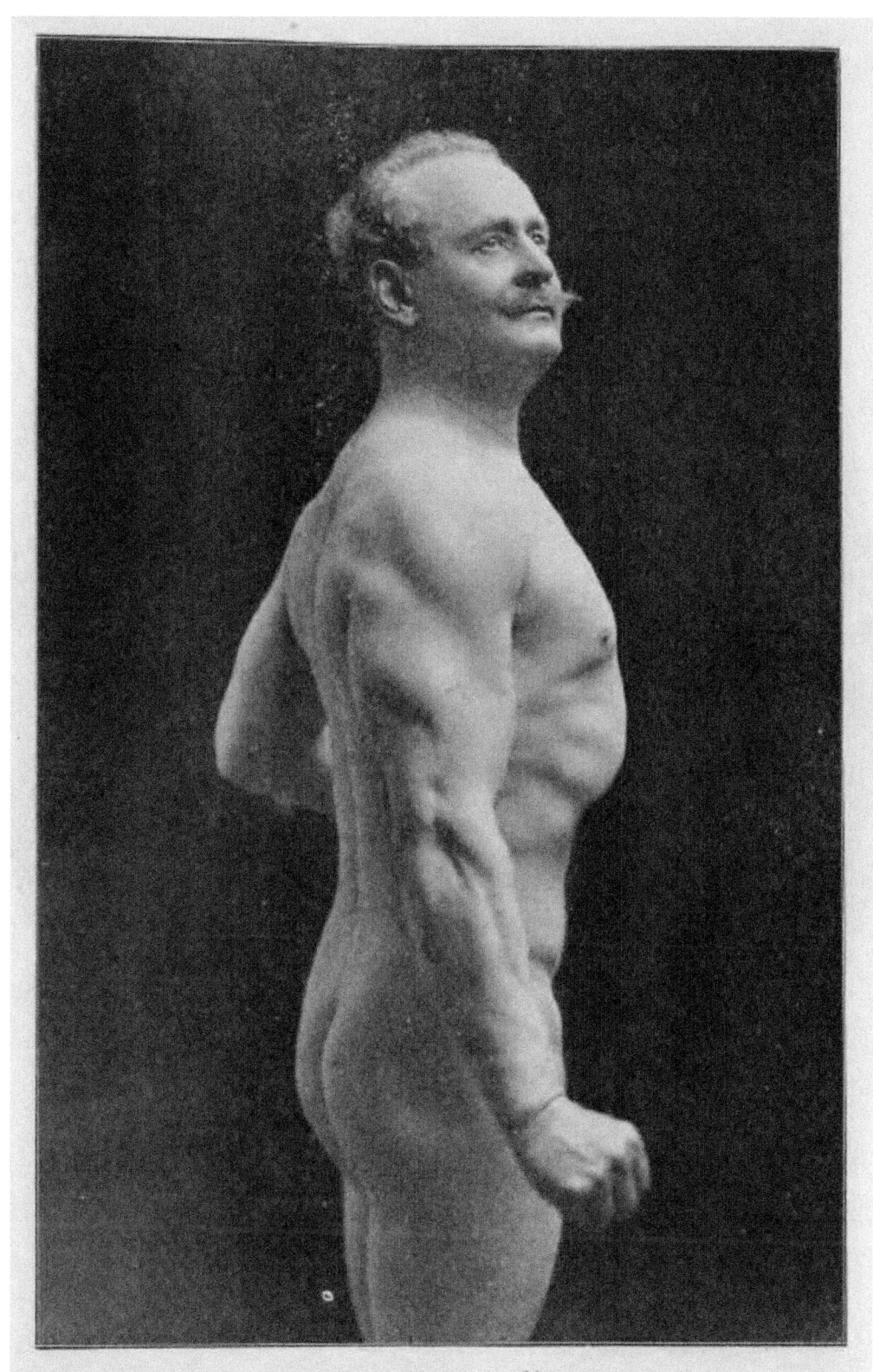

THE AUTHOR AT 52.
A convincing photographic study of the Author as he appears to-day, showing how by these methods men can, as he has done, retain their fitness until late in life, provided the physical foundation has been well and truly laid, and the muscular system—which is the corner-stone of the body—has been developed everywhere in harmony and balance.

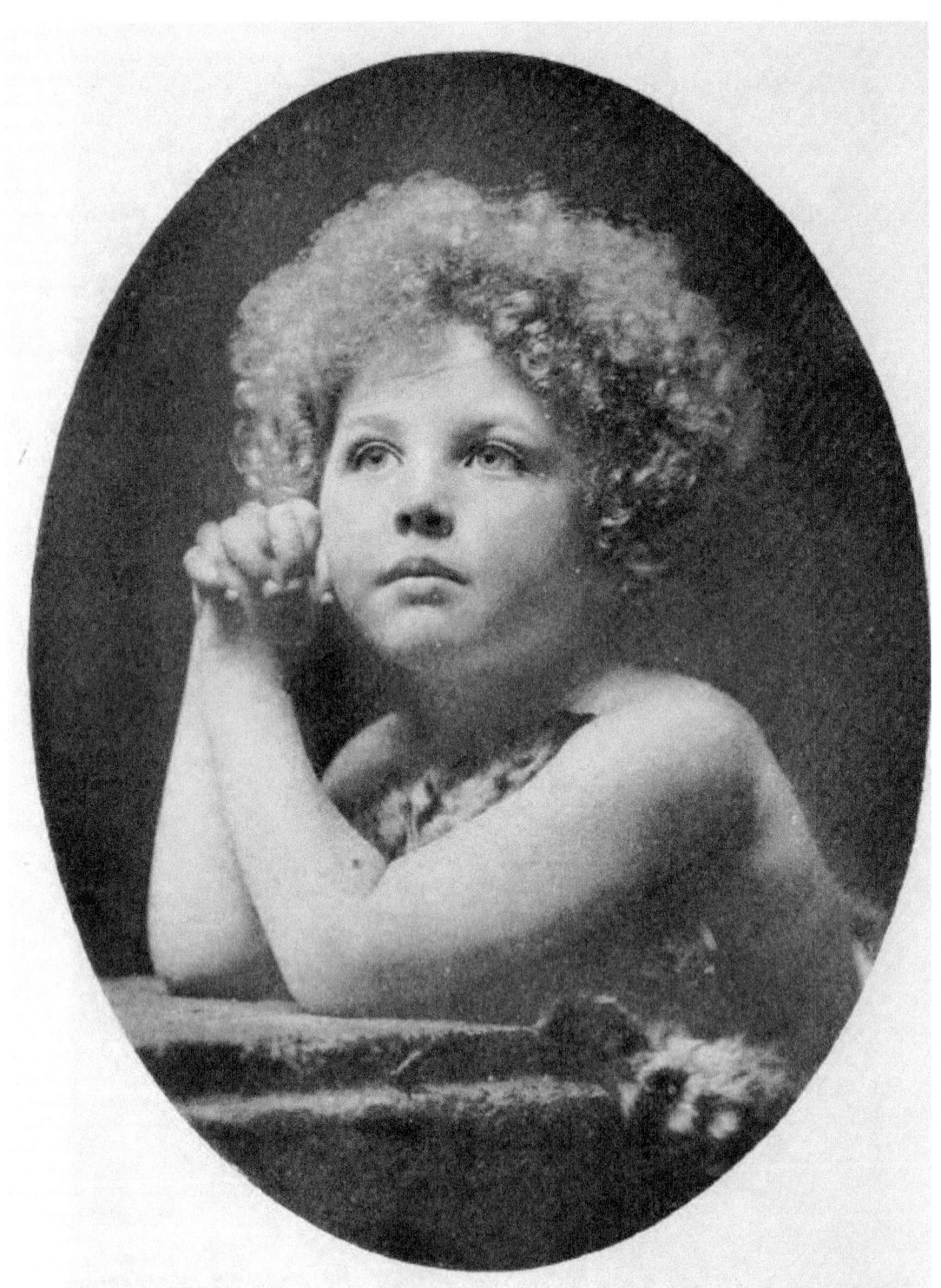

Beautiful Child-Study of one of the living Jewels which the State is asked to Treasure and Value as its Most Precious Asset, and upon the Health, Fitness and Happiness of which the Future of the whole World Depends.

WHAT IS DISEASE?

Here, surely is a prospect that must especially appeal to every medical man, for in the medical profession, with very little specialised study and training, we have the means to hand instantly to begin this great work of physical reconstruction, a work that must commence at once and continue long after the embers of strife have ceased to smoulder. In the years to come it will be the duty and pleasure of medical men not so much to cure disease as to prevent it altogether—to act upon the principle of obsta principiis, or " the resistance of the beginnings," so that we shall at least approximate to the ideal world without disease, in which, indeed, our medical men will be rewarded for its absence, and held to some degree responsible for its presence, just as we are told that the wise men of the East to-day only pay the doctor's fee so long as they remain untainted by disease.

This is a truly amazing conception—with almost illimitable possibilities—and is one opening out wide fields for research and study on the part of the medical profession. The medical profession to-day recognises, with very few exceptions, that disease is due to weakness and lack of balance somewhere in the body itself, and a consequent disturbance of organic, or rather cellular, equilibrium, chiefly through the environment of modern civilised life. Where there is destruction of tissue, this disturbance of balance is responsible for what we call organic disease, and where there is no actual injury to or destruction of the tissue-fabric of the body, it leads to functional disease and derangement.

If, then, as I am here attempting to prove, not merely by argument and medical evidence, but by actual proof and demonstration in the living human body itself, both in my own case and in the case of thousands of others, that harmony and perfect balance can again be restored, and restored only by what I call scientific physical movement, surely doctors can now learn how not only to combat and prevent disease and all suffering, but practically to eliminate it altogether, if only, as a beginning, in its grosser and more deadly forms.

To summarise briefly, the substance of my world-startling claim is that we can attain the ideal of a diseaseless world by the methods I advocate, and that where and when necessary it is possible to reconstruct the body physical in all or any of its parts as the necessities of the case demand by scientific and balanced physical movement from childhood, and the lack of which movement, through the progress of civilisation and its resultant evils inborn through generations, has hitherto doomed the world to physical degeneration and disease. To achieve all this successfully, however, the support of the State is essential, and the children must be regarded as the greatest asset of a people.

CHAPTER IV.
The State and the Child.

" OF all events here on this earth," declares Arthur Brisbane, foremost of American publicists, " the greatest is the birth of a baby."

That little bundle of plump pink flesh holds the world in its hands. It epitomises history, for all history began with the birth of a child. It contains within its little self the secret of life. It is the unsolved riddle of the world, the problem of yesterday, to-day and the unknown and unknowable future. Who guides the children steers the nation. Will the State take the helm?

Never in the history of the world was it so necessary for the State to answer in the affirmative as at present, if it is to profit by the lessons of the war, and avoid the pitfalls of weakness and disease that have so nearly ensnared us in the recent past.

REDEEMERS OF HUMANITY.

A Child born in a manger came into the world to redeem humanity. His birth we celebrate even to-day after the lapse of nearly 2,000 years, and will celebrate thousands of years hence. His sacrifice and death the nations still mourn, and will continue to mourn until the last day.

Humbler children are born every day and die daily. Except for a dry record of their births and deaths, and a brief period of parental rejoicing and mourning, their coming and their going are passed unnoticed by the State and the nation. Yet each child born to-day is a priceless jewel to the nation, an asset to the State, to some extent, indeed, a redeemer of lost humanity. Every year the State and nation should rejoice over its harvest of children and mourn for the dead, should have its national service of thanks-giving for the one and of lamentation and mourning for the other.

The State has no wealth like its children. Without them, its riches are but the barren gold of Midas. Yet millions of little ones die annually, and die, too, often avoidable and preventable deaths. The State must look to these living jewels that are its real wealth and glory.

The fiery furnace of a grim and awful war, through which we have passed, has consumed the very flower of the nation's manhood. It is scarcely too much to say that little but the embers remain. For the gallant dead we have held memorial services in our churches and cathedrals at which the whole nation has mourned. Thanksgiving services have been held for victory, and for the victors who still remain with us. Would it not be well if the State and the Churches held similar services of mourning and thanksgiving annually for the children who are added to the nation and for those who are taken away, if only as a perpetual reminder of our duty to the little ones left with us or as yet unborn, and to whom the State must look for its future prosperity and safety.

HOLDING HUMAN LIFE TOO CHEAP.

To-day, human life is the most precious thing in the world. In the past, we have held it too cheaply. For that we have paid a tragic and heavy price. Our mistake was, perhaps, excusable, because, as the author of " The Sowers " has neatly put it, " in crowded cities an excess of human life seems to vouch for the continuity of the race, where, in a teeming population, one life more or less seems of little value."

War, however, which has increased the price of everything, has also given human life a new and added value. The Empire and the State must look to the cradles of the people. For the cradle, to paraphrase Gray's lines, may well hold some mute, inglorious Milton, some village Hampden, or some dauntless Cromwell, to whom the State and the nation may yet look with pride and gratitude. Each child should, indeed, be to the State even more precious than an only child in the eyes of its mother, and watched over with the same zealous care as the child of a king. The child of peasant or artisan is not less to be mourned if lost to its country than the child of Royal birth, and the acceptance of that truth by the State will save millions of incalculably valuable lives annually, and nip revolution in the bud.

A new era is about to begin. Old shibboleths, old creeds, old ideas will have to be ruthlessly destroyed; new methods and new machinery of life must take their place. The fetish of personal liberty to the verge of license must be destroyed if we are to set our compass true and steer the Ship of State safely through the rocks and shallows of seas that even as yet are comparatively uncharted and unknown. Each of us must recognise, or be made to recognise, the stern fact that " no man liveth unto himself," and that, at least, if he be not his brother's keeper, he must not cause, menace or even, endanger another's life. The State and the nation must hitch its wagon to a star, if the people are to be saved even from themselves.

In the vital matter of public health, as the Daily Mail has well said, " the State must now step in, and this will mean interference with our vaunted liberty. We cannot have public services without public inquisitions. Our old personal liberty was the grand recruiting sergeant of our C3 civilian army. Our new creed must be that everyone, from birth, is a health soldier of the State."

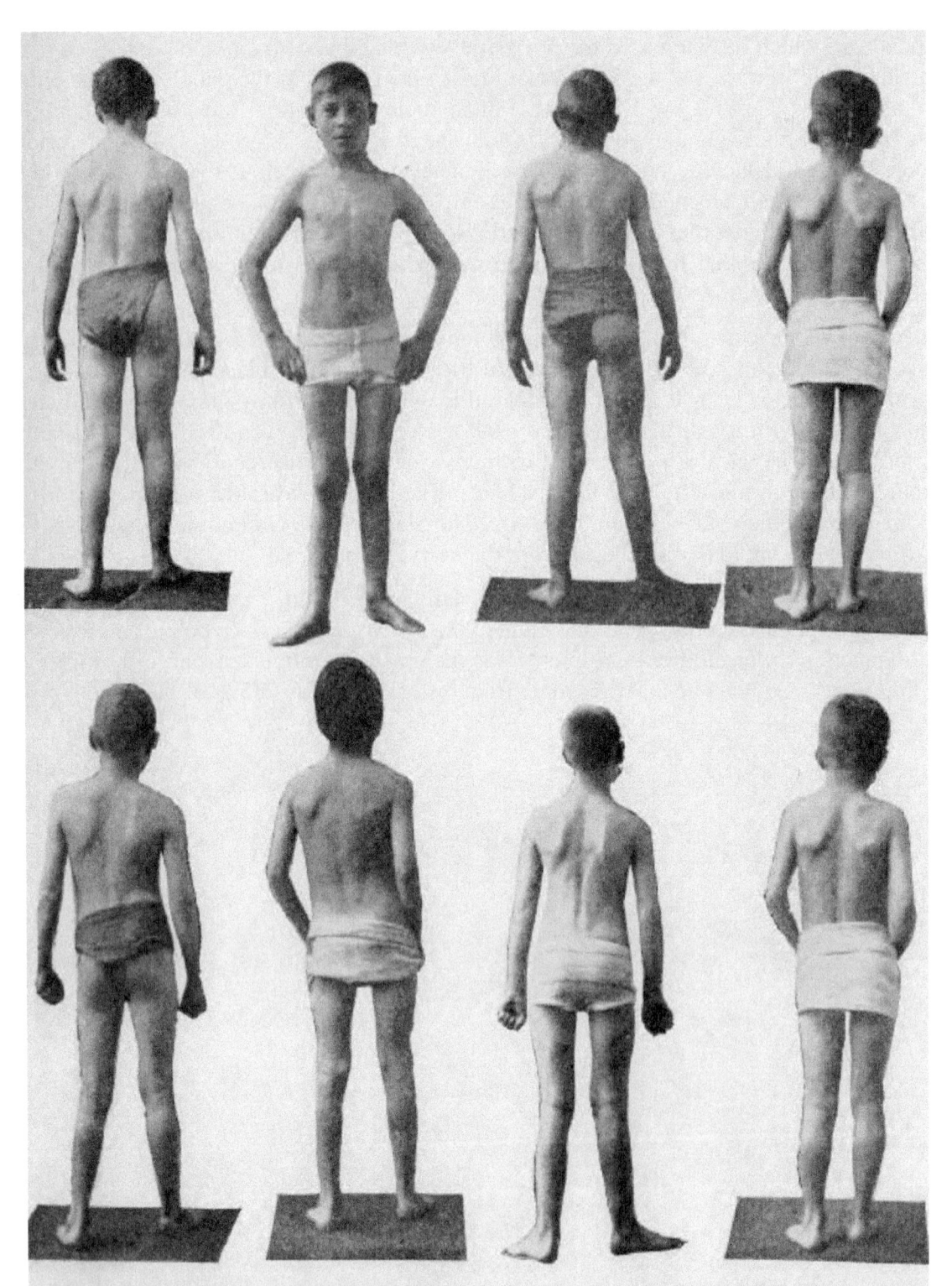

Typical children of to-day, whose poor physique, inborn from a poor parent stock, displays lack of that body-culture which has left them with the weakness and deficiency in vital resisting power to disease which, if not corrected and overcome by scientific methods of physical education such as are described in this book, must assuredly handicap them in later life, and leave them ever open to serious disease.

PHYSICAL EDUCATION COMPULSORY.

Even to-day, with all our freedom, we do not allow a sufferer from small-pox to enjoy the same liberty as a normal person free from contagious or infectious disease. The State intervenes. It must intervene more and more in a thousand ways in the life of the individual, if the nation is to be saved from other and yet graver dangers. The Government must not permit any person to neglect or abuse his or her own body, either through ignorance or other cause, to become physically unfit or diseased, and so more liable to spread disease, or, to become reduced in efficiency and economic value through weakness or illness, where educational and preventive measures can prevail. To do so, is to exhibit a tolerance that is criminal towards the whole body public. The State must, indeed, display a new and an intelligent interest in its children especially, if we are to prevent all these things.

Just as mental education, once opposed as an infringement of the liberty of the subject, has been made legal and necessary in the interests of the commonweal, so the State must make physical and hygienic education compulsory, whatever personal or powerful interests may be opposed to it, both for the well-being of the individual and of the people generally. It must, at least, watch over the upbringing of its children as zealously as the wise farmer tends to the birth and rearing of his calves or the breeding of his horses.

It is, surely, one of the greatest paradoxes of civilisation to find laws, acts, regulations and restrictions innumerable for the breeding and health preservation of horses and cattle and domestic animals generally, for their protection from ill-treatment and even from unhealthy conditions of existence, and for the propagation and preservation of their species, whilst the breeding and bringing-up of the children upon whom the whole future of a country depends, too often receives but little State attention, and such attention certainly not of a scientific or comprehensive character.

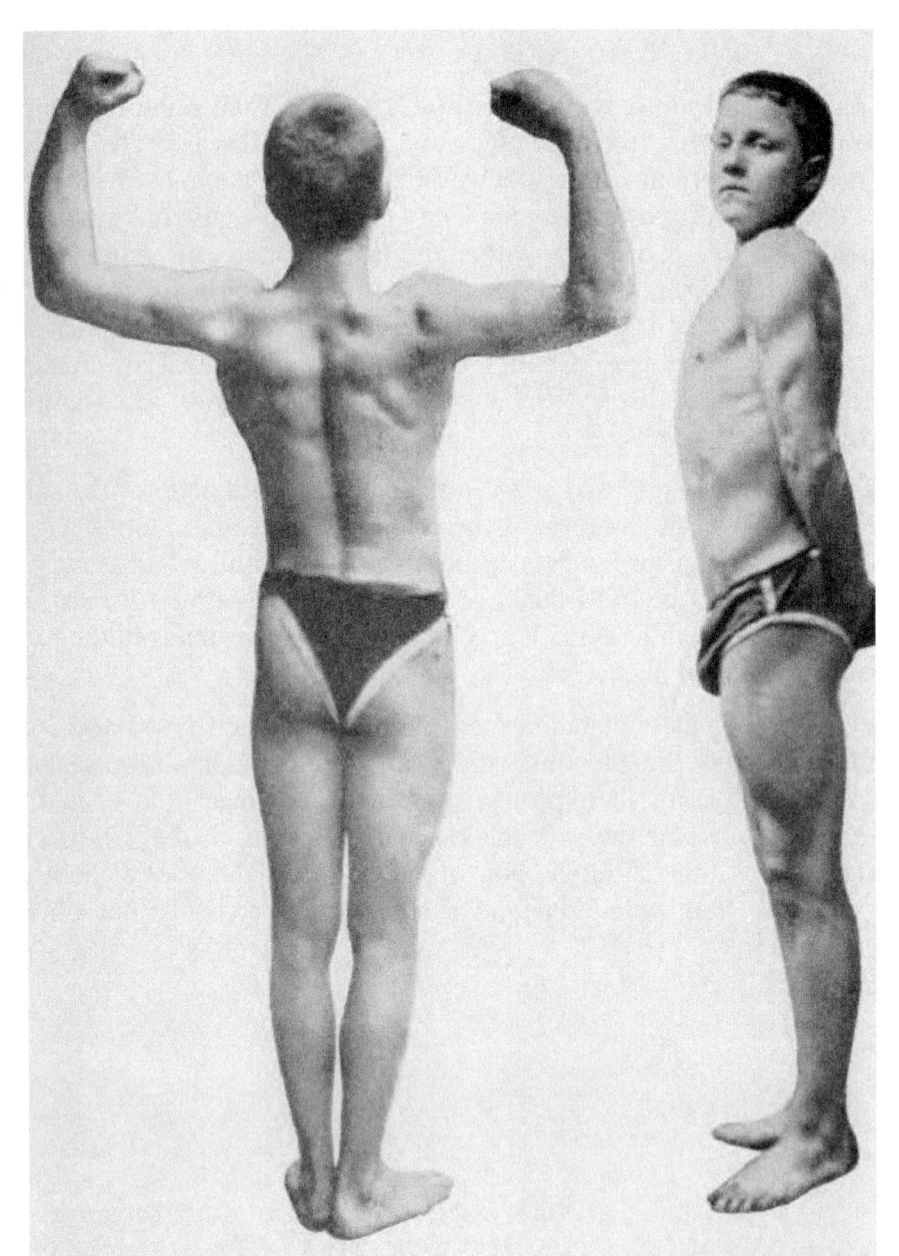

Contrast these photographs, showing back and side view of a boy who has been physically educated as described in this book. Here we have a boy with his body so fully and perfectly developed in balanced strength that it may be said to be impregnable to disease either now or in later life.

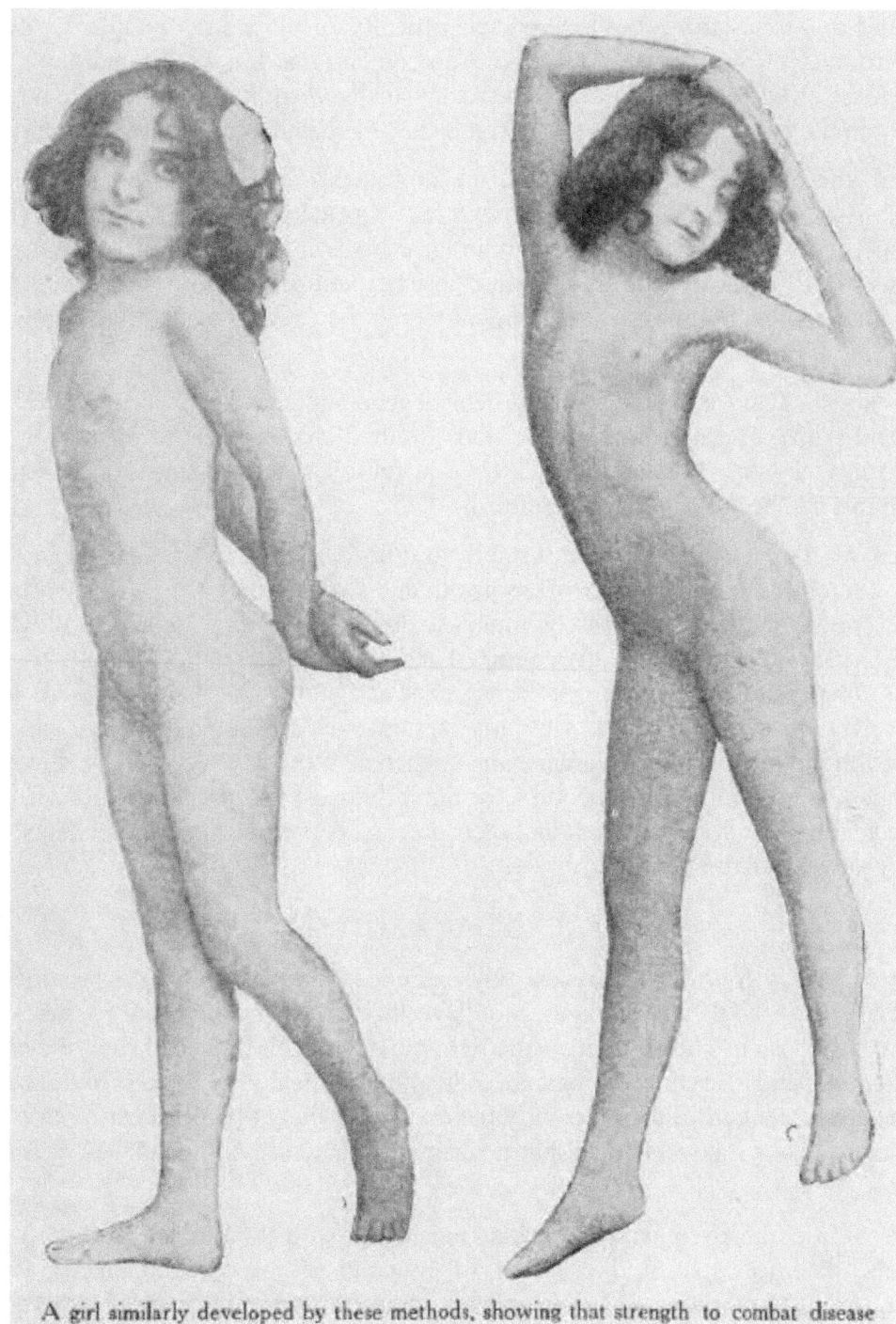

A girl similarly developed by these methods, showing that strength to combat disease need not antagonise physical beauty or interfere with symmetry and grace of contour.

THE BORDERLAND OF DISEASE.

True, much has already been done to improve upon the evil conditions existent only half a century ago, but we must hasten our forward progress both from a material and from a moral point of view. Morality, efficiency and even religion are too closely inter-related with physical fitness and bodily health, for the latter to be made secondary to any other educational development. I do not say that a healthy and scientifically developed body will necessarily make every man virtuous, efficient, or religious, but I do contend that it is easier and more natural for such a man to be or become so than it is for the physically weak, the degenerate, and those who stand always on the borderland of Disease, even if they have not actually crossed its frontiers.

The immoral, the vicious, the criminal and the inefficient are rarely to be found among the physical culturists, athletes, or any of those who take a pride in the physical body, who treat it with the respect to which it is entitled, and who have made it healthy and strong by careful and conscientious effort, because health will refuse to exist and remain long in a body debased by lack of that all-round natural physical movement which the Creator made a condition of healthy life.

It is now established and admitted that physical degeneracy and disease are prolific causes of pauperism and crime. These facts are noted and admitted chiefly because pauperism and crime are costly to any country. Why not, then, strike at these two costly burdens by removing the causes! That this can be done is easy to establish.

The children of the rich and the comfortable middle classes are, or have been, we know, individually and child for child, better off in health and strength than the poorer working classes and the very poor, and are more rarely found swelling the criminal classes. Why? Is it not because the former are better physically equipped and safeguarded against disease from birth and even before? Their parents are, as a rule, better educated, better fed, better housed, and usually come themselves of a stock that was similarly circumstanced. Their homes are situated in the healthier localities; they are more sanitary and hygienic in every way; usually they have their finely equipped bath-rooms and play-rooms for the little ones; and the family doctor, acquainted with the medical history of the children and their parents, is periodically in attendance and keeps them under pretty constant observation.

REAL SOCIAL REFORM.

As they grow up, they go to schools where physical education of some sort is provided for them daily. Most of such schools and colleges, too, have their sports, games, and pastimes under the most vigilant supervision. The children of the rich, too, have their ponies or their bicycles to ride, their tennis-courts, and everything conducive to healthy physical growth. Is it to be wondered at, then, that, as at present constituted, it is only the crust of Society that can bear minute inspection and examination, while it covers much that is unappetising and revolting as we reach the bottom of the dish?

Fortunately, we are already making progress, and it was with the utmost pleasure I read Lord Leverhulme's statement that in the North of England at least " though the children of comparatively well-to-do parents had advantages in health over middle-class children, children of poor parents living in suburban areas were now healthier than either." Such a pronouncement in any local district augurs what is possible if we take national and scientific measures to save the children of the nation.

If such a system of scientific physical education and training, as I advocate, were once in existence, there would be equal health opportunities for all, and the provocative line of demarcation which has so long existed between the health and happiness of the classes and ill-health and unhappiness of the masses would cease for ever to exist. Is not this a social reformation devoutly to be wished, especially since the war has shown us how deep-seated is the physical degeneracy and disease that consume the very vitals of a nation.

There is only one possible way to prevent disease and all its ugly spawn, viz., by making the human body too strong in each and every part to fall before them. To do that, the State must begin with the child, or, perhaps even before its birth until a better era dawns, for, as The Medical Officer, a paper representative of the Public Health Service, says, I welfare work must begin at the very commencement of life, even before birth, if its full value is to be realised."

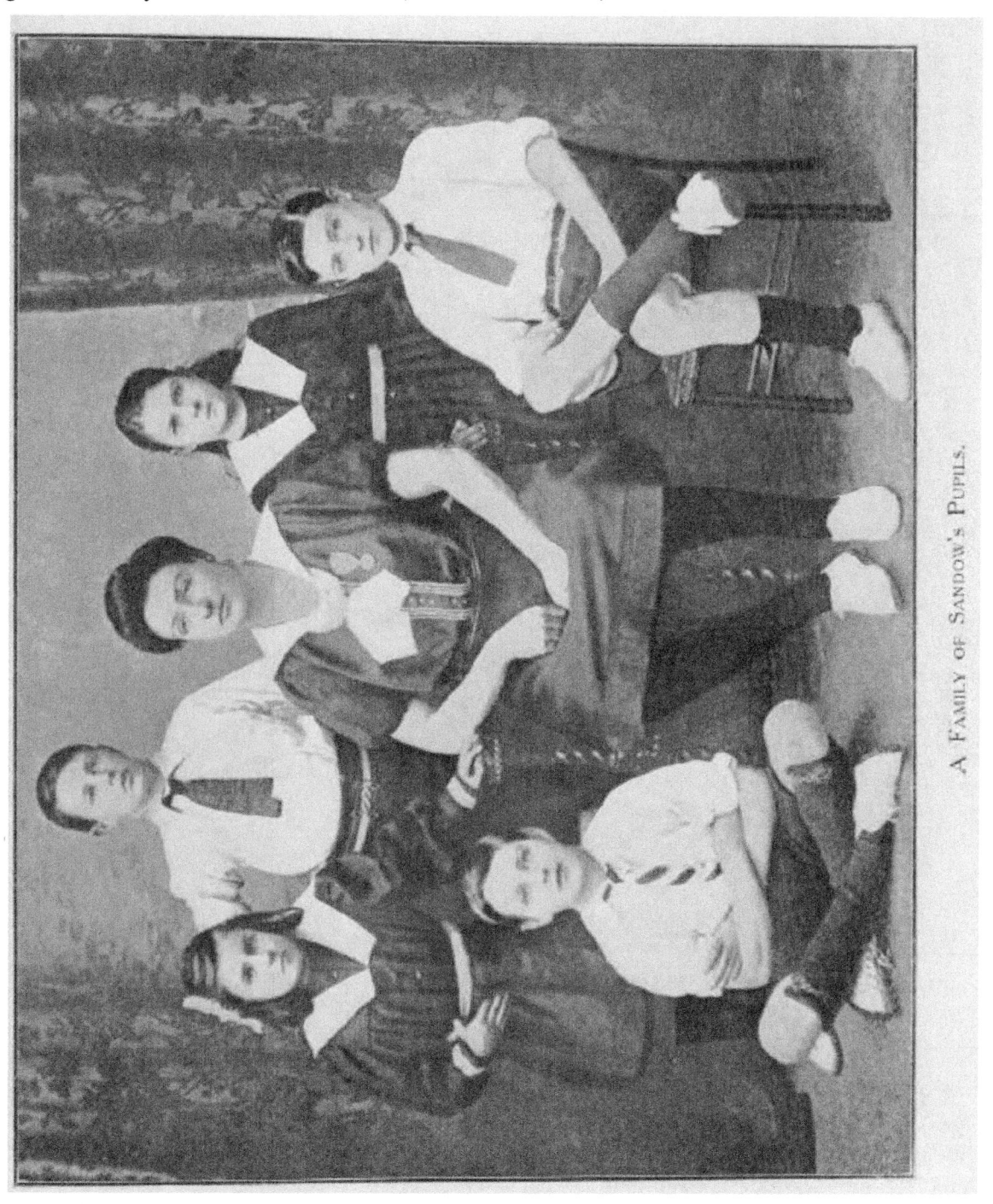

A Family of Sandow's Pupils.

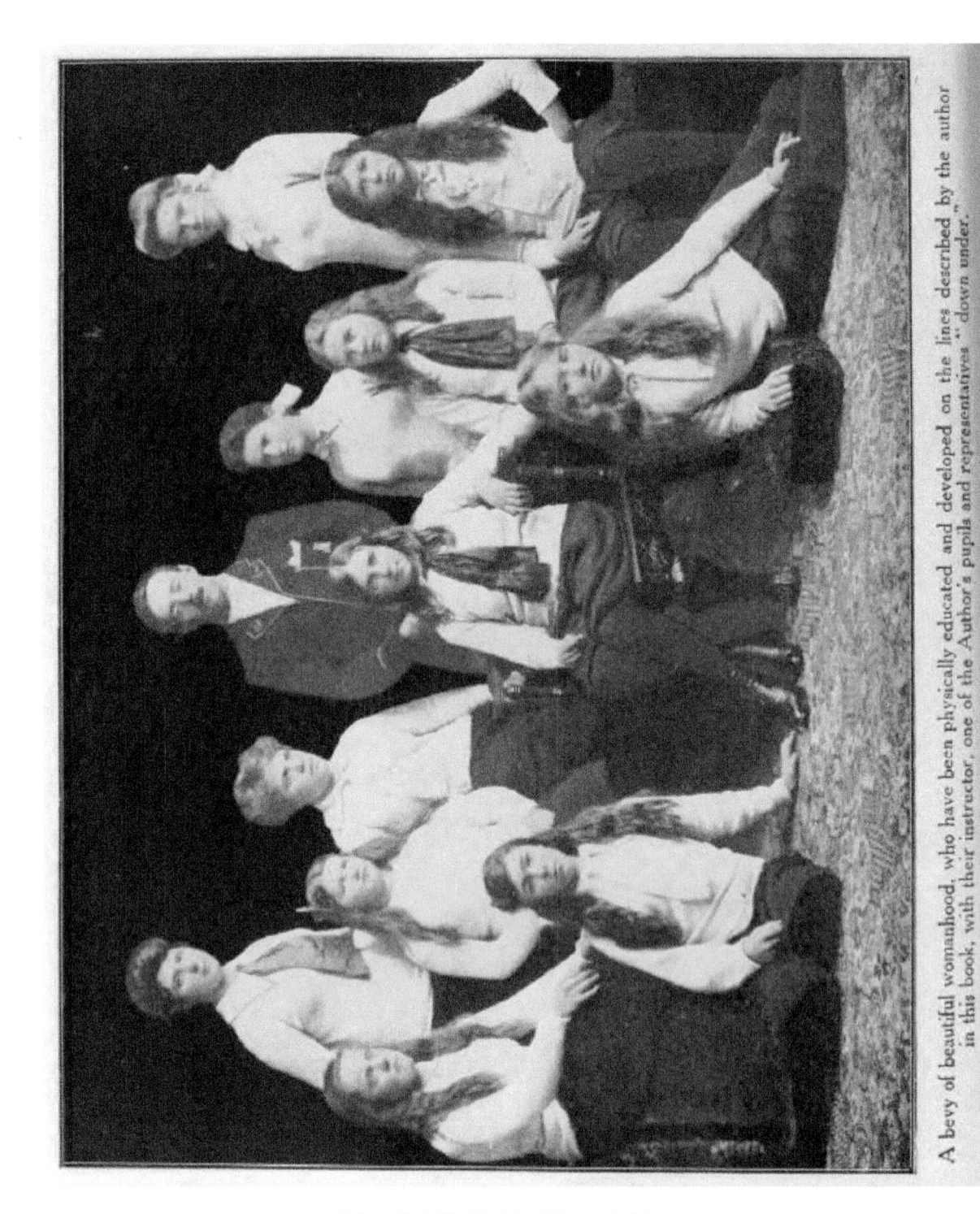

A bevy of beautiful womanhood, who have been physically educated and developed on the lines described by the author in this book, with their instructor, one of the Author's pupils and representatives "down under."

THE POWER IN THE CRADLE.

As Society is at present constituted, the first duty of the State will often be to save the child from its parents, or from the ignorance of its parents, due to the defects in past and present education, and to carefully consider the mother both before and after the birth of her child. After all, as Dr Marie C. Stopes, author of "Married Love," has well put in a trenchant article in the Sunday Chronicle, " the baby doesn't come into existence the very day it is born. It has already lived for some months previously, dependent on its mother's life and health, and to care for the pregnant mother is also to care for the child" After birth, children born of drunken, ignorant, vicious or criminal parents, dragged up amid dirt and filth, underfed because money is lacking or goes to the dramship, instead of to the butcher and the baker, must be saved from such an environment. For, every child, to adapt Napoleon's famous saying, " carries a baton in its cradle." In any cradle may rest a potential dignitary of State, of the Army, the Navy, of Commerce or Industry, or one of the learned Professions. Let us rob no child, however lowly its origin, however handicapped by its environment, at least of its birthright.

Even with the limited opportunities that are offered to-day, we have many instances of what is possible when we see men who have, by their sheer vigour of constitution and strength of character, triumphed over circumstances of birth and environment. A boy born in a London workhouse became a Privy Councillor of State. Men from the bench, the mine, the workshop and the humblest homes adorn our legislative chamber, and command the respect of the nation. If such things are possible under our present imperfect educational system what miracles are not possible under such a State system of really scientific physical and mental education and training as I have advocated now for many years, and continue to advocate in these pages.

INCREASING HAPPINESS AND EFFICIENCY.

To-day, only the exceptionally dowered in health and strength from birth can hope to win through, because our present educational methods and the unhygienic conditions of existence among the poor tend to crush and destroy all self-respect and all ambition even from childhood. The State must, in future, give each and every child an equal opportunity of health and fitness for the race of life, and believe me, the socialisation of health is a far wiser and more attainable ideal than the socialisation of wealth. The former would naturally, in time, bring the latter nearer, as the handicaps of physical unfitness, weakness, degeneracy and disease would then be removed, and from a health point of view each and all would be better human products and a credit to the State.

Further, with this better health and immunity from disease, efficiency would increase, and with it the earning power of the individual, so that the State itself as well as the individual would benefit, for individual health and efficiency would naturally mean national wealth.

If the State, in an hour of national danger can conscript the individual adults of a nation to fight for national existence and safety, why should it not, if need be, even conscript the individual child, to take it and make it a more valuable citizen in times of peaceful industry. Is a healthy and disease-free individual less valuable to a nation in times of peace than in times of war?

Millions have been spent on war, millions more have been subscribed voluntarily to help to defeat the enemy. Is it too much to ask the State and the nation to contribute as generously to defeat a far greater enemy—Disease—and, in some degree, at least, to make good the cruel losses brought about by the war? So much could be done in this way that the vision is a staggering one.

This, indeed, is a debt that every State owes to its children, a debt that would be repaid with interest by the upbuilding of the national human stock, healthy, happy, strong, and literally free from disease or the degeneracy that precedes, is associated with, or follows disease. There can be no diseaseless world until we prevent disease first in the children, and the State must lend its powerful aid to the work.

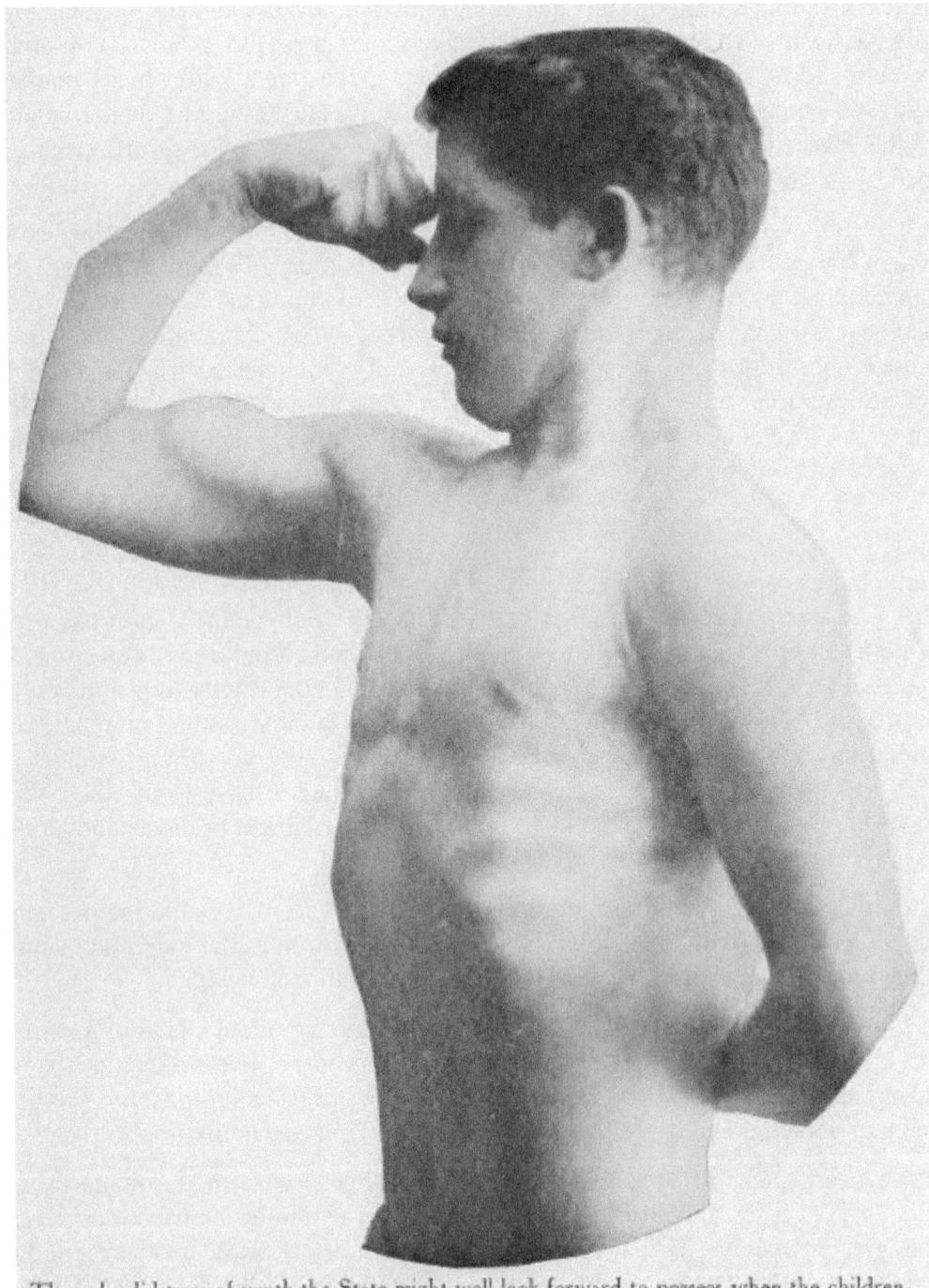

The splendid type of youth the State might well look forward to possess when the children are as scientifically educated from their schooldays as they are mentally to-day by methods such as have given this youth his finely developed and healthy body.

The State must not grapple with the question in a sporadic, unsystematic, or unorganised way. Its methods must be scientific, systematic and organised. As the Chief Medical Officer of the Board of Education said in his Annual Report for 1917:— " Measures for the promotion of healthy physical development must be preventive as well as remedial. The purposes of the School Medical Service are not the detection of defects, the discovery of child patients, and the treatment of such sick children, but the advancement of the health and physical development of the whole child population of school age. What is required is not the devotion of exclusive attention to the diseased child, much less the sporadic and intermittent handling of sick children, but a broad, carefully considered, and unified system of physical care and development of all children of school age."

After giving statistics showing the various causes and forms of physical defect and disease reported in London alone, he adds the not surprising fact that the physical condition was also reflected in a lowered mentality. " These defective children were often," says a medical correspondent of The Times, "two or more years behind their normal school standard, showing how physical weakness reacts upon mental deficiency."

Unfortunately, after carefully studying Sir George Newman's Report, in conjunction with the text of the 1918 Education Act, I still fail to see that those in authority even yet understand the true meaning of physical training carried out, as I mean it, by natural methods on truly scientific lines. In fact, they seem to think that by devoting a few minutes daily to Swedish exercises, gymnastics, games, and dancing they will be able to build up a child's body strong enough to resist disease. If that were so, the Premier would not have had to confess to 1,000,000 undesirables, in the physical sense, in an hour of danger to the Empire, and we would not have millions of unfit and diseased men, women and children in our midst to-day. For these and similar methods have now been on trial for a long time without success, and even with injury to many children, and it must not be supposed that some slight additions or alterations to them will suffice to meet the present needs. Only by the introduction of absolutely new and scientific methods such as are described in these pages can the body be built up in such balanced strength as to make it impregnable to disease, and, as Sir. George admits, the way to prevent disease is " by growing strong and resistant bodies."

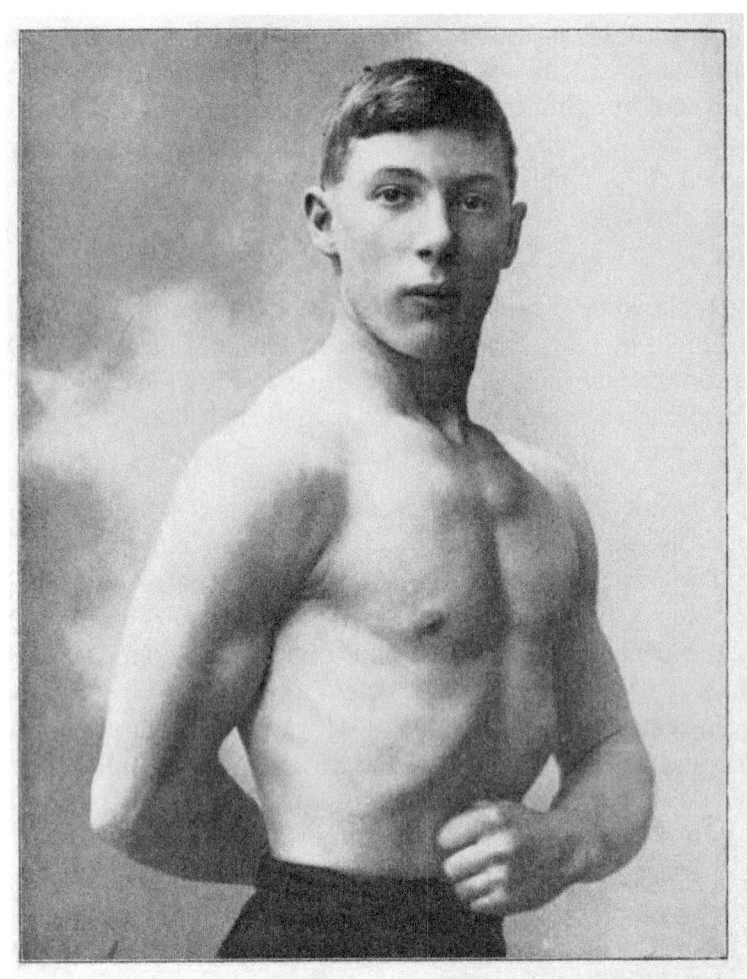

Another fine specimen of the youth the nation could easily possess if these methods of scientific physical culture were adopted and supported by the State as suggested here.

WANTED, A NEW IDEAL.

Parents, teachers, and doctors would all have a responsible and authoritative position to fill in this upward movement towards a people healthy, strong and practically disease-immune, and until a child had arrived at an age of responsibility itself, they should be held jointly to account for the health of the young.

What the nation to-day stands most in need of is a new ideal. The fetish of wealth and the idol of material prosperity have too long been blindly worshipped. Children have been given false ideals. The mind of the child must be given a new orientation, and here the State can most certainly do much to encourage the healthy ambition implanted in every child to have a body healthy, beautiful and strong, such as Nature certainly meant it to possess and maintain throughout life, but which modern ideas and habits of life have, unfortunately, made so difficult of achievement. This natural instinct has become perverted by civilisation, with its too sordid worship of wealth, position and success.

The time has come when a nobler ideal must be instilled into the youthful mind, and what better ideal could we have than that of perfect manliness and womanliness in the highest and best sense. To imbue youth with such an ideal, the State must spare no expense, no labour, no sacrifice, and there are many ways in which the State can encourage the cult of the sound mind in the sound body, that glorious ideal upon which was built the greatest Empires of the past, and upon which we can to-day erect an Empire greater even than these.

Let us give the children rather the ideal of God-like men and women, peerless in health and strength of body, and sane and sound in mind. Our children have no such ideal implanted early in their minds to-day, and national physical deterioration is the inevitable result. I have written already of the influence exerted even in the case of adults by the display of my own physical power, but how much greater results would be achieved with the children, whose minds naturally are more pliable and more receptive, if they learnt by experience and example that men diligent in something more vital to the State than even business were, indeed, thought worthy to " stand before kings."

CREATING A HEALTH APPETITE.

Every school should be stimulated to play its part in the great national work of physical reconstruction in this way. To begin with, healthy rivalry should be encouraged among the scholars, and prizes awarded to the children who took the best care of their bodies and became the healthiest and best developed of their own age. Inter-county and inter-city rivalries should also be encouraged, to still further create enthusiasm among the children, and once every year or so a great national fete or festival could be held in London, under Royal patronage, at which the children of the British Isles from all parts of the country would compete, with their relatives and friends to admire and encourage them.

A healthy hunger for physical well-being would thus be fostered, and the mind of the whole nation diverted into a channel that would lead to the new and better world which we all, like the Premier, so ardently desire, and which must come if the nation is not to sink into a fatal lethargy and apathy with regard to its most vital problem.

The days when it was the ambition of every Briton to wield bow and arrow must find a parallel in a nation to-day steering united to this goal of physical fitness and perfect health. This is the real method of building up a nation that will ever be able to defend itself against its most deadly enemies. This is the way to give us a people healthy and disease-free, a nation of men and women in which every man will be a god and every woman a queen. We spend thousands upon thousands in the erection of beautiful buildings and in the adornment of our cities with beautiful statues. Surely it would be a work with a far greater reward for the State to give us a race of men and women with beautifully developed and healthy bodies, who would themselves be " living statues " moulded on lines which the greatest artists and sculptors would be proud to copy.

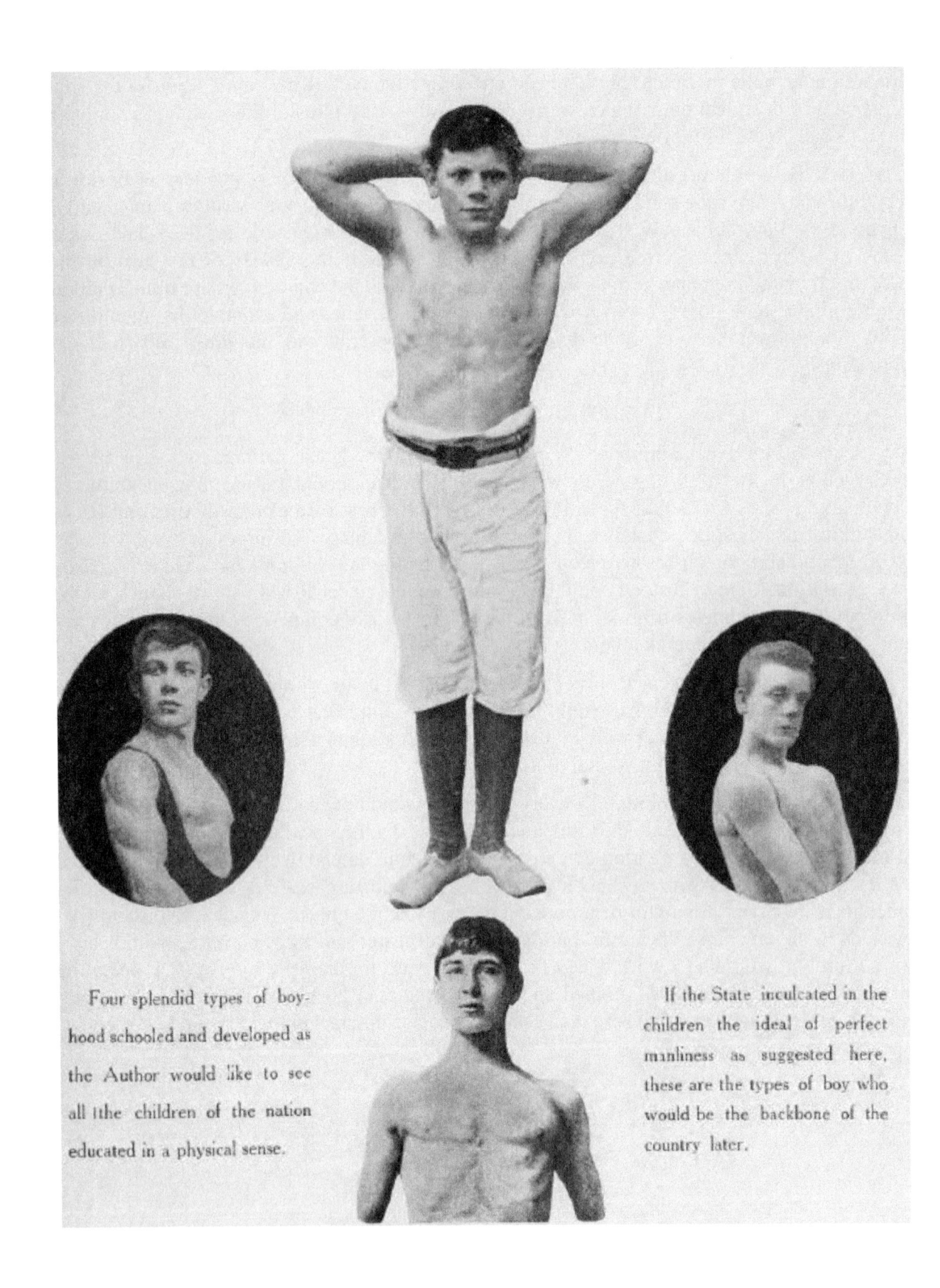

Four splendid types of boyhood schooled and developed as the Author would like to see all the children of the nation educated in a physical sense.

If the State inculcated in the children the ideal of perfect manliness as suggested here, these are the types of boy who would be the backbone of the country later.

THE REAL NOBILITY OF HEALTH.

An entirely new Order with dignities and titles was formed to do honours to those whose services, outside the fighting line, helped our brave soldiers and sailors to win the war. If a somewhat similar Order were established, with titles and dignities of its own, in times of peace for those who made and kept themselves in the most perfect physical condition, think how far-reaching would be its influence in helping in the great work of national reconstruction. It would give the children the very ideal the nation so badly needs now, and every child would look up with admiration to those who won such honours. The heroes of the youth of the nation would no longer be the famous cricketers, goalkeepers or jockeys, or the men and women who had amassed fortunes or fame in various lines of life, but the men and women whose superb physique and health had won for them such State recognition and honour.

This new nobility would constitute the real nobility of the nation, for in these men and women would course the " blue blood " of a nobility and aristocracy untainted by physical blemish or disease. The future of the race would then be in good hands, and men and women would no longer be bought or sold in marriage as they too often are to-day, but health and physical fitness for marriage and the propagation of healthy children would be the only " Open Sesame " to the portals of Hymen.

As I have already pointed out, however, we cannot, of course, consider the child without also taking into consideration at least until the new generation and type of educated mothers have arrived, the mothers to whom we must look, in the first place for the birth, maintenance and protection of the children. The mother who gives the nation healthy and sturdy children is as valuable to a country as the general who wins great battles with the aid of their muscles and sinews. There is, after all, even greater honour in saving life than in taking it, so why should not the fertile and fruitful mother be honoured for 'piloting her many young through the dangers and trials of infancy? A home, again, may be a place of safety or a danger zone according to the manner in which it is looked after and, its hygiene studied. Why not rewards for the cleanest and healthiest homes in every town and village throughout the land, with standards for the rich, the middle class and the poor.

To encourage hygiene, competitions should be held, open to all, and the rewards to be largely determined by surprise visits to the homes of the competitors, from the judges. Why not honours also for the healthiest and physically best workers, for healthy parents and for healthy school children. Why should a county not be honoured for the lowness of its death-rate and the highness of its birth-rate as well as for the bravery of its soldiers?

If we did all this and more, as I suggest, we would build up a new aristocracy, " not," as Ibsen has said, "of birth or of the purse or even of intellect, an aristocracy of character, will and mind," and, I might add, an aristocracy of physique and freedom from disease.

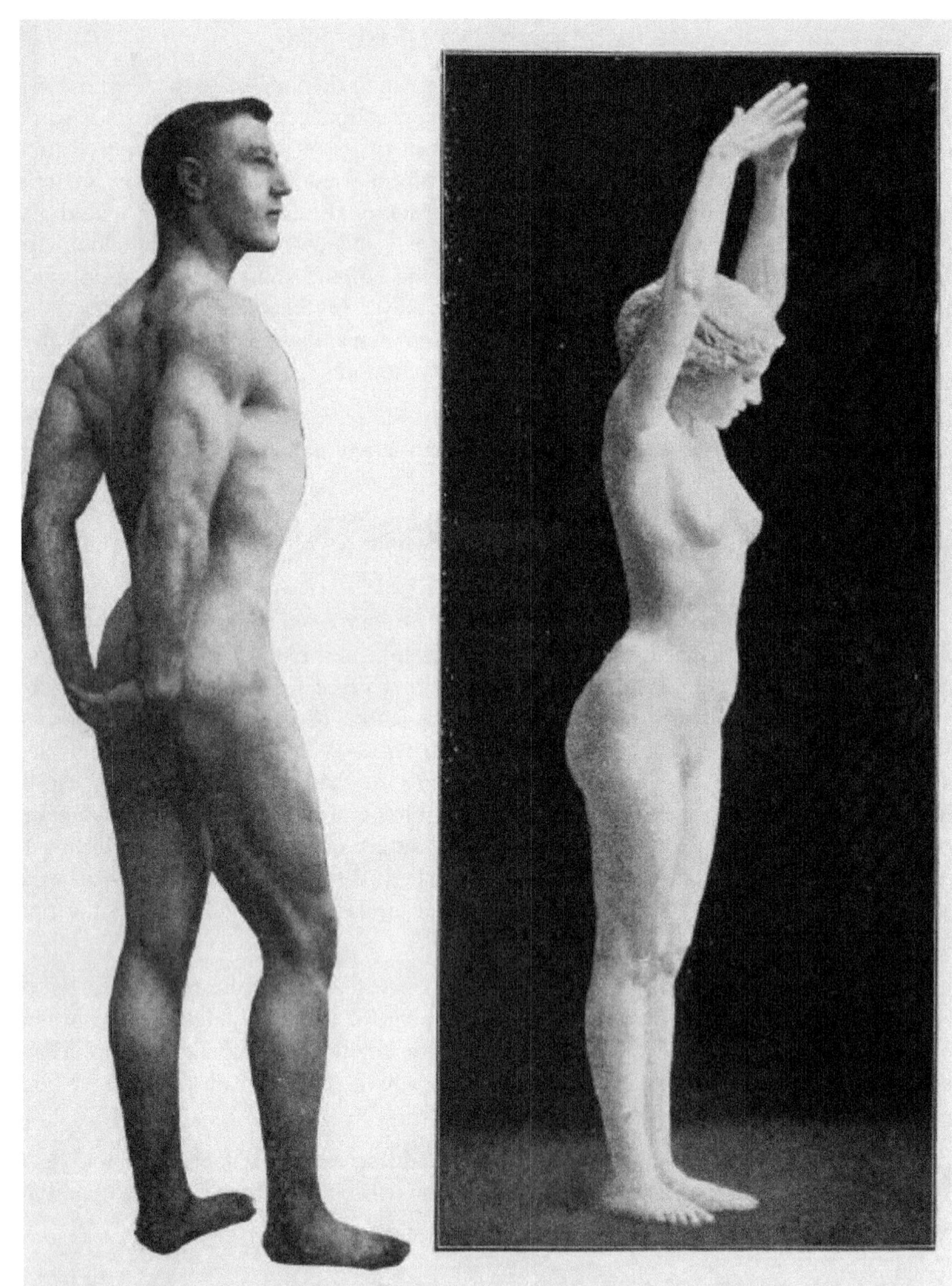

The real "living statues" which sculptors might well use as models, moulded in human flesh and blood by scientific physical movement. Such men and women may well constitute a real nobility of health, and be the real "blue blood" of the nation.

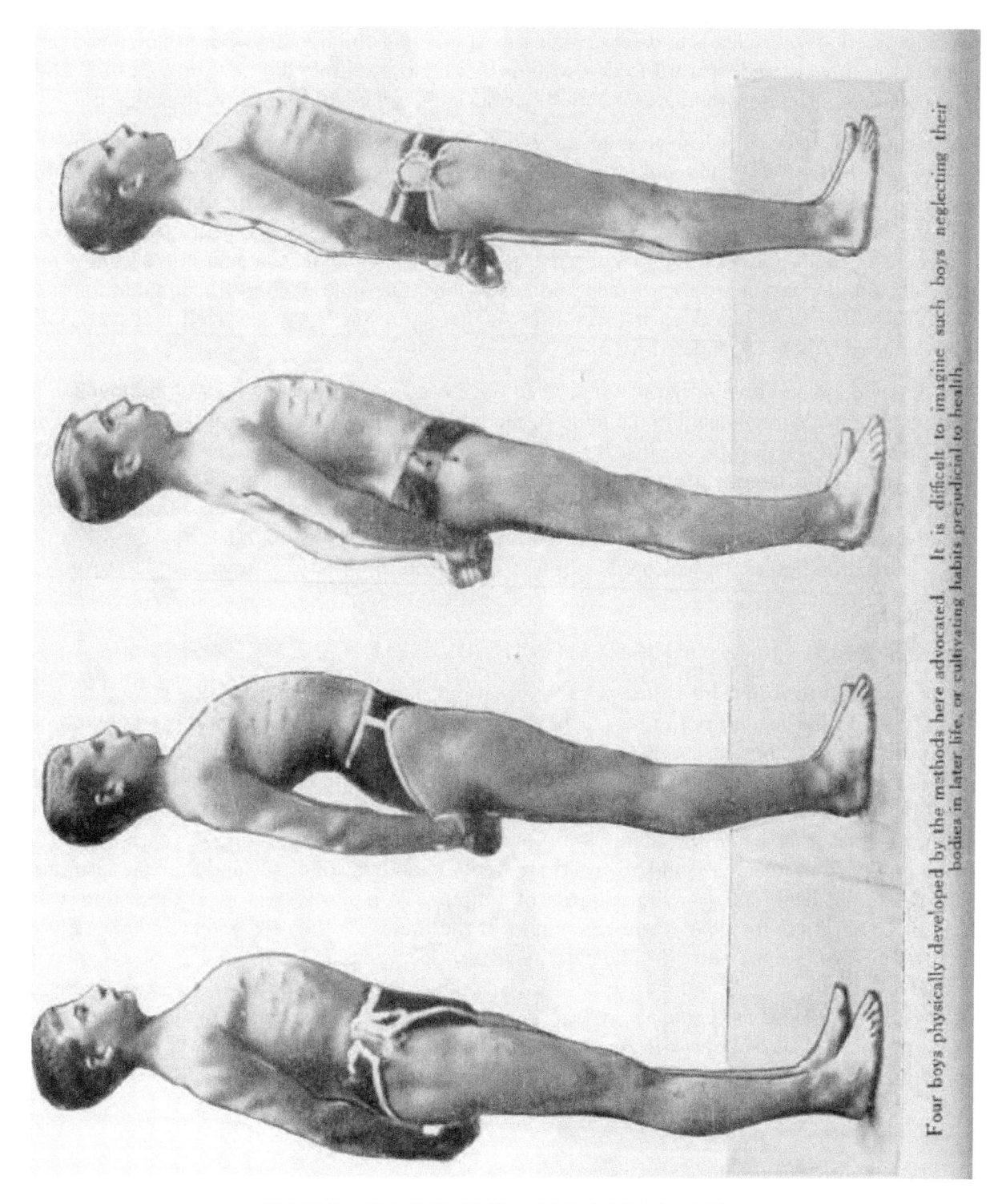

Four boys physically developed by the methods here advocated. It is difficult to imagine such boys neglecting their bodies in later life, or cultivating habits prejudicial to health.

HEALTHY BODIES IN HEALTHY HOMES.

In the children the State to-day has its greatest treasure, after the awful devastation of war. No human life is too precious to be lightly regarded or to be jeopardised where a wise foresight can prevent it. Such methods as I suggest and describe in this book would give every child a fair and equal start in life, would hold out to it alluring, prospects of rewards, would prevent disease and the weakness that surely leads to disease, and would give the children a new ambition and a new ideal to look upward and forward to that would illuminate its whole journey through life, while the State and the Empire would gleam with the reflected glory of millions of such children.

This is the real work of Reconstruction to which the State must at once put its hand, for all wealth and prosperity is contingent upon it. Machines without men and buildings without people are useless, however wonderful the machine or hygienically perfect the building. On the other hand, the State that makes human life and health its first and capital investment makes the finest investment in the world. It builds for eternal honour and fame. The State should see to it that each child should be taught to know and appreciate the value in after life of health and physical education, and to love health as it loves life. As Leonardo da Vinci has well and truly said, "knowledge of a thing engenders love of it."

When knowledge and love of its own body had once been implanted, the idea of compulsion or effort would die a natural death in the mind of the child, and the rest be comparatively easy. This very teaching, too, will promote that hygiene and knowledge of hygienic laws /in adult life, to the lack of which is largely attributable our national physical deterioration, the sacrifice of much child life and the propagation of disease. Such a health education and physical upbuilding as I now advocate would make the children when they become adults as anxious to possess healthy homes as healthy bodies, and such education is, I contend, the first step towards the prevention of disease.

FOUNDATION OF ALL REFORM.

It is not difficult to realise how great a transformation such a policy as I venture to outline here would work in the nation, not either in the far distant future but in a generation or two, and, indeed, in the generation at present in its cradle. The State would reap an immediate reward in the reduction of its hospital bill. Illness and disease would not only soon become unknown in our midst, but much of the pauperism, crime and insanity too often associated with it would also vanish. On the other hand, the State would boast a people superbly strong, a reserve fund of human power from which it could always draw freely in an hour of crisis, and the best insurance against national bankruptcy or the collapse of Empire. To attain to this ideal three things are vitally necessary; (1) the whole-hearted support of the State, (2) the unanimous endorsement of the medical profession, and, (3) the intelligent co-operation and partnership of the people themselves in every walk and sphere of life. Without this mighty triplicate effort no plans or schemes of social reconstruction or reform can be crowned with success, for all reform must have a physical basis as I show in my next chapter. To secure health and fitness is, indeed, the very beginning of all reform.

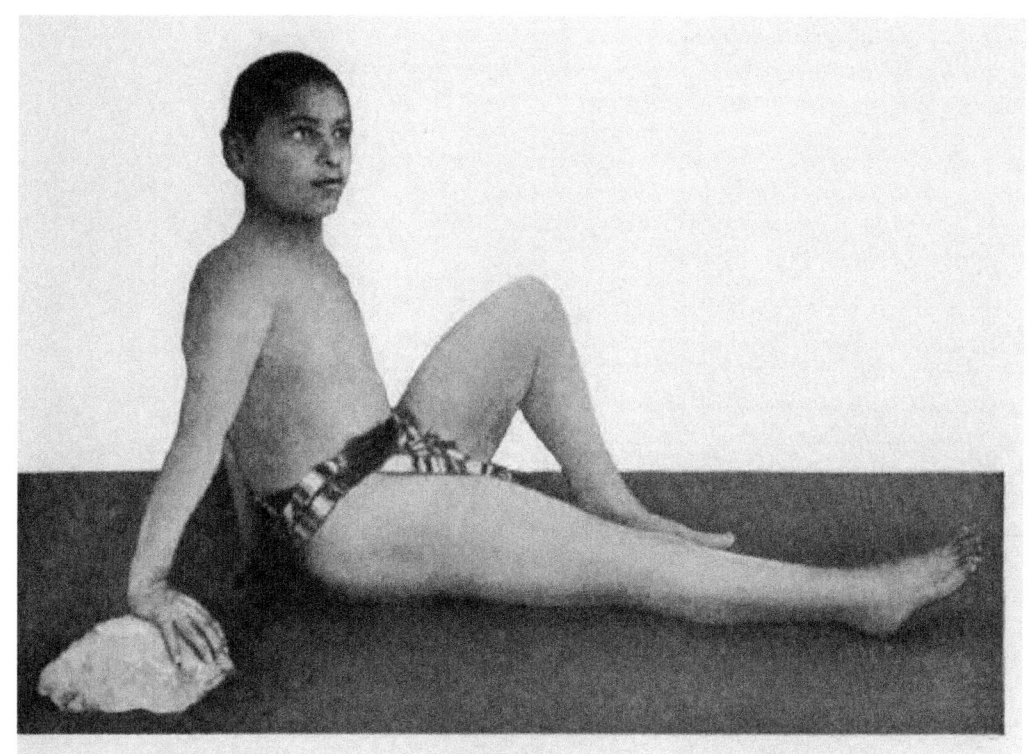

A young enthusiast from India as graceful as an Apollo.

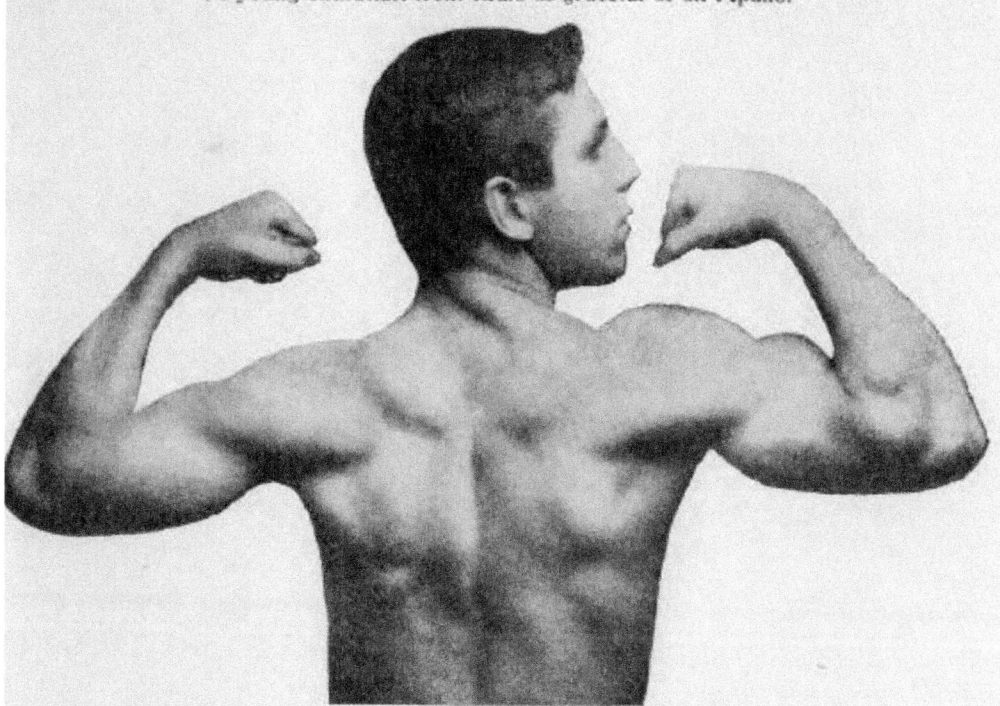

A boy of 15 who has obtained this wonderful development, with its great resistant power to disease, by the Author's methods.

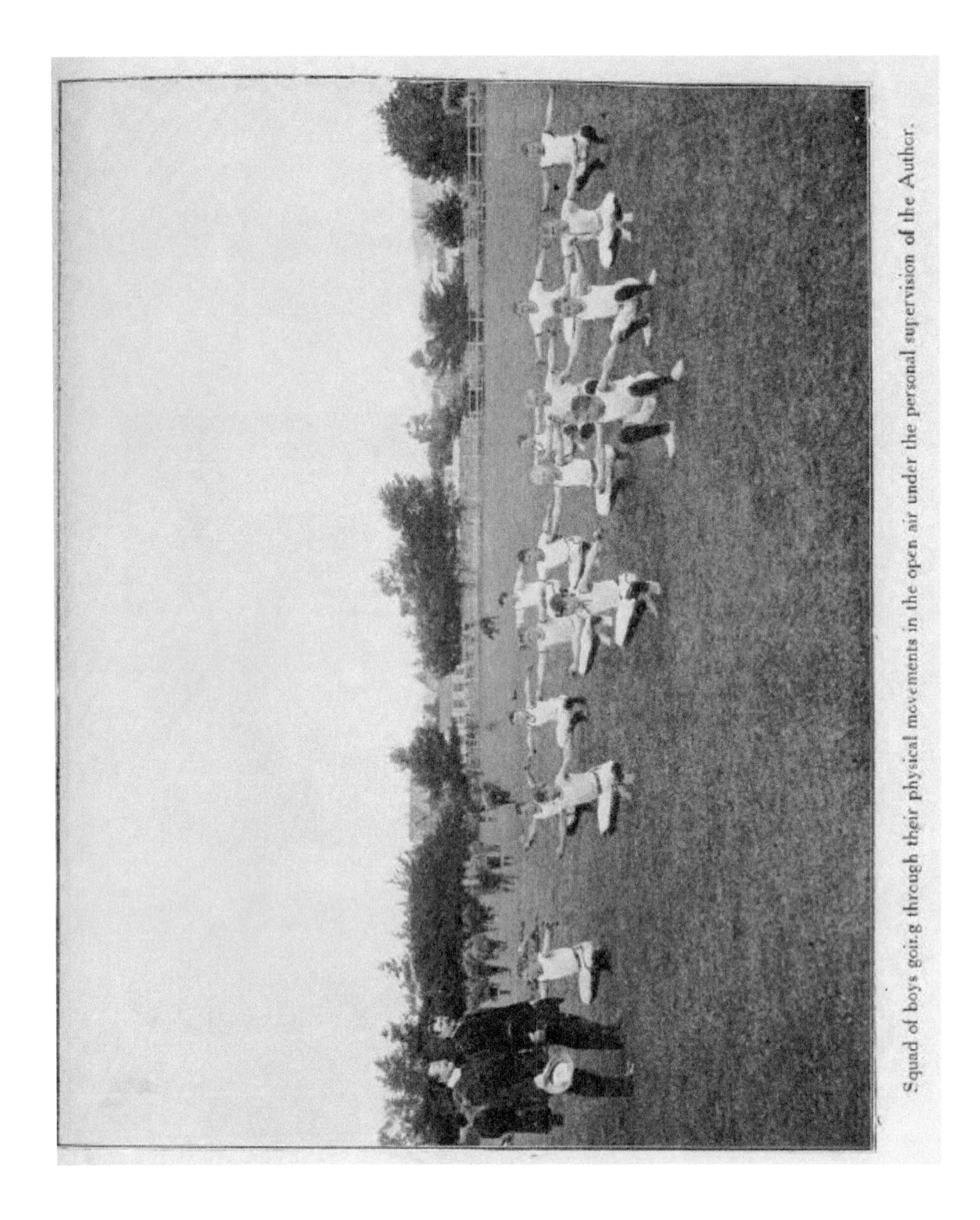

Squad of boys going through their physical movements in the open air under the personal supervision of the Author.

Photographers, Allison, Belfast.

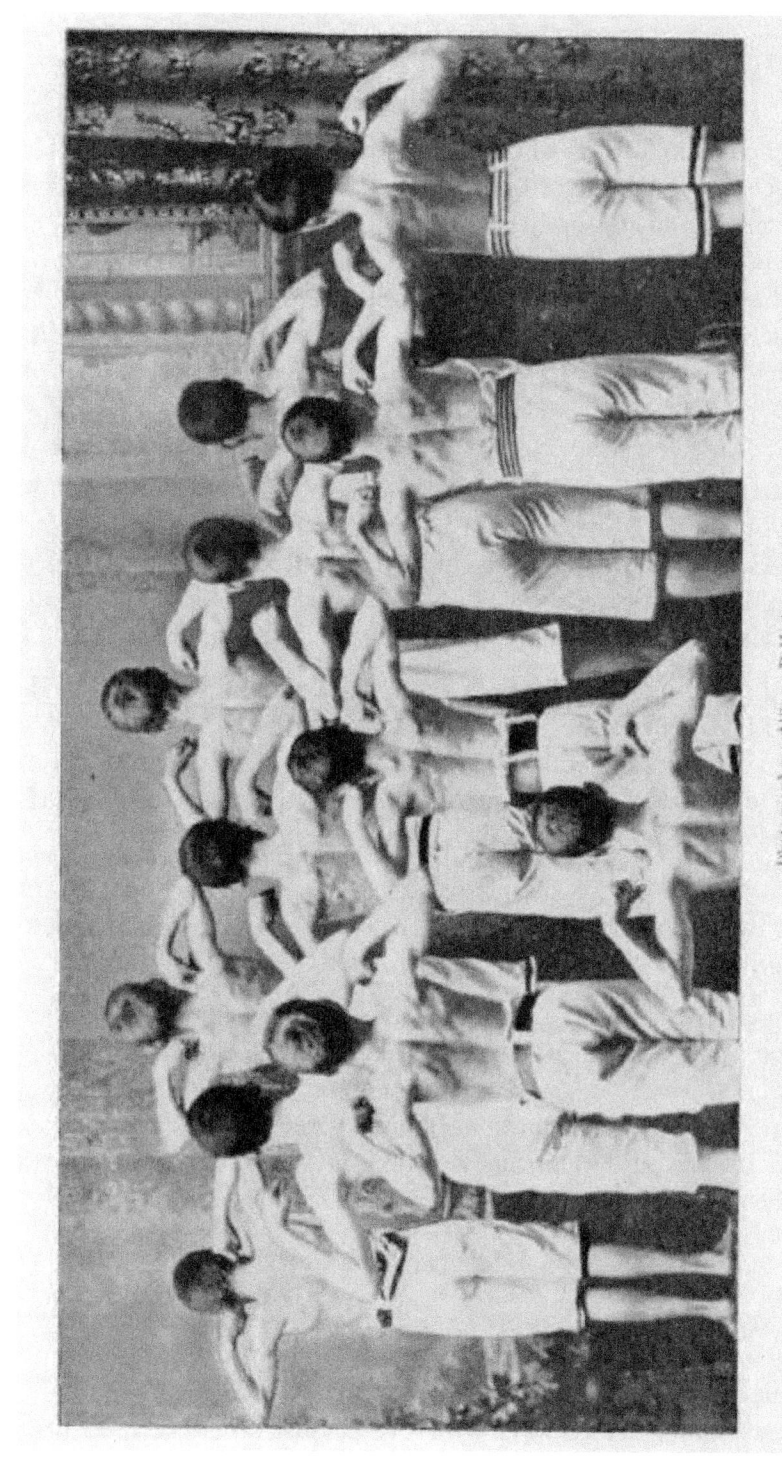

Group of boys, trained by this scientific method, showing good back development.

CHAPTER V.

The Physical Basis of all Reform.

MANY educational schemes and plans of reconstruction and social reform are already in the air and some actually in being, but the majority of these educationalists seem to forget that it is only upon the sound physical basis of the individuals comprising the nation that all educational and social reform can be built wisely and securely. The child is, then, to a nation the figure 1 in every calculation which we have to make, and it is to the physical body of the individual child that we must ultimately look in our search for all educational and social reform, and in our unending war against what is unhygienic and disease tending in civilisation.

BUILDING THE HOME OF THE SOUL.

The prudent architect or builder, when designing and erecting a building, takes into consideration every possible and probable contingency that may threaten to encompass its destruction. Its foundations are dug deep, it is safe-guarded against atmospheric changes and variations as far as is humanly possible, and it is built so as to ensure the comfort in every way of those who occupy it. Ample provision is made for light, heat, ventilation and sanitation.

So with the human bodily dwelling—" a house not made with hands "—designed and created by the great Architect and Engineer of the Universe. It was planned and erected to withstand every reasonable strain, to give the utmost comfort to the spirit and soul that must dwell within it, and with vigilance, skilful attention and respectful care it will only crumble away after many years and vicissitudes through sheer old age and " the corroding cares of Time."

When reformers of all kinds realise the dominating -fact that 'physical re-formation is the essential prelude to every other kind of reformation, they will have found a better jumping-off platform than the majority of them seem to have at present.

The utmost we can hope to do in improving the conditions attaching to modern civilisation or in modifying them will be useless, if we continue to neglect the physical body, and especially those of the children. I have no desire to decry the well-intended efforts of those who are devoting so much attention to domestic hygiene, sanitation, housing, and all other sociological, medical and humanising processes, but I would again insist on the fact that they are subsidiary to, and can only be auxiliary to, the physical education and culture of the human body itself.

GOOD HOUSES AND GOOD TENANTS.

Modern environment may, of course, be so modified as to reduce enormously the amount of disease and its vicious incidentals, and in this way many of the proposed innovations will help to diminish disease, crime and vice, as is being proved daily by the results already obtained from beneficent housing schemes, " welfare work If in large industrial concerns, advances in medical science and bacteriology, and the complete excision of many of the unhygienic surroundings of human life in large cities and towns to-day, but nothing that does not first make the human body itself a tower of strength, physically and mentally, will lead to the permanent reform and reconstruction of a nation.

The vital fact is too often forgotten, viz., that the logical first step is to devote attention to the bodily building itself (including the brain, for as Montaigne says, " it is not a mind, not a body we have to educate, it is a man of whom we are not to make two beings "), which must be made strong enough to combat an unhygienic environment at least for a time. . Our present educational methods seem to waste a lot of time and money on the steeple and roof and walls of the bodily building that might with much better results be devoted to the floors and the physical foundation.

Such methods in early and impressionable childhood, when mind and body are both alike unshaped and impressionable, can only succeed in preparing physical houses that are not likely to long retain very desirable tenants. For, one cannot expect the spirit to live and thrive in an unclean, unhealthy or diseased body. And this the body must sooner or later become unless the spiritual being who inhabits it pays at least as much attention to it as he does to his house of bricks and mortar. A house with broken windows, bad drainage, dangerously damp and dirty would not invite nor long retain desirable tenants, but a handsome, strong sanitary and comfortable dwelling-house will be found occupied by tenants who will zealously watch over it because they take a sincere and honest pride in it.

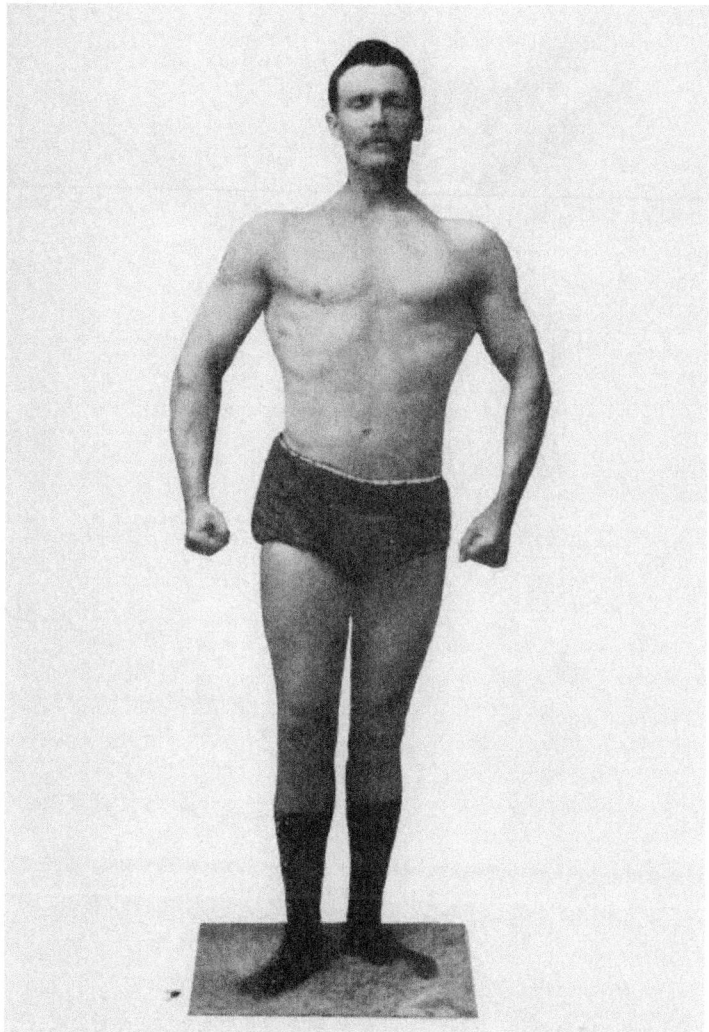

The human body in all its pristine glory, as it was intended to be, and was until man fell from his high estate by neglecting the law of life—the law of movement.

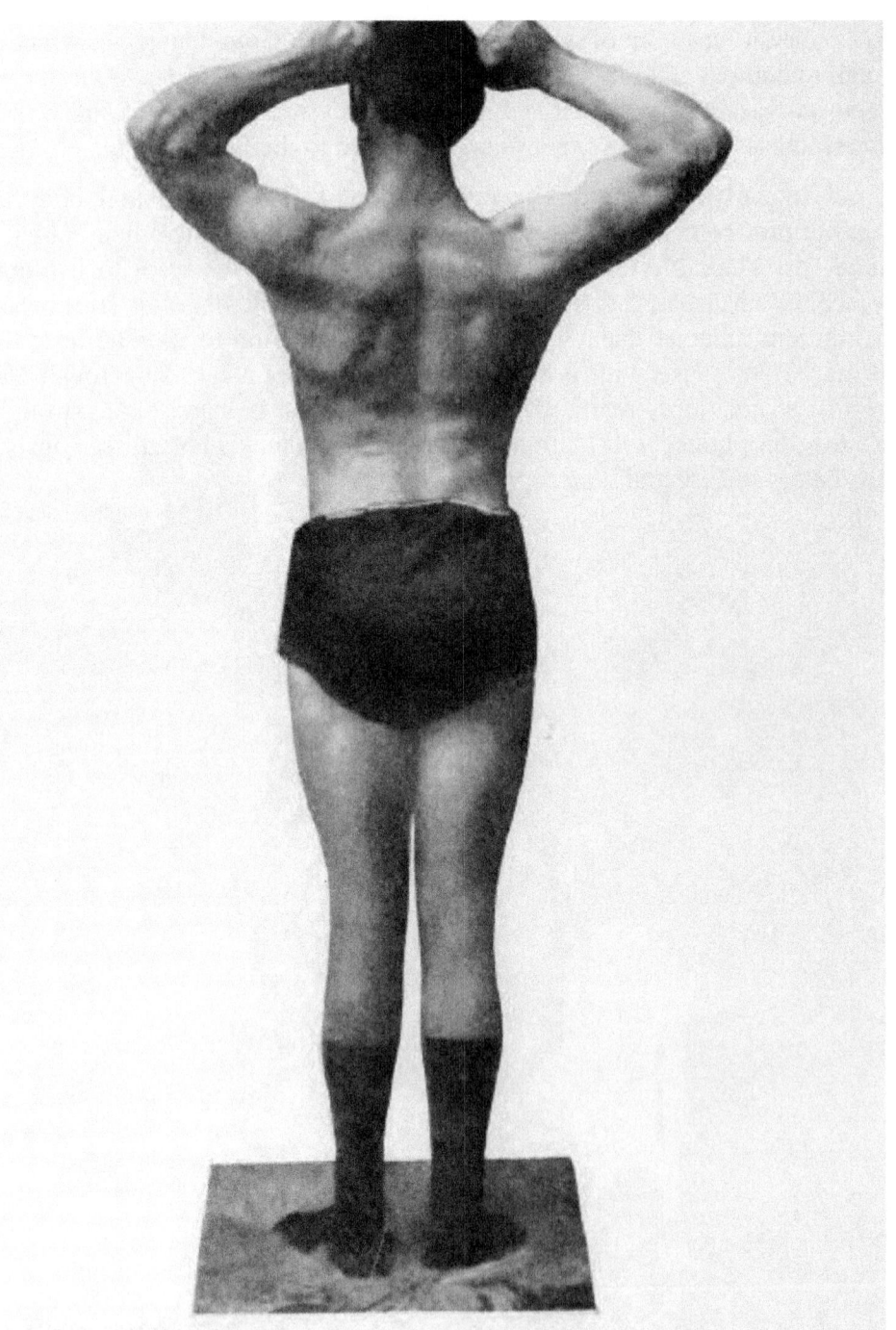

Back view of the same man, Mr. Jas. Browning, of Beaconsfield, who attributes this fine physique to the methods of body culture described in this book.

HOW WE GET OUR UNFIT.

We have now had for many years a system of education for children that has begun and still begins at the wrong end. Indeed, education, as we know it to-day, has for centuries been steadily sapping and undermining the body's physical foundation, by imposing mental strains for which the physical foundation of the bodily building had not been previously prepared. Civilisation has been ably seconded by Education in the spread of Disease. All mental work, it must never be forgotten, imposes a great strain on the physical body, and in hard study as much as from 50 to 75 per cent, of the student's vital energy may be consumed.

To replenish this, as I show in a later chapter, greater and better balanced physical movement is absolutely essential, especially in the younger children, to improve nutrition, quicken circulation and increase the oxygenation of the blood, excrete waste products, re-build better tissue, and to increase and develop the cell-population of both the body and brain. Indeed, the first steeps of all education should be 'physiological and physical rather than merely mental.

IGNORANCE AND DISEASE.

Mismanagement, especially educational mismanagement, was largely responsible for our physical decadence in the past. Our methods, or, perhaps, I should say, our lack of method, bred physical unfitness and disease. Speaking of the appalling recruiting statistics already referred to, Mr Lloyd George, in another rousing speech before the General Election, said: " On examining these statistics I was appalled to find—examining them purely for military purposes and not for any ulterior motive—that there was a much higher percentage of physical unfits in this country than in France, Germany, or any other great belligerent country. That is a disgrace to a proud and prosperous country! It is not through poverty. We were the richest country under the sun. Not through poverty, but through mismanagement! " And largely, I say, through educational mismanagement.

The country that seeks to avoid producing a race of degenerates in the future, poorer even in physique and health than the present, and devoid of the physical, mental and moral stamina, which will be necessary in every people who do not wish to sink into an obsolence like that of ancient Rome or proud and once peerless Greece, must " scrap " these mistaken and injurious educational methods, and inaugurate a new era.

Under the patronage of the State, as I have just pointed out in my previous chapter, the medical profession should have a first charge on the children of a nation, and they will then, for the first time, have a real opportunity of erecting an impregnable barrier against disease. When we have such a system of education in being, it will be worthwhile devoting more and more attention to educating the people in all the requirements of (1) a healthy body, and (2) a sound and sane mind. Such education will lead to social changes that are regarded to-day as mere Utopian dreams.

We have come, as the representative of Truth, the well-known and highly critical weekly paper, said some years ago, " to associate puniness of physical development, sloping shoulders, bowed backs, be-spectacled eyes, with the votaries of science and education," whereas our aim should be to avoid this disharmonious combination, and to teach the child to strive after the old Greek idea. In this way, every child should leave school with, at least, everything possible in its favour of growing up to be a healthy, fit and useful citizen, and with a mind so attuned to health and sanity as to be incapable of tolerating or even harbouring unclean, vicious or evil thoughts.

Perhaps the greatest and most weighty argument I can bring in favour of a compulsory elementary education in human anatomy, physiology, and hygiene, and the compulsory physical culture of the body, is to be adduced from the fact that lack of this very knowledge is, as I have already noted in the preceding chapter, one of the most fertile causes of physical deterioration and disease, and, I may add, is also responsible for much of the indifference, the neglect, the abuse, and the ill-treatment of the body, the unhygienic dwellings of the people, the insanitary and ill-ventilated workshops, etc., which still further reduce the already diminished power of bodily resistance in the people in their present physical condition, and make the body more accessible to disease, and its undesirable allies, and which are often the cause, of serious illnesses that may not make their appearance until comparatively late in life.

Photographer, Dorasawmy, Bangalore.

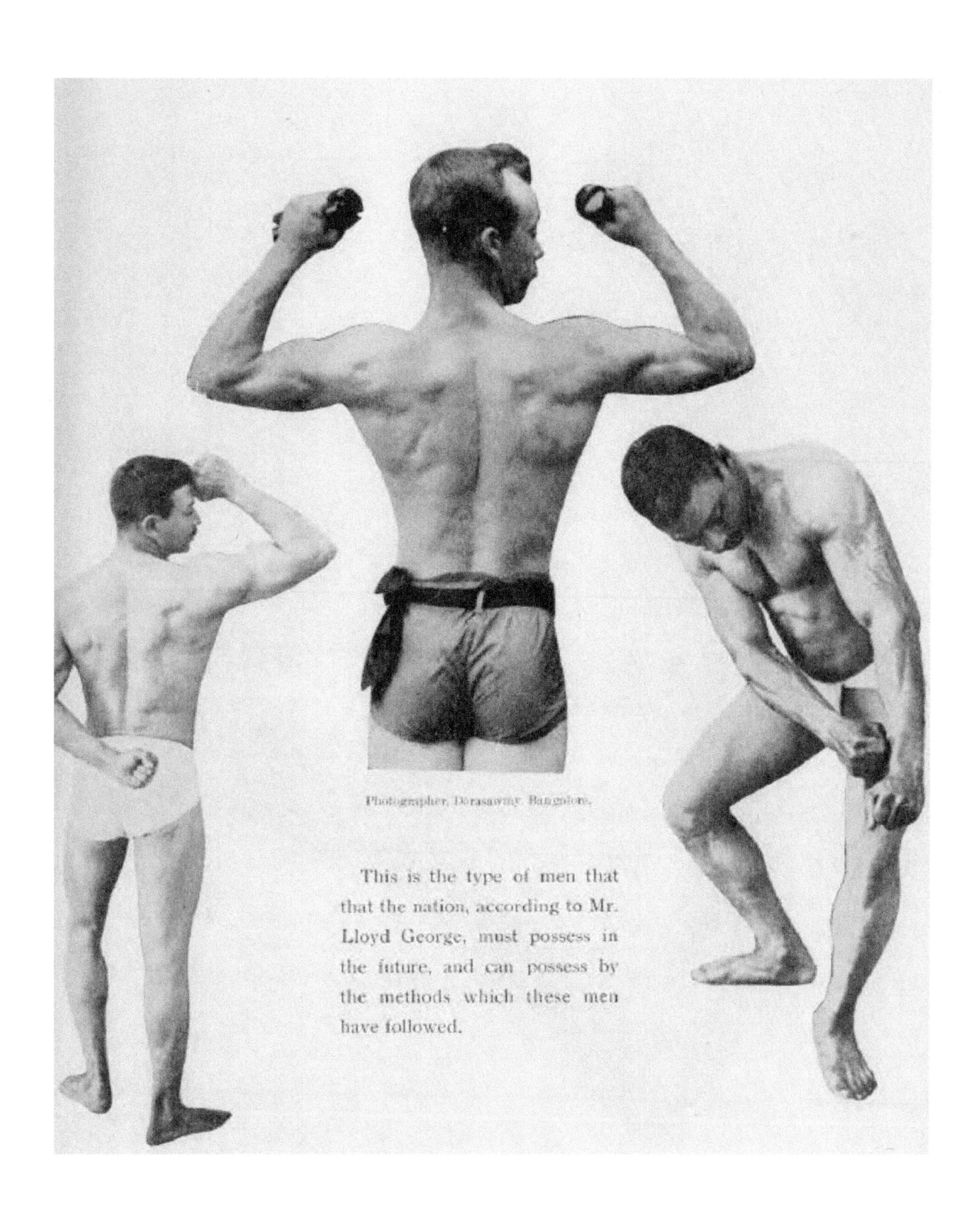

This is the type of men that that the nation, according to Mr. Lloyd George, must possess in the future, and can possess by the methods which these men have followed.

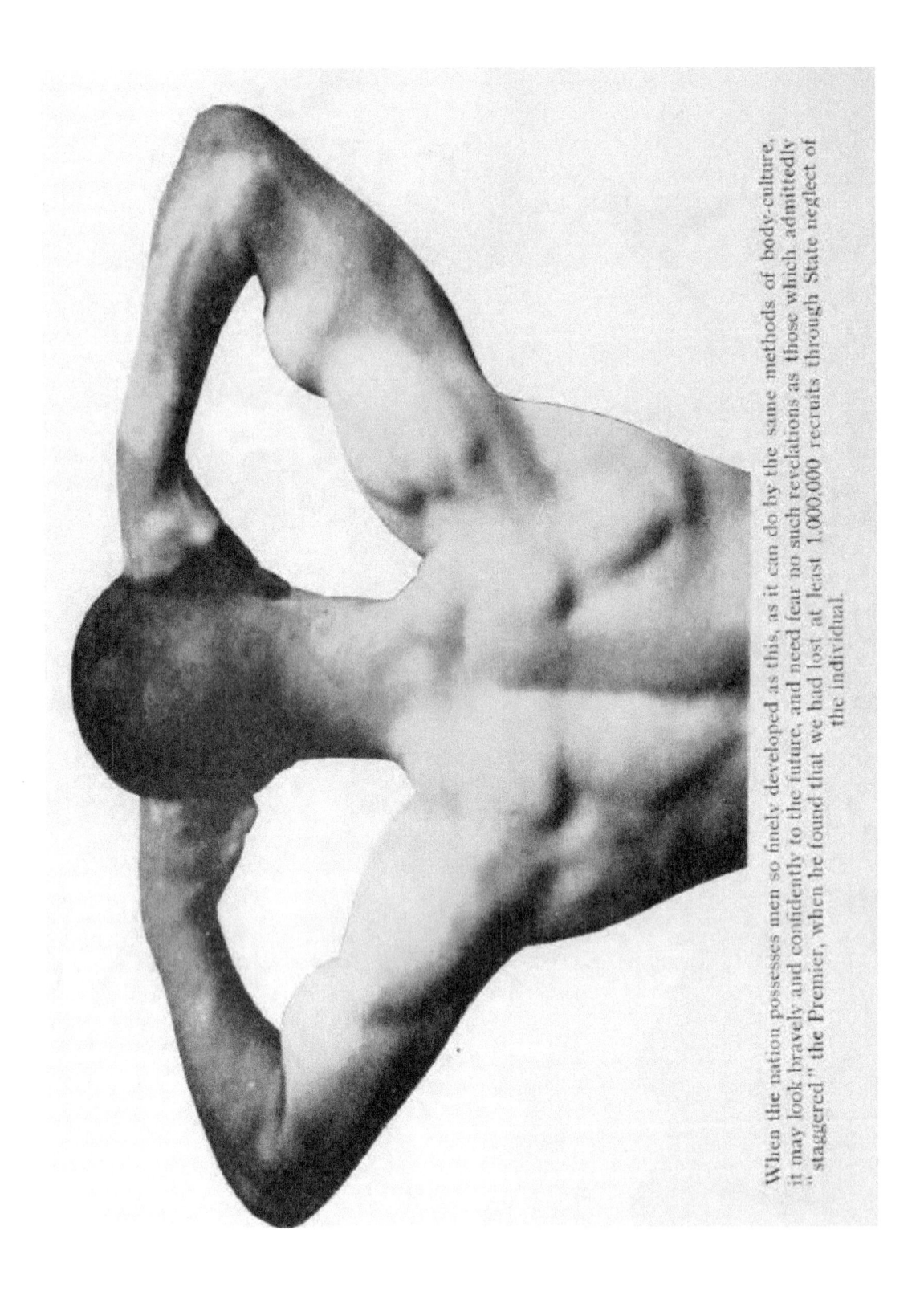

When the nation possesses men so finely developed as this, as it can do by the same methods of body-culture, it may look bravely and confidently to the future, and need fear no such revelations as those which admittedly "staggered" the Premier, when he found that we had lost at least 1,000,000 recruits through State neglect of the individual.

REDUCING THE NATIONAL HEALTH DEBT.

Every student of social reform knows how huge a part of the pauperism, insanity, vice and crime of every country can be proved by statistics to be due directly or indirectly to the sickness or disease that is so prevalent to-day. To what extent also this avoidable, and, in any really educated people, culpable, ignorance is responsible for those thousand-and-one familiar ailments which a French writer has called " the frontiers of disease," ailments arising from defective or retarded nutrition, ailments due to the generation of toxins within the body, and numerous ailments of an everyday kind arising mostly from imperfect metabolism, which, although but slight deviations from the normal, constitute no small item in the annual " hospital bill " of every nation to-day, and are the great despoilers of every nation's individual and national efficiency, only medical men are in a position to know.

The physical renaissance that I am now suggesting would erase most of them altogether from society, and the vice, immorality and crime that spring from them, because the knowledge of the body and its functions would prevent many of those " crimes of ignorance " which give birth to, invite, tolerate, foster and encourage so much disease, with its undesirable accompaniments. Such early education, too, would destroy much of the falsehood, hypocrisy and ignorance with regard to sexual relations and the reproduction of the species that are also a prolific cause of disease, immorality and vice, with their pernicious and degenerative influence on the future of any people.

No one who is acquainted with the trend of medical opinion to-day can fail to observe how sadly the " personal equation " in the whole problem of social reform is either overlooked or forgotten in the consideration of all questions of reform. We hear far too much of bad housing, of milk and meat as factors of disease, and of a thousand-and-one other questions that are but mere tributaries of the great stream which has its source and origin in the uneducated, undisciplined, uncontrolled physical body itself, in the ignorance inseparable from educational methods that do not even teach children a rudimentary knowledge of their own bodies or how to care for them, and even of the necessity of caring for them.

Such children have neither the parentage, the education, or the physical culture desirable to enable them to safeguard their health even if lodged in a palace, with all the hygienic appurtenances of modern medical science and surrounded by every protective device of civilisation. Their liability to disease would still persist. Its advent might be postponed, but that is the best for which we might hope.

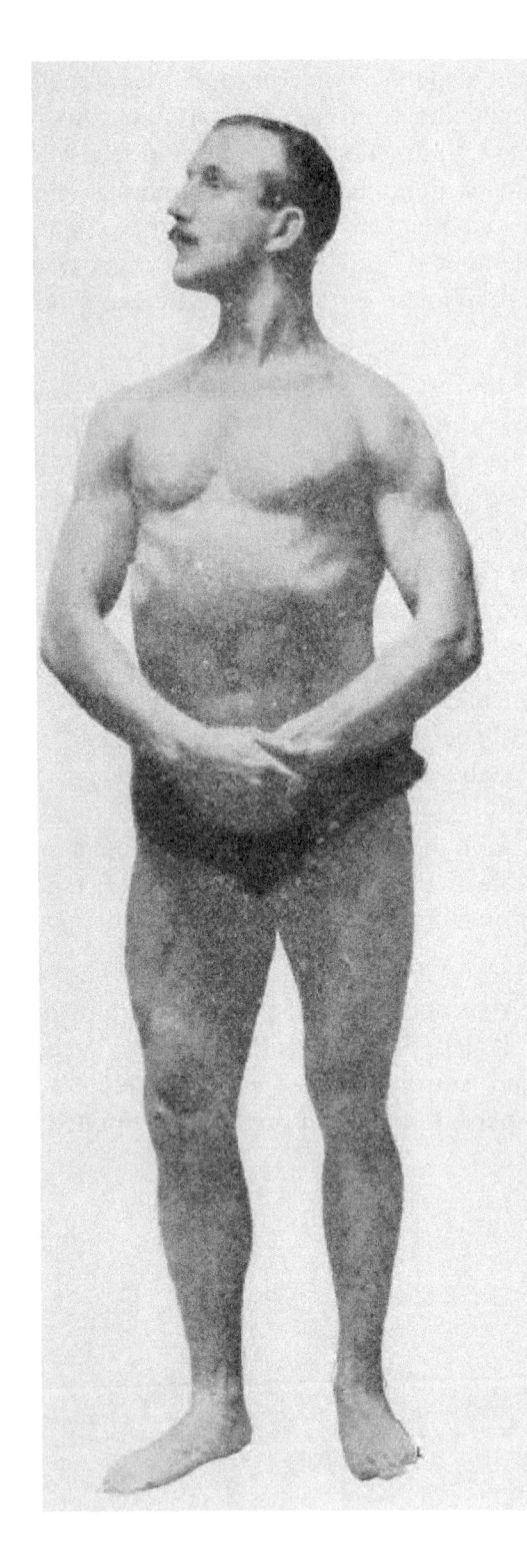

Winner of the Gold Statuette of the Author, presented by him to encourage the physical regeneration and reconstruction of the nation, and for which thousands of competitors entered from every part of the British Isles.

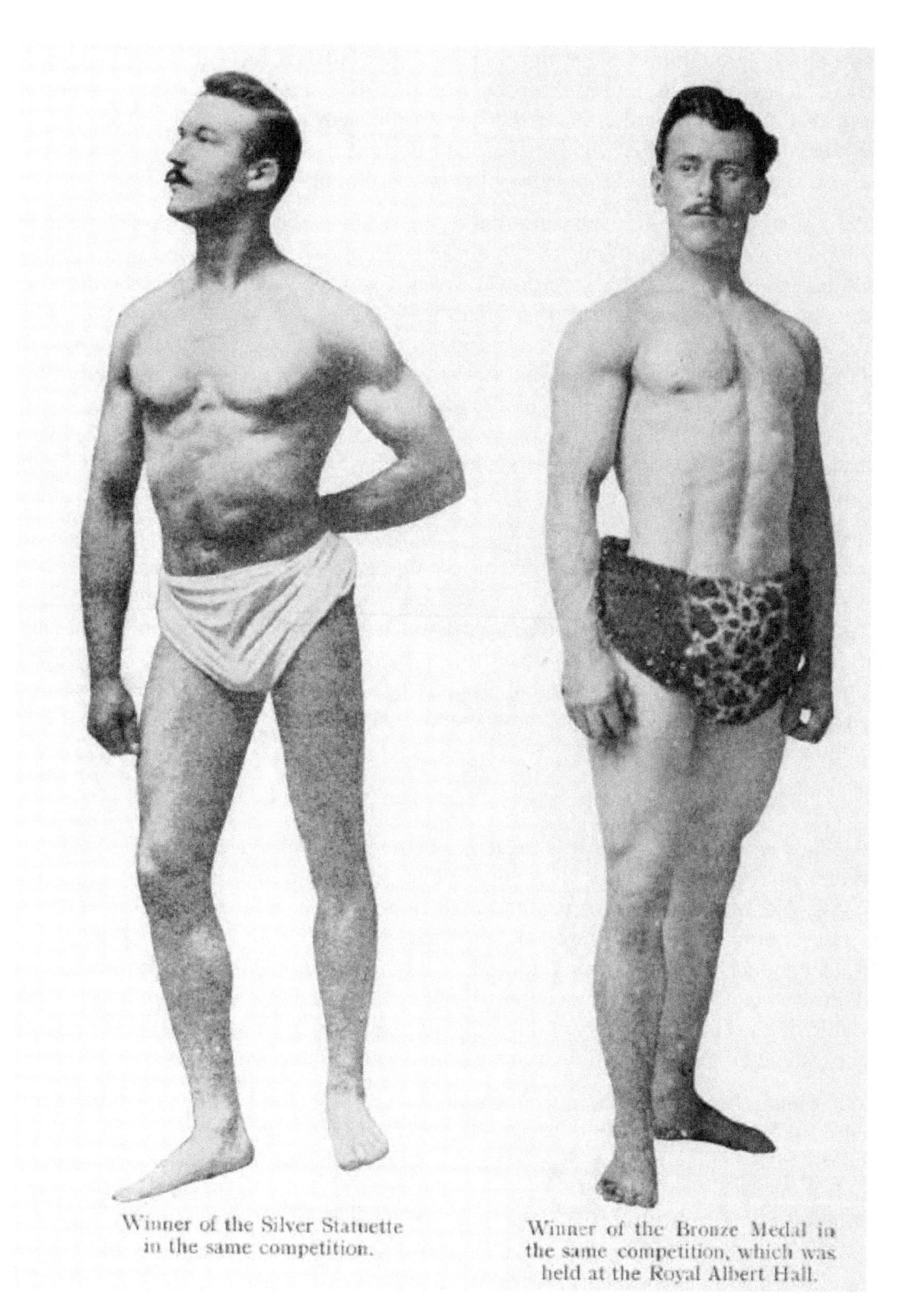

Winner of the Silver Statuette in the same competition.

Winner of the Bronze Medal in the same competition, which was held at the Royal Albert Hall.

GARDENING THE PHYSICAL PLANT.

All national reform, therefore, must begin in the physical education and training of the children just as disease can only be eradicated in the cells of the individual. Gardening of the most skilful kind may help the growth of a plant, but it cannot grow a beautiful and flourishing tree from a plant that is diseased or unsound at the root. And morality, temperance, virtue, sanity of mind, everything that the social gardeners of the human plant are anxious to cultivate to add to its health and beauty depend upon whether the plant itself is healthy and strong at the very root of its being. A diseased or unsound root cannot but produce poor foliage.

The welfare of the nation is only the sum total of the welfare of its individuals. These individuals, like the individual living cells of our own bodies, determine the health, happiness and wellbeing of the whole, and the truest and best reform is to teach and train each individual child to grow up so healthy, strong and sound in itself that it can neither succumb to internal weakness or innate constitutional tendency or even to its environment. It is not pathological but physiological reform that is required, for to reform a nation that is already mentally, morally or physically diseased is a much more difficult and costly thing than to teach and train the individual children that are the living cells of the national body and to make and keep them immune from such disease. Health, after all, is cheaper than disease, no matter what may be the cost of its maintenance and preservation.

Many of the conditions of modern life that are so badly in need of reform, and others with which we could easily and well dispense altogether, would cease to exist automatically as the natural result of such a system of physical education and training as I suggest for the people. Ignorance, indeed, is the only excuse for the presence of much that is undesirable in the social life of humanity to-day. A thing at once so beautiful, so complex, so strong, so wonderful in all its forms, operations and activities as the human body is a thing to create reverence and awe in the mind of any individual who learns to know it and understand it. Only a vandal would willingly despoil, injure or destroy it.

THE ROAD TO SELF-RESPECT.

And it depends entirely upon how it is treated, whether your body becomes your best friend and the promoter of your happiness or an enemy to cause you pain and discomfort, for disease and pain are only Nature's revenge for neglect or ill-treatment. To ill-treat it or to neglect it is not only to make one a danger to oneself but to society at large, and given a proper educational system such conduct should be made criminal, as ignorance of the law could not then be pleaded. An individual who, after such an education, allows himself to become reduced in economic value by avoidable disease inflicts a loss not only upon himself but upon society. It is then the business and duty of society to protect itself against such ignorance or negligence.

On the other hand the adult schooled from childhood to health and health habits will increase and go on increasing in value not only to himself but to the community of which he is a member. His moral worth to a nation will be even greater, because the inculcation of self-respect in the individuals that comprise the social fabric must ensure the quality of its fibre and texture. For, in the worldly-wise advice of Polonius to Laertes, " to thine ownself be true and it must follow as the night the day thou canst not then be false to any man." Self-respect is the beginning of respect and consideration for others, and wins the respect of others in return. The triple duty of the individual to his Creator, to the State and to society in general is at once performed in the mere act of doing his duty to himself.

But he must be taught that duty, and all it implies, from days of childhood, before he can be expected to do it, and to achieve this the teaching and training must be scientific and even pre-natal. His education must begin in the womb. It will only end when he dies. Through life it will be his supreme happiness to keep his body healthy and well, and with such a body it will always be easier to resist the encroachments of disease, vice and all such like. There is no wine that will exhilarate like health, to be followed by no re-action, for it gives exhilaration without intoxication.

The spirit or soul that occupies a bodily dwelling filled with the divine music of health makes a little heaven on earth within its own body. Vicious cravings, passions and tendencies cannot tarry long there. This is real re-formation, the physical re-formation and re-education of man, from which all social reformation must spring.

RICH IN MIND AND BODY.

True reformation takes place in the mental attitude of the individual, for conduct is determined not by extraneous matters so much as by a person's mental attitude towards himself, towards others and towards his Creator. That is the keynote of character and conduct. As a man sows mentally so he will reap. And though " 'tis the mind that makes the body rich," yet the physical body is the soil through the cultivation of which we must supply all the essentials for the sustenance of the mental tree, branches, leaves, and flower. Where are we most likely to find goodness, kindness, charity and love—in the mind nourished, sustained and fortified by a healthy and vigorously functioned body or in a mind diseased, tainted and deformed by the self-generated poisons of an unhealthy, stunted, ill-formed, or weakly functioned body?

To restore the human body to its pristine vigour and splendour, to make it superbly powerful to resist disease, and to make it even disease immune are the steps by which we will advance to a higher mental and moral as well as physical standard, and I am going to show now that this can only be done by a return, so far as in humanly possible in these times'., to the natural life, and especially to that all-round and balanced movement which the physical body was designed to have from the first and which sufficed for health and freedom from disease in those far-off days " when Adam delved and Eve span."

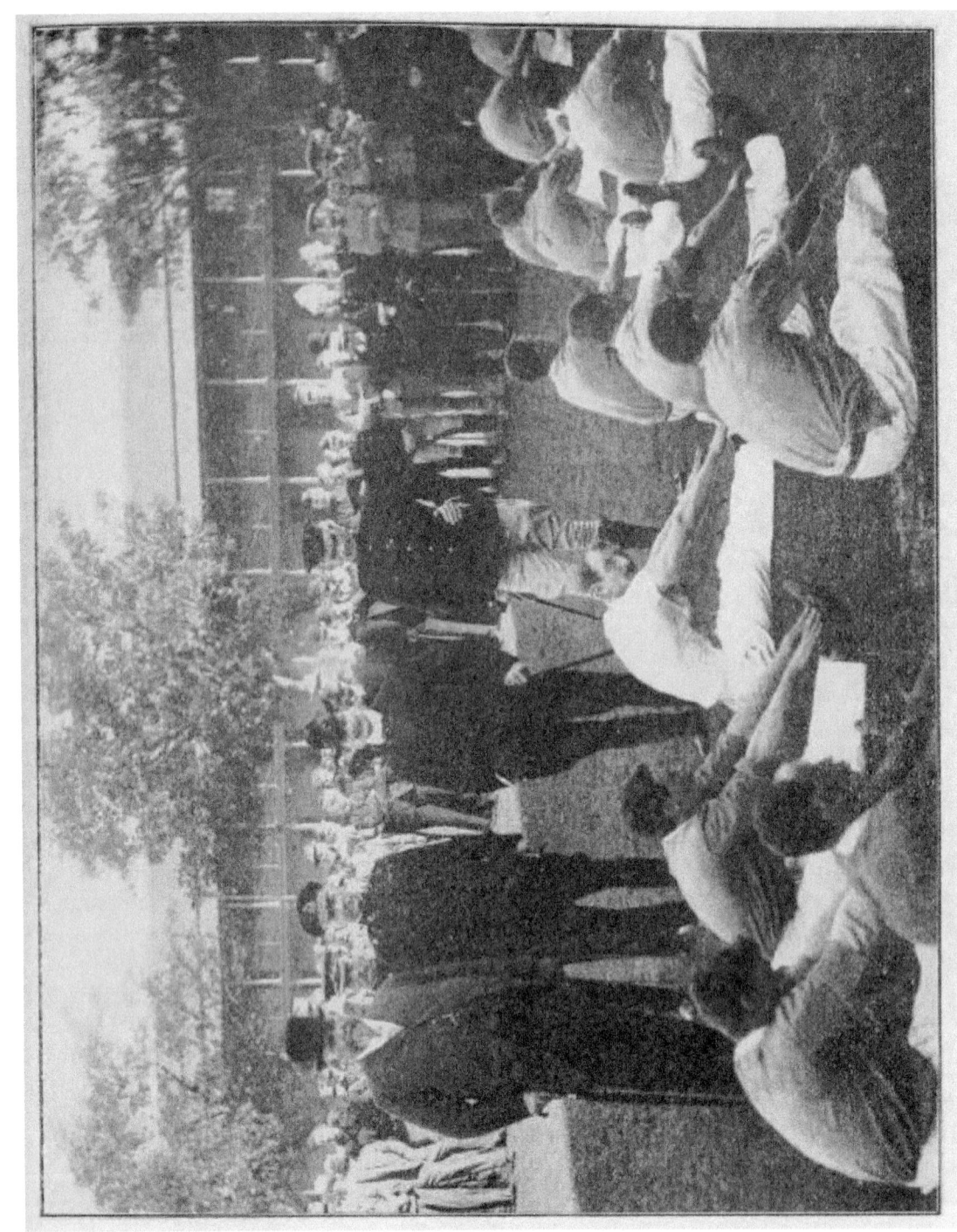

The Author inspecting a squad of Colonial soldiers carrying out physical movements on the lines described in this book.

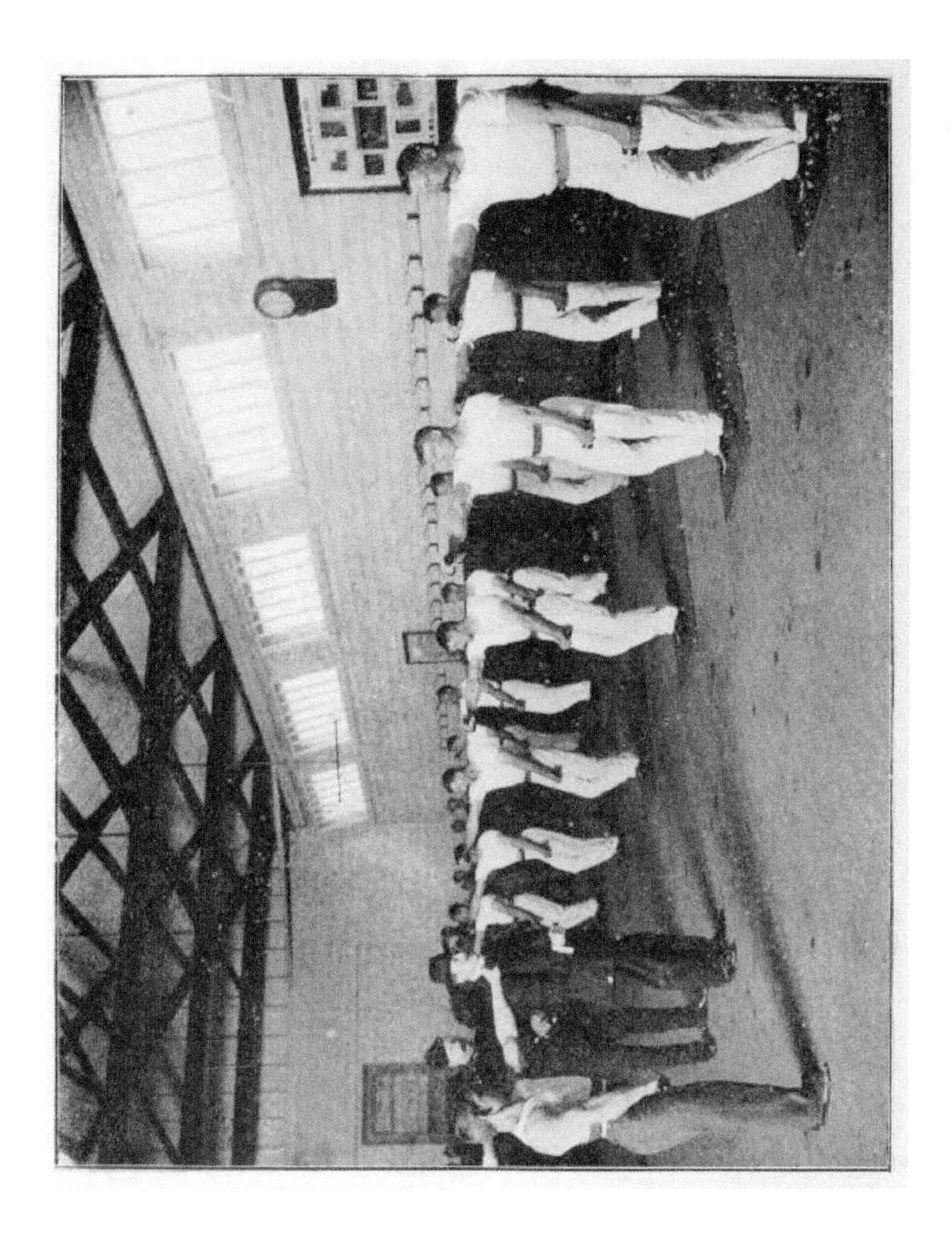

CHAPTER VI.

Life is Movement.

LIFE is movement. Movement—self-movement—is life. The fundamental phenomenon of all organic life is change of form (or movement), sometimes so slight as even to evade the microscope. Breathing, the beating of the heart, and the circulation of the blood —the three witnesses of life—are also witnesses of movement.

Life is of two kinds, animal and vegetable, and for both, movement is essential. Indeed, both animals and vegetables may be said to live by movement. Food is the fuel that supplies the motive power, the plant receiving its motive power and sustenance direct from the earth itself, the power that enables it to grow upwards even in defiance of the law of gravitation.

MAN WAS MADE TO MOVE.

Man was ordained to wrest his food from the earth by his own muscular power, and his muscular system was given him for that purpose, and also partly to convert his food into motive power by digestion and assimilation. Human life begins in the womb in some mysterious way by movement, the first throbbing of a child's heart—like a clock of which the mainspring is wound up by Divine power—announcing the advent of Life, the child afterwards keeping the clock going itself by using its own muscular system as the key. It is as if the Creator wound up the clock of Life and handed us the key in the shape of a muscular system, which has been given us for re-winding it again from time to time, so as to keep the " works " of life going smoothly, and enable the " clock " to show correct time throughout life.

The main, indeed, I may say the only, difference between living activities, visible or invisible, through which their life is expressed —nutrition, growth, function, reproduction and decay. All organised and living things grow by their own movement from within. This is characteristic not only of man or any animal, but of every living thing in general down to the earliest known form of life, which consists only of a single cell. And man, as we know him to-day, is but a bundle of cells, every organ, system, and tissue of the body being built up of living cells.

Before, however, we begin to study movement as modifying the life and health of man, let us stand in wonder when we regard movement as the fundamental law of life, animal and vegetable, the energising and governing power, as shown alike in the minutest speck of living matter as well as in the great world of systems in the firmament.

The proofs are to be found everywhere in the Universe, on land and on sea and in the air, and if we ourselves had long ago more fully realised that life is movement, that civilisation was gradually robbing us of the natural physical movement of other days, and that lack of movement in whole or in part inevitably leads to disease and death, we would not, perhaps, have so long neglected physical movement as an agent—perhaps the greatest agent—in maintaining life.

A UNIVERSE IN MOVEMENT.

Everywhere we live in the midst of movement. " Nothing," as Professor Carl Snyder says in his great work, " New Conceptions," " is at rest." There are worlds in the great firmament above that are continuously moving at speeds scarcely credible to the finite mind of man. Away up there, the invisible wind is never at rest, but whirls, speeds and performs evolutions more wonderful than anything known of on the land or in the sea.

High up above the Andes where the great condor soars, swarms of minute insects, invisible to the eye, are also carried about by the moving wind in contradistinction to the soaring eagle, whose own innate power of movement enables him to contend with and against the wind and to steer his masterly course through the air by the power and control of his own muscular and mighty wings. Movement everywhere in every element of the great Universe is essential to life. On the moon, where no evidence of life has yet been revealed by the minutest telescopic scrutiny, there is death like lack of movement in the absence of that moving sea of air and water which alone makes life possible.

On the earth the same principle exists, viz., that there is and can be no life without movement. The great rivers that " rive " the country move along fastly speeding to the sea, and so remain pure and sweet, supporting a myriad forms of life, while the sluggishly moving streams become contaminated with fermenting and poisonous matter, and are uncongenial to life. Pools, having no natural movement whatever, breed all sorts of poisonous and pestilential vapours, and foster the germs of disease. The stillness of the pool is the stillness of death. The fast moving river and the stagnant pool are two of the most striking contrasts of movement with life and stagnation with death that Nature affords. Not only are the pools dead and full of death, but they would spread death all around them if every moving current of the air did not quickly purify and dissipate the pestilent vapours and poisonous gases that arise from them.

Similarly with the land and the vegetable life of the land. The land must be moved and kept moving if the life in the seed is to become fruit, vegetable, or flower. Movement brings the land into touch with the sun, air and rain, and makes it fruitful. Left to itself and unmoved by plough, spade and harrow, it degenerates and becomes arid and sterile.

THE REAL POETRY OF MOTION.

The sea, in its perpetual and rhythmic ebb and flow, would be little more than a big cesspool filling the atmosphere with poisonous filth if it ceased to move. Life on sea and land alike would, indeed, become equally unendurable without the unceasing movement of sea and air' As it is, we bring our infirm and invalid, on the other hand, to the verge of the moving sea, or transport them for long voyages on its bosom, so that they may fill their lungs with the life- giving ozone which permeates the atmosphere above and around it. Not only is the sea a great and ever-moving mass of water containing essential life elements in itself, but it teems with an ever-moving life, a strange, unseen or rarely seen, and comparatively unknown life, so fitted and adapted to its watery environment that it can live without coming in direct contact with man's first,, last, and most vital necessity, air.

Through the whole animal world, in every element the essence of life is movement—and in all animal life movement is made by muscular power—and it is because the animals, apart from man, have been able to adhere to the law of natural physical movement more closely and continuously than man that they are consequently kept in better physical condition than him, and are less liable to disease, even when degenerated through contact with civilisation and the diminished necessity for movement.

Look at them even when held in captivity by man. What is more graceful, more truly " the poetry of motion " than the elastic tread of some lordly lion or tiger, the stealthy, measured stride of the wolf or the leopard, or the sprightly antics of the nimble and ever-active lemurs. Compared with this, the movements of most men to-day seem awkward, unnatural, and ungraceful.

The very restlessness of these animals in their cages, " cabin'd, cribb'd, confin'd," their powerful muscles rhythmically undulating beneath the skin at every step, shows the deep natural instinct implanted in what we call the " brute creation " for natural exercise and movement, the prime and primitive essentials of healthy life. In their own wild state, they never died of disease, but only through slaughter, accident, or the natural law. Why? Because they were kept disease-free, in a state of Nature, by the necessary movement and use of all their muscles, thus naturally keeping the whole organism in perfect balance, even as man himself once did.

MAN ROSE BY MOVEMENT.

All forms of life and all living organisms in the Universe, then, including man, demand movement for their very existence. They eat, breathe, digest, work, fight and have their being by movement — self-movement. " Man," says Professor W. K. Clifford, " may be described as an automaton. An automaton is a machine that goes by itself when wound up, and we go by ourselves when we have had food. There is no reason why we should not regard man as an exceedingly complicated machine which is wound up by putting food into the mouth. But the body is not merely a machine, because consciousness goes with it." And it is by the conscious movement of the voluntary muscles, as I show in another chapter, that all parts of this wonderful human automaton can be put and kept in motion, and without which, even food would be valueless.

Man rose from the primeval slime to his present conscious and erect position, his complex and altogether wonderful organism, by movement. By continuous physical processes and activities he evolved first from the jelly-like amoeba or single-celled speck of living protoplasm, and thence, by slow degrees, ever upwards to the complex multi-cellular being he is to-day, a being, truly, but a very little lower than the angels. Shakespeare—himself called "that myriad-minded man "—well and truly apostrophised this wonderful living human automaton, this self-supporting, self-propagating, self-controlling, self-propelling, self-heating, self-lubricating, self-operating and self-moving mental and physical machine, when he caused Hamlet to exclaim:—

" What a thing is Man !

How noble in reason ! How infinite In faculty! In form and moving How express and admirable !

In action how like an angel,

In apprehension how like a god."

Such was man as he was intended to be. When God created man He made the most wonderful and the most perfect thing in the world, perfect as a whole, because the human body was perfect in every part, even to the most minute and microscopic detail, and perfect in balance. There was not a weak part in it anywhere, and it was as beautiful in its design, construction and perfect balance as it was strong It was, as it should be to-day, so balanced in perfect strength everywhere that disease could make no impression upon it.

Man then was made by God in a state of perfectly balanced strength and his daily life, with its free and full physical activity, sufficed to maintain that balance. To-day, men and women after centuries of an artificial and partially inactive civilised life, are born lacking in this balance, and are, therefore, more liable to disease, from the very moment of their birth. To regain that balance which we had in primeval days is the first step in the eradication of disease, and we can only do this by returning once more to a life in which all-round physical movement is supplied to the body in a way compatible with modern habits of life. When we have restored this balance to the body, especially from childhood, ordinary games and sports will, to some extent, preserve this balance afterwards, just as the hunting and chasing of his food and the fighting of his enemies did for primitive man.

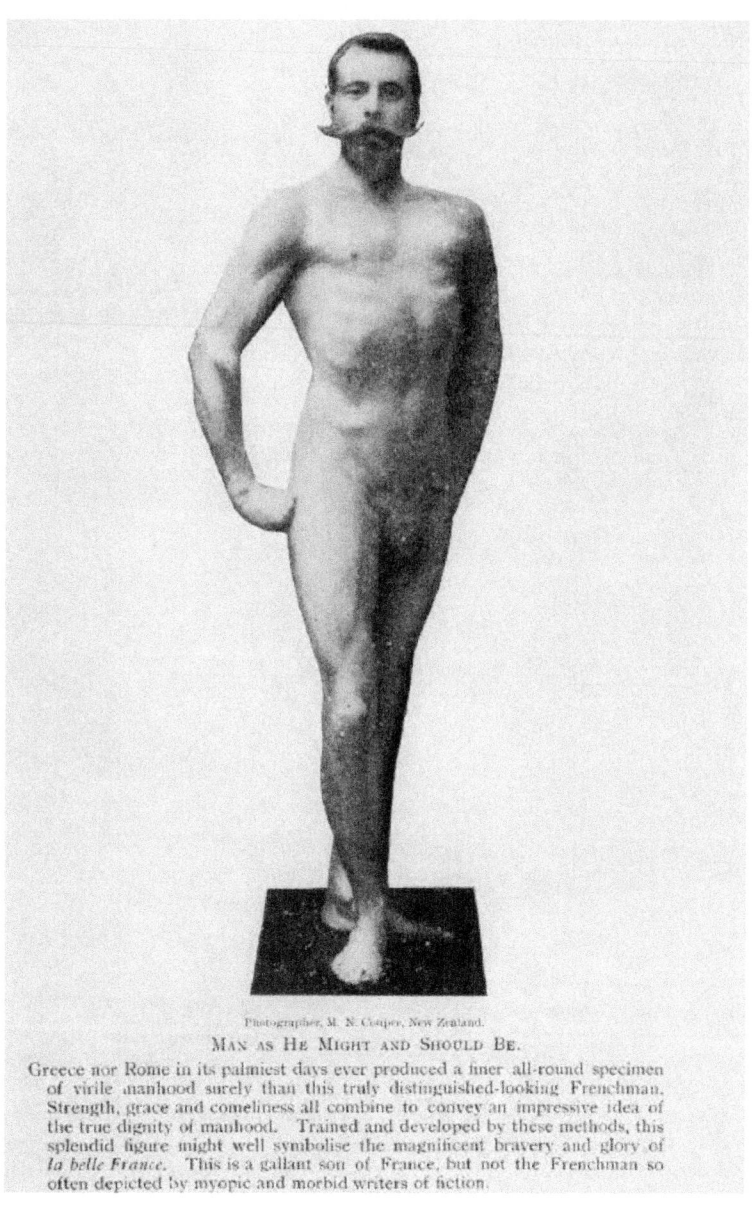

Photographer, M. N. Cooper, New Zealand.

MAN AS HE MIGHT AND SHOULD BE.

Greece nor Rome in its palmiest days ever produced a finer all-round specimen of virile manhood surely than this truly distinguished-looking Frenchman. Strength, grace and comeliness all combine to convey an impressive idea of the true dignity of manhood. Trained and developed by these methods, this splendid figure might well symbolise the magnificent bravery and glory of *la belle France*. This is a gallant son of France, but not the Frenchman so often depicted by myopic and morbid writers of fiction.

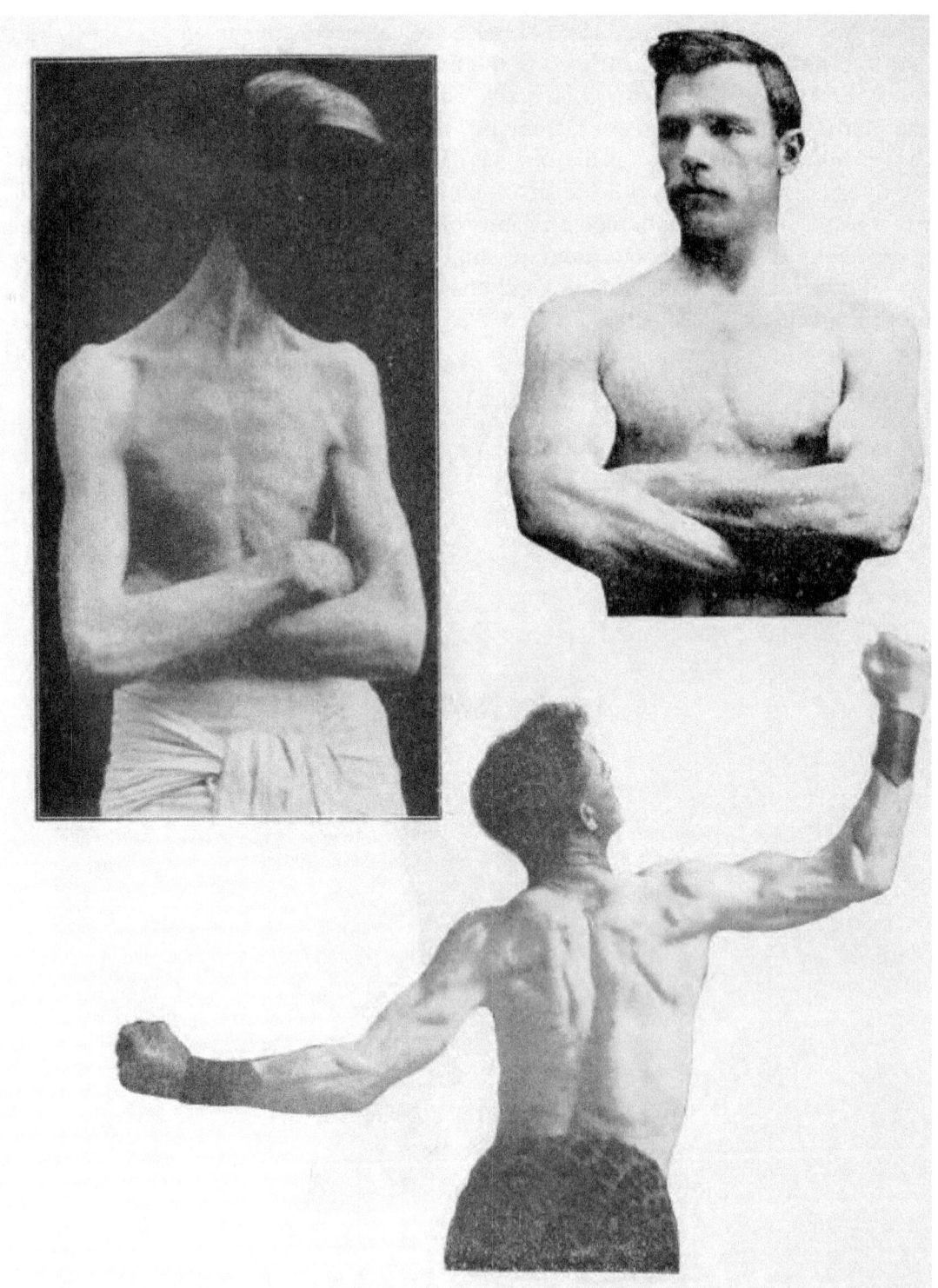

Here again, you see man as he is, and as he might be, indeed as the Creator intended he should be. The difference in physique between the pathetic figure above and the others is due to lack of scientific physical training in the one case and the application of these methods in the other two.

MAN'S WEAPONS OF DEFENCE AGAINST DISEASE.

Disease was probably co-existent with Adam, but unknown, for it could not reveal itself then because disease germs could not conquer the human body in its pristine strength, so long as it received reasonable attention and care, and that all-round physical movement which was natural and necessary in days when bodily strength and activity were absolutely essential for the provision of food and for the protection of life against fierce animals.

Man was given the possession or stewardship of a body strong enough to contend successfully against all his enemies, even what has since proved to be the greatest of all his enemies, Disease. In those early days, man was too strong and too active to succumb to disease, because each and all of his bodily cells were made and kept naturally strong enough, by daily and balanced physical movement, to resist and defeat disease. By possession of a brain and mind he was given dominion over every beast of the field and every bird of the air, and by the right use of both his body and his brain nothing could prevail against him.

At first he was compelled by Nature to use both these powerful weapons to defend himself against his enemies many and mighty. Consequently, men were giants in those days.

" The nerves that joined their limbs were firm and strong,

Their life was healthy, and their age was long,

Returning years still saw them in their prime,

They wearied e'en the wings of the measuring Time."

Gradually there dawned a more pastoral era of man's history when the peaceful tillage of the soil enabled him to live a life less strenuous, and the barter and exchange of products brought him food and clothing without the hunting and slaying of animals for himself. The days when he had to do everything by the use of his own muscles began to depart, and all-round physical movement became more and more a matter of choice rather than of necessity. Later, someone invented money, and man began to discover that money could buy almost anything without much physical effort, and that money could even make more money for him than all the work of his toiling body. So man began to neglect those wonderful muscles upon which so much depended.

Less and less physical activity now entered into his daily existence, and more and more his brain was cultivated and exploited to the neglect of the rest of his body, with the result that disease at last was able to assault him. with greater and increasingly greater prospects of success. So disease, as we know it to-day, slowly came into our everyday life with the growth of civilisation, until it has come to be regarded patiently, and even tolerantly, as an inevitable and necessary evil of modern life.

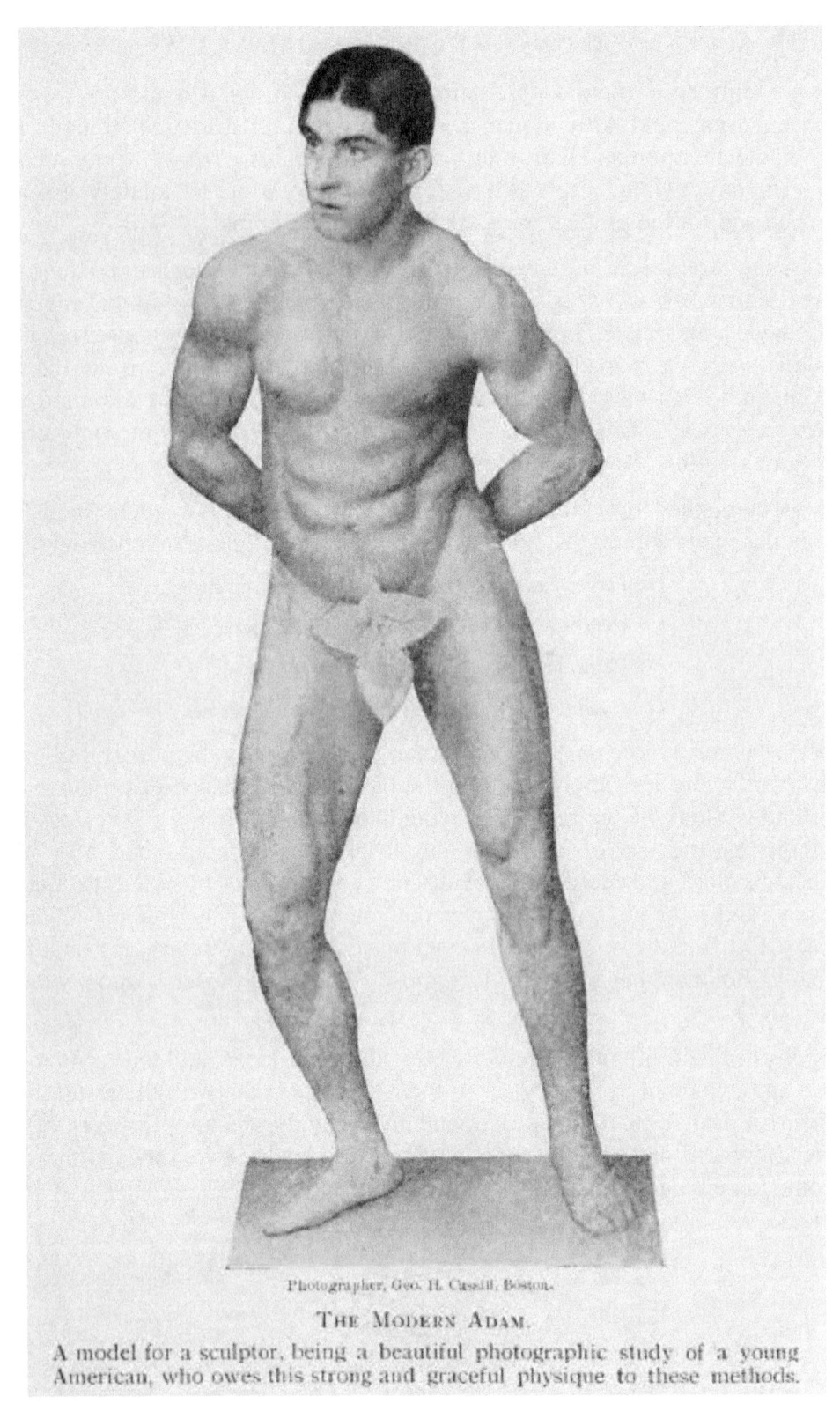

THE MODERN ADAM.
A model for a sculptor, being a beautiful photographic study of a young American, who owes this strong and graceful physique to these methods.

If we persist in this mistaken attitude towards disease, we must, with the continuing progress of civilisation, become still weaker and more diseased year after year. Man transgressed and has continued to transgress the fundamental and universal law of life, the law of movement, and thus the body was slowly but surely despoiled, to no small extent, of its own primitive weapons of offence and defence against disease, strong muscles and muscular power. Man now became like a lion stripped of its claws or a tiger without its fangs.

CLOTHES THAT CLOAK PHYSICAL SINS.

Unfortunately as civilisation advanced and education increased, man, in his search after greater ease and comfort, instead of trying once again to make his body stronger did just those very things that made it still weaker. He invented clothes to rob his skin of sun and air, he discovered the wheel and made it take the place of his nether limbs, to a great extent. He was carried forwards and backwards, upwards and downwards, instead of walking and climbing. As one humorous writer in the Daily Mail has put it, " ubiquitous cheap transport suspended our physical animation and turned us into so many bales of carted goods." Human necessity for physical movement grew still less than ever, and man grew into " the custom of shirking locomotion except on wheels." In fact, he only used his muscles and limbs when obliged to do so to earn his living or for play, which inevitably led to lack of bodily balance, physical degeneration and disease. Man had not discovered that balanced physical movement was the law of healthy life. With the inevitable loss of his primitive muscular strength and his superb natural physique and constitution he also lost his splendid immunity from disease.

Man, as the Creator intended he should appear, was a noble being, with the physique of an Apollo or a Hercules, commanding, statuesque, and awe-inspiring, like the splendid heroes of ancient Greece and Rome. Since man became a clothes-wearing animal, his body has been, like Topsy's origin, " wrapt in mystery." Civilisation and education with their ever-increasing lack of all-round physical movement, have at last sapped and undermined his physique to such a degree that to-day his clothes are often only a cloak to cover a multitude of physical sins. They are frequently so stuffed and padded that they resemble miniature " cotton plantations," the better to hide modern man's physical blemishes and shortcomings.

Handicapped as he is by the physically degenerative environment of modern civilisation, and the diminished demand for physical movement, is it to be marvelled at that disease finds in him an easy prey instead of its triumphant conqueror and master. He has invited disease to be his guest and it has arisen in the night to slay him. Civilisation has, indeed, become a slaughtering-car crowned by a grinning effigy of Comfort, before which man blindly and voluntarily hurls himself in his own ignorance.

When the mind of man invented the wheel it most rapidly accelerated his physical downfall, for the wheel of civilisation has broken more men in a physical sense than ever did the wheel of the French Revolution. As a child, he is " wheeled " in his perambulator or bassinette; as a youth, a wheeled vehicle takes him to school and home again; as a man he is |bound to the wheel " which carries him Mazeppa-like to his doom, because it has robbed him more and more of his muscular power through the comparative disuse of many of his muscles.

It is a well-established fact that disuse, or even the diminished use, of any part of an animal body leads to its deterioration and atrophy, and man became more and more liable to disease as he less and less depended upon his own muscles. We know that when man lived in primeval forests and jungles, and had to be incessantly vigilant against the fierce and savage denizens that infested those parts, and which were his unsleeping enemies, when quickness of hearing and sensitiveness to sound were as necessary for his protection and safety as among wild animals to-day, he possessed the power of moving his ears by means of muscles, just as we can see even in some of our domestic pets to-day.

As civilisation advanced, however, this keen and alert sensitiveness to sound became less and less necessary. Through continued disuse, then, he lost the power of those muscles that cause the ears to lie back or stand forth at will, and catch the slightest noise that might threaten danger, until to-day the ears of the majority of men are immovable because the muscles of movement have atrophied. True, in very rare instances, we find individuals who still possess this strange and now, to most of us, almost uncanny power.

This loss of power through use and movement is possible with all the muscles in the body. During my travels in India, I was very much interested in a wonderful old fakir, one of those devout beggars who resort to all sorts of self-mutilation to excite the sympathy of the charitable public as well as to display their fanatic willingness to sacrifice themselves for religious purposes. This grey-bearded old fellow had kept his arms for so many years in one fixed position that they had become absolutely withered and had lost all muscular power of movement. Such is the natural and inevitable result of the lack of movement anywhere and everywhere in the body.

PUTTING YOUR STOMACH IN A SLING.

Everyone knows how an arm will weaken if carried in a sling and unused. Place your own arm and keep it there motionless for sufficient length of time and its muscles will lose all their natural power to move it. When a limb has been injured or broken, and it has to be kept immovable in one position for any length of time, the power of muscular movement naturally becomes greatly reduced. It is at first only by a great effort that it can be moved at all, while such an arm, if kept long enough in a sling, would lose all muscular power and become absolutely useless. The lost power of the disused muscles can only be gradually restored by easy and graduated movement, but only so long as there is still life in the cells of the limb.

Just in the same way, the muscles of movement associated with any or every bodily organ and function will grow weaker and weaker through disuse, and unless the weak spot is strengthened and developed by use and movement, the enemy, disease, will sooner or later have the opportunity to break through at the point of least resistance.

Or, to take another instance, if you were to go without food or with very little food for a week or two, while living an active life, it will be surprising how little your bodily strength will diminish while you keep the body moving. The body will continue for some time to live on its own reserves of heat and energy, but the stomach* itself will grow weaker and demand less nourishment through lack of regular use, and will, in consequence, become a ready prey for disease. When you again commence to eat food, your food will have to be of the lightest kind at first, because the stomach has become so weak through disuse, and the food must be gradually increased in its nature and quantity until the stomach regains its former strength, which it can only do through its own daily use which means movement. It is just as if for a time you had put your stomach and digestive system in a sling until it became too weak for its work through disuse and diminished muscular movement, and has to be gradually " educated," as it were, back to it again.

In one of Mark Twain's stories, he describes how a crew of dyspeptics were wrecked on a desert island and nearly starved to death. They became, according to the genial humorist, so weak and hungry that finally they ate the leather of their boots, which proves that Mark Twain was not a physiologist. If so, he would have known that, at such a time, to have given a shipwrecked mariner even a mild chop might easily have caused his death after long starvation, because the stomach has got too weak, through disuse and lack of movement, to digest it. In such cases, feeding must begin with the lightest possible diet, being gradually increased in quantity and quality until the digestive system is strong enough to digest any kind of food.

Now, supposing, to take another instance, a person were to lie in bed and not move at all, but eat as much food as ever he desired. This time the unmoved muscles of the unused limbs would degenerate through lack of movement just as the muscles of digestion did in the previous case, because these muscles, or rather, the cells of which these muscles are composed would become enfeebled and even atrophied through disuse. These cells must have muscular movement to make them hungry, just as muscular movement increases our own appetite and makes us require more food to live. But when the limbs and the muscles of the limbs are not called upon for movement, not only do the cells of these limbs and muscles weaken and waste because they no longer are sufficiently nourished, but the cells of the digestive system also gradually weaken because less movement is now necessary on their part, and consequently they demand less food, and the whole cellular workers of the body would then have to suffer in proportion, " their services," to use a familiar expression, " being no longer required."

THE BODY AS AN HOTEL.

It might make it clearer to the reader if I used the language of metaphor. Let us imagine the body as an hotel built for the residence of some 500 busy people. The demands of all these people necessitate the maintenance of a large and efficient staff for all their needs. But suppose that some two or three hundred of these residents are thrown out of employment, and no longer can maintain themselves in the hotel, this immediately causes a cutting down of the staff and a general lowering of the standard of efficiency among those who remain. If the number of residents sank still lower the hotel must inevitably end in bankruptcy.

So with the human body and the 500 and more muscles upon whose activities it depends for existence. When all these muscles, are moved and used in balance, it means that the cell workers of the body in every system, are kept well-nourished, active, fit and efficient. The fewer of these muscles are called into play, or the less we use them in balance, the fewer the number of cell workers kept in employment and the more those that remain become lax, indifferent and inefficient until the body finally becomes weak, open to disease and, perhaps, even actually in a state of disease.

The whole body must be understood as a great organisation or establishment in which every department and system is interrelated and inter-dependent, each department being linked up with every other by the blood circulation and the nervous system. By giving movement or employment first to the voluntary muscles, all the other cells of the body are immediately and automatically set moving also, and upon this united and associated movement of all the cells in harmony and balance depends the health of the body and its power in any or every part to resist, conquer and prevent disease, as I show more fully in the following chapter.

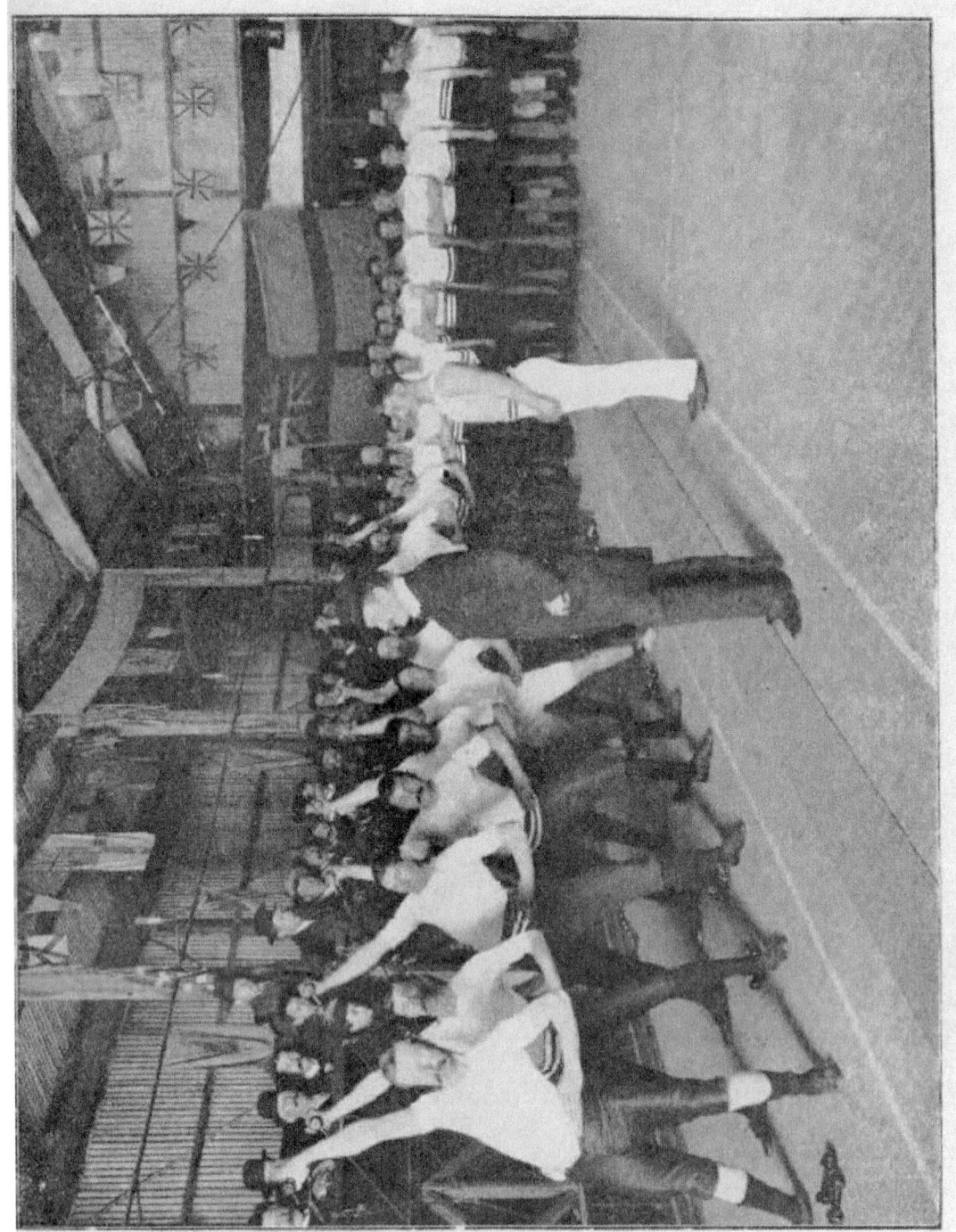

Photographers: Richards & Co. Ballarat.

A Fine Body of Men.
Dumb-bell Drill by Australians trained on these methods.

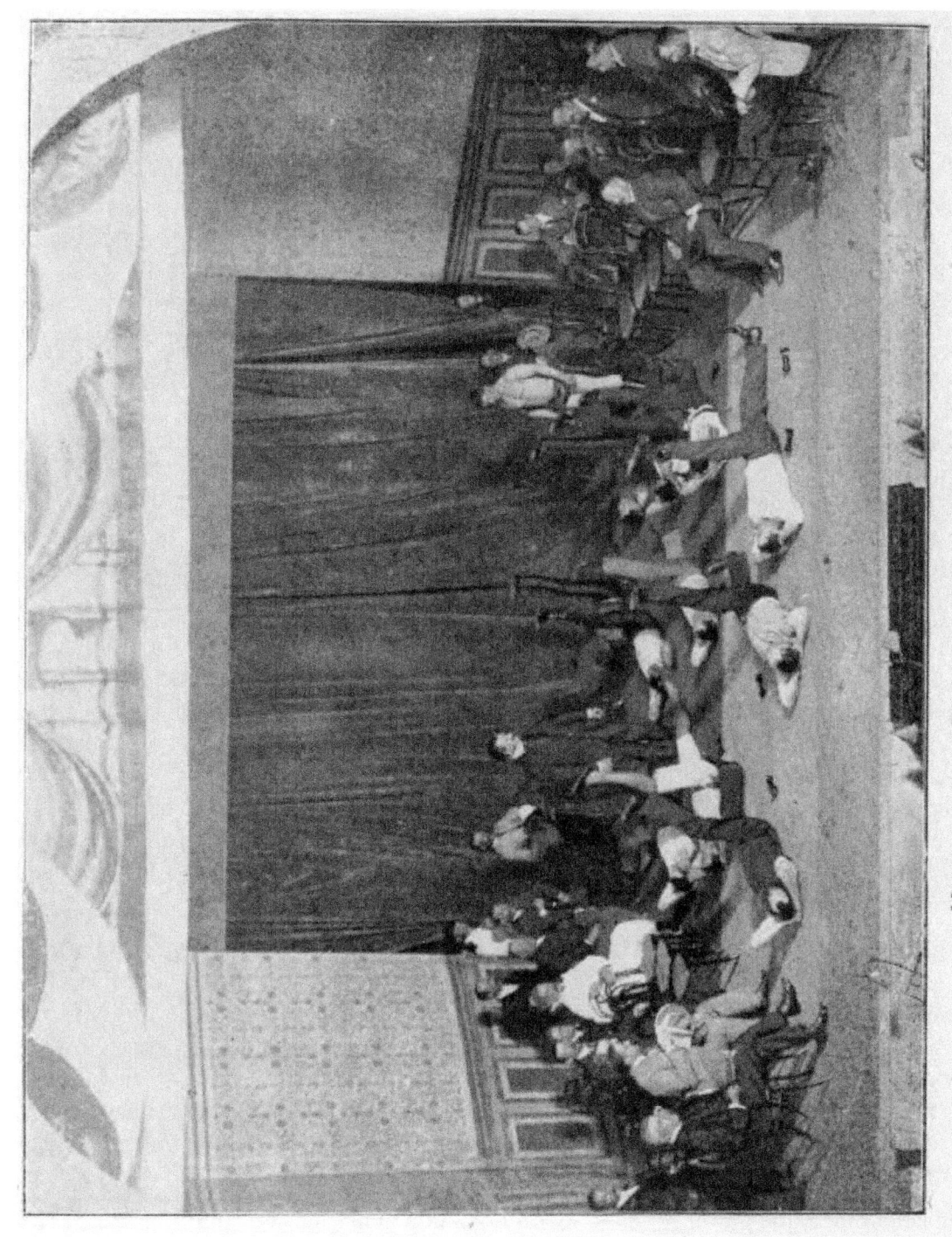

MOVEMENTS FOR STRENGTHENING ABDOMINAL MUSCLES.
As described in this book being carried out under Author's personal direction before Medical Men.

CHAPTER VII.

The Movement that Resists and Defeats Disease.

Now, man, as I have already said, is simply a bundle of cells, millions of living cells inter-dependent and inter-related each to one another.

Life in the final analysis, begins in the cell, for, as that great scientific observer, Professor Verworn, says, " everything we ourselves do is done in the individual cell. The muscle-cell gives us the cue to the nature of muscular contraction and the heart-beat, the gland-cell reveals to us the causes of secretion, the white blood cell explains to us the assimilation of food, and the secrets of the mind are to be found in the ganglion cell."

THE LIVING CELLS OF THE BODY.

We must, in short, begin with the true physiological assumption that it is to the individual cell—the unit of the multi-cellular man —that the consideration of every bodily function which regulates life and health must lead us. Through the cell and the cells of the body, therefore, we can reach, cultivate, train, develop and reconstruct every part and organ of the human body, and every cell of the body is dependent on, kept alive and maintained in health and power by the movement of the voluntary muscles, as I fully explain in my next chapter.

As it is, therefore, only movement and the power of movement that distinguish life from death—the little living organism that is the Alpha of life from the atom of inorganic and inanimate matter—so by increasing and improving or by reducing each cell's power of movement we also increase and improve or diminish its vital power, and through it reach for good or ill the whole bodily life. All the tissues of your body in all its systems and organs are composed of millions upon millions of these protoplasmic cells, creatures each of which has muscles and functions like yourself, and each of which is part and parcel of the wonderful organisation of every human being. To keep all these cells in perfectly balanced strength is the true secret of health, vitality, and resistant power to disease.

This, I contend, we can only do by the balanced physical movement of the voluntary muscles as I describe, especially as in the compelling circumstances of modern life we are deprived of the natural and all-round physical movement which made and kept our earliest ancestors superior to disease. As life became more and more artificial, new occupations, of a sedentary or semi-sedentary nature necessary for the upkeep and advance of modern civilisation, were introduced, and this natural balanced movement gradually became less and less necessary, and the consequent loss of balance in the body lowered man's resistant power and led to the ascendancy of disease over man.

The living cells supply the power for every bodily function under the control of directing cells in the brain. The cells are the component parts that go to build up the tissue of every organ and system, that form bone, blood, muscle, flesh, sinew, membrane, ligament, cartilage, nerve and brain, and they individually and collectively are responsible, therefore, for the condition of each and every organ or system, and the success or failure of its functions.

All living organisms, even these microscopic cells of the body require food as the very basis of life and growth, and the many and various cells of the body must also receive food in such a form as contains all the essentials necessary for repairing waste, brought to them, through the agency of the circulating blood.

OURSELVES IN MINIATURE.

Each of these millions on millions of cells is a living entity like ourselves. Together their bodily cells constitute us and represent us in miniature. Each eats, breathes, drinks, works, fights, sleeps, and reproduces its species just as we do. " It has no lungs and yet it breathes; no mouth, still eats; no definite shape, yet grows; no nerves, yet is sensitive; no sex, yet may give birth to endless progeny."

Each cell, too, I claim, can be made strong or weak, healthy or ill, through physical movement or lack of it. The organised cell, in short, lives much as we do, but by simpler processes, grows by assimilation, produces after its own kind, and then decays and dies. The performance of the functions of these millions of cells naturally leads to the accumulation of waste matter in the body, which the organs of elimination are only enabled to remove out of the system by muscular movement. It will be easy to understand, therefore, that physical movement by speeding up the circulation, increases the nutrition of all the bodily cells, the elimination of their waste and also the supply of their essential oxygen, at the same time developing and continuing to produce new and healthier cells in every organ and system of the body.

This most miraculous of machines, the human body, consisted at the earliest period of its existence of a single cell so small that nearly 200 of them would not measure an inch. This cell grew, developed, and reproduced other cells by division and sub-division, until its family reaches into billions, these again being distributed among various systems and organs until the complete organism we call man is developed. All these cells are divided into classes just as is society itself, some occupying more responsible positions and performing the higher duties of life, while others fill more humble spheres, and do the " hard labour " of life.

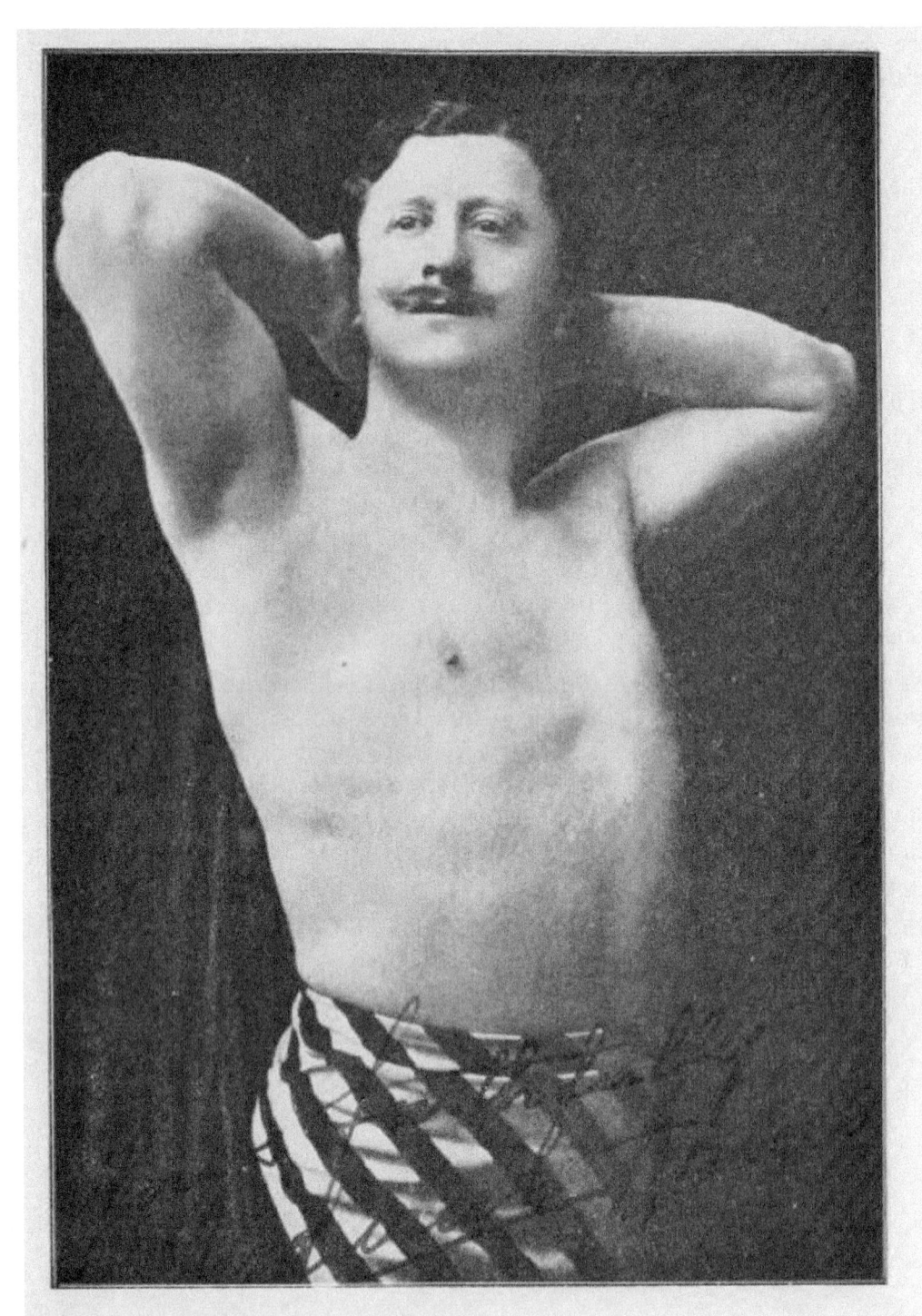

A BELGIAN APOLLO.—MAURICE ARIOSO, GOLD MEDALLIST.

The grandeur of manhood could scarcely be better illustrated than it is here from life, the original being Maurice Arioso, who hails from that country of heroes—Belgium. This figure, which might well be taken for an old master, was obtained by following out the methods described.

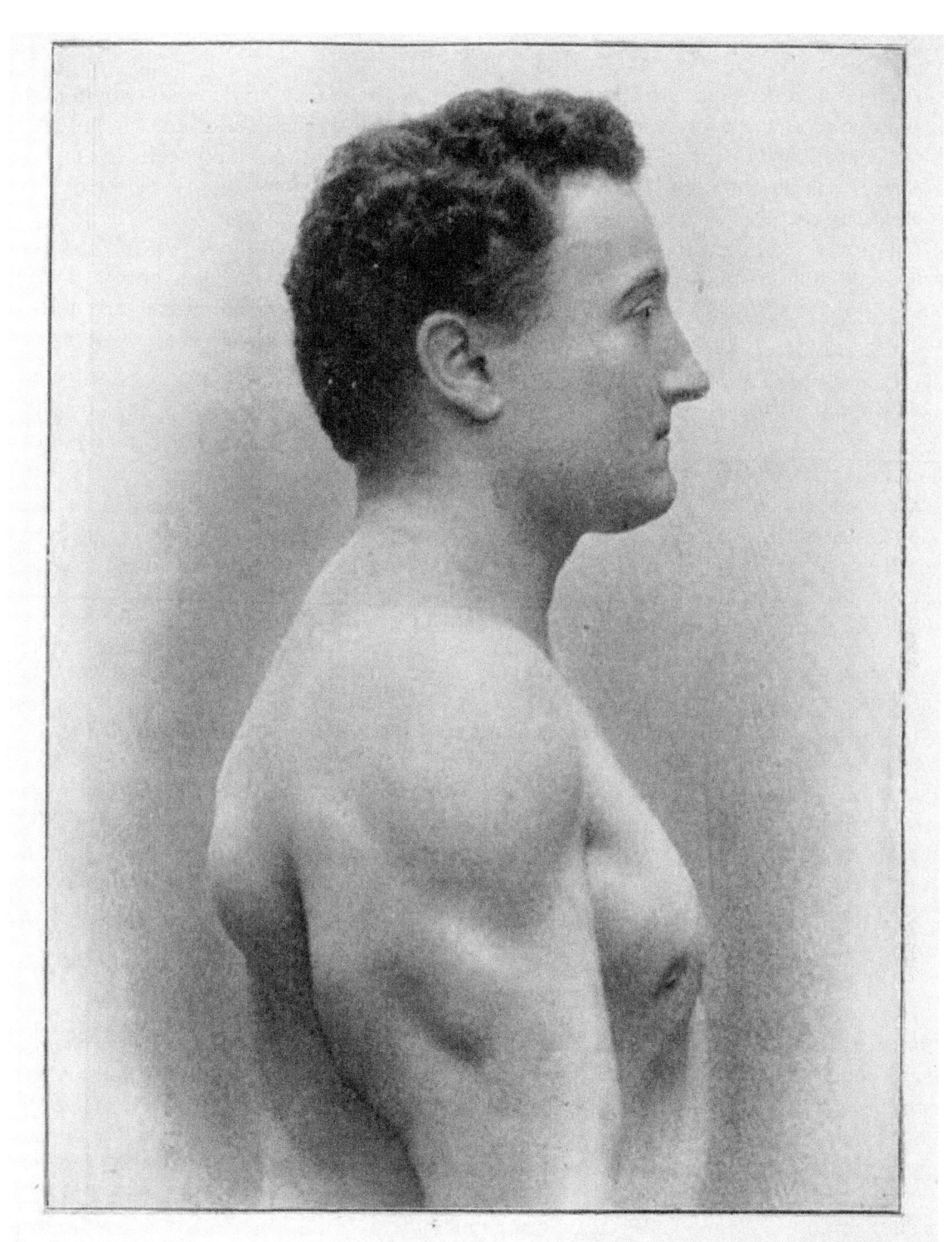

COMTE DE BOISGIRARD.
Glorious France is not behind in this great movement, as the above striking photographic study from life shows. Virility is the keynote of this study, and this young French Count owes his physique and physical power to the methods explained in these pages.

NO "WEARY WILLIES" OR "TIRED TIMS."

To go fully into a description of the various species of living cells in the body would require a volume as large as an encyclopaedia. Suffice it to say that there are cells of one kind in the brain to think, control, and direct all the operations of this wonderful community, cells in the blood to carry supplies of air and nourishment everywhere, and to fight enemy disease germs that invade the body, cell chemists in liver and lungs and kidneys, cell-stokers and engineers in the heart, cell food-producers in the stomach, cells to move our bodily dwelling at will in the brain and muscles, cell builders and masons to erect bone and tissue, and cell scavengers distributed throughout the intestines, kidneys, liver, lungs and skin to eliminate waste and poisonous products.

Each cell in the healthy body performs its duty silently, efficiently and easily, and only when any cell or group of cells grows too old, too feeble, or too diseased to carry out its duties easily and well, do we experience the discomfort which we truly call dis-ease. In this industrious community there is no room for Weary Willies or Tired Tims, nor are there any idle rich. All must work and move or die. Disaffected, old and unfit cells die quickly, if they cannot perform the duties demanded of them in the shape of rapid and strenuous activity through the united movement of all the voluntary muscles, for their waste outbalances repair under an increased and increasing physical strain beyond their power, and because they cannot assimilate the essentials necessary for their life.

Now, we ourselves are just what our cells make us, or, rather, what we make ourselves, because whether the living cells of the body do their work well or ill depends almost entirely on how we ourselves treat them. If we keep them healthfully occupied, and do not overwork them, if we feed them well and give them plenty of fresh air, if we see to their sanitation and hygiene, if, in short, we keep each and all of them healthfully active by physical movement—as I show in the following chapter we can do by moving all the voluntary muscles of the body in absolute balance—we will live better and healthier and happier lives, do our daily work more easily and more efficiently, become less liable to disease and increase our length of days in the land. To this extent, indeed, everyone can be a self-made man, the master of his own fate and the captain of his own soul.

" HALF-DEAD, WISH-TO-BE DEAD, AND UNBURIED DEAD."

All these cells must be properly nourished, given plenty of fresh air, and kept just as clean as the outward body by well regulated and balanced physical movement that keeps them bathed in a continuous stream of pure and well oxygenated blood which cleanses them of all waste and disease-generating matter. Thus the happiness of the whole bodily community and your personal immunity from disease can be assured. If, however, as I have said, some of them are starved, or ill-treated or become unfit through lack of this movement, they will fail in the performance of their duty, or do it only in a listless way, when the body itself must inevitably sicken unless steps are taken to restore the happiness, health and integrity of these cells.

Your health, in short, depends upon the health of your cells. According to the degree of physical movement—always provided there is neither excess nor too little—the state of the bodily health will generally be found to correspond. Those who live as near as possible to the natural life of movement man was meant to live are the healthier and happier, while every large community to-day, through lack of such movement, has its half-dead, wish-to-be-dead, and unburied dead who exist rather than really live.

In other words, it is only the movement of all the voluntary muscles within balance that promotes and maintains that healthy and balanced movement of all the bodily cells, which gives them individual and collective strength, linking them in harmonious cellular co-operation, and making the whole organism a single and powerful unit to resist and defeat its natural enemy, disease. Without this, of course, one may live, as so many do to-day, with a very little physical movement, but with a body weak in many parts and places tending ever towards disease in one or more of those parts and places, Another may obtain more physical movement either through his occupation or recreation and live with a body having fewer " weak spots," but still ever liable to disease. No occupation or recreation, however, can supply that perfectly balanced movement of all or nearly all the voluntary muscles which is absolutely necessary to establish perfect balance between every cell and each group of cells that alone gives the body security and immunity from disease.

On the other hand, every form of occupation in civilised life to-day, no matter how much or how little physical effort it entails, tends to aggravate the loss of balance and to lower resistant power in some part or parts, and so to make the body liable to succumb to disease in some part or parts. No occupation or sport will give the body an impregnable front against disease, because some cells will be under-nourished and under-developed and vice-versa, and some will always remain with some weakness tending towards disease. It does not, in brief, supply physical movement in a balanced and scientific way.

To make it clearer still the clerk and the agricultural labourer experience varying degrees of physical effort in their daily occupations. The latter, as a rule, lives a healthier life than the former because he lives more by the movement of his muscles, or, rather, by the movement of more of his muscles, but each is liable to disease with a liability differing only in degree, and each is most probably liable to disease in different forms or in different parts. The trained athlete, as a rule, lives a healthier average life than either, but he, too, through his specialised training, may also possess a body so unbalanced in some part or parts as to be only liable to disease in a still lesser degree, and he would be in the modern standard of civilisation the one who would most enjoy life and escape most frequently from actual disease. Indeed, such a man would possibly escape disease altogether, only if attacked by it in its gross and most deadly form, and even then his superior vitality might just enable him to pull through at great peril to his life where the others would have perished.

NO A1 BODIES WITH C3 CELLS.

Between all other forms of physical movement and the balanced movement of all the voluntary muscles there is a wide difference. It is only by such balanced movement (which I describe fully in the chapter following) that the cells of every organ and associated with every function of the body receive equal nourishment and are strengthened in equal and proportionate balance, and so are each and all brought into line as one grand defensive army and protector of the body against every assault of disease. It is because physical movement that is perfectly balanced makes every cell equally strong and fit to do its duty that it produces a perfectly disciplined and efficient cellular army of defence against disease. It is only by commencing with the children that we can really create such an army of defence as a permanently fighting force against disease for life. If we take the children in time and give them this powerful cellular army of defence, there would be no more need to lament in the future C3 men instead of an A1 people. To paraphrase Mr Lloyd George's famous words, it is impossible to have an Al body with C3 cells.

It is only when, on the other hand, from some cause or other, some of the bodily cell-workers and fighters grow weak, break down, strike, and neglect their duty that it is possible for disease to enter the bodily kingdom like an invading and conquering army. Certain cells of the body become too weak or unbalanced through lack of the physical drill necessary to make and keep them strong enough to fight off the invaders, and through lack of those supplies which only come to them in sufficient and evenly divided quantity through this balanced physical movement, they grow ever and ever weaker and less resistant to disease. And only in the body's own resistant power to disease can we look for absolute security and immunity from disease

Dr Sir George Newman, K.C.B., F.R.C.P., Chief Medical Officer of the Board of Education, in an official Report (presented to both Houses of Parliament by command of the King), that will always stand as a landmark to medical exploring parties in search of that still undiscovered country where disease is unknown, agrees that " the first line of defence is a healthy, well-nourished and resistant body." It is also, if I may use a homely expression, " the last ditch " in which the body entrenches itself against disease and death, for the medical verdict as to life or death at the last, most critical moment, is always determined by the patient's own vitality, that is, the vitality and resistant power of the living cells in one or more parts of the body.

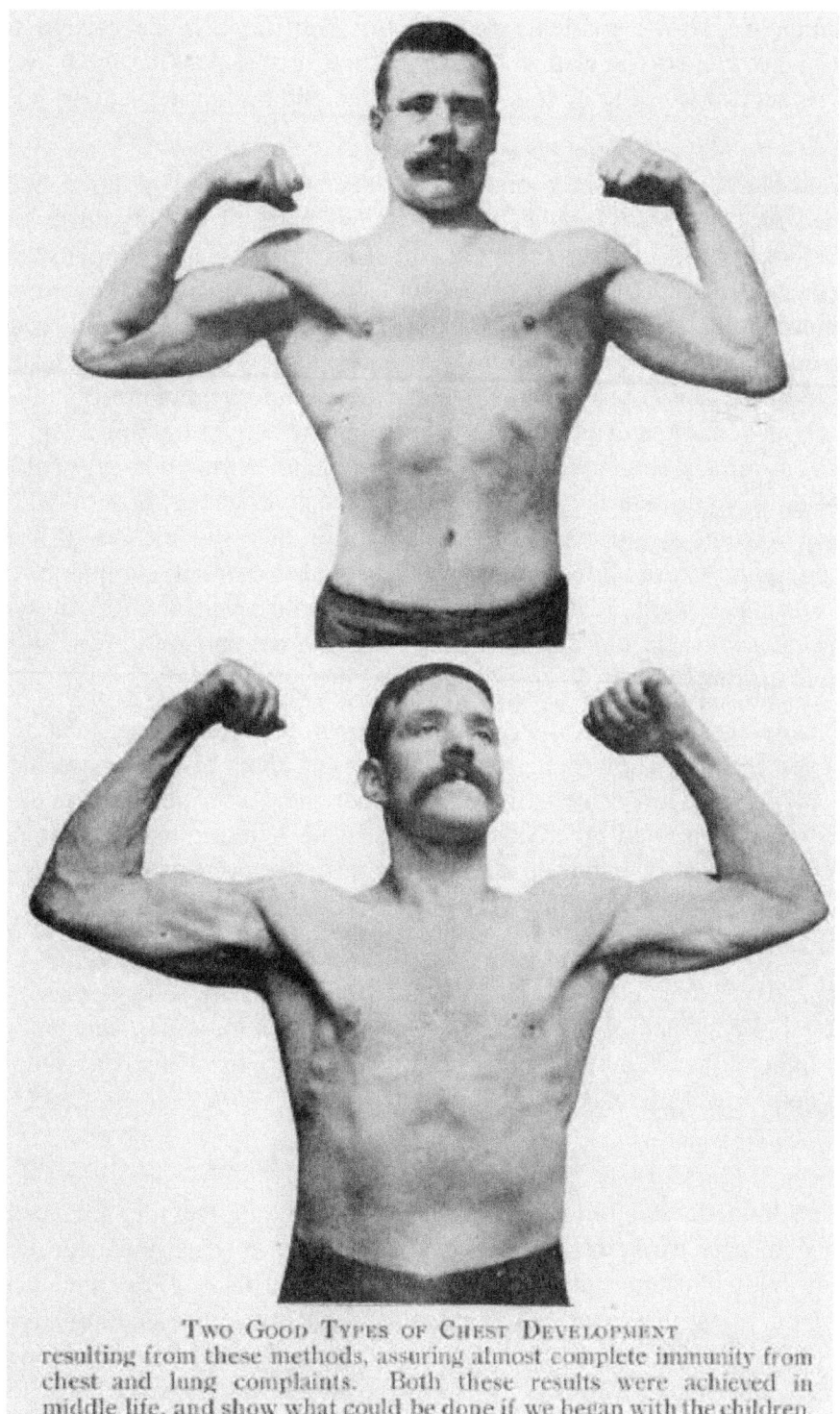

TWO GOOD TYPES OF CHEST DEVELOPMENT
resulting from these methods, assuring almost complete immunity from chest and lung complaints. Both these results were achieved in middle life, and show what could be done if we began with the children.

HOW TO INCREASE VITALITY.

Where, then, does this death-defying vitality come from? Of what does it consist? Why should one body possess it in great force and another in greatly diminished quantity and quality? What is it, in short, that makes and keeps a body " healthy, well-nourished, and resistant "? The chief sources of vitality, we know, are food and air, but both have to be carried to and equally distributed throughout every part of the body if we are to have a body well- nourished everywhere in balance, and not to have a body well-fed and strong in one part and ill-nourished and weak somewhere else.

Besides, the food has to pass through many processes before it is converted into a form from which the varied types of bodily cells in the different parts of the organism can extract and assimilate the elements essential to their nutrition and repair. The blood itself needs certain elements, bone needs others, muscle yet others, and skin, hair, nails, tendons, ligaments, etc., all need different nutrient material. How do these transformations of food and this equal distribution of supplies essential to " a healthy, well-nourished and resistant body " take place but by movement, even though sub-conscious movement. Food would lie and putrefy in a body that had no power of such movement, and air would not be taken into it, nor carbonic acid gas eliminated. And without the movement and circulation of the blood neither food nor air would be distributed to every part of the body to nourish it fairly and equally everywhere. Even while we sleep, this sub-conscious movement, in a diminished degree, goes on or we would die. If it were not so we would at last very quickly lose all resistant power essential to combat, conquer or escape disease. To make the body supremely resistant to and triumphant over disease, however, this sub-conscious movement must, in our civilised life, be supported and reinforced by conscious and balanced physical movement.

Now it is reasonable to suppose that if we can by our own free will accelerate all this internal and involuntary movement, as I show hereafter we can do, we can also increase the nutrition and aeration of every part and every cell of every part of the body, liberate greater quantities of poisonous carbonic acid gas and other waste and disease-provoking matter from the system, and thus build up a body in healthy balanced strength and resistant power in any or all of its parts and systems, so that in this way and in this way only we can have just such a body as Sir George Newman describes.

It is my chief purpose in this book to show that there is only the one way in which we can do this, and that is through the agency of the voluntary muscular system, which each and all of us have or should have under our own control, but I need not describe how this is accomplished here, as to do so would only be to anticipate my next chapter.

THE BLUE-BIRD OF HEALTH.

As all disease is admittedly due to lack of balance, and as the perfect and balanced movement of all the voluntary muscles of the body alone leads to perfect internal balance, including perfect balance between body and brain and between the body and its environment, it is evident that when such a system of national physical education and reconstruction as I am advocating is once established in our schools, we shall have begun an irresistible advance movement against the enemy of disease, which will bring us, at last, to the attainment of that long- cherished ideal, a diseaseless world. Personally, I can see no other way of arriving at that goal, but I know that we can reach it when the world awakens to a full and complete realisation of the fact that Nature's law of life is movement, and that we must obey that law or perish. A body developed in balanced strength by such a method as I describe is the only body so powerfully resistant to disease as to be immune.

This is the crucial point—the pivot—of every measure that aims at the prevention of disease, and it is just the point that is missed in every plan and scheme towards that end which I have yet seen. They revolve round it, as it were, but fail to reach the centre. The authors of such schemes are looking everywhere for the Blue-bird of Health, when all the time it is only to be found within the body itself. " A healthy, well-nourished and resistant human body " is admittedly the one and only successful preventive measure against disease, and while all the hygienic, social and even dietetic reforms advocated may be helpful to its upbuilding, they are but the scaffolding and are only essential while the physical structure itself is being erected.

When a body has been so educated and developed in harmony or what I call balance, it is built upon a sound physical foundation, for it is then so perfectly balanced in every cellular detail of its structure as to be itself resistant—successfully resistant—to disease. Movement is the law of life, and balanced movement is the first law of health. Even, for instance, if disease germs find a lodgement in a perfectly balanced body they will quickly be killed or sterilised by the body's own army of defence. Indeed, Sir George Newman himself declares that " many persons carry in their bodies the bacillus of tuberculosis without suffering from any clinical form of disease, because their bodies are resistant."

"TORPEDO NETS" AGAINST DISEASE.

It is not evident, therefore, that the health of the individual body and its immunity from or liability to disease is determined and modified by its own innate power of resistance to disease, rather than by its environment, or any particular circumstance of its environment, however opposed it may be to health or however disposed it may be towards disease. Reduced, therefore, to its logical conclusion, I think that Sir George Newman will agree when I say that we can only make the body really immune by developing and establishing within itself the fighting strength and quality of every individual living cell, and the balanced strength and efficiency of all these cells, so that these living cells will separately and conjointly defy and conquer disease either from within or from without.

To search out and destroy disease microbes, whether within or without the body is of little use, if we do not at the same time increase the resistant power of the body itself, for other microbes of the same or other diseases, and even as yet undiscovered and unrecognised microbes of disease that will assuredly reveal their presence if man is allowed to grow still weaker through advancing civilisation and diminished physical movement, will also attack it, and attack it successfully.

There, in a nutshell, you have the whole case against isolation (except to restrict and prevent the extension of a communicable disease to others for a time as, say, in the case of an epidemic), or the employment of what I may call medical " torpedo-nets " of many kinds as preventives against disease or even any particular form of disease. They do not and cannot prevent disease, so long as the body itself is not made strong enough in its own armour-plate of health and strength as to be able to defy and defeat it. They may defend it against some particular form of disease for a time, but the moment the defensive barrier is removed, the patient is liable to succumb again, or, at least, to fall a prey to some other species of disease microbes, revealed or as yet unrevealed, which are swarming in ambush everywhere, and always waiting their opportunity to overthrow a weak and feebly resistant body.

Isolation, while it will temporarily protect, does not and cannot give a man an atom of physical resistant power to combat and conquer disease. Only the individual who has attained this resistant power is safe, not only against disease germs but against the weakness within that leads to disease.

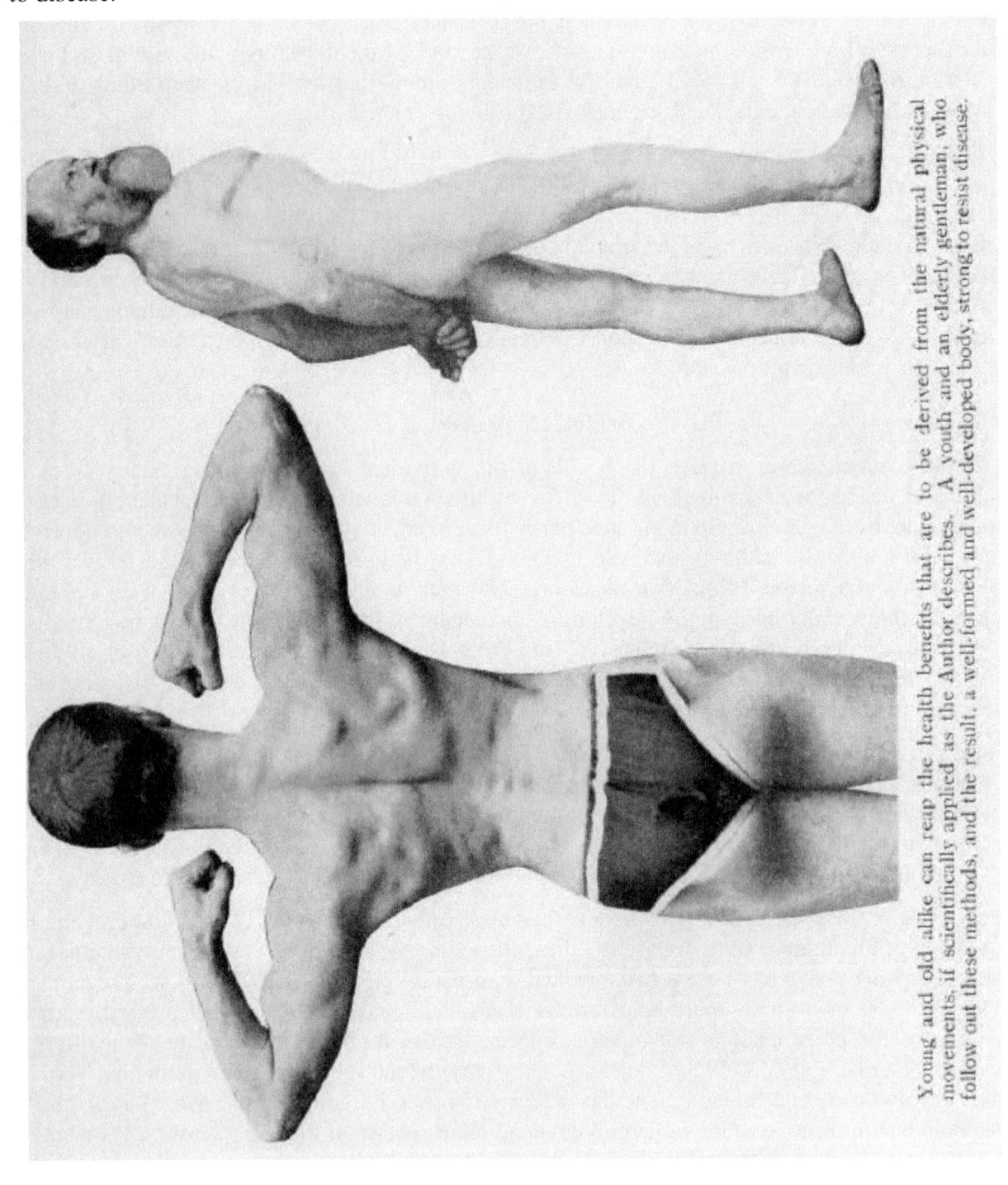

Young and old alike can reap the health benefits that are to be derived from the natural physical movements, if scientifically applied as the Author describes. A youth and an elderly gentleman, who follow out these methods, and the result, a well-formed and well-developed body, strong to resist disease.

W. HUTCHINSON.

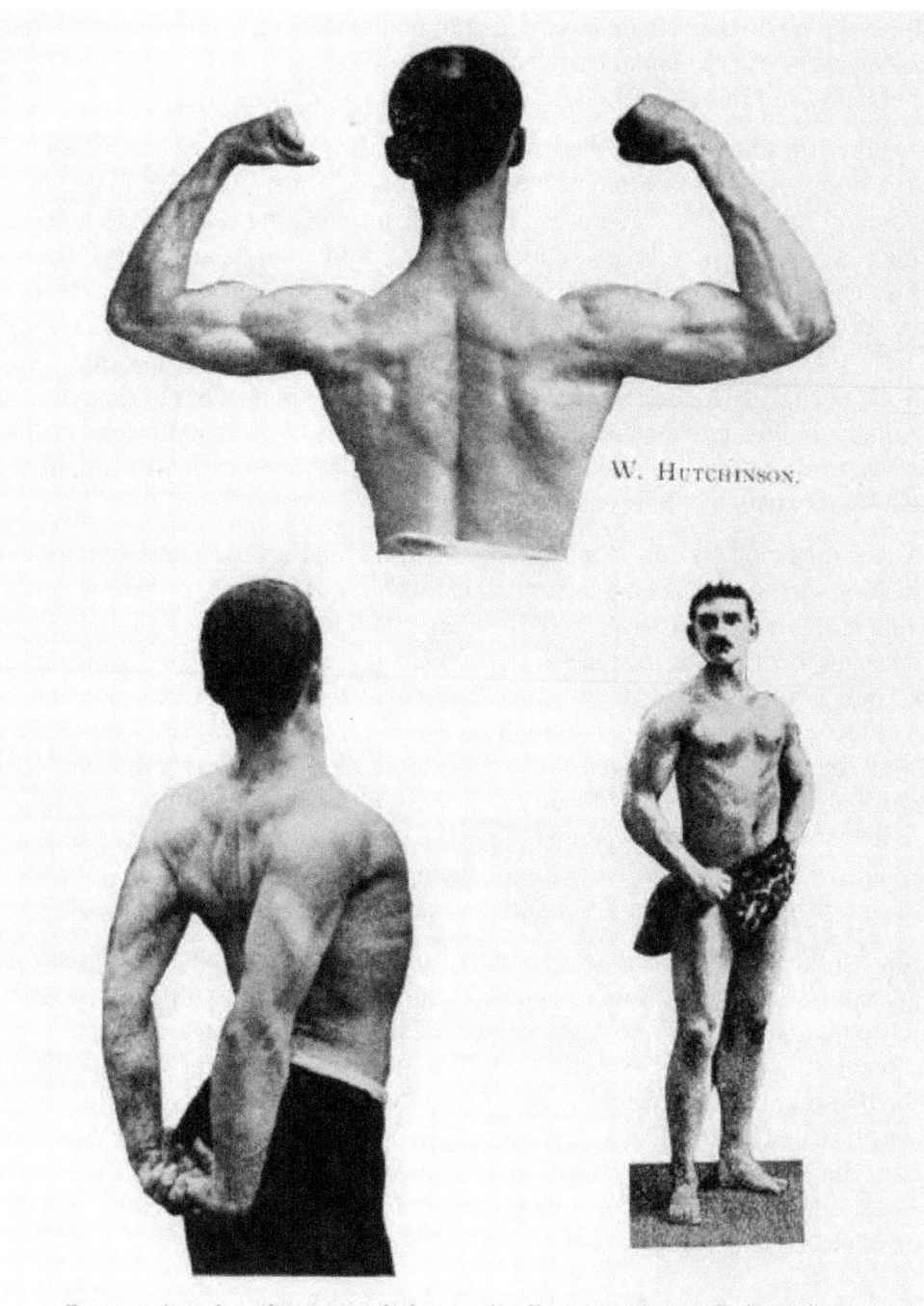

Can you imagine these men being medically rejected as unfit for military service? These men have taken the trouble to develop their bodies as Nature meant them to be developed, by natural methods such as are advocated by the Author, and there is no reason why everyone should not do the same.

THE BODY'S FIRST LINE OF DEFENCE.

That some bodies do possess this power of resistance in a high degree while others are deficient in it is the only reason why disease has not already swept mankind out of existence by now, and as civilisation tends to make the body become progressively weaker, generation after generation, new forms of disease which even yet have failed to reveal themselves have a good innings before them, unless we make every human body and every cell of the individual human body powerful enough individually and in balance collectively to resist and defeat them.

To strengthen the resistant power of the body is, on Dr Sir George Newman's own admission, to strengthen the body's first line of defence against disease. If, therefore, we make the first line of defence sufficiently strong, we can prevent disease from breaking through, so that other lines of defence, judicious though they be as supports and reinforcements, are by no means vital. The first line of defence, therefore, that is the resistant power of the body, is the paramount factor in repelling the attacks of disease. Any- thing that will not increase and strengthen this resistant force is of little value in the grim struggle between the human body and disease. Isolation cannot do it. Food cannot do it. Medicine cannot do it. I have shown wherein isolation or food are valueless without bodily movement, that, if anything, they will actually tend to lower bodily resistant power to disease by allowing some cells to become weaker than others and causing disturbance of bodily balance. This equally applies to the use of medicine or drugs.

The utmost that medicine can do is to stimulate, irritate and arouse some organ or organs into action artificially, to soothe or benumb nerves and brain, or to supply certain chemical elements that are deficient in weak or diseased cells' or elements that are destroyed quicker than they can be replaced owing to weakness in some of the cells responsible either for the elaboration of food into suitable nourishment, or for its transmission or its assimilation. But it does not and cannot give even a microscopical increase of strength to any cell or groups of cells, and it certainly does not develop the innate resistant power of the cells. Nothing but their own movement and use can do this. On the other hand, cells artificially fed or stimulated by medicine must tend to become still weaker, and snore and more dependent upon such artificial and temporary aids and supports just as a leg grown weak through lack of movement requires a crutch or stick to support it, and will never regain its natural strength except by use and movement.

Medicine, therefore, is not only not a preventive of disease— which is the great object of the medical profession to-day—but it often actually tends to cause and cultivate disease by inducing the condition of weakness and imperfect balance that permits and fosters disease in the part or parts of the body affected. To give medicine to the weak or diseased body is like lending money to a spendthrift child instead of teaching the child to be independent of such aid, and providing it with the education and training necessary to enable it to earn its own living. Scientific physical movement, on the other hand, educates a weak, helpless or diseased organ or system to be self-supporting, self-reliant and strong enough to defy and defeat its worst enemy, disease, especially if people are educated and trained to it from their earliest childhood.

THERE IS ONLY ONE DISEASE.

Disease, after all, is a unified enemy under a single command, although it assumes Protean forms. There is only one disease or cause of disease, and that is lack of balance and loss of innate resistant power somewhere in the body itself due to lack of balanced strength in any and all of its parts. What we call diseases have a common origin in the unbalanced body itself, for the body in perfect balance refuses to bow down before any form of disease, microbic or otherwise. The nosology or classification of what are really " symptoms " of disease as distinct and separate " diseases | is one of the greatest errors of medical science and has led to much confusion in the battle against the common enemy. For you cannot treat the human body, as is so often done today, as if it consisted of a series of watertight compartments or hermetically sealed chambers.

The body is also a unit, with organs and systems and functions and cells that are not to be dealt with as things distinct and apart, but as one embracing whole, for that which affects one organ or system affects the whole in some degree, just as the breakdown of one wheel in the works of a watch will stop it or cause it to show incorrect time. We must begin now to treat the body and to consider disease both as distinct entities at continuous war with one another from childhood to old age. Until we do this we may temporarily " patch up " a body diseased or weak towards disease in one or more parts, which, however, cannot bring about perfect balance and will never succeed in preventing disease or in radically eradicating it from the human body.

TO CURE ONE DISEASE IS TO CURE ALL.

That very keen observer, Dr Rush, in his " Theory of Fever," puts the case against the classification and multiplication of diseases very effectively. " Science," he says, f has much to deplore from the multiplication of diseases. It is as repugnant to truth in medicine as polytheism is to truth in religion. The physician who considers every different affection of the different systems of the body, or every affection of different parts of the same system, as distinct diseases, when they arise from one cause, resembles the

Indian or African savage, who considers water, dew, ice, frost and snow as distinct essences; while the physician who considers the morbid affections of every part of the body, however diversified they may be in their form or degrees, as derived from one cause, resembles the philosopher who considers dew, ice, frost, and snow as different modifications of water, and as derived simply from the absence of heat.

" The physician who can cure one disease by a knowledge of its principles may, by the same means, cure all the diseases of the human body, for their causes are the same." All disease, in short, springs from a common cause, lack of balance somewhere in the body itself, with inevitably lowered resistant power, and this can only be prevented and overcome by the natural and balanced movement of the muscles within and under our own control. This is the only way to correct that condition of the body that predisposes to disease by strengthening and developing the body itself, or, in other words, to prevent disease, in any of its many forms, in the individual body.

If we can prevent it in the individual we can prevent it in the nation, and, indeed, in the peoples of the world. But to do so with the greatest and most beneficial results, we must begin with the children, and see that they are from the first, safeguarded against " those minute departures from the normal which foretell the coming of disease." No man realises this more truly than Dr Sir George Newman himself, whose official position gives him unique opportunities for the study of disease in childhood, and who has seen what medical care and supervision of the children, even in a small way, can do.

A TRAMP IN A PALACE.

If we do not take the children and educate them to know how to build up and care for the human body, to respect the bodies committed to their charge during their tenure of life, and to bring their bodies into a condition of perfectly balanced strength so as to make them impregnable to disease, no medical examinations, no feeding schemes, no housing, sanitation, or other methods of reform will avail to prevent, much less eradicate, disease. One might as well take an illiterate tramp from the wayside, put him in a palatial home, dress him, and feed him well and provide him with all he desires, and expect him to forget old associations, old ideas, old habits without the necessary preliminary education and training.

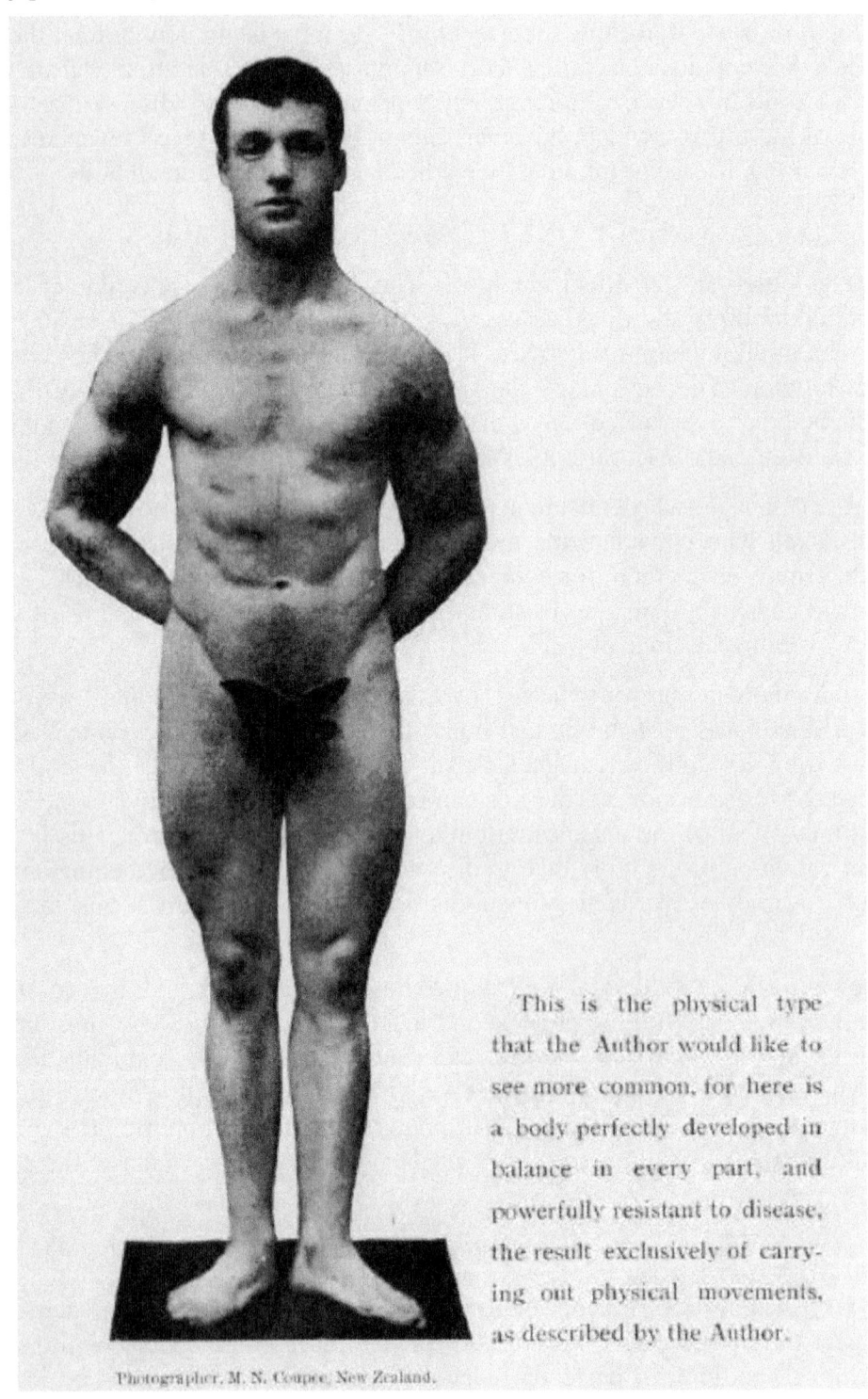

Photographer, M. N. Coupee, New Zealand.

This is the physical type that the Author would like to see more common, for here is a body perfectly developed in balance in every part, and powerfully resistant to disease, the result exclusively of carrying out physical movements, as described by the Author.

A tramp he would still remain, and he would soon be as dirty as slovenly, as improvident and as helpless as ever, no matter how hygienic or how pleasant his surroundings. The thing that would suffer most would be the temporary dwelling-place he had occupied and contaminated. So with the body of a child unschooled and untrained to healthy and hygienic rules of life and a proper sense of self-respect. The child must first be taught to appreciate, care for, and to improve its own bodily dwelling, and then all things else for health and happiness will be added unto it.

In his very thorough scheme of medical education for the prevention of disease, I am glad to note that Sir George includes physical training and " the application of physiology to physical exercise." But I would remind him that there are few schools where the children have not received or do not receive some form of physical training already, and still there remains with us disease. Why? Because physical education and physical culture, as a preventive and curative of disease, has not even yet come into its own, and while its hygienic value has been recognised since the time of Hippocrates and even before, medical men and the people in general have not yet realised that there is an actual science of remedial and preventive physical movement as well as a science of medicine, and that the former is, indeed, if anything, a more exact science than the latter.

USING EVERY BODILY MUSCLE.

For we know every voluntary muscle of the body, and it only remains for medical men to study just what is the exact physiological effect of the movement of any muscle or muscles on the organs, functions, systems and even cells of the body, and apply that knowledge in a scientific way, just as they do with medicine and drugs to-day. It is only because I have made this science an exclusive life-study and my experience is admittedly unique, that I have been able to prove these physical methods to be so successful in curing and preventing illness or disease in thousands of men, women and children.

The mistake, unfortunately, that is too often made is in the somewhat Procrustean method of forcing the individual to suit the exercise or physical movement or some special system of exercise and movements because doctors have not discovered how to supply just that balanced physical movement that would suit each individual, and especially each individual child, and as a separate and independent human entity.

UNREVEALED SECRETS OF THE BODY.

If medical men will study this subject as thoroughly, as deeply, and as scientifically as they have studied medicine and disease (as I believe they will and, indeed, must do in the future), they will be amazed at its wonderful possibilities in the treatment, cure, and prevention of disease. Physical therapeutics applied from the early days of childhood will yet play a much more prominent part in our warfare against disease, and in the prescription of physical movement the doctor of the future will study the subject of the living body, how to make and keep it healthy, and how to increase the sum of human health, rather than merely how to fight disease that might have been prevented or avoided. (Since this was written a remarkable article and letter on the value of physical treatment as a curative agent appeared in The Lancet. This is specially dealt with towards the end of this book.)

It is this study of the living body—that wonderful automatic machine, which in its marvellous intricacy, the complexity of its mechanism and its awe-inspiring mystery and grandeur, almost defies human intelligence and understanding and has still a million secrets to unfold—from a biological, physiological and psychological view-point that has been too long neglected by the medical profession, because the tradition of the profession has been mainly clinical, while pathology has, to a very considerable extent, usurped the place in the medical student's curriculum that rightly belongs to physiology.

It is my hope yet and very soon, too, to see a few more strong and independent medical thinkers, like Sir George Newman and Sir Bertrand Dawson, casting aside the burdensome impedimenta of ages-old tradition that have so long handicapped the profession, and a new orientation taking the place of the old which devoted too much attention to the dissection of the dead body and the study of a diseased one rather than to mastering the wonderful mechanism that, when properly regulated, directed and controlled, will keep the living body in health, increase its health, and give it that resistant power to disease which is its only sure and safe shield under all circumstances, in all climes and at all ages of life from the cradle to the grave.

A NEW MEDICAL STUDY.

The study of the establishment and maintenance of perfect balance of power in every part of body and brain is in itself a work of research besides which the study of medicine and disease will seem mean and insignificant to him who approaches it in a truly reverent spirit, as he must do if he is to unravel the great mystery of life and health, to fathom the secrets of this marvellous and Divinely created machine, and to woo it by patient devotion rather than to coerce it by violent methods, until it has no longer any confidences or reservations that conceal from us its real and most innermost self.

True, we are at present permitted occasionally to intrude behind the curtain, and to know something of what is going on there, but there is still a virgin mine of immeasurable and incalculable value as yet untouched, and, until now, beyond the ken of man. In physiology alone, there is much rich ore waiting to be crushed, and the exploitation of this one field will make us rich in knowledge beyond the dreams of men.

When man is taught from childhood to know and understand the many operations and activities of his body over which he can exercise a supreme and undivided control, subject only to Divine interposition and supremacy, he will have mastered one of the greatest lessons of life, and if he profits by it he need no longer remain familiar with disease, except through his own caprice, blasphemy or neglect. It is that lesson which the man of the future must be taught; and must begin to learn from early childhood at the feet of skilled, competent and experienced teachers. Our medical teachers and advisers will then have new ideals, their fundamental notions of medical science will be completely changed, they will prostrate themselves before the human body in its ascension towards the zenith of health rather than in its descent towards the nadir of disease. Thev will ask themselves not f what is disease and how can it be prevented or cured," but " what is health, how can it be attained and maintained," and they will find the answer in a full understanding of the supreme fact that life is movement, health is movement, and balanced physical movement is the prime factor in both.

In my next chapter I show, I think conclusively, how scientific physical movement as I mean it can alone give us this balance and resistant power to disease in modern times, and I explain in greater detail just what I mean by balanced and scientific movement.

CHAPTER VIII.

What is Scientific Physical Movement?

WHAT, it may naturally be asked, are the chief points of difference between scientific and unscientific methods of physical movement? What, again, is meant by balance and balanced movement?

These and similar questions will naturally arise in the mind of every inquiring reader, and it is my object here to answer them in such a way that no one can fail to follow my arguments and grasp my meaning. There are, I may say, many vital points of difference, as I will now strive to make quite clear to the reader.

The far-reaching influence and importance of the voluntary system to the economy of life and in the prevention of disease has never before been fully understood and realised, and without the primary recognition of this outstanding fact, physical exercise must fail to be scientific either in its conception or execution. Let me explain.

HEALTH BY DIVINE RIGHT.

The voluntary muscular system is the key that operates every conscious and sub-conscious bodily movement, and " winds up " what has been called " the human automaton," and it does so by the direction of our own brain and mind. It was, in fact, given to us by the Creator for the purpose of that balanced movement which is essential to healthy life, and which, as I have shown, was absolutely necessary for existence in primeval days.

Through it and through it alone we can reach and develop and strengthen in resistant power to disease every part of the body, so that each and all of us has, by Divine right, the freedom to choose for ourselves between health and disease, weakness and strength. That fact has not yet been fully grasped, and until it is, no physical exercise or training can ever succeed in building up a strong and disease-proof body. The fundamental fact of scientific and balanced physical movement may be tersely put as follows:—

The involuntary muscles and their component cells, and, indeed, all the cells of every organ of the body, are dependent entirely for their maintenance, health and well-being upon the voluntary muscular system just as a helpless child is dependent for its sustenance upon its mother. Only through it can we reach, move and make each cell and all the cells of the body equally strong, separately, collectively and in relationship to each other.

The recognition of this fact compels us, then, to the conclusion that the only certain and absolute way in which we can 'prevent disease, is to make and keep the body healthy, strong and powerfully resistant in each and all of its cells by the wise and balanced use of these voluntary muscles, because only through them can we develop and increase the strength and resistant power of all these cells against disease. By the movement of the voluntary muscles under our control we are, therefore, able to determine our own weakness or strength, and we can only build up a strong and disease-free body through the perfectly balanced and regulated physical movement of all the voluntary muscles, through this movement strengthening all the involuntary muscles and all the cells of the body in harmonious relationship. The directing and con- trolling power which we possess we also can develop and strengthen through the balanced movement and use of all the directing brain cells, employed in consciously " willing " the movement of any muscle or group of muscles, for the brain is a thing of tissue and blood just like the rest of the body, and every act of thinking or willing causes a material change in the brain cells, and develops them in power and strength.

IS DISEASE A SIN?

To no little extent, therefore, it is true to say that disease is a sin against our Creator, for our bodies have been placed entirely under our own control to make or mar them at will. That is the law which everyone should know, for ignorance of the law is no excuse and will not save a man or woman from inevitable and inexorable punishment in the form of physical weakness, ill-health or disease.

When I speak of balanced physical movement I mean, briefly, the use and development of each and every muscle or group of voluntary muscles in proportionate degree and strength, so that no muscle or muscle-cells will be stronger or weaker than others, but all will be moved, nourished and developed in harmonious balance and co-relationship. The importance of this in building up a disease-proof body cannot possibly be over-rated.

It is very important, therefore, to discriminate between physical movements conducted by scientific and exact methods and general methods of physical training or our familiar games and athletic sports, because an intelligent grasp of this distinction is essential to a full understanding of the remarkable claims I advance.

The methods that I describe here may for the sake of convenience be called a "system" (though, there is not and cannot be any strict systematising of movements, as each person must be dealt with according to individual age, needs, physical condition, etc.), of physical and constitutional education and re-education, that is intended to give us back once more that power of control over the mind, the nerves, and the voluntary muscles which man originally possessed in a state of nature, but which has largely departed from us through long civilisation and non-natural habits of life.

This self-control over our voluntary muscles was given us because by movement alone we can live healthfully, and balanced physical movement is essential to perfect constitutional health and strength and to the fortification of the body against disease. The method of utilising and developing each and all of the voluntary muscles in absolute balance, which I am advocating, will, I contend, give us back our splendid self-mastery, and is an essential feature of what I call scientific physical education and culture. The great difference between this and unscientific exercise in basic details I will show shortly.

LEARNING HOW TO BE HEALTHY.

Society in its present lowered physical condition requires some convenient and simple method of re-educating degenerate muscles and nerve centres, and of repairing and even re-constructing the somewhat dilapidated physical structure of the modern man, so as to regain perfect balance, co-ordination and control. But how? This is the question that naturally confronts us. Some of us have almost forgotten how to use and control our muscles and nerves to the best health advantage; more of us are painfully ignorant of their nature, use and possibilities; most 'people have yet to learn how they can, through the voluntary muscles, place the whole bodily system under a course of strict self-discipline, and so to bring about perfect team-work between all the cells of the body, which I show is possible only in this one way.

The muscles of the body may, for the sake of convenience, here be described as of two kinds, voluntary and involuntary, Over certain muscles of the body we have been given complete and direct mental control. Others, however, are directly beyond any effort of will. For instance, you can contract the muscles of an arm at will, increasing its substance and power by repetition of that contraction, but you cannot by the most superhuman effort of will directly increase the power of, say, the heart, which is, after all, only a large involuntary muscle.

You can, however, do so indirectly by gradually increasing its capacity to sustain effort through physical movements of the voluntary muscles, which bring into play all its involuntary muscles, including the heart. Briefly, the mere movement of any voluntary muscle brings also into play automatically other and involuntary muscles. This means that not only are the voluntary muscles directly under our own mental control developed and strengthened by movement, but that the involuntary muscles are also exercised and developed in association.

It means, however, more than this, for through the involuntary muscles again every individual cell of the body in all its parts, including the cells employed by the directing brain and the nervous system, can also be strengthened and developed in proportion by these movements, because you cannot develop one group of cells in the body without in some degree improving the physical condition of all the others.

NATURE'S "WEEDING OUT."

All the bodily cells, in short, must keep in step with the movement of the voluntary muscles or they will die through lack of movement and consequent innutrition. If, in response to the increased exertion demanded of them by the voluntary muscles, they are able to assimilate nutrition faster than they expend the force brought to them by the blood, they will become healthier and stronger and more reproductive. If waste exceeds repair, however, they will become weak and eventually die. The cells of the body must, in short, develop with the developing voluntary muscles especially when all are moved in perfect balance, or they are " weeded out " by the stern relentless laws of Nature, while the younger and fitter cells left will multiply more rapidly, producing, in their turn, still better cells of their own species, until every organ and muscle and system is perfect in every cell, and perfect balance is established and maintained between all the bodily cells.

God created man in the beginning—even the stoutest Darwinians agree that there is no such thing as spontaneous generation —but the process of evolution since his creation from the single protoplasmic cell to the many-celled man, as we know him to-day, was a process extending over incalculable thousands of years, though what may seem aeons to us would seem infinitesimal to the Creator, whose measure of Time is not a clock but Eternity.

From the very beginning, however, man was, as he still is, a being created and designed to live by movement, as was each individual cell of the billions of cells that compose his wonderful body and brain.

GIVING THE CELLS AN APPETITE.

Movement, as I have shown, is the great law of life throughout the Universe. In the human body, it may truly be said that nothing moves alone, and the slightest muscular action, voluntary or involuntary, is like the movement of a little wheel or cog of a wheel that immediately brings into action numerous other and larger wheels, or that like a pebble flung into a pond sends waves undulating even to its remotest corners. As I have already explained, the cells of the body, being mutually associated and inter-dependent, the movement of one or more implies movement in others also. For instance, you cannot flex the biceps of your arm without bringing millions of cells in various organs and systems into action.

This simple action, slight though it seems, used up the force supplied by the blood to the cells of which the muscles that made the movement are composed, and many muscles are employed in the act. Immediately, a call is made from the cells of the muscles directly moved, the circulatory and digestive systems and the blood hurry up the necessary supplies to make good this expenditure of force used in the movement. In simple English, all muscular movement sets up a demand from certain cells for food to replace waste.

To satisfy this demand, you eat, let us say, a ham sandwich. Numerous other cells are at once set moving to convert this bread and meat into an assimilable form, then to transport it by the blood not only to the voluntary muscles and muscle-cells moved, but also to the other cells of the body, which have also been called upon to work harder in preparing and transforming the food into a suitable form from which the various kinds of bodily cells can extract the nutrient suitable for the manufacture and maintenance of flesh, blood, bone and cartilage, nerve, muscle, tendon, ligament, and sinew, artery, vein and capillary, etc., in short, for each and every tissue of the various systems and organs.

In other words, the one simple voluntary movement of the muscles necessary to contract the biceps of the arm provides employment for millions and millions of living cells, that must " get busy " and " keep moving " to repair the waste caused by this apparently simple muscular effort.

WHAT MOVING A MUSCLE MEANS.

All these cells, as a result of this voluntary movement are, in short, developed, strengthened, increased in vigour and become more reproductive of other cells, because they themselves have to move more actively to do the added work, and consequently demand and receive more nourishment, air and the chemical elements essential to life. They breed faster, because more working cells are required to assist in this labour of life, and this multiplication of cells especially takes place in the voluntary muscles. In this way, the whole bodily community of cell-workers and cell-fighters is improved in individual health and vigour.

If this can be accomplished by one simple muscular movement such as that described, it is easy to understand then that when we exercise all the voluntary muscles in equal degree and balance as I suggest, 'perfectly balanced strength is established everywhere among all the cells of the body, and this perfectly balanced strength everywhere is the secret of health, resistant power, and freedom, therefore, from disease.

In such a simple act as I have described, of course, the results would scarcely be perceptible, but think what can be accomplished by a great number and variety of such movements, if applied scientifically and continually to the body from childhood, bringing into play in absolute balance every voluntary and involuntary muscle of the body and all the cells of the body in association.

Is it not evident, then, that the fine and vigorous muscular condition of the external and visible body when so developed is and must be the mirror of the internal body, and that the superficial and visible muscles of the body must give us a fair index to the internal organic condition of the body.

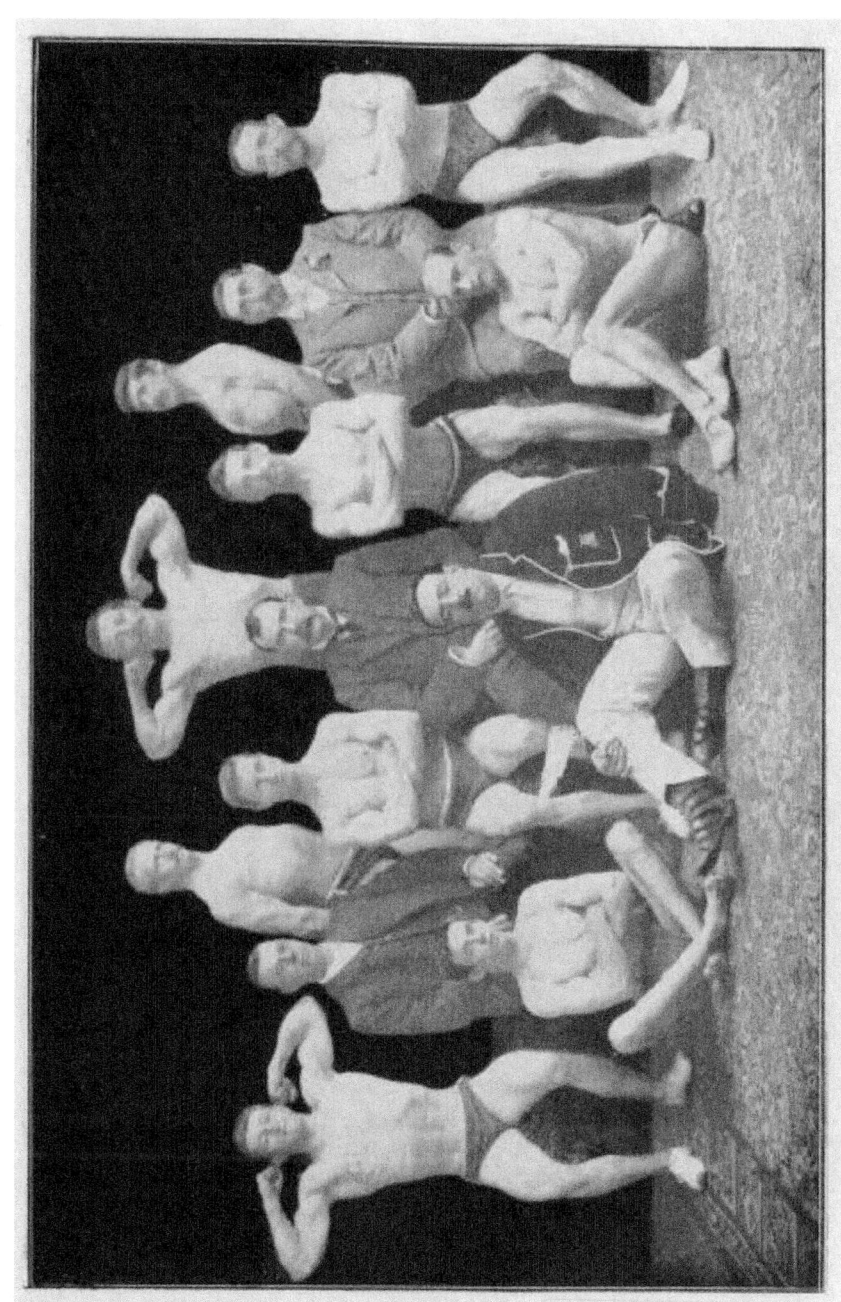

A fine class of Colonials who have been enlisted in the cause of physical progress by the example of the Author, and their instructor.

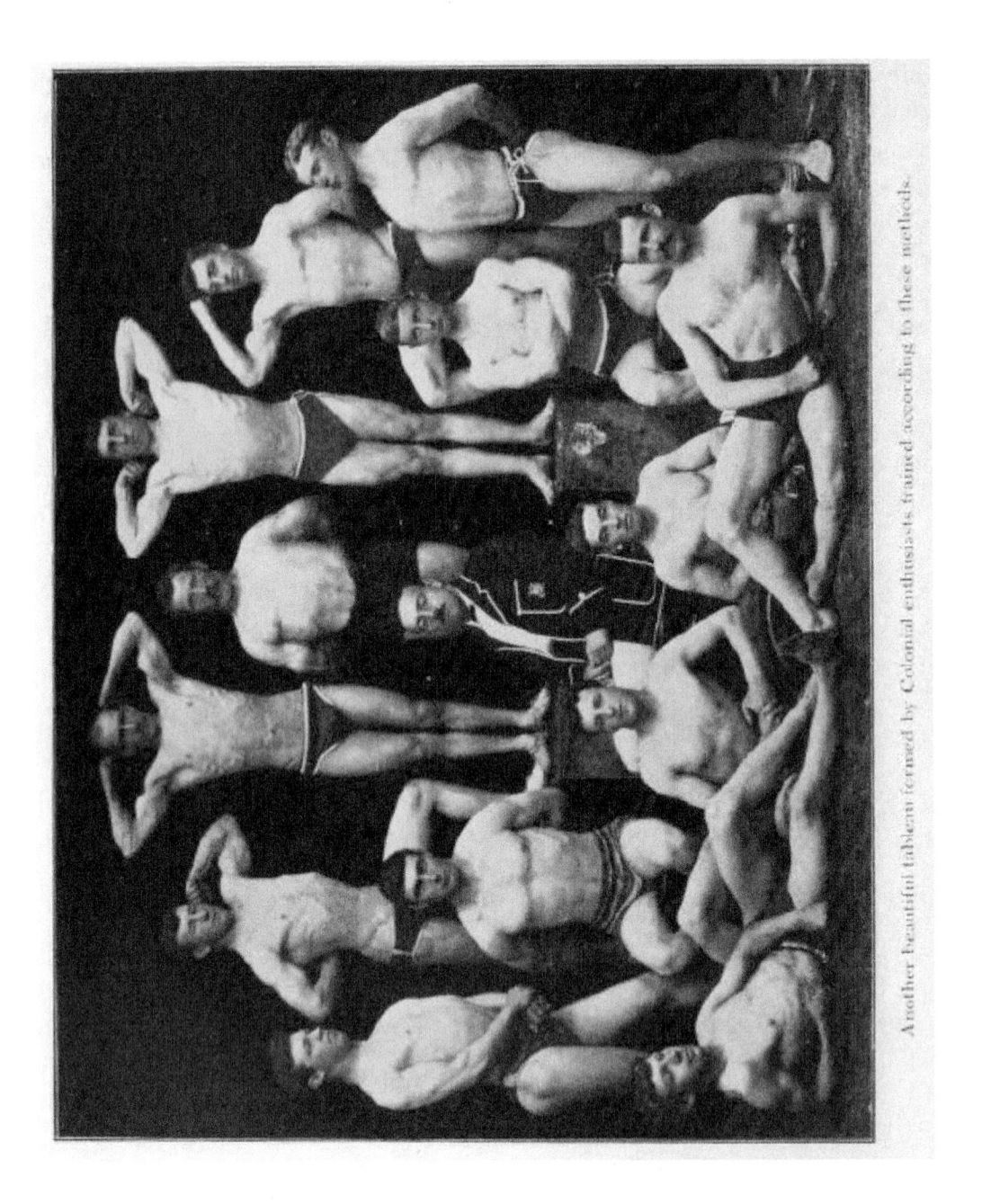

Another beautiful tableau formed by Colonial enthusiasts trained according to these methods.

BALANCED AND UNBALANCED STRENGTH.

Circumstances, of course, vary and are influenced by many considerations, and it might very easily, of course, be possible for a man with an abnormal development of some muscles to have, say, occasional functional disturbances in other parts of the body, because the excessive development of these muscles deprives, to a certain extent, these other parts of the body of their fair and equal share of nourishments. The cells of these specially developed muscles become pampered, as it were, in comparison with, and at the expense of other cells elsewhere, which explains their hyperdevelopment. This is why it is essential to the upbuilding of a really disease-proof body that all, or nearly all, the voluntary muscles are given movement in due balance and relationship, or, otherwise, there must be weak spots somewhere liable at any moment to succumb to disease.

A trained professional pugilist, or other champion in any form of sport, might, for instance, though magnificently muscular in appearance, and apparently healthy and strong, be an easy prey to disease, simply through the want of physical and organic balance, and the over-development of certain muscles to the detriment of others. What is generally regarded as a strong man might be weak in the sense I use, i.e., weak tending towards disease, unless his strength were perfectly balanced in every part; and the strongest man in some particular direction need not necessarily be the healthiest or the most disease-proof, unless his strength is in perfect balance in every part of his body.

Again, even the most perfect type of all-round muscular manhood might be prostrated with some slight functional trouble temporarily, such as, say, indigestion, through worry or tainted food, or some other cause, without any serious effect showing on his muscular development for some time, but if long continued, the superficial muscles would soon begin to lose both size and quality, as the internal organism also deteriorated through the degenerative effect of the lack of movement of certain cells in an organism that demands and needs movement for healthy existence.

OUTWARD MAN MIRRORS THE INTERNAL MAN.

On the other hand, you would never expect to; see a confirmed dyspeptic develop into a good muscular type, no matter what he were to eat or what exercise he took, until by special physical movements he first developed and strengthened the particular muscles associated with digestion and assimilation of food, or, as I explain in another chapter, until his weak and disordered digestive system were replaced by a new and healthy one.

You will agree then, that to a very considerable degree, at least, the external and visible man proclaims the internal and invisible man, and that only the carefully balanced movement of the voluntary muscles to suit each individual's special needs and physical requirements can build up an internally and externally healthy and disease-free body.

Glance, for instance, at the contrasting types of men, women and children in this book, and ask yourself which is the more likely to escape disease, those whose fine visible and balanced muscular development proclaims a life of balanced physical movement or those weak, almost muscle-less, and flabby persons who have neglected or innocently transgressed the law of healthy life, and whose photos are but typical of the average human being to-day. The grand and visible physical development in symmetry and balance of the one mirrors a body as healthy organically within as the puny and ill-balanced physique of the other may be safely assumed to indicate internal disease or weakness that tends towards disease.

Through the physical movement of the voluntary muscles, then, we can develop the individual health. Thus through voluntary and balanced physical movement, we can have a permanent cellular army of defence and offence against disease, strong both individually and collectively. And the greater the number of cells, and the greater their individual and collective strength, the more 'powerful the body is to resist and conquer disease, and the greater your vital reserves.

A PROCESS OF CELLULAR EVOLUTION.

In the case of children, such a method of physical reconstruction will not only give us healthier children in the present generation, but must progressively improve the " breed " of children in each generation, by cellular evolution, and scientific methods of training both body and mind in perfect balance will give us perfectly healthy and disease-proof men and women, physically and mentally. When the present ignorance of body and health culture has thus been dissipated, we will come to regard disease as a crime rather than a misfortune, except in very rare cases where accident or some unavoidable " act of God," to use a well-known legal phrase, intervened.

Physiologically, then, a life of physical movement and activity in harmonious bodily balance, such as man was ordained to live from the beginning, and to which we must return as far as is conformable with modern conditions of life, means the upbuilding of more and better cells in every system of the body, each and all of which are more able to resist and defeat disease. Let me now explain this, as promised, in greater physiological detail.

The movement of the voluntary muscles and their cells, for instance, consumes or destroys the force contained in the cells and at once enlists the services of the digestive cells to renew it and make good the waste, as I have just shown, because the muscle cells through this movement and expenditure of force naturally demand more nourishment and the digestive cells, for the same reason, also demand more food to enable them to do the work necessary to supply these vital essentials. To replenish the waste of the cells of the voluntary muscles, the chemical cells have also to provide chemical elements that have been consumed by the movement, and these too, must in turn, be better nourished and oxygenated. The voluntary muscular movement also calls upon the heart cells to pump the blood faster through its channels, upon the cells of the lungs to breathe quicker and deeper, and in other ways, upon the cells of the liver, kidneys, intestines, skin, and, in short, every system and organ, so that all of these, through the voluntary muscles receive that physical movement which is essential for their existence and well-being, demand and receive more food and become better nourished, stronger, and more efficient, while their waste and poisonous products are more freely excreted.

They also become more capable of multiplying their species faster, and of an ever-increasingly better quality, until the limit of physical perfection in reached in every part of the body, and the body, is made far too strong in all its cells and tissues to fall before disease. Even the directing brain and nerve cells, as I have said, are developed by this scientific muscular movement for the brain cells controlling and directing these movements have to send a message along the nerve routes to the muscles implicated, and the directing brain and nerve cells are themselves thus developed and strengthened by movement. All the brain cells, in fact, are stimulated by these movements through the increased flow of rapidly changing blood recharged continuously with fresh supplies of food and air to the brain, so that such balanced movement is beneficial alike both to mind and body.

THE POWER THAT RESISTS DISEASE.

The great value, therefore, of physical movement in balance that employs each and every voluntary muscle of the body, and certain directing cells of the brain, must be apparent after this explanation, even to one who has little or no knowledge of anatomy or physiology; while, conversely, it must be evident that lack of movement in any part leads inevitably to the decay and death of many cells, lowers the combative efficiency, individually and collectively, of the bodily community, depletes the numerical strength of the cellular army of workers and fighters, thus rendering it in time an easy prey to disease.

Health and strength, indeed, simply mean that the body has a populous and efficient community of living cells, workers and fighters, all equal in strength and vitality, sufficient in number and collectively and individually powerful enough in vitality to resist and defeat disease. In other words, health means resistant power to disease, and resistant power is simply the perfect balance and strength in every cell of the body which ensures a high reserve of vitality. Disease, on the other hand, shows that the cells &re either not sufficient in number or not sufficiently healthy and strong in themselves individually or jointly or are unbalanced in strength in one or more parts, with not sufficient vigour and fighting power to defeat the enemy in the part or parts attacked.

Without balanced physical movement and the resultant balanced physical fitness of all the cells, the body must, indeed, become " an unweeded garden," for it will also lack perfect internal and organic balance.

VALUE OF AMBIDEXTERITY.

Let me explain now what I mean by perfect physical and organic balance. I mean that first within the body itself there must be a correct balance between assimilation and elimination, between organ and function and muscle and nerve, between the mental, nervous and muscular systems, between each and every species of bodily cells, between all the cells of any particular species of cells ' between every cell in every part of the body, and, finally, that nice adjustment and total adaptation of the body to its environment all of which ensures perfect health and freedom from disease. The failure of this balance in any one or more parts means the loss of balance and imperfect adjustment to environment, and leaves the body or some part of the body open to disease.

Lack of balance in any part means, then, disproportionate development and strength between one or more species of cells and the rest, because through lack of balance the food is not equally distributed and equally consumed, which creates weakness in one part in comparison with others, and so throws the whole machinery of the body out of balance.

How or why, it may naturally be asked, is the food not equally distributed and consumed through lack of balance? In the first place, food is sent by Nature where it is most needed after any movement is carried out with inevitable expenditure of force, and the amount of supplies necessary for any cell or cells is determined by the force such cells expend in movement. The less the force spent in any physical movement by any cells the less food and air required to make good the waste. And, remember, it is not always the actual feat performed that causes the greater destruction of this force and leads to an increased supply of food and air, but rather the effort relatively necessary to perform any feat, and the force actually consumed in the movement

A trained weight-lifter can lift, say, 200 lbs. with less effort and less expenditure of force than an untrained and weaker man can lift 100 lbs., but the extra effort and expenditure of the latter would bring greater supplies to the cells used in his case than in the former to replace the extra expenditure. The relative effort and expenditure of force in the latter case is much greater than in the former, and the cells, in consequence, receive more supplies of food and air than the cells of the former, though both get food and air in proportion according to the amount of force consumed by the movement.

To make this clearer, take the muscle of the right arm as an instance. In most people to-day the right arm is naturally stronger than the left. Now, supposing exactly the same number of movements had to be performed by both arms alike. It might naturally be supposed that both would continue to develop equally, and that the right arm would always be the stronger as it was at the beginning of the movements. This, however, is not so if the movements are scientifically carried out, that is, with the maximum of effort and mental concentration on the muscles moved.

In the first place, Nature sets a limit to the development of power in a muscle. Now, the right arm being almost invariably stronger will reach that limit first, provided both arms carry out exactly the same movements and number of movements daily. Let us say there are 25 movements for each arm with a 2 lb. dumb-bell. The cells of the left arm being weaker than those of the right will have to make a far greater effort and expenditure of force to move that 2 lb. weight the same number of times than those of the right arm. In fact, the cells of the left arm are doing work and consuming force equal to the weight of lifting, say, 3, 4, or 5 lbs. compared with the effort the right arm is called upon to make, while the cells of the right arm do not need to expend force in anything like the same ratio as they, being stronger, do the work easily and with less effort and less destruction of force.

The result is that the cells of the left arm having more waste to be repaired through this extra expenditure will receive from bounteous Nature more supplies of food and air to build up more and better tissue in its place and even to build it stronger than before, through exactly the same movement or number of movements. This, too, will continue until the left arm becomes equal in power to the right. When Nature has re-established the balance between them, the cells of both arms will receive equal supplies, because the effort and expenditure of force will now be equal (as both arms are now equally strong), so long as the same movements and number of movements are continued with both arms and the same weight lifted with both.

Now this applies to every voluntary muscle of the body also and the cells of all the voluntary muscles, and we have seen how these muscles and muscle cells are the keys that wind up the whole involuntary machinery of life. When, therefore, we move all the muscles in balance the weaker muscles and cells being called upon to expend more force than the other and stronger ones are continually receiving greater supplies of food and air than the others, and are thus gradually made stronger and to multiply in greater number, producing always better cells of their own species, until all the cells of the voluntary muscles and through them the cells of every part of the body are developed, or, as it were, evolved in perfectly balanced and proportionate strength up to the limit set by Nature and as Nature intended them to be, leaving no weak spots anywhere to succumb to disease. This is what I describe here as a body developed in perfectly balanced strength, where each voluntary muscle and its cells are developed to their maximum power, as are the involuntary muscles and their cells, and all in due proportion and harmonious relationship to one another, with consequently increased resistant power to disease, and, indeed, disease-proof.

It will be seen, therefore, that the physical movement applied to any part of the body means its better nutrition, better oxygenation and greater freedom from waste and poisonous contamination, and that balanced physical movement is the pivot upon which depends the equal and balanced supply and distribution of nutriment and oxygen, and upon which every organ and system and cell rely for their healthy freedom from waste and toxic matter.

Now, I merely use the illustration of the two arms just described for the purpose of making quite clear to every reader the physiology of balanced physical movement, but, of course, this does not touch the very important question of correct diagnosis and the scientific and successful prescription of physical movement for one who is ill or diseased or weak in some part of the body towards disease. This is a much more difficult matter, for naturally the personal equation enters into the calculation. Now let me again, to simplify matters,, take the same illustration as before. As it is now evident that the cells in any muscle, organ, limb, or part of the body are nourished, developed and made to multiply more rapidly in proportion to the effort and expenditure of force made by any given number of movements, so long as these are not carried to the point of fatigue and fatigue toxins generated, the food and air taken into the body to nourish these cells would, as I have shown, be equally divided when there is the same expenditure of force. So, to accelerate both the consumption of cellular force and the consequent nutrition of the weaker cells of the left arm, it would be necessary to prescribe a greater number of movements in their case. This is what I mean when I speak in my next chapter of accelerating metabolism. The stronger cells of the right arm would have only to be given sufficient movement to keep them strong and healthy for the elimination of waste and poisonous matter, and would naturally require less nourishment in return because of their less expenditure of force. So, by careful prescription, the share of the nourishment that would otherwise go to the stronger cells of the right arm in equal proportion, can be partly diverted for the benefit of the weaker cells, in proportion to the force they are expending or destroying. This also applies to every muscle and every cell of the body as I have just explained.

Here, then, enters the delicate and difficult problem of diagnosis. No man should be better qualified for this diagnosis and prescription than a medical man, for he has already a good knowledge of diagnosing and treating disease, and a sound knowledge of anatomy, physiology and pathology, but, unfortunately, the medical profession has not given any study to the subject of physical therapeutics, which is now fully explained in these pages for the first time.

In fact, up to now, nobody has been able to explain clearly and fully the physiological and pathological value of physical movement from the cellular point of view, for the simple reason that no one has ever before made it the subject of deep and exclusive study. In a general way, the value of exercise has been appreciated and recognised for ages, but its power to promote cellular reconstruction and cellular function, with improved metabolism and the continual evolution of better and better cells, has never yet been understood. Yet it is to the cell that we must ultimately look for the prevention and eradication of disease, for it is only by making cells so uniformly strong and healthy that they will not become diseased in themselves or succumb to disease microbes from without, that we can ever hope to banish disease entirely from the human body.

The cell holds the secret of humanity's immunity from disease, and it is this microscopic speck of living matter millions of times multiplied that constitutes the human body in all its organs, parts and systems, and through which alone we can solve the riddle of the ages since the dawn of civilisation, viz., of how to again rehabilitate the human body in all its pristine physical grandeur and freedom from disease of every kind. Until medical men realise this, and understand that by physical movement alone, scientifically applied, can we reach each and every cell, give it the movement ft needs to live, and so reconstruct the whole cellular body and evolve a body disease-immune by making its every cell immune they must not expect to prescribe physical movement successfully.

Before prescribing physical movements, the patient's condition or disease must be thoroughly and most accurately diagnosed, for some diseases naturally of themselves must largely determine the nature and number of movements to be prescribed. Some knowledge of the patient's family history may also, in some cases, be advisable, for the purpose of noting any inherited weakness towards disease.

Accurate information must also be obtained as to the patient's age, occupation (very important, especially in neurasthenic cases, to regulate expenditure of energy), physical condition (with special observation of the state of the heart), blood pressure, on arteries and veins, state of the nervous system, etc., before prescribing any movements. Then, again, very great skill, experience and care is necessary, to prescribe just such movements as will exactly meet each individual's requirements, to keep such movements always subjective to the state of the heart and the nervous system, also to understand how to grade and vary the movements and the number of movements to suit each case, and in accordance with a patient's progress and improvement. The exact physiological influence and sphere of physiological influence of each and every movement on organ, function and cell must be known and understood, and, indeed, a knowledge and study of man from a biological, anatomical, physiological, pathological, and psychological viewpoint. Such a subject may well, to use Dr Sir George Newman's phrase, be in " the very vanguard of physical therapeutics," and that is why I suggest in this book that it should be added to every student's curriculum, for it is a subject which doctors and students have yet to master.

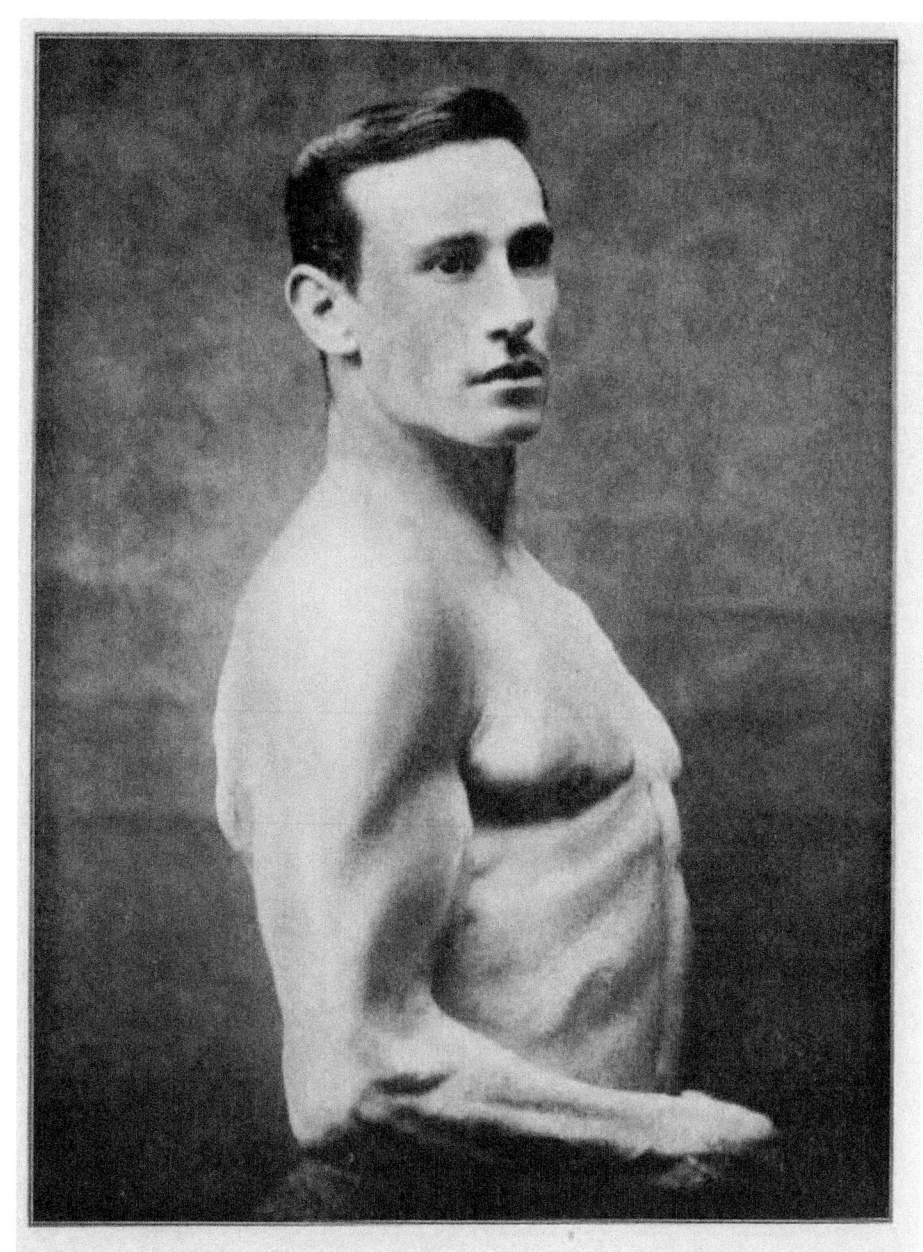

A study in balance. The type of manhood we want to see, and which we can have by the methods of physical education advocated. Weaklings are not likely to spring from such a parent stock. The photo is of Mr. E. Powell, of Dublin.

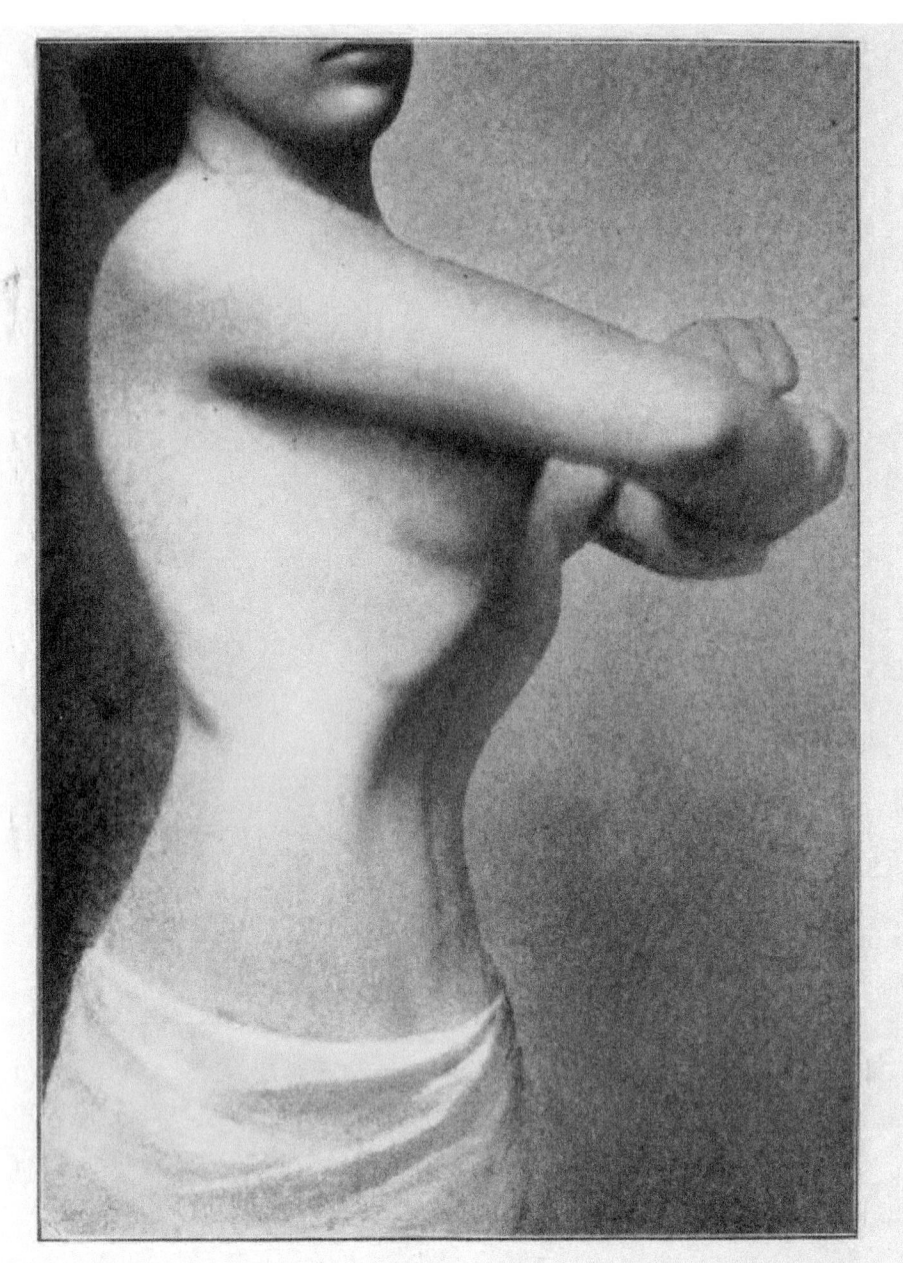

A MODERN VENUS.
Type of woman whose body has been developed in the scientific way described here. This is the feminine type the State needs for the mothering of children who will be a credit and a source of strength to the nation.

MOVEMENT MUST NOT BE SUB-CONSCIOUS.

Physical education and bodily culture such as is described here, demands, in the first place, organised knowledge of the living body and all its requirements, at least in a strictly physical sense, with the skilful application of such knowledge by qualified and competent persons, preferably by medical men themselves or under trained medical direction, and the intelligent employment by the individual of muscles under his own control, so as to cause them to act upon the involuntary muscles that are responsible for all those internal bodily activities and movements, which are implied in the word function.

The doctor who employs this method of physical therapeutics must know the exact number and relationship of movements necessary for any muscle or group of muscles to secure or restore perfect balance internally and externally.

The human body has only so, many voluntary muscles, each having its own special duty in the body, capable of a certain number and variety of movements (though these, of course, can be blended in many combinations) and it should always be possible, therefore, for any qualified medical man, with a little study and experience, to select, vary and combine any or all of these movements of the voluntary muscles as required to suit each or any individual, and to teach and develop every individual cell of the body, or specific groups of cells to restore balance. It will thus be seen how far-reaching must the study of this subject be.

These voluntary movements can be applied locally or generally as needed in each individual case, for no two individuals are alike owing to the varied conditions of civilised life. The movements must be selected, combined, varied and graduated, and so applied as to ensure a healthy balance everywhere, while at the same time enabling the pupil or patient to put by a sufficient and ample reserve of vitality to meet unexpected demands and emergencies.

When physical movement is thus prescribed to suit each individual, and afterwards carried out as I describe, it cannot fail to lead to life on a higher, healthier, and, therefore, happier plane. By such physical movement, we can regain lost weight, lost muscular power, lost nerve tone, improve every bodily function, and toughen the bodily tissue and fibre so as to make it impregnable against disease.

But voluntary physical movement may be carried to the point of fatigue, overstrain and exhaustion, or movements may be ill-chosen, ill-arranged, and too severe for the physical condition of the pupil or patient. This makes the most exact individual study and diagnosis always advisable before physical movement is prescribed for either adults or children, and explains why remedial or curative movements, at least, should preferably be prescribed by one who has thoroughly studied and mastered the whole subject of producing a perfectly balanced organism by balanced physical movement.

When we realise then, how important it is to obtain and maintain balanced strength among all the cells not only of the body but of the brain, it is scarcely necessary to point out the value of training either a child or an adult to the equal use of both arms and legs and to the equal employment and development of all the muscles on both sides of the body. Ambidextrous development, indeed, is absolutely necessary in establishing perfect balance between the body and the cells of both lobes of the brain, for unless both sides of the body are equally developed both the brain and the body must be imperfectly developed and balanced.

The training of the muscles of both the right and left sides of the body not only helps to ensure better bodily balance everywhere, but means the development physically of a stronger and better balanced brain, making the acquisition and assimilation of knowledge and the exercise of self-control, both easier and more perfect. However, this important phase of educational physical culture I have dealt with at greater length in another chapter of this book.

IMPORTANCE OF INDIVIDUAL TREATMENT.

The scientific education of the voluntary muscles must be carried out so gradually that progress is almost imperceptible.

Milo learnt to lift the ox, because he first began to lift it when it was a new-born calf and continued to lift it daily as it grew and increased in weight. An athlete does not attempt to win a long-distance race without a course of carefully graduated training to improve his strength, pace and stamina if he expects to prove a victor. And muscle or muscular power, never for a moment forget, is just as essential for life and perfect health as for feats of strength, speed and stamina, and can only be developed in balance by the judiciously balanced movement of all or nearly all the voluntary muscles.

It is most important that these voluntary movements are never allowed to become automatic or sub-conscious, as they would lose their effect, just like work repeated in a mechanical way day after day. The pupil or patient must be taught and trained to concentrate his or her mind on the muscle or muscles brought into play by each movement or movements, and to put his or her utmost effort into each and every moment as it. is made, and also to understand the object and results of such movement, for this also develops the directing power of the mind and teaches a person how to regain complete control over the muscle or muscles moved. (The reader will find this subject very fully explained from the curative point of view in the chapter entitled "How and Why Scientific Physical Movement Cures Disease.")

EXERCISING MIND AND MUSCLE.

I want particularly to emphasise the importance of this intense mental concentration on the muscle or muscles employed while making any movement, and also of exerting the maximum of possible muscular power in making it, for this is what I may call the ABC of such a system as I am now advocating for general use.

To make quite clear, then, what I mean by the maximum of effort when contracting any muscle or muscles, let me give a homely example, one which, indeed, gave me the germinal idea from which the methods I advocate have only been extended and elaborated.

Watch a baby as it awakes from sleep. Its first movements are to stretch and yawn, putting every ounce of unrestricted effort into the movement. Probably this is done once or twice before it is fully awake, and its little arms tremble from the amount of effort put forth in the sub-conscious contraction of practically every muscle in its body. Indeed, it is not too much to say that every voluntary muscle is contracted to the fullest extent.

Now, why does Nature give us this instinct even from childhood? There must be a reason, for Nature is essentially logical and never trusts to guesswork. The reason is this. During the night, waste and toxic matter has accumulated in the system, and Nature prompts this natural contraction or exercise of all the muscles, to help in its elimination. That natural and involuntary contraction of all the muscles, though only carried out once or twice, achieves Nature's object by squeezing all this toxic matter and helping in its elimination.

But that contraction was sub-conscious and was directed by Nature. I want to see men and women taught from childhood how to contract their muscles consciously in the same way, and with full mental concentration upon the muscles or set of muscles moved, and how to do it on a much larger scale, employing all the muscles or any muscle or separate group of muscles as desired, to bring the body into perfect balance in and between all its parts. I have no " system " in the meaning of that word, as generally understood when applied to physical exercise. What, for convenience, I call a " system " is based entirely on Nature and Nature's laws, and my part is only the enlargement and broader application of the simple and instructive act performed by the baby in its cradle.

The " system " I advocate is simply the outcome of this and similar observations and of a life-long study of Nature and especially of human nature, and I am merely doing what modern engineers have done with the waters of Niagara, harnessing Nature for the benefit of humanity, and finding in a baby's cradle the secret of health just as Newton discovered the law of gravitation in the simple falling of an apple from the tree.

HEALTHY ACTIVITY IN "TABLOID" FORM.

Moreover, it is only in this way that it is possible to provide mankind to-day with the equivalent of his primeval physical activity in a compressed or tabloid form just as Nature provides it for the baby.

Taking my cue, as it were from Nature, I have studied Nature's methods and laws and applied Nature's lessons in a scientific way. Man has not yet surpassed Nature in any sphere of life, and just as our greatest inventions have been anticipated by Nature so in the prevention and healing of disease the doctor must learn from Nature and adapt and utilise her methods. When medical men know and understand how to employ natural physical movement either locally or generally as required so as to build up a body in perfect balance everywhere or to restore an ill-balanced one, they will know and understand how to conquer, prevent, and eliminate disease.

When men and women have re-learnt the very old lesson of contracting and relaxing any or all of the voluntary muscles in the manner I have described, the contraction being made with the maximum of effort, as Nature prompts in the cradled baby, they will have mastered the true secret of health and the best method of combating disease in a natural and tabloid form. They will have learnt how to extend still further and apply the great natural law which is the basis of healthy life, and to provide compensation for the physical inactivity inseparable from modern civilised habits.

Only in this way, too, can a person be taught to regain lost control over the muscles and the nervous system, and only in this way can he or she learn how to completely relax muscles and nerves in equal degree to the contraction as thoroughly as does the healthy baby when it lies down to sleep. For, as the relaxation of a muscle should be equal in degree to its contraction, it will be seen at once how important is this intense mental concentration and muscular effort in teaching one also how to completely relax a muscle or group of muscles completely, or all the muscles when and as desired, while it is only by such fully conscious mental and muscular effort that we can also reach and develop the brain cells controlling and directing the muscles, and sympathetically the cells and nerve-centres which give us control over the nervous system, thus leading to the reestablishment of that complete control over the whole body which has almost become extinct in the human species.

Children, of course, must be most carefully educated to this power of maximum effort and mental concentration on the muscles moved, as I describe later in the chapter on " The Machinery of National Physical Training." In this way, both children and adults can be taught to completely relax muscles and nerves at the direction of their mind and will, and attain to that condition of repose and serenity which is the high-tide mark of health.

THE REPOSE OF PERFECT HEALTH.

Tennyson was something of a physiologist, and when he spoke of " that repose which stamps the class of Vere de Vere," he uttered a deep physiological truth, for such self-mastery indicated the possession of a standard of health rarely to be found in the poor or even in the nouveau riche, but which comes from centuries-old habits and standards of healthful living and life, such as I hope may yet become the common inheritance of all.

Let me now show by a simple illustration the value of conscious movement, such as I describe, as distinct from comparatively sub-conscious and imperfect physical movement which is the kind of physical exercise usually taught and practised to-day. The blacksmith whose daily labour calls upon him to swing the heavy hammer which, in the familiar words of the poet, makes " the muscles of his brawny arms as strong as iron bands," does so sub-consciously, because his mind is not concentrated on the muscles moved in the operation but is engrossed wholly with the work that has to be accomplished.

The movements, therefore, are sub-conscious, and the cells of the muscles employed are only developed in strength sufficient to perform that work. As a result, the strength of the blacksmith remains stationary, after a certain stage has been reached, and the cells of the muscles used do not continue increasing in number, youthfulness or vigour, because they are allowed to live long after they have reached and passed their highest standard of efficiency.

PUTTING YOUR MIND INTO YOUR MUSCLES.

On the other hand, if another man carried out similar movements, even for a much shorter time, with a much lighter hammer, or even without any hammer or other weight, but with his mind fully concentrated on the muscles moved and full muscular effort throughout each movement, this conscious movement would develop and go on developing his muscles until he became stronger even than the blacksmith. In his case, there would be the continual birth of new, younger and stronger cells, and this would continue just as long as he continued this conscious movement as I have described, until he reached his highest possible physical standard so far as these particular muscles were concerned. After a time he would be able to wield a much heavier hammer than the blacksmith, because there would be a continuous supply of young and more vigorous cells each better and stronger in their generation than the preceding one. This is what I refer to when I speak of cellular evolution.

But if this man, in turn, began to carry out these movements sub-consciously like the blacksmith this would no longer be the case, and his strength would decline to just sufficient to carry out the work automatically. The conscious movement of the muscles keeps the cells always in their youthful prime, and keeps " breeding," as it were, cells of an ever-increasing vigour and quality.

In both these cases, however, this particular development of one set of muscles while others are neglected must result in lack of balance both externally and internally, as I have already explained, and it is only when all the voluntary muscles are thus moved consciously and in balance that we can produce the perfectly balanced and disease-free body.

Of course, once this natural and perfect balance has been obtained, games, sports and even physical labour will, to some extent, go far to maintain this balance, especially if one has been so schooled from childhood as I suggest. But it is always preferable in modern life that, in addition, each and all of the voluntary muscles should be given a few contractions daily in turn, no matter what the nature of one's sports or occupation may be.

WHERE GAMES AND SPORTS FAIL.

You will see, then, how vitally important this conscious concentration on the muscle or muscles used is in any system of physical education, for without it there can be no truly scientific foundation. Here, too, is another difference between the training I am advocating and physical exercise in which the movements are carried out in a sub-conscious and ineffective manner. In the same way does the method I advocate differentiate scientific physical education and training for games and sports in which the mind is centred mainly on the game itself or on the winning of the game and not on the movements that the individual is performing in the game or the muscles that are performing the movements. The movements, in fact, are not carried out consciously as physical exercise, and so the cells do not develop in balance as they would do by the scientific and balanced movement of all the voluntary muscles.

In games, only such muscles as are necessary in the games are called into play, and, consequently, certain cells employed in the muscles more moved than others are better nourished and developed while others suffer neglect. Thus certain cells, as in the case of the blacksmith, remain stationary, while others through lack of movement are deprived of necessary nourishment and exercise. Conscious and balanced movement of all the muscles alone, or, at least, nearly all those muscles under our control, will develop the body in harmonious balance and so make it impregnable to disease. It is not for me to condemn games or gymnastics, but merely to say that helpful though all or any of these may be, as a recreation for those who are physically fit to take part in them, they are not to be recommended either for adults or children, until at least a child or adolescent has reached a certain physical and constitutional standard of fitness and health, as harm may result in many cases through over-strain and physical efforts of an unbalanced nature. In modern life, time does not permit the expenditure of time necessary to indulge in games sufficiently varied to exercise all the bodily muscles, and indeed the physical body to-day would not be able to stand the physical strain.

REBUILDING THE NATION'S CHILDREN.

All that we can do, therefore, is to enlist scientific knowledge, thought and experience, and to adopt methods by which each individual citizen, from childhood to old age, can obtain balanced physical movement, easily and without interference with his or her daily circumstances of life, and atone, as far as in humanly possible, for the deficiency due to the enforced conditions of modern civilised life. Such a method must be scientific in its conception, organisation and administration. It must be based on a sound knowledge of anatomy, physiology, and pathology, and it must be State encouraged, if not, indeed, State endowed, as I have already pointed out, and have behind it the loyal support and service of the whole medical profession, and, indeed, of the whole nation.

It must take a liberal and sweeping view, not only of the actual physical welfare of citizens, but also of those well-meaning efforts for the better conditioning of the people in every way which are auxiliary to it. Over and above all, however, those responsible for such a system of education must ever keep in mind the outstanding fact that man himself only lives, moves and has his being by and through muscular movement, that lack of balanced movement means physical deterioration and disease, and that to approximate more and more closely as far as possible to natural primitive life and physical activity is to diminish and prevent disease and finally to eliminate it altogether.

By these means, too, it is, I argue, possible to literally and actually rebuild a new body, a new system, organ, muscle or limb by operating in conjunction with the natural changes ever going on in the body, as described in the following chapter.

CHAPTER IX.
The Physiology of Bodily Re-construction.

As everyone with even a slight knowledge of physiology knows, all the cells and tissues of the body are in a state of perpetual unrest and change, so much so that we are literally re-born every few years by the regular and continuous birth of new bodily cells. Our whole future health and well-being are dependent entirely on the nature and character of the new cells to which birth is ever being given.

It is my purpose now to show that by the application of specific and balanced voluntary muscular movements, in a scientific way such as I have just described, we can steadily improve all these cells in quality and increase them in number and efficiency until we attain to a cellular perfection that makes the whole body in all or any of its parts free from disease or any weakness that would make it a victim to disease.

The lightest thought, the slightest movement, the most casual feeling or emotion causes waste in the brain or body, and this waste has to be removed from the system or it would remain and putrefy, tending towards illness and disease through what medical men call auto-toxication, while new material also has to be supplied in its place. This work of elimination, like all the work of the body, has to be done by muscles or muscular cells, partly under our direct control and partly reached only through the involuntary muscles. In its place, food and air supply, or should supply through the blood, new material containing all the elements of which the cells are composed in equal if not greater quantity, to repair and make good the waste. For we now know that the cell itself is not destroyed by muscular movement, but only the force contained in and brought to it by the blood.

THE RECONSTRUCTION OF THE BODY.

Now I am going to demonstrate my truly amazing claim, viz., that by balanced physical movement of the voluntary muscles, scientifically applied, we can re-build not only a new but a better body in every part, but also a better body than we actually had at birth, and quite as strong in every way as when man was first created in the very prime of Jus existence. Mow ! By building the new body with better cells through what I may call conscious evolution—that is, the conscious application of all our knowledge and experience gained through the centuries, and scientifically organised—to these ever-changing cells of the body. I hope also to be able to show that it is now possible for us to build up better, healthier and disease-defying bodies with much less and more agreeable physical effort than our ancestors, because our present knowledge enables us to apply physical movements far more effectively than those of primitive life casually performed without any particular objective except the immediate one of fighting enemies or securing food.

This method, which I discovered (and am still studying), after careful observation and study, unremitting thought and a unique experience, I have tested and proved in the case of tens of thousands of men, women and children whom I have cured of weakness and disease by the scientific application of this fundamental law of life, the law of movement.

By means of the scientific physical education and training of the body, especially in the young, we can so modify and regulate the changes of the body to which I have referred, as to accelerate the cellular birth-rate, improve the cell-species of every part of the body, eradicate disease, or the weakness that alone makes disease triumphant, from any body, and make that body so strong that it will be able to ward off all attacks of disease—in other words, both cure and prevent disease.

These metabolistic changes or processes, as they are called, constitute the real life of every individual, and regulate his health in every way, for defective metabolism leads to loss of balance and so to disease.

All or practically all the ailments and diseases with which we are so familiar to-day may be ultimately traced to this cause, that is, to the retardation, arrest, or diversion of nutrition the imperfect elimination of waste and poisonous matter and, consequently, lack of balance between certain cells of the body, or between these cells and other cells. These evils arise almost invariably from the loss of natural and balanced physical movement as a consequence of our modern and sedentary civilised life through many centuries.

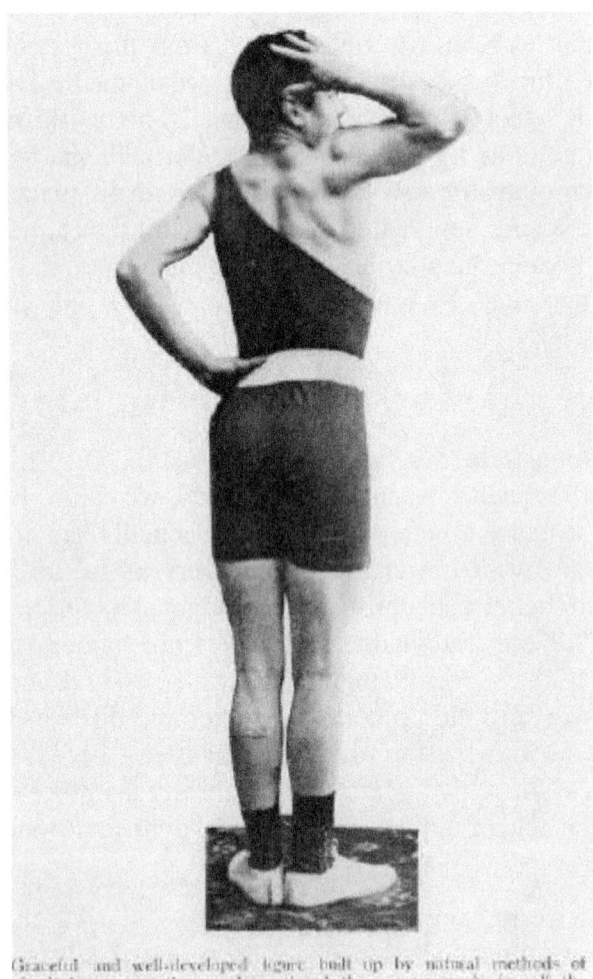

Graceful and well-developed figure built up by natural methods of physical reconstruction, such as the Author recommends for all the children of the nation as a State system of physical education and reconstruction.

CELLS THAT DIE AND ARE BORN DAILY.

Through the natural and normal bodily changes our soul and spirit may, to some extent, be said to inhabit a new bodily building every few years, and the hygiene or otherwise of this bodily dwelling is dependent on movement. Even after we have lain down to sleep at night many of these vital changes continue to go on. Old cells die off and new cells take their place, so that we may be said to awake, to some extent, quite a different person to the individual that lay down. By modifying, regulating and accelerating in balance these processes of change, the application or administration of physical movement in a scientific way will literally re-create a new and better body in all or any of its parts as desired.

As I have said, with our present knowledge and experience there lies to our hand, indeed, the means by which we can actually " breed " new and better cells in any body on an ever-ascending scale to an ultimate state of physical perfection, so that modern man may even yet actually surpass in physical fitness and power of resistance to disease the man of primitive times. This, too, without the incessant physical activity that was necessary for man in primitive times, every hour of his waking life. By these means, we can achieve better results through a few minutes of physical movement, without interference with the occupations of civilised life, because we now possess knowledge and experience that enables us to obtain the equivalent of this all-day-long physical movement in a scientifically compressed and concentrated form.

By carrying out the movements with conscious and concentrated mental and physical effort the results of a few simple movements are equal to the day-long activities of our ancestors. We can, as it were, " touch the spot " or spots in any body that is or are weak or ailing, and apply balanced physical movements in the best way and in a manner that is truly scientific, to such a body or any part or parts of such a body.

" SPEEDING UP " BODILY CHANCES.

Balanced physical movement thus scientifically applied, as I have fully explained in the previous chapter, means that weak or diseased cells must either grow out of their weakness by the physical movement of the voluntary muscles or die through lack of movement and consequently lack of nutrition. It means also that the cells multiply in number more quickly even than in an active state of nature. It will not allow even healthy cells to become too old or degenerate in the body or to propagate weak or inefficient cells of their own species.

It will enable us to modify the chemical changes that convert what you eat and drink into the living cells that make up bone and muscle, nerve and sinew, tendon and ligament. It will strengthen the great heart muscle, which will then send the blood more quickly flowing through arteries, veins and capillaries, distributing copious supplies of air and nourishment everywhere, and hurrying all waste and poisonous matter out of the system, thus increasing nutrition, respiration, and excretion. It will increase lung capacity, enriching the blood and purifying it, thus striking at the very root of anaemia and other blood disorders. It will stimulate the sluggish liver and cause it to rouse itself from its torpor. It will, in short, speed up all the bodily processes of waste and repair, compelling nutrition and growth to exceed waste and decay, and will, indeed, as the familiar saying puts it, " make a new man of you."

To revert again to the individual cell which gives us the basis for all physiological argument and deduction. Man was, as we have seen, once only a single cell which fed itself and ejected its waste by simple muscular contraction, drawing into itself the food it required and excreting its waste. The single-celled animal takes in body-building material and ejects its own waste by a sort of muscular contraction. In man, a multi-cellular being, this power of internal contraction is supplied by that part of the muscular system beyond our voluntary control, but which, as I have shown, can be reached and to an extent regulated by the movement of the voluntary muscles. Man, unlike the single-celled being, has special organs for carrying out the functions of digestion, assimilation, nutrition, respiration, circulation, secretion, and excretion, and the cells that make up the working population of these organs are responsible for these varied functions.

"BREEDING" BETTER CELLS.

This means that the whole body is in a state of perpetual movement, and upon this movement, which has its origin in muscle, depends the whole health. Anything that naturally stimulates and accelerates this movement must inevitably lead to the better nutrition of every cell of the body, and this is why perfectly balanced movement of the voluntary muscles, directed and employed in an absolutely scientific way, has such a beneficial influence upon these internal bodily movements of the millions of cells of which we are composed.

By increasing the nutrition of the body and hastening the elimination of all waste products in this way the new cells that are continually being " born " in the body are better fed, better nourished, have more air, and so thrive and reproduce even healthier young of their own species, just as do human beings living a healthy life in a healthy environment, so that every organ and system becomes better, healthier, more efficient to carry out its functions and more resistant to disease. In most cases this is effected directly by these muscles actually under our own control, but in others, it is accomplished indirectly by these muscles acting through the agency of the great sympathetic nervous system, upon muscles beyond our direct control.

HOW BETTER TISSUE IS BUILT.

As all the tissues of every organ and bodily system are built up by the living cells, and as these cells are steadily increased in number and liveliness, with great reproductive power and the reproduction of progressively better and better cells in each succeeding generation, the effect of balanced physical movement must be to build up and keep building up better tissue in every part of the system, so that structurally and organically, at least, we must have certainly a better as well as a new bodily fabric in time, with the perfectly healthy performance of all the bodily functions.

I might summarise the structural effect of such a natural and scientific system of physical movement as I have described upon the whole body as follows:—

> 1. Life is movement. Death is stagnation. Health swings between these two poles, and is modified and determined by movement. Perfect health is perfect movement in all parts and of every individual cell of the body in absolute balance. It follows logically, therefore, that if we can make the human body a perfectly balanced moving machine in all its parts, we can have perfect health and freedom from disease, so long as we receive nourishing food, pure air, and the essentials that sustain life through this perpetual movement of and in muscles, organs, blood, bone, cells and tissue of every kind.

2.　All tissue is composed of cells, each cell being a living entity like yourself, requiring air and nourishment to thrive, producing and causing to accumulate waste matter by its activities, and with the power of reproducing its own species. That air and nourishment can only reach it by muscular movement, working through the circulation of the blood, and its waste be similarly removed.

3.　Each cell has to have the air and nourishment necessary to its existence brought to it by the blood, and depends also upon the blood to carry off its waste matter which would otherwise accumulate, decay, and ferment in the body and tend to cause disease.

4.　But the blood and the cells of the blood, which are the distributing agents for this air and nourishment to these millions of living microscoplic cells of the body, and which carries away 'their "refuse," depend for their activity and continuity of movement upon muscular motive power, the heart itself being but a large muscle that distributes the blood through the body, and the arteries and capillaries having also the power of muscular contractility to propel the blood onward. Balanced physical movement, if scientifically applied, causes the blood to flow faster in every part of the body, and the cells it contains to travel faster, bringing more and better supplies of food and air to each living cell of the body, and also ensuring the freer elimination of all waste and poisonous matter, so that with every sweep of the blood through the system better tissue replaces the old and effete.

5.　This, in turn, means that each cell becomes individually more healthy, more muscular, more vigorous, and more active, having a greater reproductive power, and reproducing better cells until perfect cells only remain, the cells being, as it were, kept always in a condition of perpetual youth. All the organs and systems of the body will then be better protected in every way as a result of the greater bodily movement, because they will have more and better working and fighting cells to safeguard their interests, until finally they possess cells that will neither be weak in themselves nor tolerate disease, and much stronger than those of the preceding generation.

6.　Thus structurally and organically, physical movements, scientifically applied, re-build newer, better, and healthier tissue in every part of the body, and as tissue is the living fabric of which the human body is made, and upon which the healthy performance of every function depends, really scientific physical education will thus build up a new, better and disease-free body.

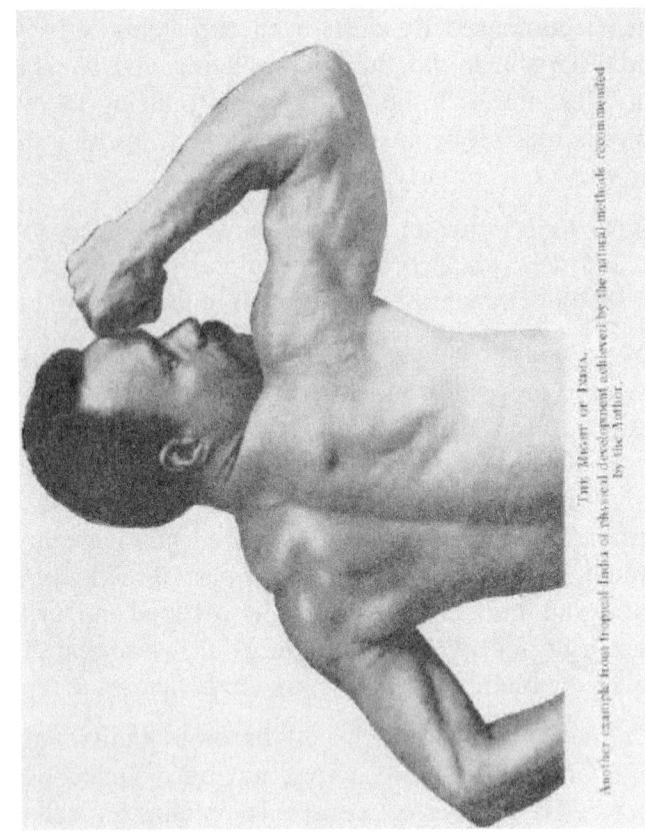

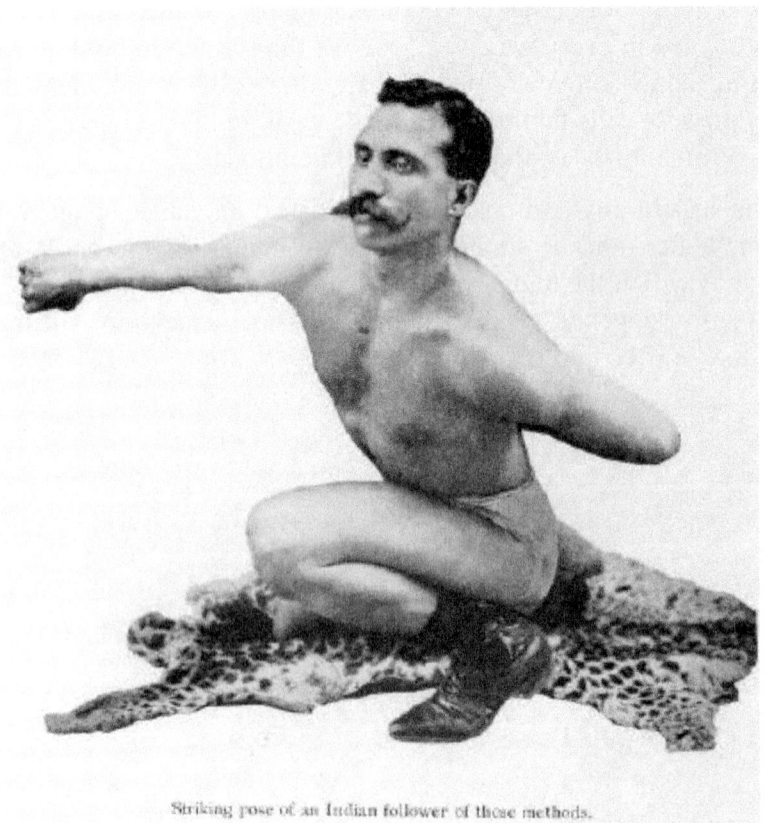

THE MOUNT OF JUNO.
Another example from tropical India of physical development achieved by the natural methods recommended by the Author.

Striking pose of an Indian follower of these methods.

Let us now show briefly how this physical and structural reconstruction affects and improves the functioning of the body:

1. Life is movement, and all human movement, including organic function, is muscular, for muscle has been well defined as " crystallised function."

2. Owing to civilisation, the natural movement which is necessary for the healthy life of the body has become less and less, until lack of movement or insufficient movement in balance has permitted disease to enter.

3. With the aid of the knowledge and experience humanity has gathered and acquired through centuries of investigation and education, I claim that we can now compress and concentrate the physical movement necessary for healthy life into a " tabloid " form to suit modern conditions of life. This movement can be applied locally or generally as desired by scientific methods such as I have already described.

4. Such physical movement will improve the " breed," as it were, of the bodily cells by evolving a better and better type until physical perfection is attained.

5. How? Because, in the ordinary way, the cells are continually dying, others being born. The more balanced the physical movement, scientifically controlled and regulated, the more rapidly too old or feeble cells die. Only the better cells are left, and these reproduce a better offspring even than themselves.

6. Why? Because the more we move all the voluntary muscles of the body in balance the more air and food all the cells of the body receive, the more equal is both the distribution and consumption of this air and food, the better nourished they are, and the healthier their environment. The cells of every part of the body have to move in balance with this movement of the voluntary muscles, thus developing their muscles and improving their functioning. The cells of the digestive system, for instance, supply better nourishment, the cells of the various secretory glands secrete more of their essential fluids, the cells of the lungs, the skin, the intestines, the kidneys, and of every muscle, nerve, organ and system do their work more easily and more efficiently. In other words, all the bodily functions will in time, be better performed by fitter cells through the balanced movement of the voluntary muscles.

7. Weak and unfit or diseased cells are ruthlessly weeded out as the physical movement is increased and the strain upon each cell becomes greater. Only fit cells remain to perpetuate their species, and this process goes on until through generation of cells after generation, physically perfect cells are evolved, to carry on the functions of life healthfully and vigorously. This is, in short, a beneficent application of the doctrine of the survival of the fittest to the cells of each individual body rather than to the individual himself or herself, thus " breeding " better cells until perfection is attained and we have a body that is like a perfectly balanced engine and a faultless machine.

(This is the effect of balanced physical movement upon the structure and function of every organ and system of the body, and its value, then, from the curative point of view, will be apparent. Those who are more especially interested in the effect of such movement upon pathological or diseased conditions should read my chapter on " How and Why Scientific Physical Movement Cures Disease," in conjunction with this chapter.)

In conclusion, I may explain that the structural effect of such movement by a simple illustration, taking the case of a man who wishes to perform an athletic feat like, say, running 100 yards in ten seconds. Now if he were foolish enough to attempt such a feat without the special training of all the muscles employed in such a feat he would overstrain and might possibly kill himself, while he would most assuredly fail.

Why does specialised training enable him later to achieve his object? Because, better and better cells are "bred," as I have described, in those particular muscles he exercises and develops until the muscles become absolutely new muscles, far fitter and with a greater capacity than the old, having been consciously " evolved i by graduated and progressive training methods to the standard of physical perfection necessary for the performance of this feat.

Some, of course, would never be able to achieve such a feat no matter how long and assiduously they trained, for there will always be standards and degrees, with limitations, of individual excellence, though in generations hence these differences must become less and less, until they will disappear, if such a system as I advocate be adopted in our schools. A few men, on the other hand, might become able to run a 100 yards even in a shade less than ten seconds.

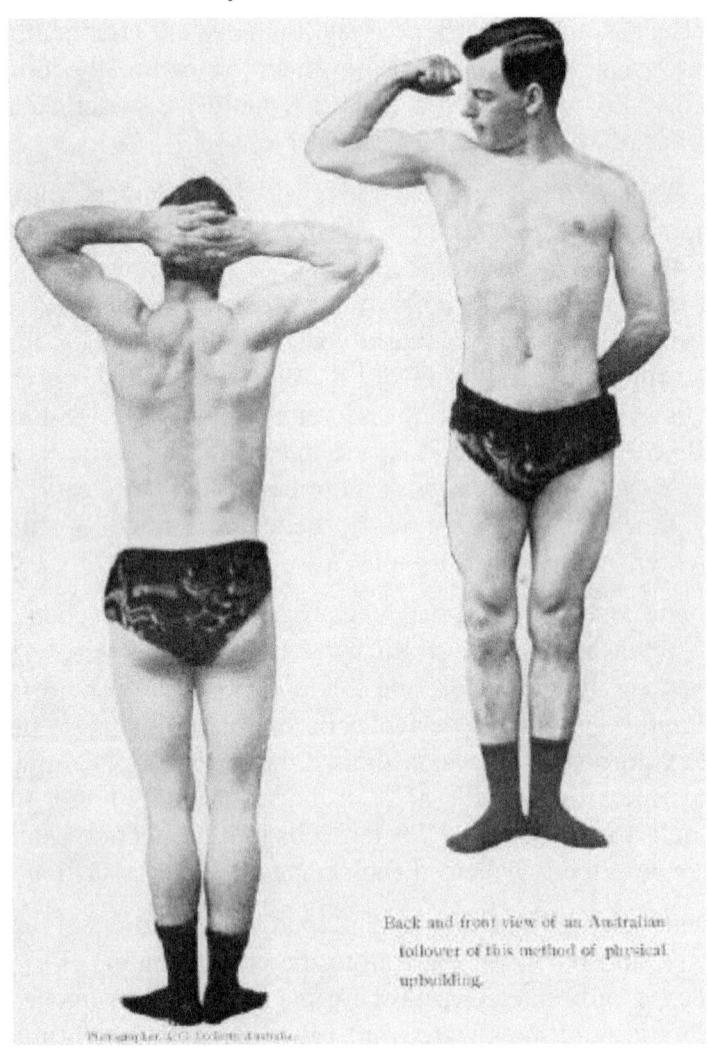

Back and front view of an Australian follower of this method of physical upbuilding.

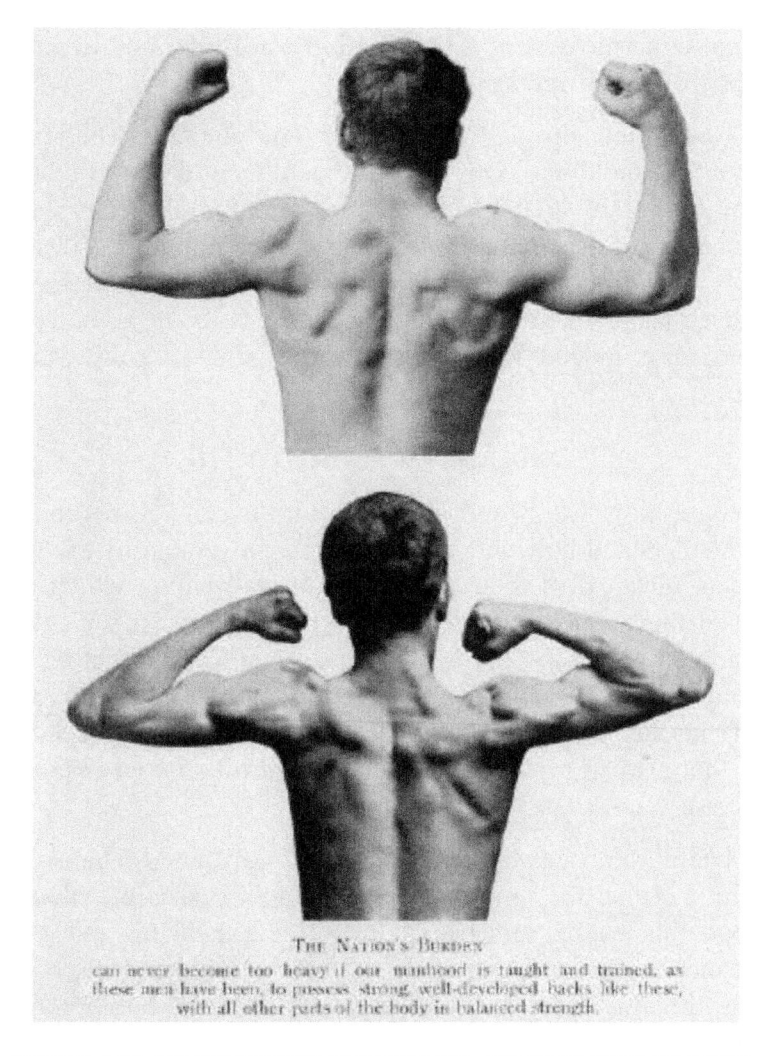

THE NATION'S BURDEN
can never become too heavy if our manhood is taught and trained, as
these men have been, to possess strong, well-developed backs like these,
with all other parts of the body in balanced strength.

WHY AN ATHLETE'S MUSCLES GROW STRONGER.

But in this training the athlete had not only to " breed " better muscle cells of certain muscles to perform this feat. The same training caused other cells of his body to cry out for more nourishment, so the cells of the whole digestive system had to work harder and to move faster, and they themselves were better developed and nourished through this greater movement and activity. The athlete had to eat more or assimilate more nourishment to enable the cells, of the muscles specially developed to get the nourishment sufficient to do the extra work. This meant more movement for the cells of the digestive system, and they, too, became better nourished and stronger by this movement.

In the same way, the cell-chemists of the body were called upon to deal with the chemical transformation of this additional food, and had to move faster and work harder. They, too, were consequently developed and strengthened by the movement, in the first place, of the voluntary muscles used by the athlete. The cell- scavengers of the eliminatory organs, the cell-workers of the heart, of the lungs, of the skin, of every system and organ of the whole body were proportionately developed to meet the increased effect put upon them through the increased and increasing effort put upon the athlete's voluntary muscles. They received more food and more air, through this greater muscular movement. They lived in a healthier bodily atmosphere because of the greater elimination of waste from the system.

This happy colony of industrial cells grew fruitful and multiplied more and more under their new bodily surroundings, their " children " grew up still healthier and more vigorous, until every cell employed directly or indirectly in this athletic feat become stronger and better developed, including the directing cells of the brain employed. But such unbalanced training as this, though it admittedly exercises a healthful influence upon certain muscles and systems of the body, does not and cannot produce that perfect balance among all the cells of the body which alone makes the body superior to disease, indeed, tends rather by special and local developments to increase disturbance of balance.

EXERCISES AND GROWTH.

It is only when we realise how closely and intimately all the cells of the body are associated and inter-related, that we understand how and why balanced movement of the voluntary muscles or lack of such movement must affect their joint life and well-being, which is the life and well-being of the individual they separately and conjointly represent. It will, therefore, be easy to realise from the illustration I have just given how, by applying and directing muscular movement of all the voluntary muscles of the body and not in a limited or drastic fashion to some particular number and group of muscles, we can make and keep each and every cell of the body not only fit and healthy in itself, but also so powerful and strong and all so well balanced as to be able to defy and conquer disease.

While any muscle is being exercised waste is going on rapidly, and the muscle might waste away altogether, but for the fact that the moment the movement ceases the blood begins at once to repair and make good this waste, renews all the force expended, and adds to its bulk and substance so that the more a muscle is exercised the bigger, stronger, and better it grows. When, as I have pointed out, the muscular system is responsible for the functioning of every organ, it will at once be seen how important is this development of muscle in a scientific way, and how profound is the influence of balanced muscular movement and development on the health of the whole body. For this power of growth and development also takes place, proportionately, in all the tissues of the body as the result of the movement, in the first place, of all the voluntary muscles which causes the simultaneous movement of each and every cell of the body.

NO UNNECESSARY MUSCLES IN THE BODY.

The human body is no mere chance accumulation of atoms, but was divinely designed and created with organs and muscles and cells, each having a specific and pre-determined duty to perform in the general scheme of bodily operations and activities. The fact that there are over 500 muscles in the body makes it self-evident, then, that each and every muscle was placed there by the Creator with and for a distinct purpose, and it is flat blasphemy to argue that any muscle or group of muscles can be allowed to fall into disuse and inactivity without prejudice to the vital functioning of the whole human machine in which every part is so closely interrelated and inter-dependent. Each separate muscle has its allotted duty to perform and also plays a part in the whole inter-dependent operation of the human machine, and if it is allowed to shirk that duty it is not only injurious to itself but handicaps or prevents the Smooth and easy working of the whole bodily Organisation. There is no muscle in the human body that cannot be moved and exercised either directly or indirectly in the manner I have described, and through the joint and balanced movement of the voluntary muscles, all the involuntary muscles and every cell of the body are also reached, moved and developed in balanced strength. The results of such a system of balanced physical movement in our schools to-day would be amazing, and would quickly be evident in the prevention or eradication of that weakness or lack of balance which is the true cause of all disease.

The full realisation of this fact by the medical profession will, as I have said, mean a complete revolution in the healing art. It will, as I point out elsewhere, lead more and more to the study of man rather than of disease or medicine, and still more it will lead to the study of that humble speck of protoplasm, the cell, of which man is made, and from which, by incessant movement, he evolved from the primeval slime. If we begin with the child we may yet achieve what, will seem miracles to the present generation. Just as the child is father of the man so the cell is father of the child, and just as it is only by movement that a single Cell multiples and increases until it is a fully formed and organised living child, so the process is only continued by movement until the child becomes a full-sized and fully-developed adult.

The more these cells are made to increase and multiply by movement—the movement which is their only means of life,, and which only can come to all of them in equal balance through the balanced movement of the voluntary muscles—the better nourished, more healthy, and more resistant to disease they must become. It should be, then, the supreme duty of the future medical man to discover how to select and apply perfectly balanced movements of the voluntary muscles, so as to develop all these ever-multiplying cells in such perfect balance from childhood, or to correct any lack of balance in any particular group of cells, in this way making the body so perfectly developed and balanced everywhere as to prevent breakdown or to permit the intrusion of disease germs from without. I myself have done this in thousands of instances as will be perceived from the splendidly cellular-developed and balanced specimens of men, women and children in many of the illustrations in this book.

In my next chapter, I show how essential it is that all physical movement be based on the condition and state of the heart, and why the heart must be made the pivot of the whole machinery of scientific physical culture.

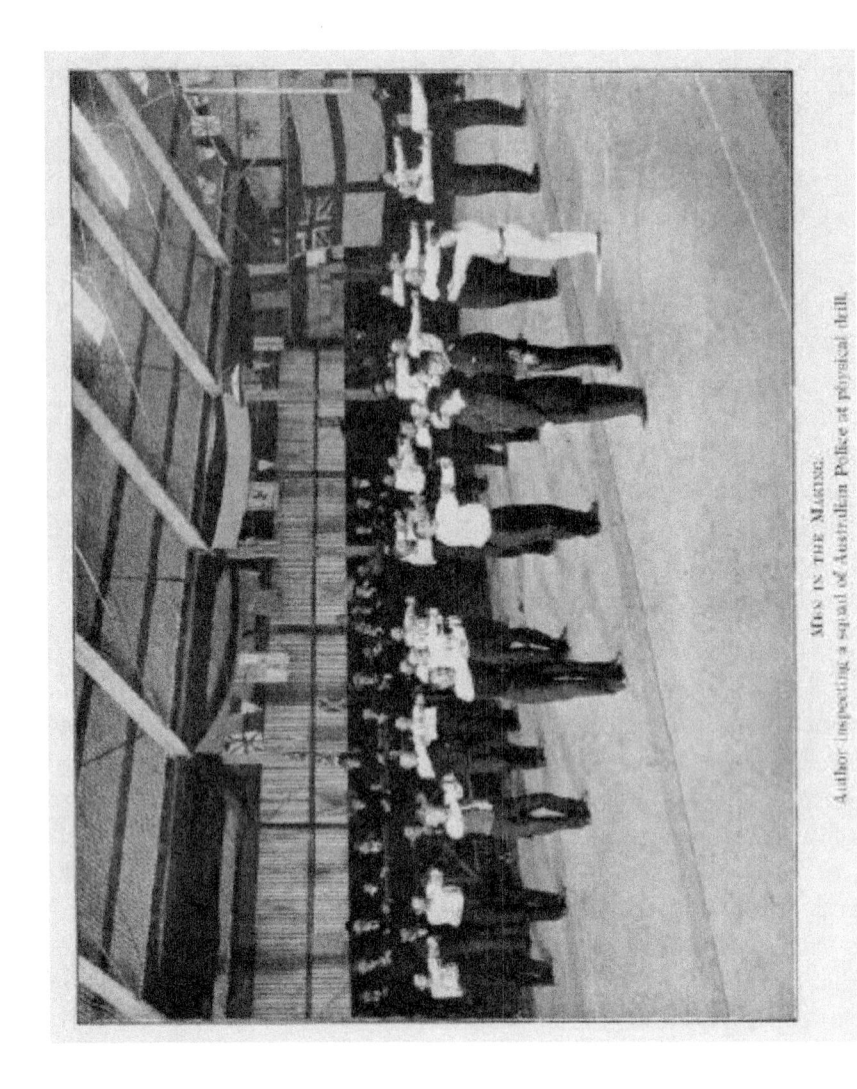

MEN IN THE MAKING.
Author inspecting a squad of Australian Police at physical drill.

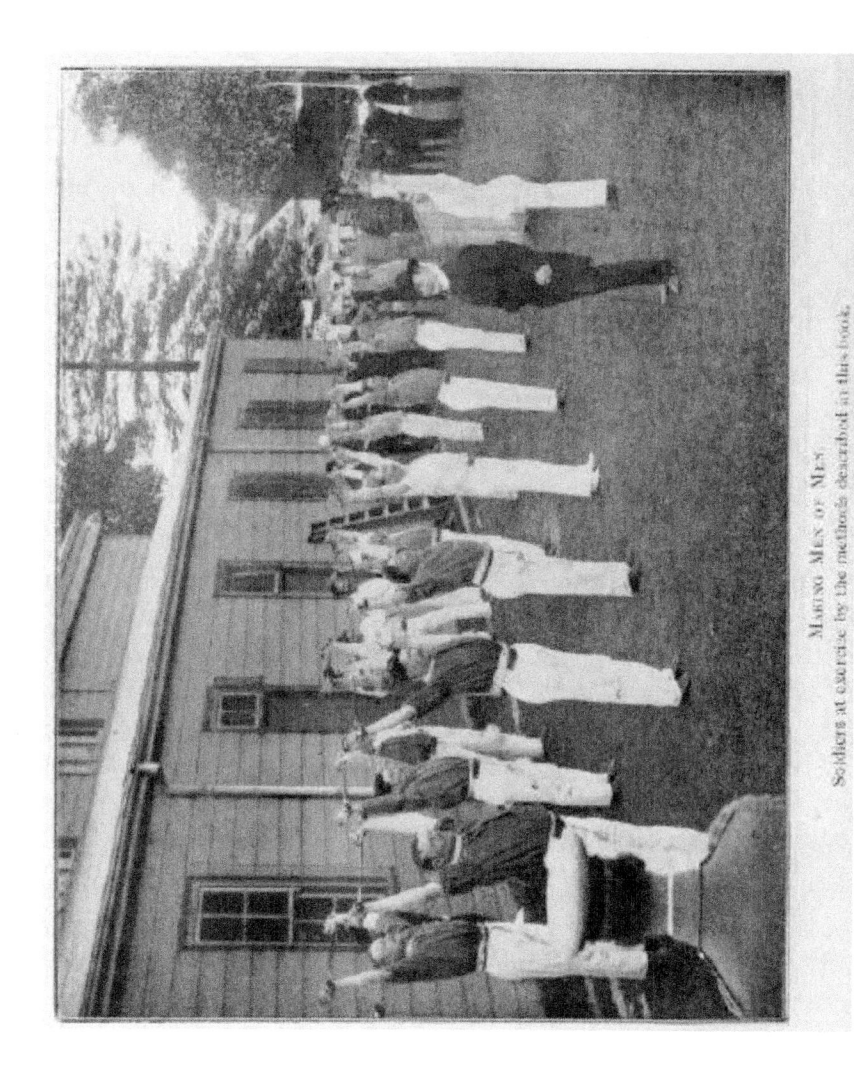

MAKING MEN OF MEN
Soldiers at exercise by the methods described in this book.

CHAPTER X.

The Heart the Pivot of Remedial or Preventive Physical Culture.

THE heart, the most vital of all organs, being itself nothing little more than a mighty muscle, and most responsive to the movement or movements of those muscles within our own control, must be regarded as the pivot of all physical movement of a remedial or a preventive character, and all such physical movement must be determined and regulated by the condition of the heart.

WORKS NIGHT AND DAY FOR LIFE.

The heart begins its labours from the very moment that life signifies its advent in the unborn child, and continues, day after day and year after year, until death, with no rest or with only a very brief interval of rest between the heart-beats, that is, between its own contraction and relaxation.

The heart, which is only about the size of a man's closed fist, is, then, the most important muscle in the body and should be the strongest, for its work is never done, waking or sleeping. It contracts automatically for about half a second, and each beat is followed by a rest of about the same duration. At each beat, the ventricles lift into the arteries about 2½ ounces of blood, and this even under the most favourable circumstances. " Let anyone," says Dr A. T. Schofield, " firmly clench his fist seventy-two times a minute for only ten minutes, and see how he feels, and then remember the heart does this day and night without ceasing,, with a force stronger than that it would take to lift itself each hour higher than Mont Blanc."

Exercise or physical movement of any kind naturally increases this work of the heart, and for this reason it is imperative in prescribing physical movements to any person to regulate such movements entirely according to the strength of the heart, and to keep all physical movement in the strictest subjection to that organ.

Before any physical movement then is prescribed, especially where there is existent or suspected weakness to disease, and always in the case of children, the condition of the heart should be ascertained by the most painstaking examination, and if the heart be weak or impaired in its functions, this condition must be attended to in precedence of everything else, and the action of the heart rectified and strengthened. This is the only way to secure pupil or patient against physical injury, and to prevent the " medicine," as the saying is, from being worse than the disease.

The prescription of physical movement, or even of deep breathing movements in heart cases must never, therefore, be undertaken m any perfunctory manner or without considerable study, knowledge and experience, in the selection of such physical movements as will impose no excessive strain or tax the heart beyond its own strength. These movements should be most carefully graduated both in the number and the degree of effort required, and time should not be spared in arranging these gradations, while continuous re-examination and tests should take place from time to time.

THE HEART AS THE INDEX.

When this is done the heart muscles will be developed consistently, and in balance with the developing voluntary muscles. In other words, the effort demanded of the voluntary muscles, under the patient's direct mental control, must be regulated entirely by the muscular power of the heart, for only in this way can that great vital muscle be developed proportionately and in harmonious balance with the other muscles and organs of the body. Even where the heart's action is normal, this is the only safe rule to follow, because, unless the heart is taken as the index of the muscular strain placed upon the voluntary muscles, there will always be danger of dilation or enlargement—what is known as athlete's heart—if not even more serious structural and valvular troubles.

This great care and skill in diagnosis and in the prescription of balanced physical movements, especially where there is actual heart weakness or disease, is another of the fundamental features that distinguish physical culture which is scientific, curative or preventive from exercise that is mere play or physical movement that is unscientific and likely to prove dangerous or even fatal, and this is why I am so emphatic in advising that, especially in the case of children, games, sports and competitive athletic contests, should only follow physical education and training on scientific lines, and then only after medical examination and on the doctor's recommendation.

Otherwise there is always the grave danger of overstraining in early life, and lack of that nicely adjusted and balanced physique and organism towards which all scientific physical movement ever aims and tends. It is just this lack of balance in any organ or system that causes the weakness somewhere which lays the body open to any form of disease, and which may even cause organic heart disease. The prescription of physical movement, therefore, is a matter demanding serious study and attention from the medical profession.

Professor Ballet, the distinguished French savant and neurologist, says, " it is not enough to prescribe muscular exercise in a vague manner, leaving to the patient the work of finding out what kind and amount of exercise are suited to him; to do so would be to lay oneself open to cruel disappointments. It is not uncommon to see a patient who has aggravated his condition by indulging in excessive or badly regulated muscular work. The choice and regulation of the form of exercise require the whole attention of the 'physician."

PHYSICAL MOVEMENT IN HEART CASES.

The immediate effects of physical exercise on the heart itself and the vascular system are known, in a general way, to every physician. It quickens the heart beat, balances the distribution of blood in the body, increases consumption of oxygen, generates heat, makes the passage of the blood through the valves of the venous system easier. But exercise may be beneficial or injurious accordingly as it is prescribed and carried out in a balanced and scientific way, or simply indulged in at random without knowledge of its possibilities and its limitations. It can be used, when carefully prescribed and carried out, to strengthen a weak, and even to reconstruct a diseased heart, or it may prove more dangerous than the most potent drug if carelessly prescribed and faultily carried out.

The work that is being done at Nauheim in morbid heart conditions is well-known to medical men, but I do not think that even there there is a clear understanding of the how and the why of the beneficent influence of physical movement on the heart and the action of the heart, or a full realisation of the possibilities of physical movement in heart troubles. Doctors know and have been compelled to admit the curative and preventive value of physical therapeutics, by the results already achieved, but it is my object in this book to give them a physiological reason for the faith that is in them.

Indeed, the value of physical movement in heart cases has been proved at Nauheim over and over again, but even greater results will be accomplished when the doctors who select and prescribe physical movements have themselves passed through a long course of study and actual personal experience in physical culture and physical development before being considered fully qualified to prescribe the physical movements best calculated to improve the condition of their patients, especially in cases where there is even a suspicion of heart trouble.

A far more careful and exact diagnosis will be necessary in prescribing physical movements than in prescribing medicine whenever there is any heart trouble or even pseudo heart trouble, and the movements must, as I would again emphasise, be most carefully selected and varied, taking great care to prescribe the right sort of movements according to the individual circumstances of each case. Physical movements, including breathing and balancing exercises, so selected and applied, will be wonderfully successful in many functional heart troubles, and in organic heart disease, if taken in time, except where there is serious structural malformation. In fact, the time may come when, thanks to the careful and scientific physical education of the people from childhood heart disease will be a thing of the past or nearly so.

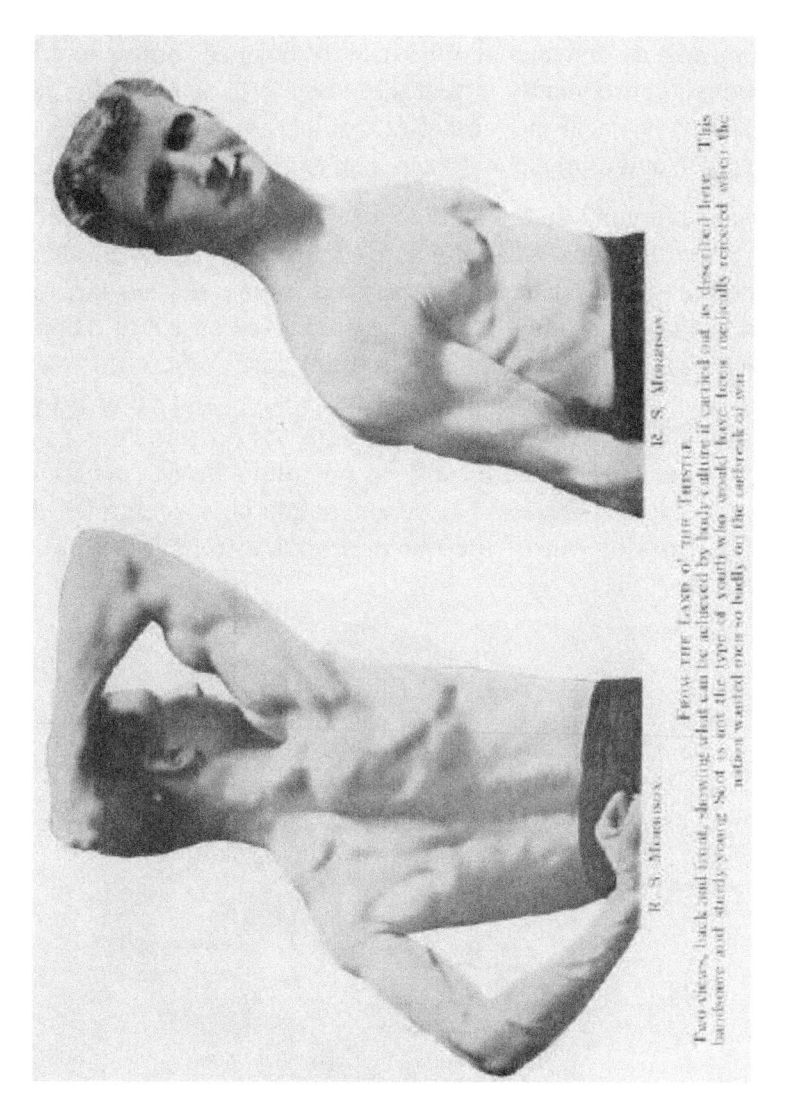

DEVELOPING WEAK HEARTS.

The first effect of physical movement on the heart, provided it is prescribed and carried out as I point out, is to develop and strengthen it just as any other muscle of the body is developed and strengthened by use and movement, and a great deal of the heart weakness and disease of to-day is the inevitable result of lack of balanced physical movement, as naturally the less we use the voluntary muscles in balance the less we develop the heart, because the action of the heart can only be strengthened and improved by the exercise and movement of muscles under our control.

Without such movement the heart becomes weaker and weaker like an unused limb until it is liable to succumb to serious organic disease, especially in a boy already weak and imperfectly balanced. Only through re-educating it gradually by the use and movement of the voluntary muscles can we bring back its normal and healthy action, and make it even stronger than it was before!

It is, moreover, only by securing perfect balance in these voluntary physical movements that we can secure the best results, for we cannot and must not consider the heart as an independent organ but as one of many organs all closely inter-related and interdependent. Imperfectly balanced movement means, as I have explained, lack of balance somewhere in the organism, and this lack of balance must, consequently, affect the whole organism, including the heart. For this reason, perfectly balanced physical movement is absolutely necessary to reconstruct a heart that has been weak or diseased and to make and keep it strong and disease-free in every cell.

It must not., of course, be thought that even the most scientific application of physical movement in heart disease will effect miracles in cases where the sufferer has reached a stage where he may, perhaps, die at any moment, and where the disease has progressed too far, for the heart can only be re-educated to its work very gradually, and the process of cure and reconstruction takes time even under the most favourable circumstances. In many cases where this treatment would prove effective, too, the sufferer loses patience at a very early stage and gives it up, and so, of course, there is never really any opportunity of effecting a cure. As doctors know, especially in cases of this kind, it takes two to effect a cure, and co-operation between patient and physician is absolutely essential to complete success. No treatment can be successful if the sufferer does not submit patiently to the carrying out of the doctor's advice from first to last, however slow or tedious progress may seem to be.

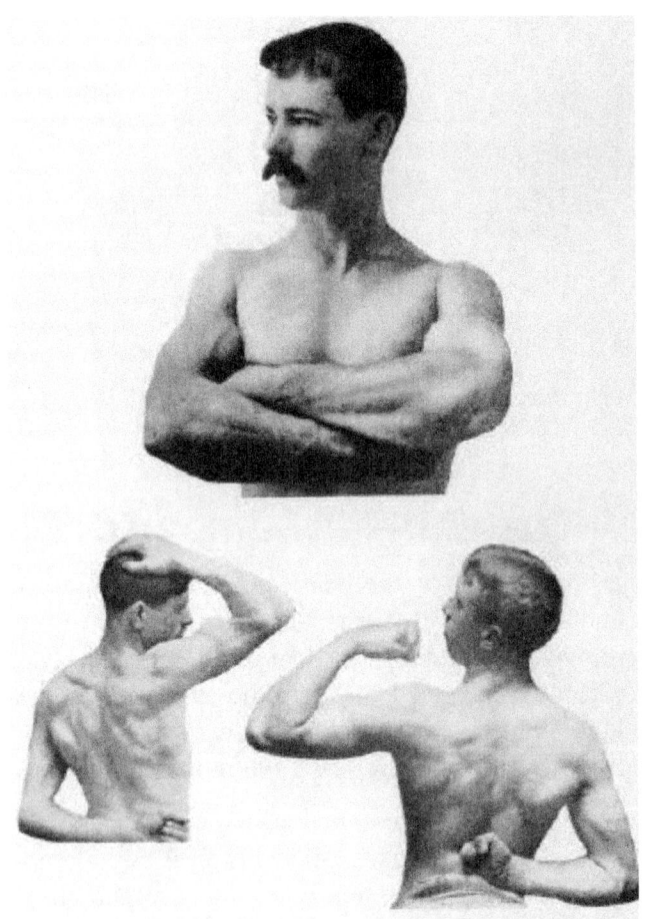

Three Models for the Youth of the Nation.
Every boy can do the same as these three young men have done if they follow out the same methods, which are fully explained here.

THE PHYSIOLOGY OF EXERCISE.

Not only in heart disease, but in the treatment of nearly every form of disease, this holds good, because the state and condition of the heart must dictate the nature and progress of all treatment by means of natural physical movement. The heart must first be got into condition, and the patient can only travel at a rate or progress towards cure that must be determined and regulated by the actual state of the heart, which organ must not be jeopardised however anxious the sufferer be to get well in other ways. It is because the patient rarely realises this that he becomes impatient, declines to continue the treatment, and so sacrifices his last hope of recovery.

Let me now enter more fully into the physiological effect of muscular movement, especially as it affects the heart and the circulatory system, while we must never forget that it is through this muscular movement that the whole organism in each and all of its cells can be reached, cleansed, nourished and developed. When any muscle is exercised, the muscular cells and fibres are made to contract and relax, and in doing so the stale and poisoned venous blood in the system is squeezed out by the act of contraction and afterwards eliminated, while fresh and well-oxygenated blood, with copious supplies, takes its place immediately the muscles are relaxed, and does so in greater quantity.

In this way the muscles themselves are first benefited, their vital activities quickened and, as a result, their size and bulk increased and quality improved. As any muscle or set of muscles is contracted the blood is quickened in its journey to that muscle or muscles, but the moment it is relaxed the blood is pumped more quickly and vigorously to the lungs, where it is relieved of much of its poisonous matter and takes in fresh supplies of oxygen. This, of course, means faster breathing and increased consumption of oxygen, so that the blood is, in consequence, purified and enriched. By this muscular activity the heart muscles themselves are developed just as the biceps is developed by repeated contraction and relaxation.

SPEED AND VIGOUR OF CONTRACTION.

Of course, much depends on the quality and nature of the contraction, the amount and regulation of the effort, and the conscious concentration of the mind upon the muscle or muscles moved, as I very fully explain in my chapter on " The Machinery of National Physical Training." It is here that the medical man of the future will be called upon to exercise his utmost skill when it comes to prescription of physical movement, especially where there is heart weakness or disease and still more so in the case of children.

Equally, too, the utmost care will be necessary as to the speed at which such movements are carried out, because the faster the movements are made, even if sub-consciously carried out, the greater the work thrown upon the heart and the less benefit derived in pro-portion. The speed of the movements will require the most exact regulation, according to the state of the heart, or the gravest results may ensue. An athlete training to run 100 yards in ten seconds only does so by increasing his pace very gradually, but an ordinary individual might do himself serious and even fatal heart injury if he attempted to run 100 yards even in 20 or 30 seconds. The pace of all physical movement as the vigour of effort should always be determined and modified by the state of the heart, being graduated only according to the improvement shown and maintained in the heart. This, indeed, should be a guiding principle in every case whether there is any heart trouble or not.

I have explained in an earlier chapter that when all the voluntary muscles are moved in balance many involuntary muscles and cells are also set in motion, so that the benefit of this movement though at first local is ultimately general, leading to the better nutrition and aeration not only of the muscle cells directly moved, but of all the bodily cells, thus bringing about their greater purification and nutrition, and the rapid multiplication and maintenance of younger and more healthy cells in every part of the system, including the heart itself while old, feeble and diseased cells die because they are unable to keep pace with the movement of the voluntary muscles, and because their waste outbalances nutrition and repair. In this way, too, I assert, we can give a man a new limb or even a new organ or system and even greatly improve a malformed heart organically diseased by improving the quality of all its cellular constituents.

PREVENTING HEART TROUBLES.

With the effect of balanced physical movement on the circulation I have already dealt. It is also the best and surest preventive of that hardening of the arteries known as arterio-sclerosis, and its faithful attendant cardiac hypertrophy or enlargement of the heart. In the same way, physical movement, when balanced as I suggest, prevents or disperses fatty and gaseous accumulation in the abdominal region, with consequent venous dilatation, and disturbance of the circulation, which may, if neglected, lead to valvular disease of the heart.

The heart, however, can not only be consciously influenced directly and indirectly by the balanced movement of all the voluntary muscles, but it is also susceptible to mental influence through the nervous system and its action may be readily affected, as we know, by any strong emotion, passion or sensation, such as anger, love, fear, shock or acute grief. Such control as we can exercise over it is physical, and only through the correct and balanced use of the voluntary muscles can we develop and adjust it to bear still greater strains and to become stronger in itself and in its functioning.

The complexity of the heart's mechanism, the wonderful delicacy of its structure and the exact nicety of its operations might convey the impression that it would be easy of derangement or would quickly wear itself out by its increasing labours. Yet in an octogenarian it goes on night and day for 80 years at the rate of 100,000 strokes every 24 hours, while at every beat it has to overcome a great resistance, and as a rule, without derangement or weariness. It contracts over 4,000 times in an hour, and there passes through it every hour nearly 8,000 ounces or nearly 700 lbs. of blood.

As the whole mass of blood in an average adult body is nearly one-tenth that of the whole weight of the body (one-fourth of the quantity being contained in the muscles alone), a heavy quantity of blood equal to the whole mass of blood in the body passes through the heart over 28 times an hour, or once in every two minutes. Such a feat is super-human and the power to perform it would only come from a Divine source beyond the finite understanding of the human mind. Indeed, the wisdom of the Creator is seen in these marvellous operations and activities of the human heart, and it is well that the absolute control of this tremendous force is placed beyond our volition. For, if we had to control it by our own volition we could never know the refreshing balm of sleep, as we should have to keep watch over this wonderful human engine night and day, for fear it might cease to beat even for a few seconds and we would die. As a great anatomist has truly said, fortunately it is so made, and "the power of the Creator in so constructing it can in nothing be exceeded but His wisdom."

CHAPTER XI.

The Machinery of National Physical Training.

BEFORE I attempt to outline my ideal method of applying balanced physical movements, especially to children, in a scientific manner— for merely to give anything like the complete details of such a comprehensive scheme would require a volume for itself quite as large as this, and is not, therefore, to be attempted here—I may at once anticipate what I know will be one of the first arguments advanced, viz., that of expense.

CUTTING DOWN THE HOSPITAL BILL.

Apart from the fact that in a time of national crisis the British Empire had to find as much as £8,000,000 a day for purposes of defence in war-time, and that it would scarcely be too much to ask for even so large an amount to avert another and even greater crisis, or, at least, to give the country a physical backbone that would make war too grave a responsibility for the most audacious statesmen to incur rashly, I contend that the cost would be more than met by the tremendous reduction that would be effected in the present charge made annually for hospitals, infirmaries and clinics, police, reformatories, asylums, penal and charitable institutions of every kind, the care and after care of the diseased, the weak, the criminal and the insane poor, and a thousand other channels of wealth wastage due mainly to disease and physical unfitness.

However, let me go into this matter in proper sequence, and name only some of the methods by which we might employ a well- conceived system of natural and scientific physical education and culture for the gradual elimination of physical weakness, ill-health and disease, with all their immoral spawn in the form of degeneracy, vice, crime and insanity, from a world intended by the Creator to furnish us with every rational pleasure that the heart of man might desire, provided we, on our part, do our duty to ourselves and by so doing begin a great pioneer work in the re-construction of a nation.

THE DUTY OF THE STATE.

It should be the first duty, as it is the interest of the State— that is, the Government chosen by and representing the people—to give every child, rich and poor alike, an equal opportunity of possessing a sound body as well as a sound and educated mind. To do this is essential to the very existence of a people, for weakness and disease are in direct antagonism to Nature, a conflict that can only end disastrously to any individual or community of individuals. Every child born into the world ought surely to receive at least as much attention to the development of its physical power and its whole bodily well-being as a pedigree puppy or a thoroughbred colt or filly.

A really sound and scientific scheme of physical education and bodily reconstruction ought to be drafted by a responsible authority, preferably the Ministry of Health, assisted by a Medical Council of eminent medical men. For, as I have pointed out, so grave a matter should not be left, as at present, in the hands of the educational authorities. It is a matter first and foremost of ensuring and establishing a good physical basis for our little ones instead of still further sapping their vitality and physique by overeducation of the mind in a weak, diseased and unbalanced physical body, for, as Mr Arnold Rowntree, M.P., the famous sociologist, told the House of Commons, " healthy childhood was the foundation of all education." The policy of the past has been a mistaken one. If we pursue that policy further it will lead to a more grave crisis still, for it is madness to think you can produce a people able to win and keep commercial power and prestige if their minds are educated while their bodies are being neglected. Physical education has too long been made secondary and subsidiary to mental education, whereas I contend, on the contrary, that physical education should come first, and be carried out in a really scientific way and under medical direction and supervision.

A recognised programme and plan of national physical education and health culture should be drawn up, medical officers appointed to carry it out, and all the doctors placed under one Central Authority to whom they would be responsible. Physical instructors of experience and high qualification should be appointed to assist in the carrying out of this great work of national physical reconstruction, and we should then be in a position for the first time to formulate a system of health and physical education really worthy of being called scientific.

SCIENTIFIC v. UNSCIENTIFIC METHODS.

I am, of course, prepared to hear many object that already the majority of our schools and educational institutions are devoting considerable attention to the physical education and training of children, which, to a certain extent, is true. But my contention is that, as a present carried out, the methods are unscientific, and, in many cases, even injurious because they do not take into consideration the weakness that may be apparent or latent in each individual, or aim, from the outset, at the physical and constitutional upbuilding of the young in perfect balance.

Indeed, in many of the methods in vogue to-day the child has itself to be naturally very strong in every part to bear them, and not to injure heart, lungs, or other vital organs, the condition of which has not first been taken into consideration. A weak child may be injured for life, and even the strong given a badly balanced physique and organism by any method of physical culture that is not scientific in its conception, organisation and execution.

In many methods, there are serious faults to be found. The aim of the instructor is too often to produce a series of nicely fitting and smoothly changing movements in mass so as to form a pretty tableau on examination days or at public demonstrations, while the individual weakness of each individual child are overlooked or forgotten. The physical movements, too, are only carried out in a sub-conscious way, and are utterly useless to train the will, improve muscular and mental co-ordination, in order to acquire complete control over each and every voluntary muscle, or build up a really balanced physical, organic and mental organisation.

What I mean when I speak of scientific physical education is as far removed from such immature methods as the educational system of a modern 'Varsity or public school is from the old " hedge-school " teaching of an unmourned past. I would have physical education conducted on just as scientific lines as mental education already is, separating the children at first into classes, categories or standards according to age, constitution, family history, etc., the younger and weaker children in the lowest class and only winning their way to higher classes and standards by examinations and actual improvement in physique and health.

Where there is incipient weakness or evidence of any weakness inherited by the child (per the parents' own medical history already in the hands of the doctor, as I explain later), actual disease or malformation, the child should, at first, receive special and individual attention and physical treatment until it has attained a physical standard to qualify it for classification. Above all, no effort should be spared to give such a child a well-balanced body and brain with every muscle, organ and even cell developed in proportionate power and vigour.

SAFEGUARDING THE WEAK, DELICATE, AND DISEASED.

The present methods are most unfair to weak or delicate or backward children, apart from being too drastic, and can never build up a body in physical and organic balance. Indeed, it is no exaggeration to say, on the other hand, that there are tens of thousands of the men and women to-day who have grown up to suffer all their lives from injury received during their youthful physical training and games at school. Many unable to trace this to its real cause, attribute it to family weakness. This, however, is not always so, but it more often the result of allowing children to enter into competitive games and sports before they are physically fit to do so. Only when the doctor passes them as physically fit for games should they be permitted to indulge in them.

Just as scientific mental education not only sorts out the children according to their mental standards, so it also aims to rectify all mental and moral defects, and to develop the brain and mind gradually until it is solidly, firmly and permanently established. This is exactly what I want to see done in a physical sense as well, a system of physical education that would gradually and harmoniously develop every muscle (voluntary and involuntary), every organ and every system and every cell, building the body, as it were; in storeys upon a solid, firm and secure foundation, which would continue to the end of a person's days. And just as the brain is most receptive in the young, so the youthful body is best adapted for this physical education, training and development of every cell, organ and system, for the establishment of a harmonious and perfect balance between physique, constitution and brain, of, in short, healthy mental and muscular co-ordination.

GRADING THE CHILDREN.

For, after all, the process in brain and body is very much the same. The physical brain, like the physical body, is simply a community of individual living cells, partly independent yet all inter-dependent, with muscles and activities like ourselves, although these muscles and activities are naturally more simplified in the cell. Mental education consists of developing each of these individual living cells by mental use and activity, so improving its health and muscular quality and increasing its faculty of multiplication, because the more numerous and better developed they become the more intelligent will be the individual.

If you can so educate, train, develop and increase the number of these living cells of the brain by mental use, exercise and daily activity, so similarly you can develop and strengthen the cells of all parts of the body by what I describe as their balanced physical movement.

In other words, the body must be educated scientifically, as we train the mind, if we are to build up a people healthy, strong, courageous and self-reliant, and we must proceed in much the same way to grade the children from the very outset, according to their physical and organic condition, as we do mentally to-day. This work, of course, must be the work of an expert, and none should be better qualified for it than the members of the medical profession. It would be for these medical men to see that each and every child has its body trained to the highest standard of physical excellence in every cell, rather than that its little mind is crammed and overdeveloped at the cost of bodily strength.

STATE MEDICAL EXAMINATION AND SUPERVISION.

Every school should have its doctor or medical staff, according to its size, whose duty it should be to look after the bodily welfare of the children and to supervise and direct the scientific physical education of every child. This would be a position of great responsibility and prestige, and the greatest care should be exercised to select physicians and surgeons with a strong and sympathetic personality, likely to command at once the respect of the teachers and the affection and regard of both the children and their parents. This is a basic essential of such a system as I advocate, and it is of paramount importance. Every country boasts such medical men in profusion, who follow the noblest of all human professions not for lucre, but are animated by a truly sublime spirit of unselfishness, service and even sacrifice.

It would be the work of such men to "sift" the children medically and physically, and to prescribe movements to suit each individual pupil or patient, taking, as I have just said, age, sex, temperament, constitution, personal idiosyncracies, physical defects, family history and other individual detail into full consideration. The rectification of individual defects whether physical or organic or functional, the establishment and preservation of physical and organic balance, the co-ordination of mind and nerve and muscle, would be some of the chief aims of the medical men.

All this, of course, will be a matter requiring the utmost care and attention on the part of medical men, as yet comparatively inexperienced in this matter, but in a few years after its establishment we would have quite a new generation and type of doctors, men who have made a special study of curative and preventive physical movements in their University or College, and who will have themselves gone through a course of special physical education and training, and passed examinations as to their own physical standard of fitness, making them physically as well as mentally fit for their duties.

The admission of a child to any school or other educational institution should be equivalent to a guarantee to the parents of the safe custody of the child's health and physical body during school hours, and a child should enter school much as a recruit enters the army only after passing a thorough medical examination. On the other hand, the parents would be reasonably held responsible to the State for the child's health out of school hours up to a certain age fixed by legal statute.

Before a child was admitted the parents should be obliged to fill up a printed form containing questions regarding the child's and its parent's health history, somewhat similar to those asked of applicants by insurance companies, but even more stringent and far-reaching in their details.

The answers would supply valuable information as to the cause of the grandparents' death, the age, and medical history of the parents themselves, whether they had any disease or physical shortcomings, etc., etc. The answers to these questions would be a kind of index to the doctor before he examined the child personally, to help him more readily to discover any inherited weakness or tendency towards disease.

Charts for each child would then be prepared, to unfold, showing the various bones, muscles, organs, nerves, etc., of the body, and on this chart the medical man would be able to mark all local weaknesses and derangements, to make notes of any lack of muscular, mental or organic balance, and also to record any improvement in the child from time to time.

Especial attention would be paid to lung capacity, for no function stands so near to the centre of vitality as respiration. For, as medical men are aware, the ratio of the lung capacity to the bodily weight is considered the vital index of a person's general vigour and power of endurance. Where there were narrow chests or weak lungs from family history, round shoulders, or anything likely to invite or induce consumption, such an examination would be invaluable, and movements to improve the carriage, strengthen the muscles of the spine, square the shoulders, enlarge the chest cavity, deepen and broaden the chest, increase lung capacity and strengthen the cells of the lungs would be a powerful preventive measure against deadly consumption.

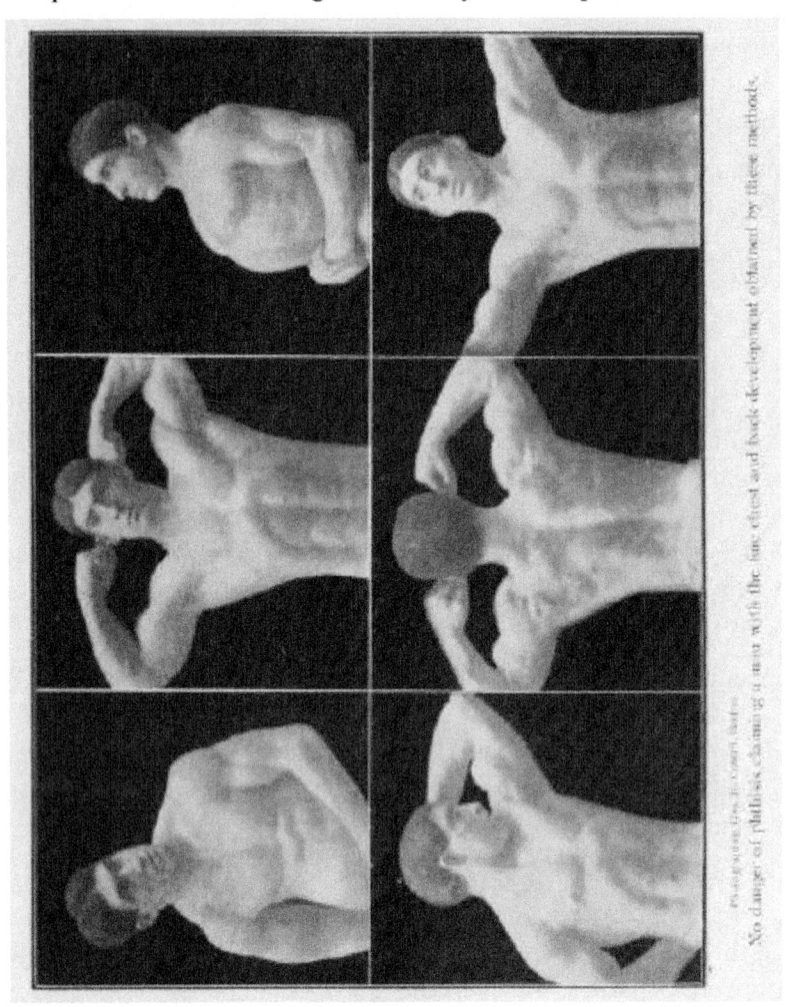

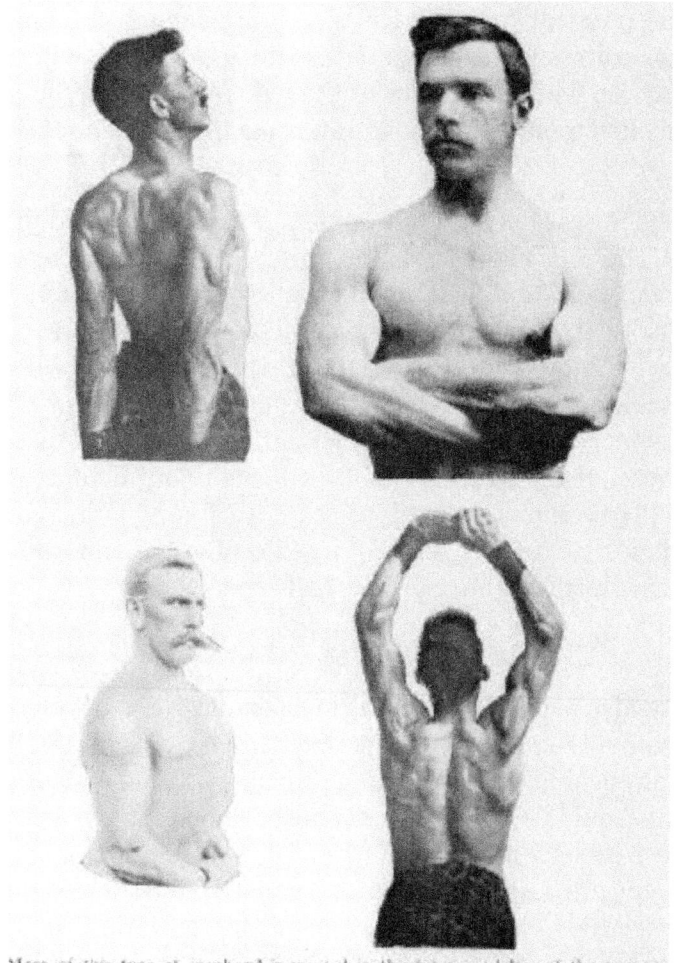

More of this type of manhood is wanted in the future and less of the narrow chested, flabby, undeveloped and disease-introducing type too prevalent in our midst to-day. To the methods of physical rebuilding described here all these men owe their fine bodies and developed physique.

PHYSICAL EDUCATION BEFORE MENTAL.

The doctor should be attached to the school, just as much as the schoolmaster, and it should be part of his duty to give popular lectures to the children on anatomy and physiology, to instruct them in the value and effect of exercise, to explain to them the reason of its absolute necessity, to make clear to them its influence upon the anatomy and physiology of the body, to describe its value as an aid to mental work, and especially to warn them against the self-abuse and pollution of the body by self-drugging, alcohol, smoking in early life, and other evil practices and habits. Just as there are annual mental examinations so there should be an annual examination and inspection of all the children to ascertain their knowledge of anatomy, physiology and hygiene, and prizes awarded.

Physically and organically the children should be examined periodically, reports made and careful records preserved. Competitions could be inaugurated, and prizes awarded for physique and health, and altogether at least one-fifth of the time devoted to mental training should be set aside for health education and the building up of the physical body in the case of physically normal children, and as much time as the doctor thinks necessary for delicate and diseased children, while the doctor should even have power to order a total cessation of mental training in extreme cases, until the physical body was made strong enough to support the mental effort. Reports on the child's health should be forwarded to the parents with the customary school reports, with medical advice when necessary to the parents, while in the more serious cases the parents should be compelled to attend personally for medical advice regarding the requirements of the child or children.

Under the present system, disease is often allowed to develop unnoticed in a child at school until it is firmly established, and precautions such as these will go far to prevent disease, instead of merely waiting until it develops and then attempting to cure it with more or less success; or, as Sir Kingsley Wood puts it, " building a hospital at the bottom of a cliff instead of erecting a rail at the top." Fortunately, with the education of those who themselves will be parents of another generation, a double check on disease will be added, and all this will lead to the total defeat and rout of the enemy. It is, at least, certain that such ailments as heart disease, adenoids, and all ailments to which children are especially liable, consumption, debility, rupture, and physical deformities, defects and weakness towards disease of every kind, can thus be practically obliterated if the children have such a really scientific physical education and training as this, with the conjoint State and medical supervision of all schools.

THE DUTY OF THE INSTRUCTORS.

Every large school would have its own department exclusively devoted to health culture by physical movements, with all the necessary apparata, and its staff of highly trained, experienced and carefully selected physical instructors with a proved knowledge of anatomy, physiology and hygiene. Smaller schools could be similarly catered for under one control. These instructors will be as vital to the success of such a scheme as I propose as the doctors, and they must be dealt with financially in no niggard fashion. On the other hand, they must not only be handsomely remunerated for their services, but must receive every encouragement for their study and research, for they will be, to no little extent, the working builders of the nation, and indeed of the Empire.

The instructor would stand in relation to the doctor much as the chemist does to-day. Just as the chemist has to understand chemistry, the nature, use and action on the body of the many medicines in his store, and the doctor prescribes from these such as are required in proper proportions, doses and combinations to suit the individual pupil or patient, so the instructor should have a thorough knowledge of the body and bodily hygiene, of anatomy and physiology, and of the effect of every muscle and its movement on the body, to see that the exercises prescribed by the medical officer after careful diagnosis of each case, are carried out correctly and successfully. This diagnosis would be, of course, the supreme duty of the doctor, for only the medical officer himself would be allowed to diagnose and prescribe.

While the children should be taught to take a pride in the size, substance, and quality of their muscles and of their body as a whole —a natural thing for every healthy boy at least—they should be given an intelligent idea of exactly what muscular development meant to them in health as well as in physical appearance, and girls should be shown how it helps to improve their carriage, their gait, their figure, and even their complexion and their health. Special prizes should be offered to those with the finest physique, carriage, and gait.

All the exercises, however, should be selected and grouped with the one main object of always developing the muscle necessary for the healthy functioning of the vital organs (and of developing both the voluntary and involuntary muscles in balance) that are jeopardised by lack of balanced physical movement under modern and civilised conditions of life, on the part of their parents or ancestors.

WHY APPARATA ARE HELPFUL.

The classification that we need for guidance in our labour for the all-round and balanced development of the individual in which health plays the chief part, must be founded upon the effects of the exercises upon the organs and their functions. An ideal classification would be one which grouped together in indissoluble union such exercises as affected a given function in a definite manner. That is the ideal at which really scientific physical training must ever aim.

Before the children begin their systematic exercises they should have their own interest aroused, and have impressed upon them the result of every movement they perform, or otherwise they may be inclined to regard the physical training as mere labour and carry out the movements without concentrating their mind upon them, the latter one of the most vital essentials to the success of what I call physical reconstruction. To help them to concentrate their mind in this way it is always better at first to use some apparatus (for some children have not sufficient power of muscular and mental co-ordination, and having an apparatus to carry and control gradually schools them to perfect self-control not only of the muscles but of the nerves and brain).

Apparata may or may not be dispensed with afterwards, but I maintain that an apparatus of some kind is desirable if only that the medical man has an agent by which he can measure, check and regulate the 'progress of each child and protect it against over-effort. Moreover, the use of apparata in the form of light dumb-bells in contracting the muscles of the forearm and biceps will help the children to see these muscles contracting and to understand what is meant by the contraction of muscles that they cannot see. I might add also that I am not in favour of the movements being performed to the accompaniment of music except for exhibition purposes or merely for a display of the children's ability. Where physical movement, indeed, is meant to be educational, corrective, or remedial it is by no means necessary for it to be made pleasant or to be regarded merely as a pastime. The mind must be totally engrossed with the movement or movements and concentrated on the parts moved.

CARRIAGE, POSTURE, AND GAIT.

In every case, particular attention should be paid to the development of the muscles associated with the vital function of respiration, the abdominal and groin muscles which influence elimination, and all the muscles whose perfect balance holds and supports the spine and the spinal cord, and weakness or faults of these should be corrected as they are closely allied with the most vital functions of life. After any prescribed course of exercises is finished, the children should, at first, be again medically examined, the state of the heart, the pulse and the temperature noted, and occasionally even the blood and the urine should be tested. This medical examination would become less necessary and less frequent as the child progressed.

Simple as it may seem the children should be taught how to sit, stand, and walk correctly, for faulty attitude, either in sitting or standing or walking causes enormous wastage of vital energy, and indeed, saps more of the individual vital force than any other factor. It throws the whole spine out of alignment, it disturbs the spinal cord, and through it many important functions, it interferes with the heart's action, decreases respiration and the influence of respiration on the circulation. It prevents that important muscle, the diaphragm, from performing the natural massage of the viscera and leads to constipation, it robs many organs of their natural support, and it is responsible in general for unfavourable conditions of the organs of nutrition, secretion, circulation, respiration and elimination. To prevent this ought to be one of the first duties of the doctors, teachers, and instructors.

What makes the average physical training lesson at present of little actual educational value is the fact that the brain is not employed as it should be. The pupil is taught to go through a series of movements, without even thinking of the muscles or parts being moved, so that all this effort is of little value in developing either the muscles or the brain centres, because it is purely sub-conscious. It is most important that the mind be concentrated on the muscle or muscles moved, for this not only means an increased flow of blood to such muscle or muscles, but develop and strengthen the directing cells of the brain employed in the movement. It also develops mental and muscular co-ordination and teaches control over the muscles and through them over brain and nerves, as I more fully explain later.

Nor is the question of balance taken into consideration by teachers or pupils, for balance in the body is everything. The flexors must be balanced with the extensors, and each muscle or group of muscles, organ and group of organs, proportionately balanced, with perfect balance between the brain that directs and the body that is directed. Mere physical movement without conscious effort and the concentration of the mind on the muscles moved is only recreative and pretty to look upon and should always be regarded as secondary only to movement that is intended to develop a body and brain in equal and perfect balance.

The child should always be taught to contract and relax the muscles with equal thoroughness if it is to acquire that perfection of direct control over the voluntary muscles which is necessary to have perfect and equal control over contraction and relaxation. This is of greater importance than may be thought, and is, indeed, a vital feature of such a system as I now propose.

1.—CONTRACTION MOVEMENTS.

These, of course, are the very beginning of all physical training, for contractility is the peculiar and especial characteristic of muscle. Indeed, if the tendon of a muscle is out, the muscle at once contracts like a piece of stretched rubber, showing that it is always, when at rest, a little stretched. Contraction movements should be carried out with the concentration of the mind upon the muscles or groups of muscles contracted with full muscular effort. The concentration should continue right through the entire movement with full maximum pressure and mental concentration, and so should be continued during the entire number of movements prescribed, the breathing being normal and natural. This only constitutes the ideal contraction, but, of course, is only possible for those who are physically sound and well.

The teacher should also explain to the child which muscles are brought into play by any and every such movement in order that the child knows upon which muscle or muscles to concentrate. Movements so performed will increase the power, size, and quality of muscle, and benefit all internal parts in proportion, and will also increase a child's control over the muscles by the brain which supplies the directing power.

The child should be taught to keep its mind exclusively centred on the muscles or parts moved at the time, and so through each of any series of movements, as this develops its will-power and causes a greater flow of blood to the muscle or muscles affected, and to the whole area they influence, while the reaction of the blood means a better flow of blood and supplies to the brain and its greater nourishment and oxygenation, strengthening the brain and making good the waste previously expended in mental learning, while also adding to its receptive capacity. Contraction movements should always be performed slowly.

(Here, again, I would direct the attention of the adult reader to my chapter on " How and Why Scientific Physical Movement Cures Disease," with its appendix in the form of a reply to an article in The Lancet). This chapter explains most fully just why labour involving muscular movement, general exercises, games, sports and pastimes or massage, electricity and hydropathy cannot compare from a curative point of view with the natural and balanced physical movement of all the bodily muscles in a scientific way, where there is disease or the weakness tending towards disease. It explains the reason why conscious and concentrated muscular movement alone has a remedial and curative value, in the treatment of all sickness and disease, and this chapter and the appendix should be carefully read and studied by all who are personally interested, for what applies here to children as a preventive equally applies to adults for curative purposes.)

2.—RELAXATION MOVEMENTS.

It is just as important for the child to be taught how to relax the muscles during each movement as how to contract them, for above all things else, a perfect balance must be observed between contraction and relaxation whilst carrying out each and every movement to prevent the pupil from becoming muscle-bound, and to train the child also to swiftness of action.

Perfect balance between power of contraction and power of relaxation movement means that the reaction when the muscles are relaxed is equal to the action by which they were contracted, and when this balance is ensured strength and speed will alike characterise muscular action. The practising of contraction and relaxation movements for swiftness and power of movement will, as I have already shown, also develop the motor areas of the brain, and when this mental and muscular balance is established we are approximating to physical perfection, especially if, at the same time, there is exhibited an organic and physical balance between all the various organs and functions and the muscles responsible for those functions.

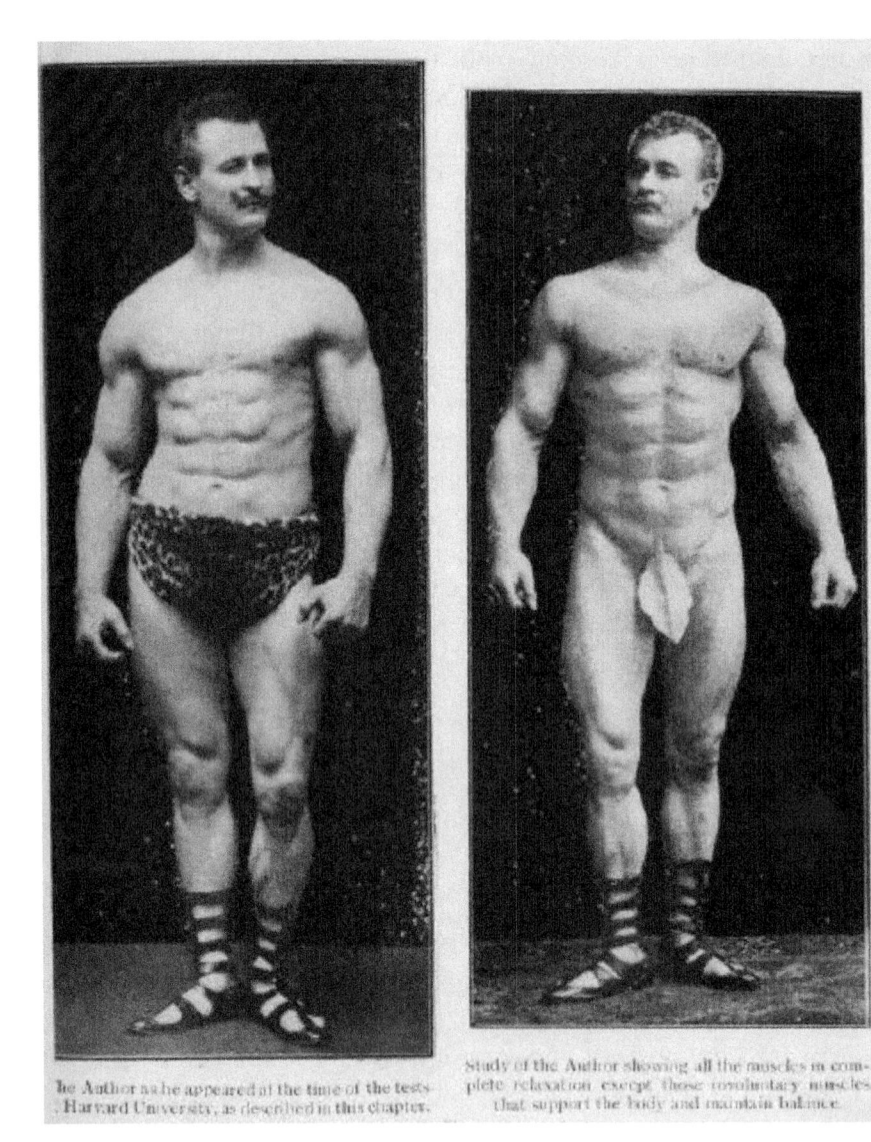

The Author as he appeared at the time of the tests, Harvard University, as described in this chapter.

Study of the Author showing all the muscles in complete relaxation except those involuntary muscles that support the body and maintain balance.

It will also give that perfect control over the nerve and brain which most of us, as I explain elsewhere, have lost through the diminution of natural physical activity through successive generations of civilisation, and which we can only regain by such a system of physical education and re-education as I have outlined. (See also chapter on " Muscle, Mind and Nerve.") Such training will bring about quickness of judgment and decision, swiftness and power of action, and will fit a person for success in any business or sport where such qualities are essential. Relaxation movements, unlike those of contraction, should be performed quickly, thus relaxing from the very beginning of the movement.

We see a splendid example of combined speed and power both in thinking and acting in the case of a well-trained boxer, and where two opponents have an equal knowledge of and facility in all the tricks of the game, the winner is always the man who can strike most swiftly and with most power, that is, with the most powerful muscle or muscles behind the blow and the swifter execution of an order from the brain. Where there is this splendid balance between contraction and relaxation in this movement and between the brain and the associated muscles employed, decision and action are almost instantaneous and simultaneous.

Indeed, if I may again intrude a little personal experience of my own, it will help to prove this. While on tour in America, Dr D. A. Sargent, M.A., the world-famed medical director of the Harvard University athletes, was amazed to find that I was as speedy in action as strong, because, like so many others. Dr Sargent expected to find in a strong man that the power of contraction had been developed at the expense of the power of relaxation, and that what I had gained in strength and power had been at the price of agility and speed.

Before a group of athletes, which included a famous boxing instructor, Mr Michael Donovan, of New York, a man noted for Iris speed in striking a blow, I was put through a series of speed tests with this specialist in boxing, and it was proved that I was almost as swift in striking as Mr Donovan, notwithstanding all his greater 'practice and experience, and the fact that his mind had been so much better educated and trained for such a performance than mine. It was shown in 16 trials by means of an ingenious electrical apparatus that the average time occupied by my fist In travelling a distance of 15 75.100 inches was 11-100th of a second. Mr Donovan's speed in 10 trials averaged 8-100 of a second.

In another test I proved to be Mr Donovan's superior, my average time between making up my mind to strike and beginning to strike being 22-100 of a second, while Mr Donovan's was 23-100, or just 1-100 of a second slower. This was because I had trained my muscles to contract and relax in perfect harmony, and my mind co-ordinated perfectly with both.

IMPORTANCE OF FULL CONTRACTION.

With children, the movements of contraction and relaxation should be practised alternately, and the child should be taught to be able to contract or relax each muscle or all the muscles at will, while its capacity for both these acts should be tested at each physical examination. Of course, the child cannot learn to relax until it intelligently understands how to contract, so that contraction is the keynote of successful physical training. The teaching of intelligent relaxation will bring increased power of recuperation, for the more complete the relaxation of the mental, nervous and muscular systems, as in sleep, the better the re-building of the muscular system and the whole body will be.

Complete relaxation without movement of any kind should also be taught, for it is surprising how few there are even among grown-up people to-day, who can utterly relax the muscles of the body when they desire, and so obtain that complete and re-invigorating rest of a healthy babe, as yet unspoiled by its association with a degenerative civilisation. The children should be taught how to relax the muscles either when standing up, sitting down or lying down. When they have been given the intelligent understanding of how to control the contraction of the muscles, they will then more quickly be taught to understand how to completely relax any muscle or group of muscles. This should be practised, with each limb alternately, also with the body as a whole.

Such practice from children would undoubtedly be of great benefit in preventing and eradicating functional nervous troubles and disorders, as it would gradually develop self-control and the inhibition of such purposeless and unnecessary activity of a morbid nature which is responsible for a great wastage and prodigal expenditure of nervous energy.

The teaching of this valuable lesson of total and equal contraction and relaxation must be most thorough and most careful, and it would be best always in the case of children—especially where there is the slightest heart trouble—to teach the child first to contract and relax only one muscle or group of muscles at a time while performing a movement. As a simple example, let us take the biceps. At first, the one arm only should be employed at a time, and the child taught to contract and relax the biceps, with its mind only concentrated on that muscle, and with its fullest effort, the rest of the body being relaxed as fully and as far as possible. The triceps would, of course, also be brought into play automatically, but its movement would only be sub-conscious and of a relaxed character.

The child should be taught at this time to feel with its own free hand the contraction and relaxation of the biceps in turn, keeping the hand there during the performance of the movement or movements, thus having sensory evidence of the hardening of the muscle in contraction and its softening under relaxation. It should also be informed that the harder the muscle when contracted and the greater its softness when relaxed the better the quality of the muscle. All this would not only have an excellent educational value, but it would teach the child to fully concentrate its mind only on any muscle or muscles moved, and so to derive real benefit both from contraction or relaxation. Instead of the mind being divided in its attention between several muscles it would be concentrated for the time entirely on a certain group of muscles so that the results in this way would be still further enhanced.

Above all, the strain put upon the heart by the maximum of muscular and mental effort in one muscle or group of muscles, or in one limb or one side of the body instead of two, would be lessened, so that in every case of heart trouble the child should begin any treatment for its heart only in this way. This illustration is only given as an example, and holds good with regard to every other voluntary muscle or group of muscles, the child being taught to feel the muscle or muscles moved where possible, hardening or softening during contraction and relaxation wherever possible. When I say that the maximum of effort and complete concentration of the mind are essential to achieve the best results, I would point out, however, that it is best to attain this ideal by gradual stages, especially in the case of children or when there is any suspicion of organic weakness or disease or tendency to disease. This gradual increase of effort and mental concentration should be obligatory with children, and is preferable even in the case of adults to avoid the possibility of overstrain or injury at the outset. The same also holds good with regard to the speed at which the physical movements are performed, and these should only be accelerated gradually as the heart grows stronger, as I point out in Chapter X.

The complete relaxation of the muscles will teach children to acquire control over the brain itself, and to regulate their nervous expenditure, a most valuable lesson at a time when nervous troubles are so painfully in evidence. It will also be of the greatest benefit for those who are afflicted with sleeplessness, a formidable sapper of vital and nervous energy, and it will help men and women of the future to regain that serenity and calm equipoise of health so marked in contrast to the over-strung, restless fidgety type with which we are all too familiar to-day.

BREATHING EXERCISES.

Breathing exercises must, of course, receive most painstaking attention, for breathing is the first and last act of life and the most vitally essential of all bodily functions, except, perhaps, the beating of the heart. The teaching of proper breathing at school would undoubtedly help very much by strengthening each and every cell of the lungs to completely eliminate the terrible disease of consumption, and all that fearful train of lung and chest complaints, such as asthma, bronchitis, etc., which levy so heavy a toll upon human life to-day.

Children should all be taught the health value of breathing through the nostrils instead of the mouth, a practice that warms the air on its passage to the bronchial tubes and the lungs, and helps to check germs of disease from gaining entrance there. They should be taught to make each inspiration slowly in this way, and equally to exhale fastly, freely and fully by the mouth. Deep breathing must be done very gradually,, especially where there is any heart or lung trouble or weakness tending towards such, and the state of the heart noted after all such exercises.

Deep nasal breathing fills the lungs with the oxygen that the Hindoo Yogis call prana or life itself, and full exhalation, of course, means the free expulsion of carbonic acid gas and much gaseous filth that would otherwise be retained in greater quantity in the system, very much to the prejudice of the bodily health.

The children should be taught upper-chest breathing, abdominal breathing and costal-breathing in turns, filling the lungs to their fullest air capacity at each inspiration, and to realise the difference in these forms of breathing by placing their hands where the muscles of respiration in each case can be felt moving in inspiration and expiration.

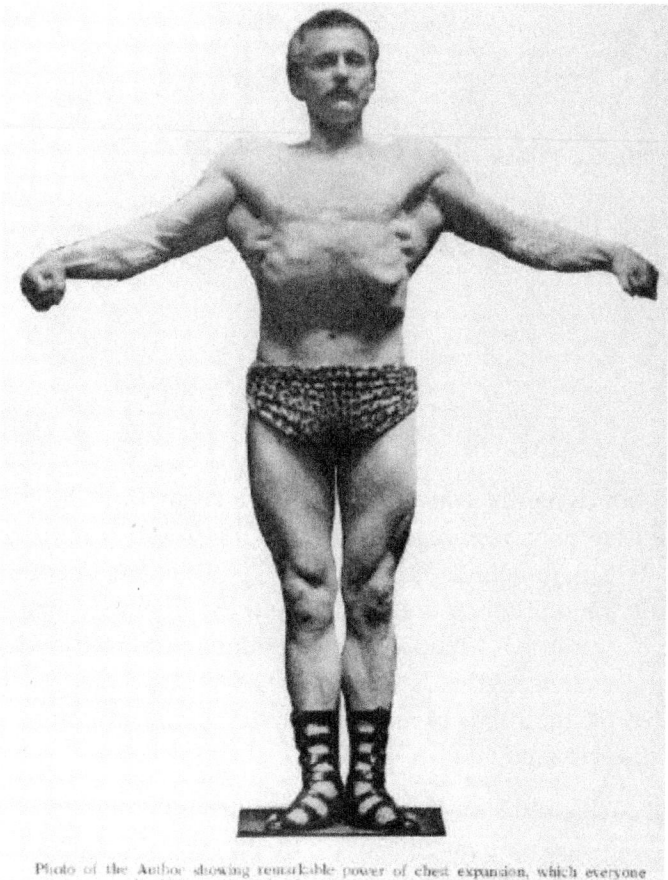

Photo of the Author showing remarkable power of chest expansion, which everyone should be taught and trained to possess by the same methods.

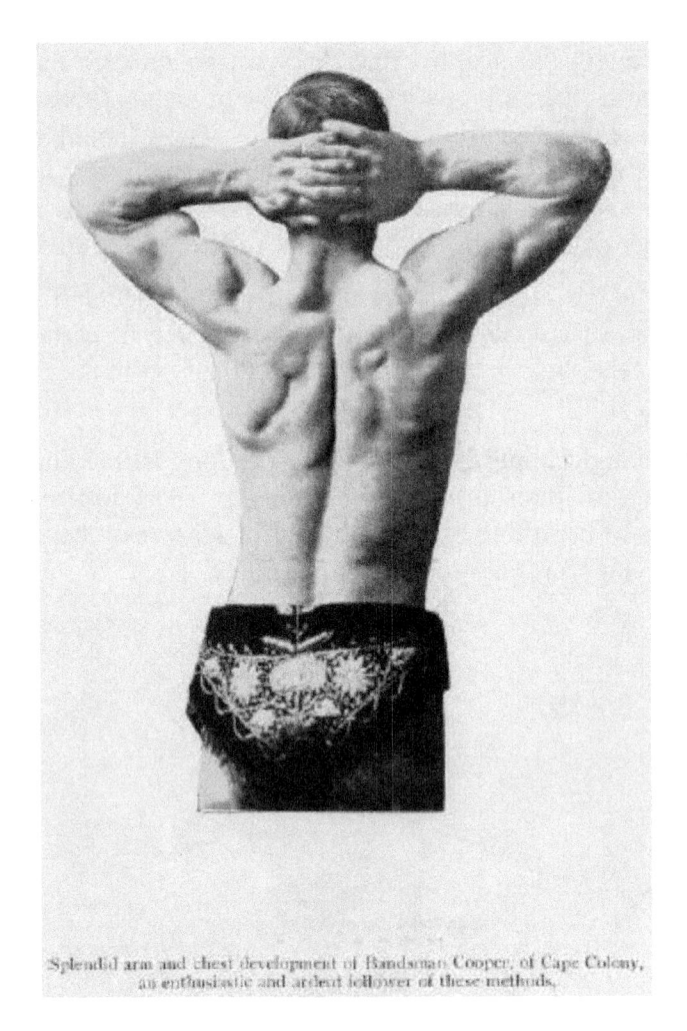

Splendid arm and chest development of Bandsman Cooper, of Cape Colony, an enthusiastic and ardent follower of these methods.

USE OF MODELS AND CHARTS.

Above all, they should be vigilantly watched to prevent them from holding in the breath while carrying out these breathing exercises, and all this teaching will train them to breathe naturally and deeply and to exhale fully in later life, while it must, of course, deepen and broaden the chest, increase the lung capacity, and toughen the tissue of all the organs of respiration. As the cells of the respiratory system can only be directly and separately exercised and developed in resistant power by such breathing exercises, this is the only way that we can reach them and bring into balance with the cells of all the other organs and systems, the importance of deep and natural breathing cannot be over-estimated.

It is important, too, that each child should be made to thoroughly understand the exact nature and meaning of every physical movement employed in its education and training, the muscle or muscles influenced by it, and the bodily organs and functions also affected. A pupil of exceptional development and possessing perfect co-ordination of mind and muscle might be used as a model and anatomical charts should be employed and teachers or instructor should point out the exact result of every movement as the model makes them.

I cannot, of course, go into all the details that I consider essential in such a system of scientific physical education and training as I advocate as a necessary step to the eradication and prevention of disease and the restoration of that physical movement and activity so lacking from modern life yet so essential to life and health. To do so would mean my writing another volume quite as large as the present on the practical side of this question alone, and it may be that if I find the whole question taken up and supported by those in authority and the people themselves, I may yet find time to prepare such a book for the press, and to do my share to assist the doctors, the physical instructors, the teachers and the State in this most important part of modern education. I might just add here that, of course, my whole scheme presupposes the proper feeding of the children, for no scheme, as I enlarge upon elsewhere, can ever be effective that is not based on the unchangeable and unchanging fact that a hungry child needs food to assimilate before it can assimilate either knowledge or wisdom, or build up a healthy physical organism.

In conclusion, as a leader writer in the Daily Mail has said very truly, " the making of the next generation is the greatest reform of all. If we can ensure that every child shall have a chance of growing up with a sound physique and a solid groundwork of health knowledge, we shall have taken some considerable step towards transforming our whole national life."

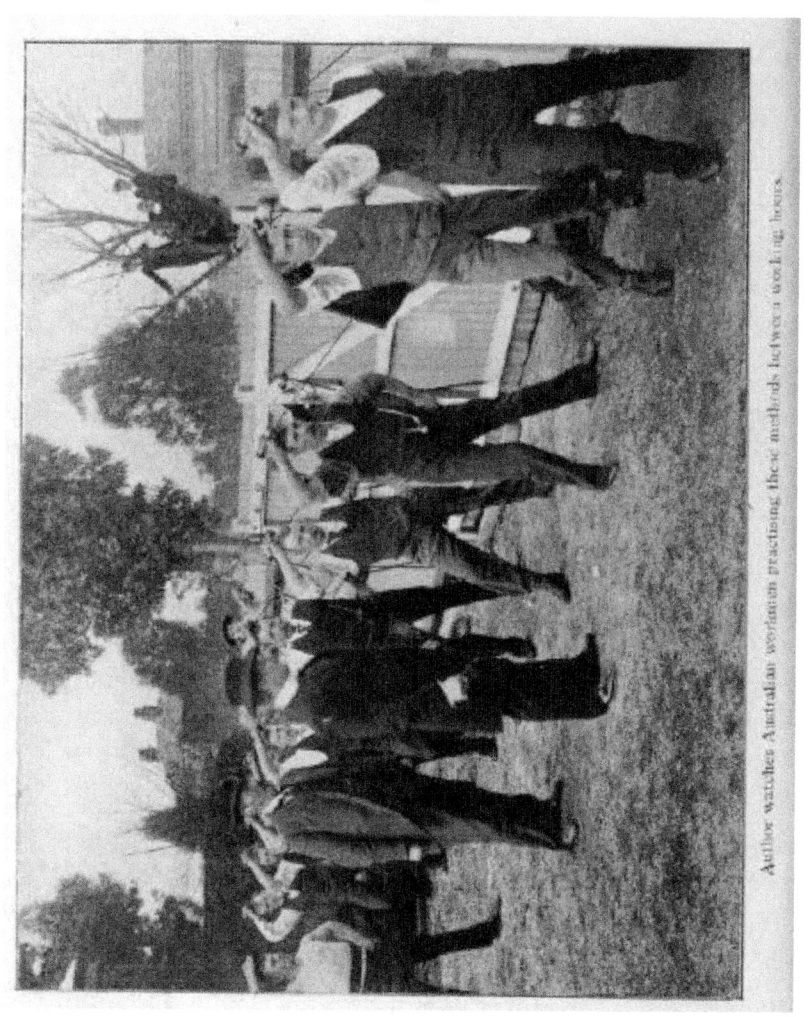

Author watches Australian workmen practising these methods between working hours.

CHAPTER XII.

A Well-nourished Body the First Step in Education.

THE stomach is the furnace of the human engine, and the food taken into it the fuel.

It is impossible to raise steam without fuel, and what coal is to the steam-engine food is to the human engine, the prime source of all power. It will be impossible ever to successfully educate starved or starving children, either mentally or physically, any more than you could train a Derby winner on short rations or while feeding it on chaff. This is so self-evident a truism that it almost insults the intelligence of my readers to give expression to it. Yet it is necessary for me to emphasise it, because any such scheme of physical education and reconstruction as I propose falls to. the ground if the children, from any cause, are underfed.

We want "thoroughbred" human beings even more than thoroughbred horses, and nothing breeds disease and deterioration, mental and physical, like privation or starvation, because nothing more quickly lowers bodily resistant power, as was painfully evident during the war period when every country suffered in degree, and Germany endured quite an epidemic of " hunger-typhus " and consumption. In Belgium 40 per cent, of the patients in hospital were victims of phthisis through starvation, and the mortality in Vienna, through the same cause, was appalling.

Even neutral countries like Sweden and Spain were devastated by disease, several epidemics arising from privation. It leads to in-nutrition and mal-nutrition, diminishes resistant power and undermines all the bodily defences. So, if we seek to eliminate disease and build up a stronger and better people, it is at once evident that we must grapple seriously with the food problem which is responsible for so much disease, especially in the young.

One of France's most gifted writers, after a visit to London, ironically remarked of our well-worn boast that all men had equal rights under British law, that there was nothing whatever to prevent a rich man from sleeping away a winter's night on the Embankment any more than a poor one.

Both would probably be arrested and fined; there the equality would end. The rich man would pay the fine, the poor man, being unable to do so, would go to prison. The one was, however, driven by necessity, the other his own free-will.

THE DEVIL OR THE STATE?

The children of the rich may not get the food necessary for their health and well-being, the poor often cannot. The parents of a rich child may be cruel, avaricious, mean, or they may be dissipated, drunken and neglectful. In many cases, the same holds good, of course, with the parents of poor children, for even the poor or comparatively poor are not always paragons of virtue. Both rich and poor parents can starve or under-feed their children if they desire. Both, however, if detected, can, and should, be punished except where poverty justifies or excuses.

The punishment, however, must always fall heaviest on the poor, and always it is the child that suffers most. Before the parents are detected and punished a child may even be starved to death. We must not wait until either rich or poor parents commit the offence. We must make it impossible for either of them to do so.

Here, too, I wish to express my agreement with the Premier, who said in his first election speech in 1918, " wages must not be permitted to drop to the point where the strength of the worker cannot be maintained in efficiency, and where the mother cannot discharge her sacred functions of bringing up children to undertake the burden of Empire in the next generation. The health of the people must especially be the concern of the State." Better wages, better food and better health should now be the watchwords of the nation.

If, as we are so often told to-day, no child wholly belongs to its parents but in part also to the State, then we must have fatherly, if not grandfatherly, legislation, to protect every child from even the possibility of starvation. It will, of course, cost money, but you cannot buy good citizenship if you are not prepared to pay the price. The Devil will outbid the State if the latter bids meanly or grudgingly for its children.

It matters not however, how or whence the money comes, the children must be fed with really nourishing food, if any scheme of any kind for their physical reconstruction and salvation is to bear fruit. If the parents are able to afford to pay for it well and good. They must do so. If they fail to do so, the State must punish them and save the children. If the parents, from " any just cause or impediment," as we say in another place, are unable to do so, either permanently or temporarily, the local educational authorities must do so, and failing them, the State itself.

THE HEADQUARTERS OF HAPPINESS.

The stomach is the real headquarters of the body, and all human happiness or misery springs from that source. If this applies to adults, how much more truly does it apply to children who need food more because they are growing, and who, by their natural activities, consume vitality at an enormous rate.

A child has two arms, two legs, two lungs, two kidneys, even two brains. It has only one stomach, and that stomach ultimately may decide the fate of a people or of an army. It will certainly decide a child's view of life for good or evil. As Dr B. W. Richardson well said, " the centre of the emotion of felicity is not in the brain." The centre is in the vital nervous system, in the great ganglia of the sympathetic, lying not in the cerebro-spinal cavities but in the cavities of the body itself, near the stomach and on the heart. Everybody who has felt felicity has felt it as from within the body. We know, again, where the depression of misery is located; our physicians of all times have defined that and have named the disease of misery from its local seat. The man who is always miserable is a ' hypochondriac '—his affection is seated under the lower ribs."

Or, again, as a distinguished ex-Army surgeon puts it:—" You may cut off a man's leg or his arm, you may knock out a teacupful of his brains, you may cut and carve him pretty freely, still he will sing and laugh and keep up his pluck, so long as stomach and liver are on duty. Let them fail, and the man will sneak or lie down and whine."

That was how a soldier spoke of soldiers. What, however, must be the sufferings of a child who, with an empty paunch, is asked to master the rule of three or follow the labyrinthine mazes of grammar.

Every city, town and village should have its communal kitchen and dining hall, and the food should be selected, prepared and cooked by skilful cooks, under medical supervision and direction, so that only the most nourishing foods should be provided and cooked in the most hygienic way. At least one good meal a day should be guaranteed to every child whether its parents are able to meet the cost or not, for a workless father should never mean a starving child. For, as Sir George Newman has pointed out, over and over again, all lessons must be lost on a child that is hungry or insufficiently nourished, and the money spent on education in this way is simply wasted.

CHILDREN MORE PRECIOUS THAN CONVICTS.

Children at school should be weighed on entrance, and at least once a month subsequently, and any declination of weight, or any child not of normal weight, should be immediately brought under the notice of a doctor, who would then order it such a diet or special diet as he thought desirable. Of course, any standard of weight must be, to some extent, elastic according to the build, condition and temperament of the individual child. No child should be permitted to lose weight, for even a convict in a prison is not allowed to lose weight to any reasonable extent without immediate medical attention, and it is not surely asking too much to ensure that innocent children should at least be as well treated in this matter as the inmates of a convict settlement.

Any system of free meals is, of course, open to abuse, and inspectors should be appointed to see that drunken or avaricious parents do not attempt to take advantage of such a scheme. Just as most public hospitals have almoners to inquire into the financial status of persons seeking admission, so every school or every local authority should have an official, whose duty it would be to check all applications for the free feeding of children, to ensure that only genuinely deserving cases received benefits under such a scheme, and to prosecute those whose neglect or voluntary idleness threw their children on the public funds, or who attempted to obtain relief by fraud in any way.

Free meals should only be allotted on application, except in rare cases, where medical recommendation would be sufficient, or otherwise, or many mothers might, through false pride, allow their children to suffer rather than apply for gratuitous assistance from the authorities or the State. The school doctor should have the power to order free meals in every case where he considered a child undernourished, while the almoner should make it his business to discover whether the parents were culpably responsible or not.

EVERY MOTHER HER OWN COOK.

The proper feeding of growing children is too grave a matter to be left to chance, for all money spent either on mental or physical education is money thrown away if the little ones are not supplied with sufficient nourishing food to support " each constituent and natural force" of the body. At present, the majority of parents have but the slightest knowledge of dietetics or food values, and are equally untrained in that culinary skill which enables a good cook to conserve all the valuable food essences, oils and salts which are so often lost in cooking by evaporation.

A better system of education will change all this, as we realise more and more that food is a most vital factor in the physique and health of a nation, the fuel that " stokes up " the body and energises the brain. Parents will be better informed as to the value of different articles of food and better trained in the art of cooking, for, under the system I suggest, mothers would receive a book from the State on the choice, preparation and cooking of food, which is, after all, the great question of paramount national importance in the dieting of both children and adults. Whether the State, the school or local authorities or the parents feed the children is not so much the question as whether they are fed properly and well fed or not.

Poor or improper feeding cannot but lower that innate resistant power of the body which is the only true and absolute preventive of disease. In this respect I may quote from the report of Dr E, Wyche, senior medical officer of the Nottingham Educational Committee. " The statistics," he says, speaking of his own district, "indicate a remarkable aggregate of ill-health, much of which is preventable, and should never have been permitted to occur. These children, handicapped by malnutrition and disease, during the most susceptible and plastic period of life, are thereby condemned to grow up with so much per cent, permanently knocked off their value to their native city and the community at large. As are our children so must our future be; as they grow up dirty, ill-nourished, diseased and inefficient, so will be our future place among the nations." This is wholesome talking and worthy of permanent record, while this very intelligent medical officer emphasises the value of " a successful offensive against the entrenched enemies of childhood, dirt, delicacy, and disease," malnutrition being a prolific cause of the latter.

METHODS THAT OUT-HEROD HEROD.

The experiment of issuing valuable nutritive foods and preparations to delicate children has already been made on a limited scale in certain districts, and this, again, is another area of service in which the school medical officer can exercise a most beneficial influence on the future men and women of the nation.

All this work of child welfare should not be left under different bodies as at present, but should be co-ordinated and centralised under a Ministry of Health, as I have before pointed out, if only that a continuous record of every child's physical life up till a certain age fixed by law should be preserved, and the statistics thus gleaned would be of the utmost value in combating and conquering national weakness, inefficiency and disease for the future. Even after the children leave school and begin work, such records should still be kept under one authority so that we would be able to have a consecutive story of the nation's individual physical life recorded, as it were, in yearly chapters.

Infant feeding is almost a problem by itself. Tainted and impure milk is an admittedly generous contributor to the cemetery through tuberculosis and other wasting diseases. Many mothers are unconsciously " baby killers " through ignorance as to the correct food for* infants and children.

As a writer in the Daily Mail has trenchantly remarked, " the law of life for multitudes of babies who have not nursemaids and ' mail-carts " is the harsh law of the survival of the fittest. They are the babies who are given long-brewed tea as a stimulant, whose milk, polluted before it is delivered, is left uncovered for hours in crowded dwelling rooms, into whose mouths germ-laden ' comforters ' are thrust when they cry with pain," the poor mites, unfortunately, having " no language but a cry." " This is why," continues the writer, " ten in every hundred of the babies who are born in Great Britain do not live twelve months." And it is important to bear in mind that the greatest harm to the human race through faulty feeding is not merely the loss of precious infant life, but the fact that even those who survive must grow up with weak, unhealthy or even diseased bodies. We shall never get rid of national inefficiency until we have taught every mother how to feed her children.

Our efforts at present to stamp out disease are severely handicapped by our want of organisation and co-ordination. A child is attacked, say, with phthisis, contracted through tainted milk. It is admitted to a hospital or sanatorium and either recovers or dies. A few questions are asked as to family history, habits, etc., and the case duly recorded, but no further steps are taken to bring what is really a crime against the public home to the guilty ones.

What I would like to see is a Ministry of Health with similarly organised powers and forces to fight disease and disease germs as Scotland Yard has to fight crime and criminals. Such a

Ministry of Health would have a wonderful disease-detective and police system in the medical profession, with special offices to investigate the various forms of health-crimes, and staffs to hunt down disease to its lair and arrest it. The " evidence " of the victim should be taken and by a highly-trained and experienced officer.

A SCOTLAND YARD OF HEALTH.

Let us suppose, for instance, a patient's statement made it quite evident that the tubercle bacillus was introduced through drinking infected milk. Every effort should then be made by the medical detective system to trace that milk supply to its source, to locate the exact cause of the infection and to determine responsibility. Was the cow tuberculous and why? Were the byres clean and sanitary and well ventilated? Was there any dereliction of duty on the part of the inspectors? Was anyone who came in contact with the milk tuberculous? Or did it get tainted in transit between farm and dairy and retailer, or retailer and consumer? Such questions as these pursued painstakingly and conscientiously would, in many cases seal the doom of the guilty person or persons, and should also ensure his, her, or their punishment, for to supply tuberculous milk consciously to anyone is as criminal and culpable as to administer poison, and, if the victim should die, the responsible person is as guilty of manslaughter or even murder as if the victim had been killed by knife or bullet.

A Ministry of Health carrying out its work on such lines as these in every case of deadly disease would soon be able to bring to punishment many malefactors and be in possession of the most valuable information for the prevention and suppression of health crimes against the body, whether self-inflicted or otherwise. Such measures would also make people more careful, as they would be warned in time of the punishment their conduct would bring. In this way, too, many industrial diseases due to unhygienic and unsanitary workshops would be " rounded up," those responsible punished, and the annual hospital bill of the nation greatly diminished.

EVERY CRADLE A CRADLE OF EMPIRE.

The time has arrived when there must be an increasing public desire to cherish our children. They hold the future in their chubby little hands. Their cradles are the cradles of Empire. The occupant of the cradle to-day may be the first Minister of State some day. The biggest telescope ever made cannot see the far-off future of to-day's infant-in-arms. It is no excuse for us to say that it is the duty of the parents to feed their children. Admittedly that is so, but it is also the duty of the State which looks to its children to defend it in an hour of danger to see that the children are fed, whether there is parental neglect or not. Thousands may be neglectful, but tens of thousands find it most difficult, if not impossible to make ends meet. Let neglectful parents be punished by all means, but do not let the State and the community be robbed of efficient units because parents are either neglectful or poor.

The time has come for big, broad views on this subject, for if we punish those who would attempt to rob the State of a soldier, as the law does at present, is it not worse for the State itself to permit the sacrifice of a child through lack of food, for that child is the citizen in embryo to whom the State must look for prosperity in peace or victory in war.

He who said " feed My lambs " regarded the children not merely as the component units of a country or even an Empire, but reminded us rightly that " of such are the Kingdom of Heaven."- Let us, therefore, treat the children as we would an angel from Heaven.

GOOD FOOD, GOOD DIGESTION, GOOD HEALTH.

If we see to it that every child is assured of the food necessary to nourish, strengthen and maintain it, and keep its digestive system in healthy working order by such methods as I describe, the money and time spent on the mental education of children would quickly return a much higher dividend. As I have pointed out, movement is essential to life, for food without movement remains undigested and badly assimilated, lowering the resistant power of the body, disturbing the whole bodily equilibrium, and opening the door to disease, while, at the same time, debilitating the brain and nervous system by the accumulation of waste and poisonous matter, thus nullifying the best efforts to cultivate intelligence and understanding in such a child.

To avert malnutrition is to strengthen both body and mind, and to wipe out at one stroke a whole family of diseases and disorders. Scientific physical education and reconstruction will undoubtedly succeed in this if it be carried out carefully, thoroughly and courageously from the first day a child enters school. The school, too, will no longer be regarded with something akin to horror as it is so often by the children to-day, for under the new regime they will find full scope for the instinctive and natural desire in the young to display their physical capacity as well as their mental, and a welcome break to the monotony of mental work.

MAKING GOOD DIGESTION WAIT ON APPETITE.

To give the children good food and a good digestive system is to facilitate educational progress in every direction. I am glad to see that the subject is receiving considerable attention both in the medical and the educational press, and also to note that medical officers of health in every part of the country are directing attention to this important aspect of the whole educational problem.

Dr G. W. N. Joseph, of Warrington, says in his report that " One of the great problems of the future will be to see that all children receive suitable and ample nourishment if a strong and healthy race is to grow up." A very distinguished physician in Dr Eicholtz declares that " food is at the base of most of the evils of child degeneracy, and if we can take steps to ensure the proper and adequate feeding of children these evils will rapidly cease." I could go on quoting similar expressions of opinion by the thousand, all of which are straws showing in which way the wind is blowing. If the nation and the State sees to it that the children have good food such a system of national physical education as I am now advocating will give them the good digestion that should wait on it if it is to be converted into useful human energy and power. One cannot build up a body with a plentiful reserve of nervous energy and muscular power without good food, and the marvellous muscles of the body, which play so important a part in every bodily function, as I show in the following chapter, depend upon food well digested for the necessary supplies to sustain them and make good their waste.

CHAPTER XIII.
The Marvels of the Muscular System.

How important is the part that muscle plays in the life of an individual must at once be evident from the fact that for the mere act of living muscular power is essential. Logically, therefore, we may deduce the additional fact that the quality and amount of muscle one has, modifies and even determines, to no small extent, one's life and health, the degree to which we may be said to live and even the length and happiness or otherwise of our days in the land.

Quality of muscle is of even more importance than bulk, and, of course, one often finds wonderful strength and vitality in a person who does not carry any very exceptional show of muscle. Some will always have a greater bulk of muscle just as some will always grow taller than others. Each person has a different standard of muscular development, and when that is attained the quality of the muscle cells is then the determining factor. When each muscle cell is developed to its highest possible standard both in size and quality a small muscle-development may be quite consistent with strength, vitality and resistant power to disease, for ten of such cells have quite as much value as twenty of an inferior quality, just as ten strong men could lift a greater weight than twenty weak men. But where there is both great bulk and the same high quality there must be still more strength and more vitality because, to use a sporting expression, "a good big 'un is always better than a good little 'un."

Vitality or nerve-force is the motive power of the body (although some physiologists contend that muscle tissue has contracting power even without nervous stimuli), acting through the muscular system, but it must not be forgotten that it is through the muscular system that this nervous energy is generated, for upon the muscular system largely depends the digestion and assimilation of food and the circulation of the blood that carries the vital supplies of air and food necessary to nourish and support the nervous system, to free it from poisonous and waste matter, and to replenish its continually decreasing reserve of nervous energy.

THE UNITED STATES OF THE BODY.

It is surprising, indeed, even in these days, how little is understood of the value and importance of muscular power in the maintenance, protection and preservation of the nervous force and all the vital functions and processes of life, and how frequently it is still regarded as essential only for the performance of feats of strength or endurance. So much is this so at times that I remember a haughty young man, whose right arm had grown very weak and almost helpless, as a result of a long confinement to bed following an accident, saying to me when I told him that he would only be able to use it with assistance, and as he used it, it would gradually regain its lost muscular power; " Oh, Mr Sandow, I don't want to be muscular, you know." How he expected ever to move his arms without muscular power surprised me, so I told him that if he wanted to use his arms without muscles, he would need someone with him always to move them for him. For, as I show in another chapter, disuse of any part of the body must lead to deterioration and atrophy, because of the lack of movement that maintains life. Ignorance such as that referred to seems incredible in the twentieth century, yet there are many who are almost equally in the dark as to the real value and necessity of muscular movement.

The superficial muscles they can see are the only muscles they recognise, for many people, to use Emerson's phrase, are only " eye- wise," recognising and admitting only that of which they have visible evidence. They do not pause to consider that in the mysterious wonder-world of the body there are other invisible but important muscles associated with every vital act of life—respiration, digestion, circulation, secretion and excretion. We have not only muscles to move us about from place to place and to move the various parts of the body, but muscles also that help each organ to perform its functions in the body, either under the control of the mind and will or through association with these involuntary muscles and through sympathy in a body so closely inter-related and interdependent, where every system is linked up with every other system in what may truly be called the United States of the body.

THE LANGUAGE OF THE MUSCLES.

Each of us has certain muscles directly under our own control, and others are operated sub-consciously independent of our will. Others again, are partly under our control and partly beyond it, as, for instance, the muscles employed in breathing, which move even while we sleep, but which, however, we can, to some degree, control by an effort of will, breathing slowly or quickly as desired. Some muscles are capable of movement sub-consciously through the emotions and passions and feelings, without conscious effort of will on our part—often, indeed, in defiance of it, as, for instance, the muscles employed in laughing or crying, and in the various passions which act so strongly at times as to overcome the will. Control over these muscles can, to some extent, be developed by training, as I prove elsewhere, especially in children. Some have it more strongly developed than others, and by closely observing a child's degree of control in this way, a valuable index as to its mentality and moral trend may be obtained by the doctor or teacher.

Man, then, is a machine capable of motion and locomotion by means of muscle, voluntary and involuntary, and it is most important to recognise as a bed-rock fact how essential muscles are to our very existence and how much our health and immunity from disease depend upon muscular fitness and tone, and also how dependent is the mental structure upon the physical and muscular sub-structure.

We could not open or close an eye but for muscle. We could not move a finger without muscle. We could not laugh, cry, smile, scowl or frown without muscle. We could not even speak, sing, chew, swallow or digest our food without muscle. We could not breathe " the breath of life," our heart could not even beat, and our blood would stagnate and grow cold, without muscular power.

All the bodily muscles can be set in motion either by the direction of our own will or sub-consciously. The facial muscles, however, are usually moved only in response to some emotion, thought, feeling or passion. It is the muscles that give expression to our feelings and emotions, and, therefore, interpret often our most secret thoughts.

WHY SOME LOOK OLD SOONER THAN OTHERS.

The question is often asked why does one man look older than another of exactly the same age. I will answer this in the Irish way by asking another question, viz., why does a healthy child look younger than a man of middle age? The answer to both is simply that in the one case the muscles of the face are kept in more constant movement than the other by the more frequent expression of varying thoughts, feelings, or emotions.

The child naturally allows its emotions and feelings to express themselves more fully through the movement of the facial muscles than an adult. Its every thought is freely expressed by the muscles of its face, the muscles that move it so quickly to laughter or tears. The facial muscles being thus, as it were, constantly exercised and developed by its more emotional life, its freedom from responsibility, care and worry, its innocence and its carelessness of consequence, its skin is kept healthy, clear and well-nourished, while the firmness and chubbiness of its cheeks give the whole face that angelic experience of youth which we older folk so often envy and covet. This is entirely due to the fact that the muscles underneath are well developed and keep the skin fully" stretched.

As the child grows up it is taught to exercise self-control, to hide or dissemble its thoughts, emotions, and passions, to stifle its feelings, and so these facial muscles become less and less brought into active daily use. The result is that the face begins to lose its firmness, roundness and smoothness, and the muscles being little used grow weaker and smaller until the flesh hangs loosely and sags between the bones, because there is less muscle to fill up the intervening space or spaces.

Now take the case of two business men of the same age in exactly similar business circumstances. Both are in good physical trim, but one looks facially years older than the other. The one, as the saying is, " wears his heart upon his sleeve," takes the whole world into his confidence, accepts " Fortune's buffets and rewards " alike with smiling face, and does not even attempt to conceal or disguise his thoughts or suppress his emotions.

The other, of sterner mould, has cultivated an almost Indian reserve, has carefully trained himself to repress any facial expression that might reveal his real self behind a face that has become merely a mask, and the muscles of his face have consequently almost atrophied leaving deep hollows and furrows and " crows' feet." Probably the only exercise his facial muscles ever get is when Nature compels him to the act of yawning or when he occasionally unbends in private life. Is it any wonder, then, that the former man preserves an appearance of youth long after the latter?

WHY WRINKLES COME WITH AGE.

The middle-aged, and the old, who are still less susceptible to the passions, emotions, and thrills of youth slowly cease to exercise their facial muscles altogether, and their faces become wrinkled, cadaverous, and gnarled because the unused muscles and fatty tissue have shrunk to nothingness and there is little left but skin and bone Were it not for the act of yawning, through Nature's demand for more oxygen, which frequently brings their facial, throat and neck muscles into play, the bones might almost pierce the skin through lack of muscular protection.

Muscle, again, when fully developed in balance, gives the body its symmetry of form and grace and dignity of carriage and movement. It smoothes over the bony angularities and rounds off the figure, and this outward harmony and symmetry in a healthy and developed human body is but the visible expression of a similar but invisible harmony in the internal body, where all the cells have also been fully developed in true proportion and balance to one another.

What many, including even the medical profession—with some rare and gratifying exceptions—have not yet fully recognised is that it is necessary to build up the whole internal body in perfect proportion and balanced strength if we are to possess a body outwardly and visibly strong, symmetrical, graceful and balanced, the outward body being but the reflection of the body within. Because, balanced movements of the voluntary muscles, in the way I have explained, will also cause all the involuntary muscles and all the bodily cells also to move and develop in co-operation as described, with the result that any or every organ, system and function of the body can be developed, strengthened and improved thereby.

YOU LOOK AS YOU REALLY ARE.

In a sound and scientific system of physical education and training for children, the children would be taught to realise this, and to develop a healthy and well-balanced body in every way, internally and externally. With this internal and external bodily culture, a child would grow up to possess an exterior physical appearance of health, beauty and strength with an internal organism to correspond, and would be little likely to fall a prey to disease either then or in later life, for muscle once developed, especially while young, remains, in some degree, for life. Medical men will, I think, agree with me then that muscular strength and organic and, functional health are not things in antagonism or even apart. These must, on the other hand, go together. They are inseparable. They are one, in the natural order of things.

The scientific physical training of the muscular system, including, as it does, all the muscles of the body—the involuntary as well as the voluntary—will produce better balance and proportion of the whole organism, because it will develop and strengthen every organ by giving it just the movement that is necessary to its wellbeing, and thus bring about the better performance of its function or functions, and make the body both stronger and healthier in all its minutest parts.

In short, an individual1 s health is mainly contingent on his muscle-power, for as I have shown,, the nervous system, which regulates all the functions of the body, depends for its supplies upon the muscular system, and the better developed and balanced his muscular system, visible and invisible, the healthier and better functioned the nervous system must be. This muscle-power and balance can only be obtained and developed through balanced movement of the voluntary muscles in a scientific way.

OVER 500 MUSCLES IN THE BODY.

There are in the human body over 500 muscles of various shapes and sizes, some flat and ring-shaped, some spindle-shaped, some fan-shaped, some that look like little feathers, and some that have the appearance of small fish. When, again, one thinks of the many varieties and degrees of muscle from the brawny biceps and triceps of the blacksmith's arm to the tiny throat and chest muscles regulating the musical trills, the crescendoes and the diminuendoes of a Melba or a Tettrazini, it is possible for us to realise that muscle should command as much respect as, if not even more than, brain and nerve, for it plays an even more important part in the general scheme of things, as nerve and brain and every organ are dependent entirely on the muscles of the digestive, circulatory and eliminatory systems for their nutrition, aeration and purification-

Yet many still look upon " mere muscle," as it is sometimes called, as vulgar. This is a popular delusion that must be crushed by education, for it is a most dangerous attitude and especially unfair to the young, while it is a belief that has been and is to be held largely responsible for the physical deterioration of the people. People have been foolishly taught to use and develop the mental rather than the muscular system, because mental work is more highly remunerated or is considered more "respectable," but they have not been taught, what is far more important, that only by muscular movement can the body be made and kept strong enough to support the increased labour of the brain, or to obtain that exact balance between the mental and the muscular systems without which there must be the ever-present danger of mental breakdown.

Muscle, indeed, is just as essential to the brain-worker if he is to reap the best results from that organ, as it is to the manual worker, and must not, therefore, be despised or regarded as a non-essential.

FUNCTION DEPENDENT ON MUSCLE.

A man or woman will faint or grow pale as the blood flows away from a cut or a blow, or will be quite alarmed at any appreciable loss of nerve, but will watch his or her muscles grow weak and flabby almost to helplessness without a qualm. Why? Because even yet the health value of muscle is not fully understood nor the fact realised and recognised that it is the muscular power of the body that maintains both life and health.

Neglect, abuse or ill-treatment of the muscles brings its own revenge, because all or at least some of the functions will become weak and impaired if the muscular system is not well-nourished, well-treated and well-trained, and thus the balance of the body will be disturbed and its resistant power to disease diminished.

In the human body not the least important work of the muscles is to regulate nutrition, and to supply and maintain heat. The 500 muscles themselves consume a great part of the food we eat. Whatever food is not immediately used is stored away as a reserve in the form of tissue. By carefully regulating one's exercise and daily food the weight of the body may be maintained practically at an equilibrium, an important fact which all doctors, teachers and instructors at school should continually bear in mind.

VALUE OF AMBIDEXTROUS TRAINING.

Here, too, I would impress upon them also the great value of ambidextrous teaching and training for children. Such a system of scientific education in the care and culture of the body as I am describing naturally demands, as an essential feature to obtain perfect physical and mental balance, the equal education of the muscles of both sides of the body. If this were not so, it would not only be impossible to obtain perfect physical balance, but it would also, as I show later, still further aggravate the disturbance of balance between brain and body that is already an inevitable result of our present methods of education. In very few schools, for instance, are the children educated and trained to use even both hands alone with equal facility.

In the methods of physical education and training which I propose, the children must be trained to develop the muscles not only of both hands and arms in equal balance, but every muscle of both sides of the body, for in no other way is it possible ever to arrive at what I call perfect physical and organic balance such as is absolutely necessary if we are to make the body so powerfully resistant to disease as to be disease-immune.

To further support this, I am a strong advocate of ambidextrous education in every way, and I see no reason whatever why this method of teaching should not be introduced conjunctively with my proposed national scheme of physical and hygienic education. There is no reason why any and every child should not be taught to write, say, equally as well with the left as with the right hand, and to do many other things with both hands, with equal facility. The average child is just as awkward when it begins to write with the right hand as with the left, and, indeed, it seems ridiculous not to train them to use both as there is no extra trouble or cost, while it would help to maintain better mental and muscular balance which, I contend, is necessary for perfect health and freedom from disease.

Nature, after all, gives us two arms, two legs, two eyes, two ears, two kidneys, and two lungs, so that if we lost one the other would still be left us as compensation. A wise Creator has placed nothing in the body without its specific object, and we have two arms so that we should be able to use either if the other became injured or destroyed. Yet how few to-day could use the left hand and arm if, say, they were unfortunate enough to lose the right.

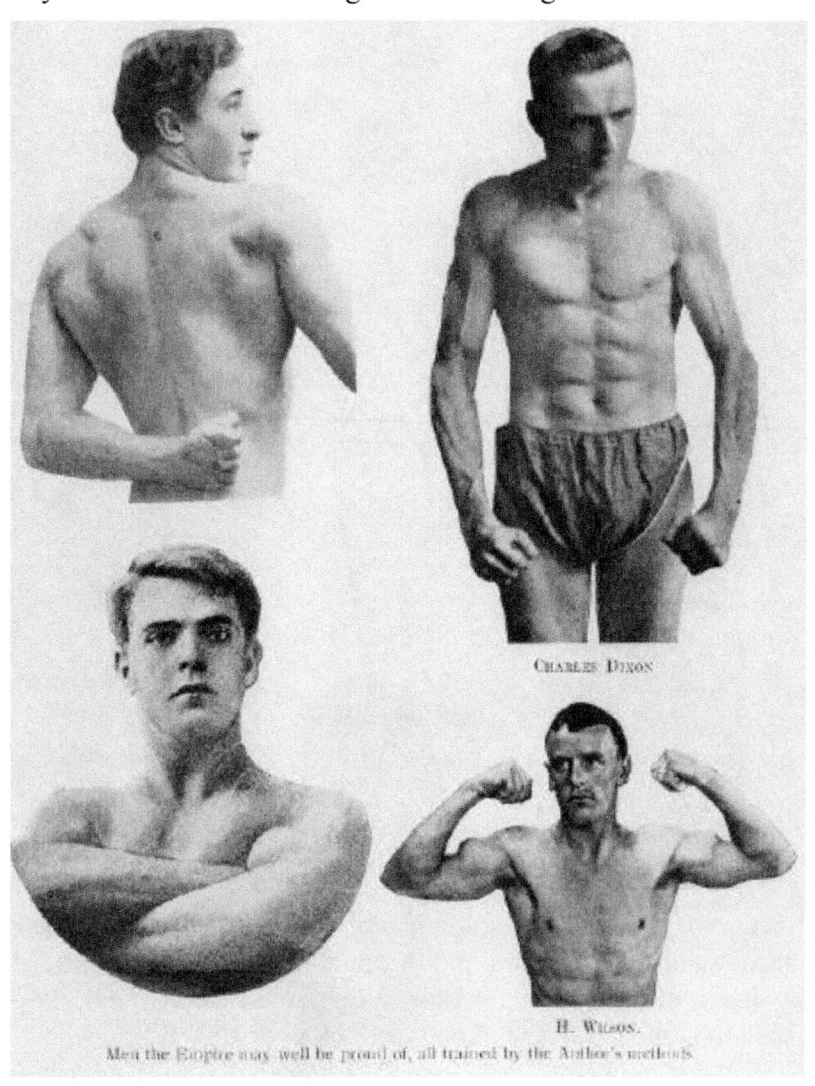

CHARLES DIXON.

H. WIGGS.

Men the Empire may well be proud of, all trained by the Author's methods.

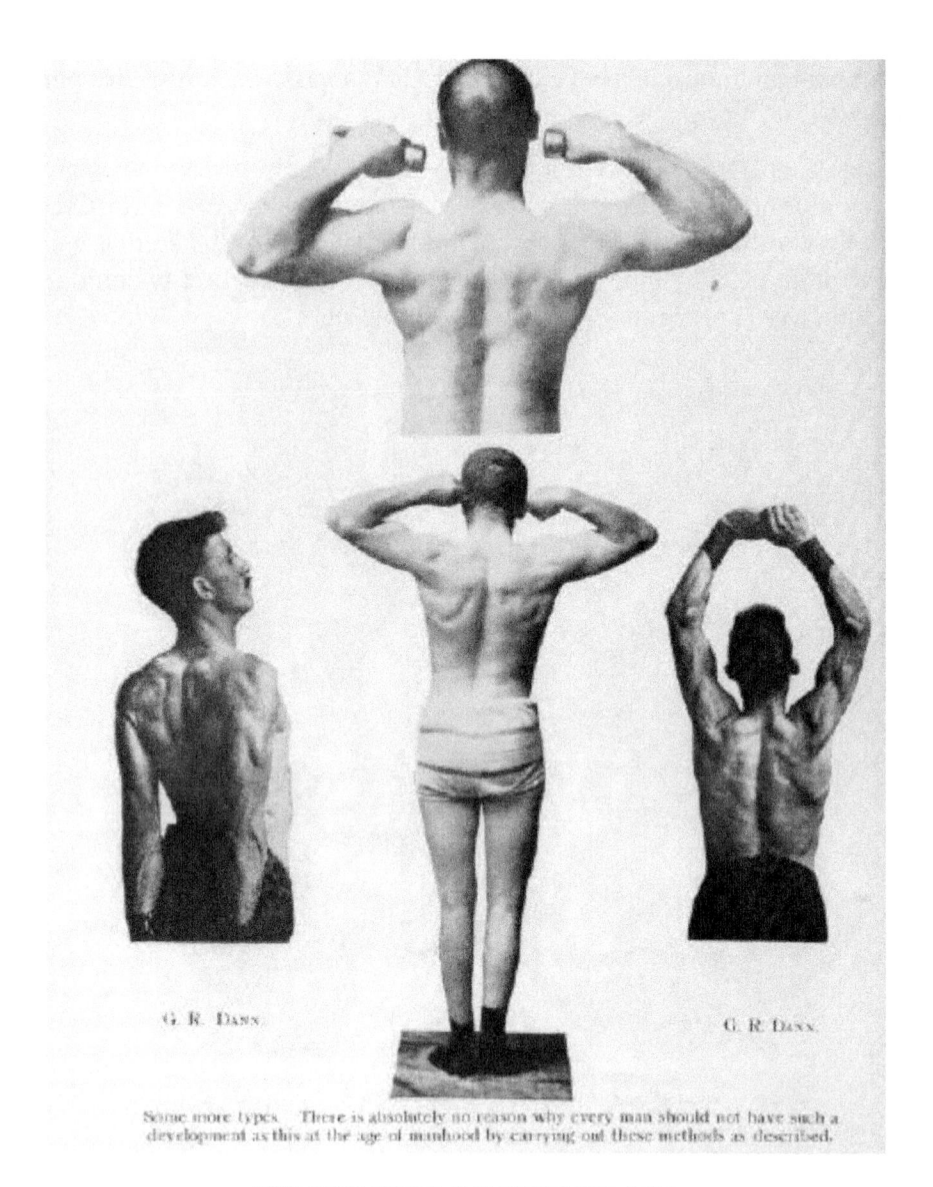

Some more types. There is absolutely no reason why every man should not have such a development as this at the age of manhood by carrying out these methods as described.

ITS EFFECTS ON THE BRAIN.

Think how much better off thousands of soldiers who have lost arms in the war would be to-day if they had only been taught in childhood and throughout life to use their left hand and arm, as easily, as naturally and as skilfully as their right. What an advantage, too, they would have had over a less educated opponent in actual conflict. In everyday life, again, diseases such as " writer's cramp " or " telegraphist's " or " typist's cramp," due to overwork of the right hand, would never exist if all were taught to use with equal facility both hands.

Every child should be taught at school to use the two hands equally well—write, work and play with the left as well as with the right. Such training would be excellent to teach the child all-round mental and muscular co-ordination in balance and would be especially beneficial in the case of either mentally or physically defective children. I have seen wonderful specimens of work produced by children so trained. In scientific physical education such as I am describing this use and exercise of the muscles of both sides of the body in perfect balance is absolutely necessary to obtain the best results. Afterwards, children should be taught to play games equally well with the limbs of both sides. The value of such muscular education and training on brain and mind can scarcely be over-emphasised.

It is known now that all the voluntary muscles of the body are under the influence and control of certain areas in the brain known as motor areas, and the nerve communications between these motor areas and muscles merge into, meet and cross one another at the point where the spinal column and brain meet. Thus the muscles on the left-hand side are influenced and controlled by motor areas in the right lobe of the brain, and vice-versa. As these areas of the brain can, in turn, be reached and developed through the movement of the muscles on the opposite side of the body, it will readily be seen how the all-round and two-sided training and development of the body will also develop, strengthen and balance the brain power in its various manifestations.

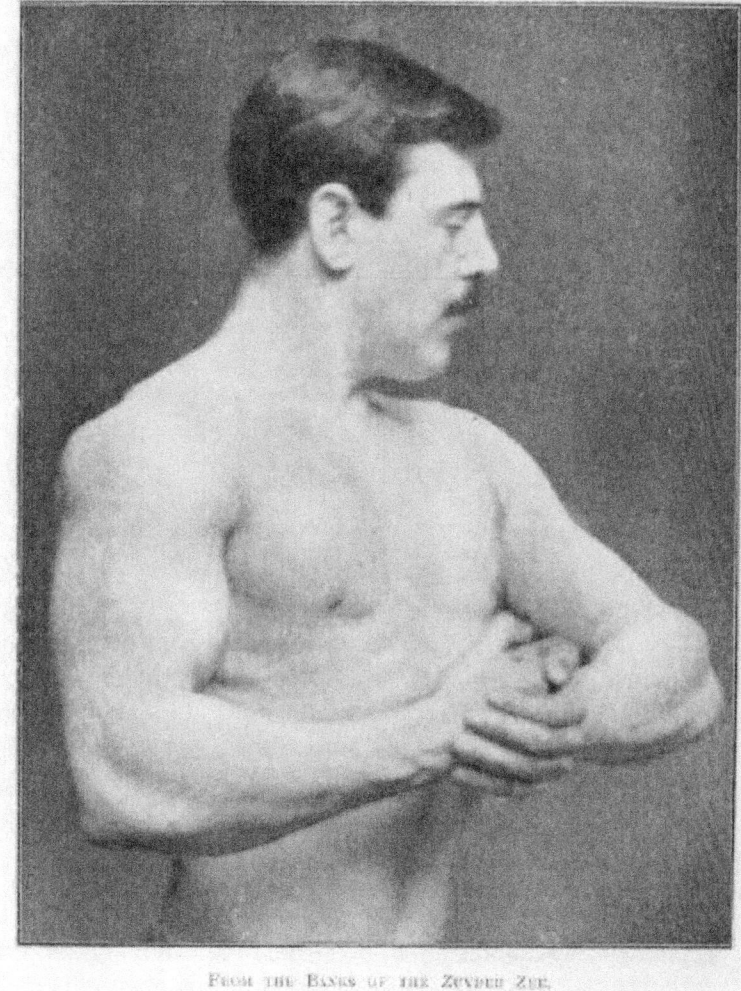

FROM THE BANKS OF THE ZUYDER ZEE.
Even in Holland these methods of physical development are winning many followers, and this is a fine type of the young Dutchmen they are producing.

MUSCLES THAT EXERCISE BRAIN AND NERVE.

Of the influence of muscular movement on the mental and nervous system Dr Sir James Crichton Browne speaks strongly and with the voice of authority. He argues from the fact that " the stimulus to muscular contraction is conveyed by motor nerves, the stimulus in the case of voluntary movement, originating in a certain region of the brain, called the motor area, whose business it is to preside over muscular movement, and from the fact that the muscular movement stimulates sensory nerves, which convey the impression made upon them to other centres in the brain. The exercise of the muscles means, consequently, the exercise of nerves, of nerve-centres also, and of part of the brain itself,

" The training by which a child, acquires the ability to perform certain movements with rapidity, regularity, energy and precision, is a training not of muscles only but of nerve-centres also, of the nerve-centres set apart to reign over these special muscles. The actions which stimulate the growth and development of certain muscles stimulate also the growth and development of certain associated parts of the nervous system. Just as a muscle or group of muscles will show weakness and also wasting if the movements, for the performance of which they are designed are not practised, so also will the associated nerve-centres fail to develop or waste— atrophy—for want of exercise of their corresponding muscles."

The human body may be likened to a great travelling workshop, moved about and operated entirely by the employment of many voluntary and involuntary muscles, which, in turn, receive their commands direct from the brain or through the sympathetic nervous system, according to whether the muscles needed at the moment are voluntary or involuntary. But, as demonstrated elsewhere, balanced movement of the voluntary muscles and the cells composing them also causes the movement and development of the involuntary muscles and their component cells and of the brain cells directing them, while it also caused a greater flow of better oxygenated blood to the latter and the better elimination of waste, so that not only a better developed body but also a better developed and more receptive brain will be the result of harmonised physical movements when scientifically carried out in any educational institution.

PHYSICAL AND MUSCULAR MORALITY.

And, just as all the elements of the soil are brought into being in the crops and the fruit so all the physical qualities of man are the feeders of his intellectual and even his spiritual and moral life. All education, in short, should begin with the physical and muscular part of the body, whitfh is the sole support and source of supplies of that rare trinity of Spirit, Mind, and Matter which we call Man. For the brain into which copious supplies are brought daily by rich, red and well-aerated blood through movement—the movement, purity and richness of which again, are all dependent on muscular power—is bound to be better nourished, healthier, stronger, clearer and more receptive than the brain that rests unsteadily upon a body neglected, ill-cared for, or undeveloped. Through the physical body all that is noblest in man can be reached, and the body instead of being despised or humiliated by those men aspiring to saintliness of character, should be respected and reverenced by all as a true fount of spiritual, mental and moral inspiration.

Physical decadence or physical degeneracy will be almost invariably accompanied by mental and moral deterioration, for as Herbert Spencer well said, " we must never forget that there is such a thing as physical morality." Nature demands, both physically and mentally, that you must go forward or backward, upward or downward. There is no possibility of remaining stationary, for all life is movement, depends on movement, and movement is a necessity of life. Physical development means moving upwards, physical deterioration means moving down.

Scientific physical development means physical and mental balance, and perfect physical and mental balance is mankind's best policy of insurance against disease, degeneracy, vice, insanity and crime. The influence of muscle on brain, mind and nerve is more fully dealt with in my next chapter.

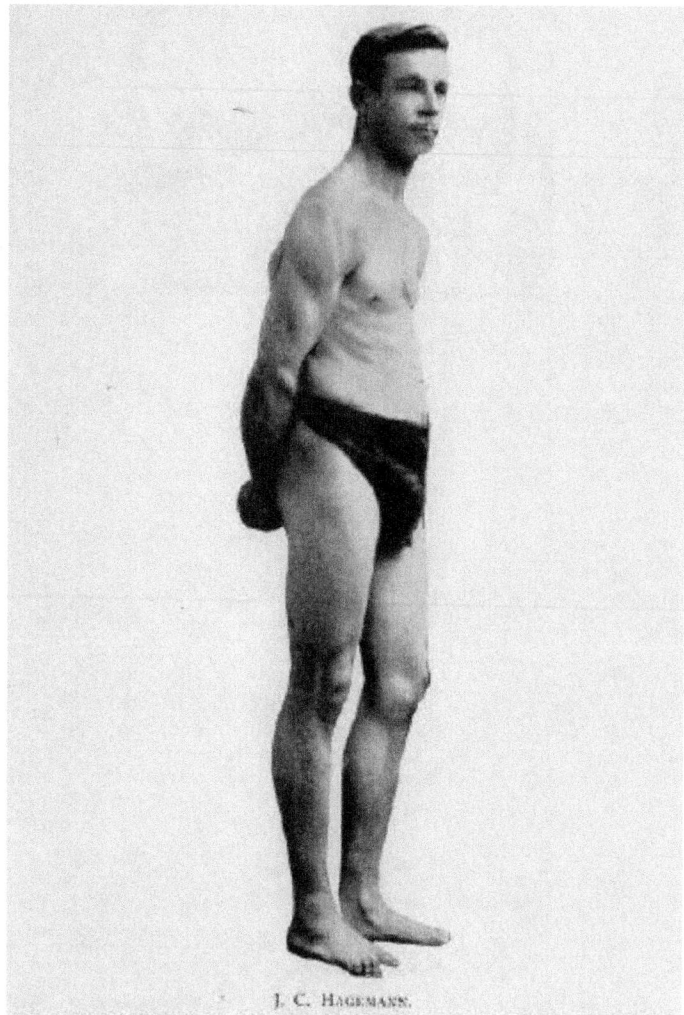

J. C. HAGEMANN.
Front view of a well-developed youth, the sound-mind-in-the-sound-body type that is produced by scientific physical movement, and not the bar-lounging, cigarette whiffing youth which swell the army of C3 unfits.

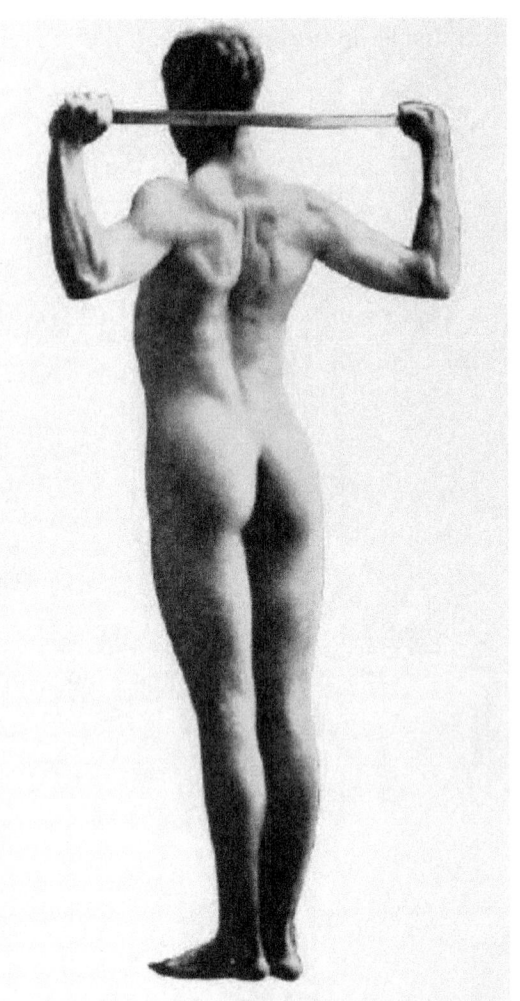

J. C. Hagemann.
Back view of the same youth as on preceding page.

CHAPTER XIV.

Muscle, Mind and Nerve.

THE relationship of muscle and nerve and mind is a subject into which it is necessary to enter if we are to have a true appreciation of the importance of muscular movement in schooling and disciplining the mental and nervous as well as the muscular man. Much has been said and written of late concerning the effect of mind on matter, of the curious influence mental and nervous phenomena often exert upon the physical organism, as if the mind and the nervous system were something apart and distinct from the purely physical man. But it is too apt to be overlooked that what we call mental force and nervous energy are merely the expression and functioning of material and physical things, and that the brain and the nerves, of which mental and nervous force are only manifestations, are themselves things of tissue and blood very much like the muscles and other parts of the body in many ways. In other words, the physical brain and nervous system, while, perhaps, of a higher type and quality than muscle, and possessing distinct and peculiar properties and powers, exclusively their own, have yet much in common with the rest of the organism.

In other words, the manifestations and workings of the nervous system and the brain, wonderful and still mysterious as they are, are not things that transcend human understanding and defy human research, elusive as they admittedly have been so far, but things, rather, having a common physical and material origin and means of subsistence, things, too, that can and have been developed by use, and that will deteriorate through abuse or disuse, and things which must ultimately yield up their as yet unrevealed secrets and mysteries to the eternal inquisitiveness of scientific research. Indeed, the worship of the mind as something transcendent above and beyond the merely physical body has been one of the greatest of human errors, and an idolatry for which humanity has paid a great price.

INFLUENCE OF MATTER ON MIND.

Though there have been and are exceptions to the general rule, it will be conceded that the brain and nervous system lodged in a healthy body are more likely to thrive and flourish than a brain and nervous system located in a body physically debased, debilitated, or diseased. For just as it is the sap within the tree that gives the leaves and the flowers their rich verdure and colour, so it is the vital force generated within the physical body that gives the brain and nervous system their freshness, flexibility and tone. On the other hand, a body robbed of some of its vital energy by a sluggish or torpid liver, will throw a pall of desolation over the clearest and strongest brain until the normal functional movement of that large bodily organ is restored.

Indigestion, as we have seen in the case of even so great an intellect as Carlyle, will tinge the mind with the sable hue of melancholy, set the nerves a-quiver like aspen leaves, and give to utterance a bitterness and an acidity that will make the most brilliant dyspeptic a very Ishmaelite among his fellows. The body, meant to be the temple of the soul, can, if allowed to deteriorate and decay, become instead the tomb of the spirit.

It was a distorted perspective that led man, in days gone by, to humiliate his physical body by irritating it with "hair shirts," and other devices designed to glorify the Creator by assaults upon His handiwork. The body was given to each and all of us, by the Creator of all things, not to despise, neglect, abuse or humiliate, but to know, honour, respect and even reverence.

Asceticism can never be a substitute for athleticism, for muscular activity in one form or another is as necessary for the culture of spirit, mind and nerve as it is for the development of muscle and the healthy functioning of the humbler but not less vital organs upon whose well-being all the higher attributes of man are dependent.

NERVES BECOME REBELLIOUS.

The very word nervous, as we use it to-day, has a meaning very much perverted from that originally intended. In the original it meant strong in nerve. As understood at present, it generally indicates a condition in which the nerves are weak, irritable and beyond control. The fact is that the gradual adaptation of man to a civilised environment, through the ages that separates us from primitive man, and which has introduced so many new factors into human life, has robbed the nerves of their pristine vigour because modern conditions of life and modern educational methods have shorn man of his nerves as well as his muscular grandeur. Primitive man knew not neurasthenia or nervous disorders, because his nerves were kept in subjection and well sustained by his life of incessant and general physical activity from childhood. To-day, we are educated from childhood to other habits of life, in which the muscular system receives the scantiest consideration or attention, and the result is that too many have become slaves of their nerves rather than their masters. Our whole training and habits of life have reacted injuriously upon the nerves—the most sensitive of all human things—and they have become sullen, rebellious, uncontrolled, and, in many cases, uncontrollable.

Each nerve-cell, like every other cell of the body, is a living thing, and depends for its existence and maintenance upon physical movement. Even if its power of movement be limited to that change of form which takes place by nutrition and excretion, such movement is essential to its very being. But we cannot voluntarily command a nerve to move and give it exercise as we can command a voluntary muscle to contract, and so we can only increase the movement of the nerve-cells indirectly, bringing to them, as a result, greater supplies of food and air, and securing for them the free and continuous ejection and elimination of their waste matter.

"EXERCISING" THE NERVES.

This, I say, we can only do through the use and movement in balance of all, or nearly all, the voluntary muscles that are, or should be, under our control. Every time we consciously, and by an effort of our own will, move a voluntary muscle we also move certain nerve- cells and certain cells of the brain. It is not too much, therefore, to say that all muscular exercise and education is, to some extent, also mental and nervous exercise and education. Indeed, because of this, it is only through the movement of a great number of voluntary muscles that we can reach, exercise and develop certain cells of the brain and nervous system, viz., the cells of those centres in the brain that give the orders for these muscles to be set in motion, and those cells employed in the transmission of those orders and in arousing the muscles into action.

Though we speak of the nervous system as being beyond the power of human volition, this is only partially true. By " willing " a muscle to move, for instance, we do, to a certain extent, exercise also control over the nerves that link that muscle with the brain. If we cannot thus command a muscle to move at will, it is evidence that there is something wrong either in the ganglion cell or in the nerve- cells and nerve-fibres that form the lines of communication between brain and muscles, or weakness and atrophy of the muscle itself. If it be only degeneration or weakness of brain or nerve tissue, and there is no actual lesion or destruction of the tissue, the repeated effort of will to move a particular muscle will gradually restore strength and tone to the deteriorated brain or nerve-cell as well as to the muscle. This, surely, is both drill and discipline for the mind, the will and the nervous system just as much physical training for the muscle.

This close relationship between the nervous and the muscular systems is evidenced in many ways. The disturbance of the nervous system often reveals itself in a host of muscular movements that are tardily, stumblingly, or, perhaps, too rapidly performed. Often, indeed, the power of inhibition is so feeble in such cases that it gives rise to what are called " motor habits," such as fumbling with a button, twirling one's moustache or watch-chain, tremors and twitchings and other little individual muscular movements that are done without conscious effort. How easily may such people pass to a stage amounting almost to mental and nervous collapse if the nerve-centres are not re-educated through the agency of the voluntary muscular system.

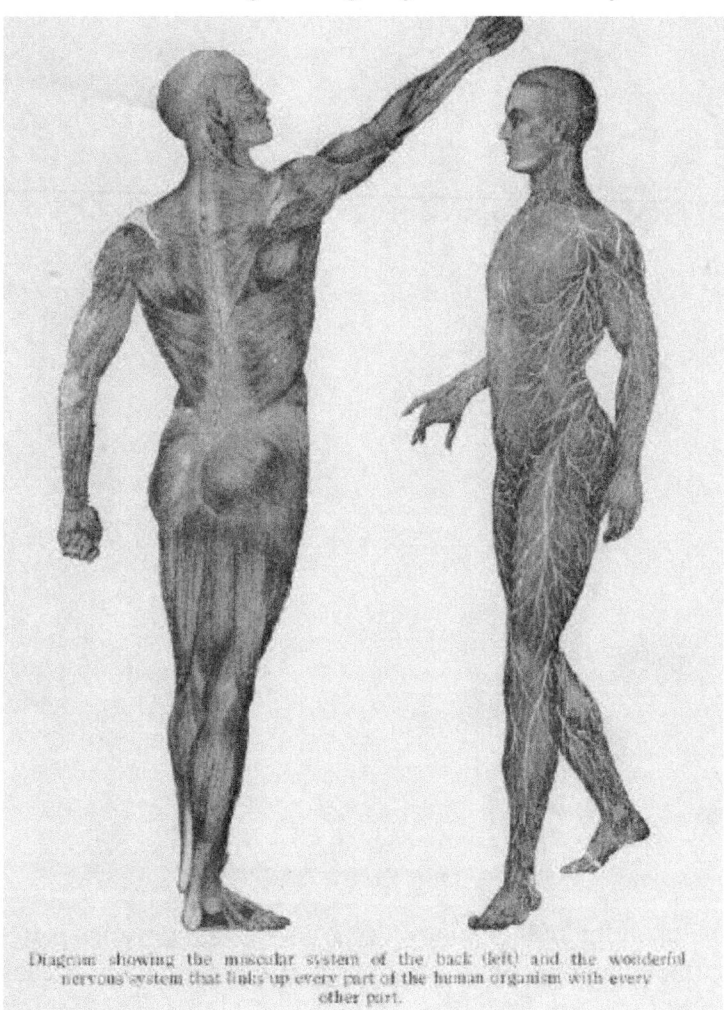

Diagram showing the muscular system of the back (left) and the wonderful nervous system that links up every part of the human organism with every other part.

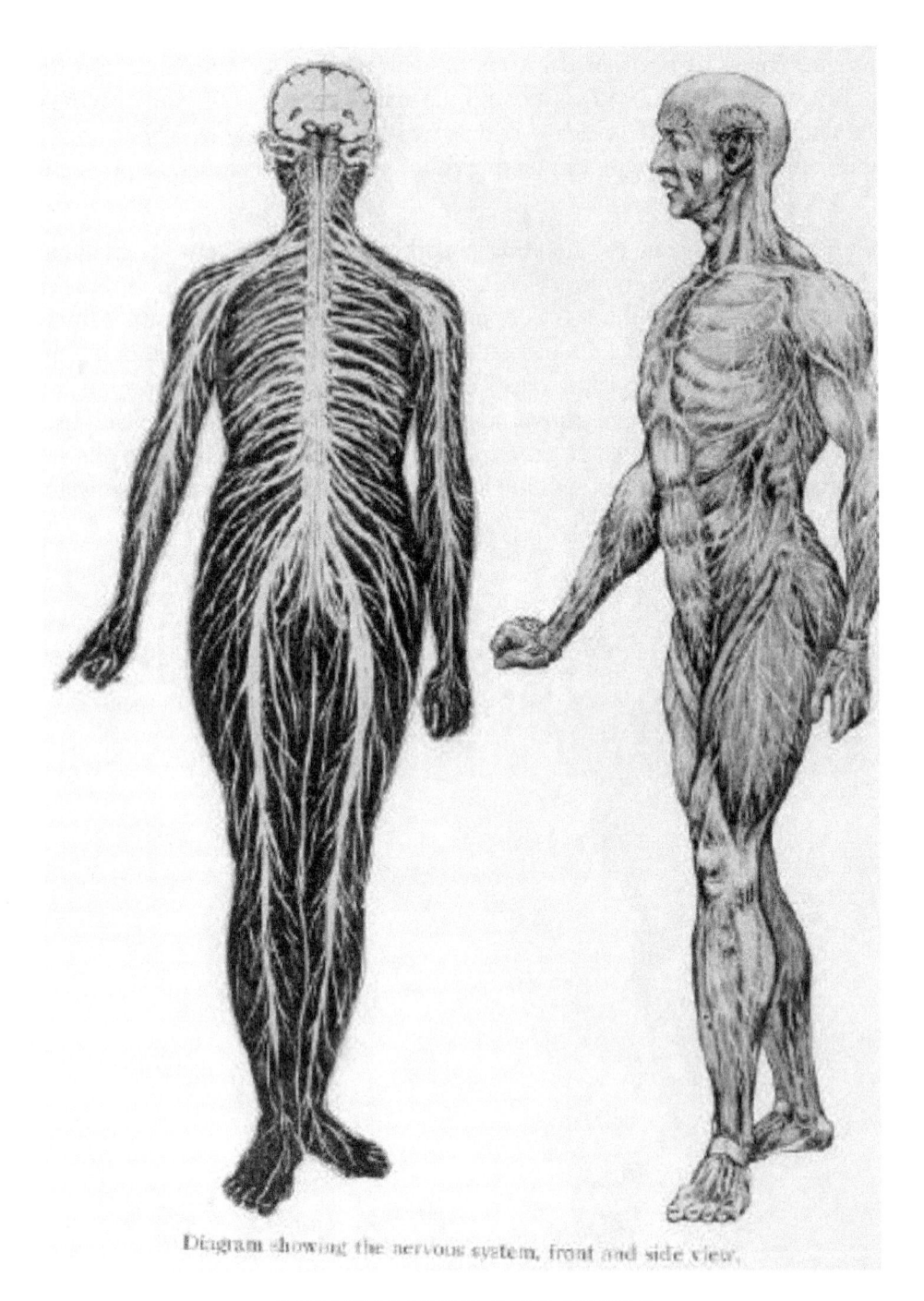

Diagram showing the nervous system, front and side view.

WHAT IS NERVE TENSION?

In the imbecile, again, the utter lack of control over nerves and muscles is to be seen in his abject limplessness and diminution of all muscular power. His arms droop, his legs drag along, often his head falls weakly towards his shoulders, and his chin drops. Through training the voluntary muscles of his body that are associated with certain directing cells of his brain—which in his case are too weak to direct and control—we can develop and strengthen these brain cells and thus teach him not only to control his muscles, but to develop and strengthen the brain and nerve-cells directing the movement of these muscles.

The cells of the nervous system that link up these muscles and brain cells are developed in association, and in this way he can often be taught to regain the lost power over brain, nerves and muscles. From this extreme case it can be safely argued that the degrees of muscular and mental power are relatively in proportion, and through the balanced movement of the voluntary muscles we can also develop, strengthen, and literally reconstruct associated brain and nerve cells.

Just to what extent modern man can be said to possess such direct control over his nerves as he possesses over his muscles is a nice point for argumentation which I prefer to leave to students of minute physiology and psychology. Over the nerves that regulate the vital functions it is a wise provision of the Creator that removes them beyond our direct control, though we certainly can influence these functions by the physical condition in which we maintain the nerves. Nervous disturbance will cause a simulation of heart disease, and disordered nerves will disorganise the whole establishment of the body. As the nervous system is the dynamo in which is generated the vital energy necessary for the functioning of the -organism, it is very evident that to keep the nervous system well- nourished, well-oxygenated and free from the accumulations of waste and poisonous matter is to bring it under better control and to improve the functioning of the organs dependent upon it.

UNABLE TO RELAX TENSED NERVES.

But, as I have shown, it is only through the balanced use of all the voluntary muscles of the body that we can keep all the cells of the body, including all the nerve cells, in this healthy and tractable physical' state by bringing to them the movement that ensures life, and it is through our neglect of such movement in present-day life that our nerves have become intractable, undisciplined, ill-nourished, causing a condition of general anarchy in every organ and system, and disturbing, to some degree, all the functions of life. Naturally, the brain cells are directly or sympathetically affected, and a vicious circle is established in which all the organs and cells, instead of operating harmoniously together, become engaged in a bitter internecine strife. There can be no control over nervous expenditure or income in such a body, and this is the condition of the neurasthenic, as I have more fully described and explained in my chapter on " Neurasthenia."

Nerve-tissue, according to recognised physiologists, does not possess the property of contractility like muscle. Yet it possesses something very much akin, something which even yet has eluded precise identification. A nerve can become tense just as a muscle can become contracted to a degree of pain, and probably the familiar nervous headache is the result of this over-tension through mental and nervous overwork and overstrain. As man has for centuries been living by his brain and nerves rather than his muscles, and as his brain and nervous system have been taxed to a far greater degree than his muscular system for centuries, with the result that the nerve-cells have been kept, and are being kept, in a high state of conscious or sub-conscious tension without any compensation, and have become hypersensitive, we have arrived at the age of neurasthenia. To-day, many men and women, to use figurative language, have nerves so over-tensed that they are like elastic that has lost its elasticity, or, in other words, they have lost their power of relaxation. The neurasthenic cannot obtain this relaxation of the nerves, strive as he will, and can only regain this power of relaxation through learning how to completely relax the muscles of the body.

CONSCIOUS AND SUB-CONSCIOUS RELAXATION.

Only by regaining complete control over the voluntary muscles can man regain the power to relax his nerves at will, the power that man had sub-consciously in the days when physical activity was his only means of living, and this one protection against his enemies. To-day the majority of people have to learn how to do consciously what primitive man did automatically or sub-consciously as the result of his active physical life. Let me make the difference between conscious and sub-conscious relaxation of the nerves clear by a couple of simple illustrations. Supposing that you have some great trouble hanging over you, the greater is the mental and nervous strain you have to combat through the excessive and long-continued over-tension of the nerve-cells. Your mind and nerves are wrought up, as we say, to a great tension. Finally, one day the good news comes to you that all danger has passed away, and the tension begins to depart at once, because the brain and nerve-cells relax sub-consciously as a result of all trouble and danger having passed away, and this relaxation is in equal degree to the degree of over-tension. That is what I mean by sub-conscious relaxation.

HOW TO RELAX OVER-TIRED NERVES.

Now take another case. You receive bad news of some kind that comes as a terrible shock to you. A friend, say, in whom you placed every confidence has betrayed you. A faithful servant has proved false and caused you heavy financial loss. The shock causes the nerves unconsciously to become so tensed that there may be even a temporary suspense of vital functions. You may collapse or faint. On recovery, however, by one great effort of your own will you determine to forget the betrayer and the betrayal, to thrust the incident from your mind, and to forget or laugh at the whole affair. Again, the nerve-cells relax, but this time consciously at the direction and dictation of your own mind and will, and not through circumstances beyond your control. This is what I mean by conscious relaxation, but few fully possess this power to-day.

To be able to relax the nerves consciously in this way requires a method of training that will literally re-educate the nerve-centres, for just as most people have, to a great degree, lost their power of full muscular control, so they have lost all command of their nerves.

The nervous system is a wonderful, a delicate, a complex and intricate machine which we must teach people from childhood to understand, regulate, direct and care for. When they can do this, they will learn how to modify the expenditure of nervous energy and prevent the waste of nervous power, and it is because they lack this self-control that so many spend nervous energy faster than they can make it, which is the chief cause of neurasthenia and the many nervous disorders so prevalent.

The method that I so strenuously advocate, which I alone advocated nearly thirty years ago, and which I have since then been continually advocating all over the world, will teach us to regain this comparatively lost mastery of both our nerves and muscles. When one has this perfect self-mastery over body, mind and nerves it will react on every act of life and every phase of the conduct of life. It will give one greater efficiency, greater directing power and authority over others, greater self-confidence and self-control, and make one feel better, kinder and more tolerant to others. For self- knowledge leads to self-respect and self-respect implies respect of others and respect and veneration for our Creator.

INDIA'S SPLENDID EXAMPLE.

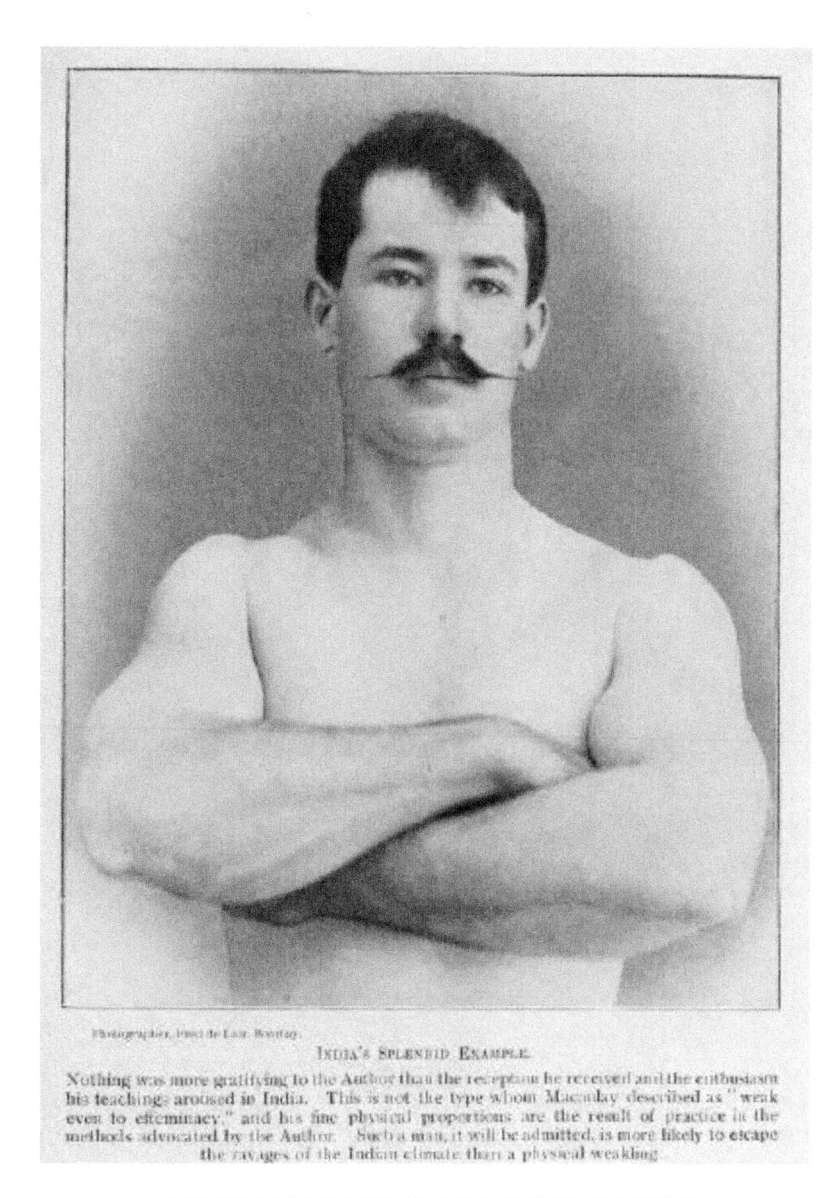

Nothing was more gratifying to the Author than the reception he received and the enthusiasm his teachings aroused in India. This is not the type whom Macaulay described as "weak even to effeminacy," and his fine physical proportions are the result of practice in the methods advocated by the Author. Such a man, it will be admitted, is more likely to escape the ravages of the Indian climate than a physical weakling.

WHEN MEN KNEW NOT " NERVES."

Without such self-mastery of one's own body, mind and nerves, on the other hand, the child will be handicapped through life, and lacking self-control will lose all self-respect, respect for others and even respect for its Creator. Its salvation will probably be the exception and not the rule, and it will be exposed to risks, temptations and disasters that it might otherwise escape or avoid.

Nothing was more gratifying to the Author than the reception he received and the enthusiasm his teachings aroused in India. This is not the type whom Macaulay described as " weak even to effeminacy," and his fine physical proportions are the result of practice in the methods advocated by the Author. Such a man, it will be admitted, is more likely to escape the ravages of the Indian climate than a physical weakling.

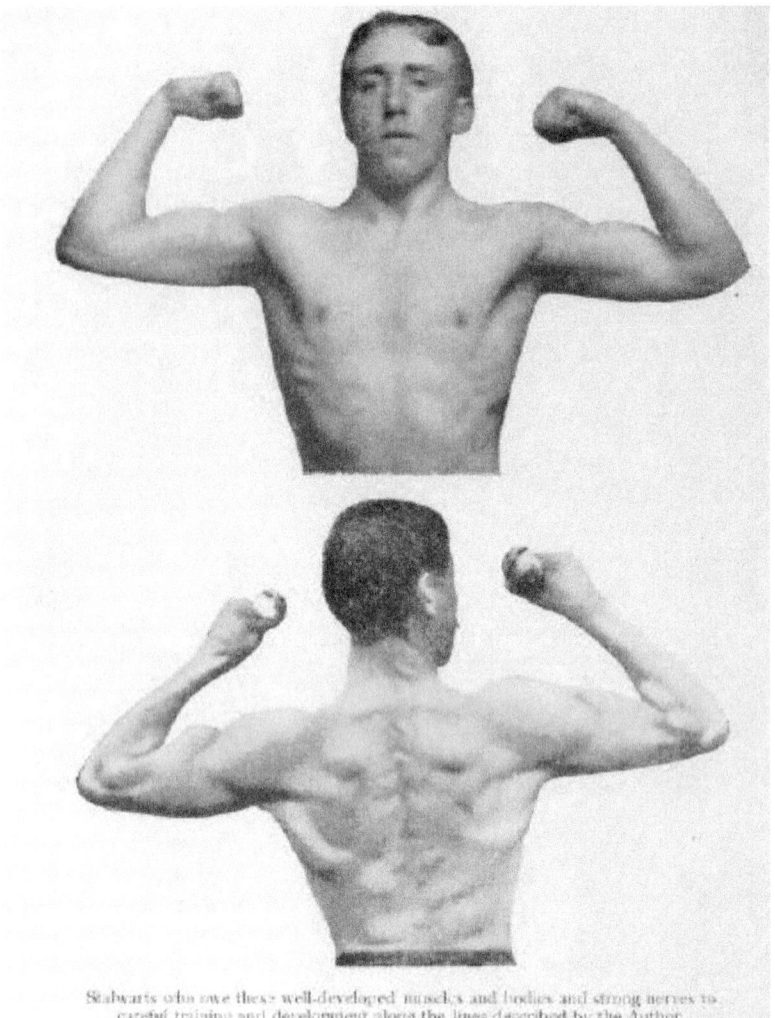

Stalwarts who owe these well-developed muscles and bodies and strong nerves to careful training and development along the lines described by the Author.

With scientific physical education and reconstruction, giving the physical precedence over the mental, beginning in early childhood, and its influence persisting through adult life, may we not hope with certainty to be able yet to give any and every individual the complete freedom from what is called " nerves " or " nervousness " our ancestors had in the dim and distant past, when man knew not " nerves " because his nervous system was established on a sound and stable physical basis and operated so smoothly and so efficiently as to be free from all discomforts or pain.

The re-education of the nerves through the muscles can, however, not be achieved by physical exercise that is not carried out in an absolute scientific way (in the little time that can be devoted to it to-day), and exercise that is sub-consciously performed, or which is carried out without mental concentration on the muscle or muscles moved, can have little or no educational, disciplinary or therapeutic value under modern conditions of life, because sufficient time cannot be given to it to exercise all the muscles as required.

NERVE-TENSION AND INSOMNIA.

Even where physical training of some kind or other is at present practised in our schools, the movements are only performed in a sub-conscious and certainly unscientific way without having any influence for good on the mental and nervous system, or for obtaining bodily balance everywhere, for movements to benefit brain and nervous system and to lead to better control and co-ordination must be performed with complete concentration of mind on the muscles moved with the thoughts fixed firmly on the movement and the specific end in view, and with the maximum of physical effort, for without full effort, mentally and physically, there cannot be full and complete contraction. Only by such a method will those who have lost their nerve-power learn to r<4ax the nerve-cells, obtain the mastery of nerves and muscles, and break down the habit of subconscious tension of the nerve-cells, when not actually in use, a habit which, in some, persists even when asleep, and which often causes people to wake up more tired than when they lay down, because their nerve-cells are kept in a condition of constant tension, consciously or sub-consciously§ until they grow over-tensed through all kinds of worrying thoughts and disturbing dreams just as the muscles over which we have control would stiffen in an arm if the biceps were held in a continuous state of flexion.

To tell them to " make their mind a blank " is no doubt well-meaning advice, but that is just the very thing they cannot do, except after patient practice. The mind—the apex and crown of the nervous system—has got beyond their control. They are restless, " fidgety," impulsive, while there is a continuous leakage of nervous energy through the incessant tension of the nerves, until, to quote Victor Hugo's words, in some extreme cases, it " tumbles down in veritable avalanches."

THE SERENITY OF THE NERVES.

In such cases it is possible to reach all the nerve-centres through the balanced movement of the voluntary muscles, to re-educate them, and gradually to regain that control over both muscles and nerves which enables a person to enjoy complete relaxation, and to be able, at a command of the will, to shut out every thought from the mind. It was this power of complete self-control and the ability to relax completely at will that enabled and enables men like Wellington and Napoleon, Foch and Haig to snatch a few minutes' sleep at any moment, even in times of the utmost crisis, and enables the great leaders of all nations to support mental and nervous strain and to be supreme master over circumstances and conditions that would overthrow weaker men. The serenity and self-control of all such men is in marked contrast to the incessant and often aimless restlessness that characterises so many men and women of a neurasthenic disposition to-day.

MUSCULAR WORK AND MENTAL TRAIN INC.

The child at school should be taught to regard its physical body as its spiritual dwelling-place. It should be shown how to keep its bodily house in order, it should be initiated into the wonders of its system of ventilation, its sanitation, its healthy installation and everything that is provided by the Creator for its comfort and well-being. It should be taught to take such a pride in its own body that it would be practically impossible for anything so foul as disease even to cross its threshold.

The value of such a system of scientific physical education and reconstruction and culture as I suggest to the mind must be assessed by the fact that every muscular act, however trivial, requires the action also of brains and nerves to produce it. Even the hammering in of a nail calls into play mental effort, or the blow would either miss its object altogether or strike it clumsily. Every act of physical movement implies, too, resistance and the breaking down of resistance and, therefore, it necessitates an effort of will-power to overcome the resistance. Thus in the simplest physical action we find the two valuable faculties of concentration and will-power being exercised and consequently developed. If, in such simple acts these higher faculties are employed and strengthened, how easy is it to realise the value of schooling the youthful physical body in such a way that every voluntary muscle of the body will be called upon and made able to do its special service in that body, and perfect balance also be obtained between the physical and the mental and nervous life of every individual. This important subject, however, I leave to my next chapter.

CHAPTER XV.
Perfect Physical and Mental Balance.

THE attainment of perfect physical, mental and nervous balance ought to be the goal of any system of education for the children, if we are to erect a sound mental and moral as well as a physically strong structure. For, as Canon Kingsley said years ago, " wherever you have a population generally weakly, stunted or scrofulous, you will find in them a corresponding type of brain which cannot be trusted to do good work."

SLUM MINDS AND SLUM BODIES.

Quite recently, too, The Times truly pointed out that " if we cannot make the generation now in the schools healthy, the slum- mind will not disappear," and the slum-mind will always and inevitably lead to the slum body under any circumstances or conditions of life. The writer also added that to secure the abolition of the slum body we must secure " the periodical medical examination of all children, the following up of all serious cases, the adequate nourishing and cleaning of all mal-nourished and verminous children, the use of organised physical exercises for all children, and the abolition of evil employment of children for profit. At a comparatively small cost we can do all these things for those who need it. We have never tried to do these things except in a sporadic fashion."

Any system of education that does not make the mental training of the child subordinate, at least at first, to the physical, and does not lead to balance and proportionate mental and physical power stands condemned already. Such education in the past has done much harm.

Where there is a lack of balance between the physical and the mental man two things are likely to occur. The purely physical man may overbalance the mental, or vice versa. In the one case we would have what George R Sims has humorously described as a race of " robust nobodies," in the other, a breed of homuncles with brains out of all proportion to their bodies.

The splendid physical and mental balance so admirably exemplified in our own " Grand Old Man," the late Mr Gladstone, in Mr Lloyd George, in M. Clemenceau, that splendidly virile type of Frenchman, in President Wilson, ex-president Roosevelt, and many living statesmen and public men, ought to be the type towards which all our education must aim. If such men had been physically educated and trained from childhood in the manner I describe in this book, their splendid gifts and talents might even have been exploited to greater advantage still, and their great life-work done with less anxiety and effort, for they would have had a still better physique to support their strong and active brains and to bring out the very best that was in them.

BALANCING THE NATIONAL ENGINE.

What I want to see established in every educational institution, is a system of mental and physical education so harmonious that it will give us neither " robust nobodies " nor " intellectual pigmies," a system not only more in accord with the ideal training of the youth of ancient Greece but even above and beyond it, as we might naturally expect to find possible to-day considering our tremendous progress in every branch of knowledge and science since those days. I contend that it is possible for every country to have such a system, that it is vital to the future of any nation to have it, and that unless a country in the near future adopts such a system that country will, and must, " go under " as the weakling in a fight or the illiterate in a Civil Service examination.

Engineers know that the balancing of an engine is their most difficult task, and the most vital to obtain 100 per cent, efficiency, and yet they are able to see and handle all the parts of that engine and take them to pieces if necessary. But those upon whom devolves the task of balancing all the parts, visible and invisible, tangible and intangible, of the wonderful living human engine have a much more difficult and infinitely more responsible work to perform, a work, indeed, not merely of national but of universal importance.

Great skill, great knowledge and great experience will be necessary on the part of those who aim at producing the perfect physical and mental balance of the human organism. It is not a duty lightly to be undertaken or imposed, but the reward of those upon whom it devolves and who attain success in its performance will be exceeding great, and it is in this internal scientific research of the human body itself that I hope to see millions spent in the near future that are now being spent and have been spent for years in other and less profitable fields.

A perfectly balanced bodily system, mentally and physically, implies the harmonious development and symmetrical equality of every part of the body and the brain and of every cell of both. Mind and muscle must be in complete co-ordination as in a business firm where the employees, directors and employer or employers work together in efficient harmony.

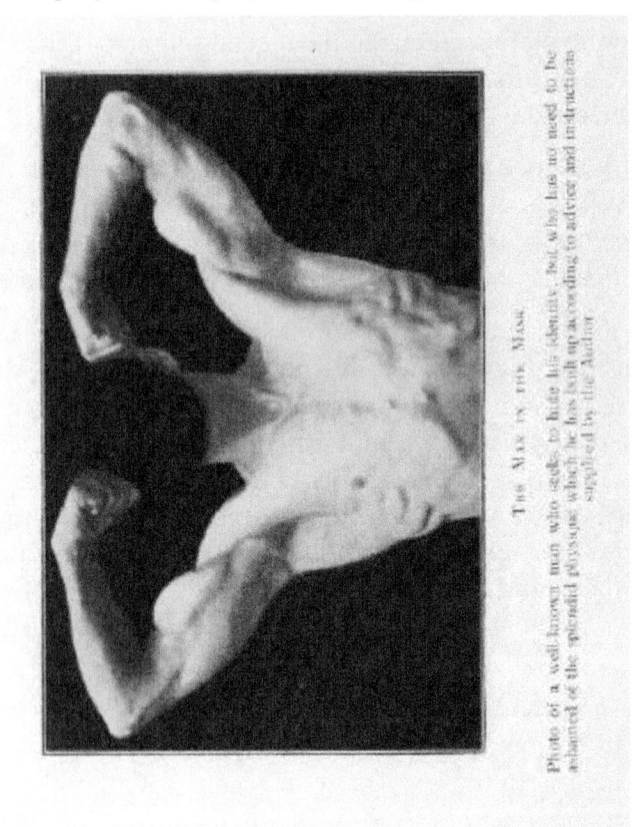

The Man in the Mask.

Photo of a well-known man who seeks to hide his identity, but who has no need to be ashamed of the splendid physique which he has built up according to advice and instructions supplied by the Author.

TEAM WORK IN THE BODY.

There would then be no confliction of interests, no unfriendly rivalries in the human body thus schooled and developed, but a body in which there was harmonious " team work " of all the organs, systems and cells. The voluntary and the involuntary muscles would work together for the bodily commonweal, and while the voluntary muscles would be in subjection to the authority of the brain, mental prosperity would not, however, be sought to the detriment of the " labouring classes " (the muscular cells) of the body. Organs and muscles, functions and nerves and senses will all, in the scientifically balanced body, have the nicest relationship to each other according to the duties they are individually called upon to perform.

The attainment of this perfect bodily and mental balance is, of course, an ideal, but I see absolutely no logical reason why it should not be attained, in the case of any child ushered into the world under favourable and obtainable conditions of birth.

Who, among us, has not been acquainted with young students whose mental studies have been prosecuted with such utter disregard of the physical body that supports the brain that they have broken down, mentally or physically, or both, under this unfair division of labour. It is thus that neurasthenics, the hysterical, and even the insane are often manufactured in the school, the college, the study and the class-room, and I have myself known a senior wrangler who was for ever hovering on that shadowy borderland that dimly separates the sane from the insane because of a body neglected, ill- treated and not developed in balance commensurate with his hyper-developed brain.

How many " broken columns " stand erected in cemeteries everywhere throughout the world, monuments sacred to youths cut off before they had scarcely tasted of the sweets of life, hurled to an early death through lack of that muscular and organic balance without which the brain becomes little better than a vampire, sucking the life-blood from the body it inhabits until the exhausted body at last fails to support either itself or its dependant brain any longer.

BRAIN CELLS WELL HOUSED.

I do not, of course, claim that balanced physical movement will develop all the cells of the brain—as mental exercise and practice only can develop the muscular action of all the brain—but that it will certainly provide all the cells of the brain with better living conditions, with better nourishment, while the cells in the motor area controlling the muscular movement will directly be developed in power by their use and exercise. In short, balanced physical movement enables all the brain cells to live in a hygienic and sanitary dwelling, and to do their work under the most favourable conditions possible, certainly under conditions that are lacking in a brain deprived of necessary supplies, or congested through the accumulation of waste products arising from mental overwork and insufficiency of physical movement.

Dr Sir James Crichton Browne, M.D., instances the case of a student or person engaged on sedentary and mental work who, when his brain becomes tired and confused, takes a gentle walk up and down his room until the exercise restores mental power. Now, why does the student's brain weaken and become confused? Because he has been using up brain power faster than it can be replaced, and the brain cells, through their activity, have caused the accumulation of waste matter. The blood is contaminated and the brain becomes congested, in consequence, because the blood is too impure and moves too slowly either to cleanse the brain of this waste matter, or to bring up fresh supplies in sufficient quantity to nourish and sustain it in its work.

Nature instinctively prompts the student to physical movement, in the form of a gentle walk, and soon the heart begins to pump the blood faster, and the waste matter is swept out of brain and body, while greater supplies of nourishment are also brought to the organ of mind, and it immediately reasserts its power through this reinvigoration brought about by the movement of the student's muscles.

Now, if a gentle walk, carried out involuntarily, will benefit the brain, as Dr Sir James Crichton Browne admits it does, even to this slight extent; it is easy to realise how much more mentally efficient would such a student be if his brain and body were developed in perfect balance as I show they can be by the perfect and balanced movement of all his voluntary muscles.

TRAGEDIES OF GENIUS.

There can, indeed, be no sound, sane and stable mentality that is not based on a perfectly balanced physical and organic foundation, and the mental can only be, to a very considerable degree, the mirror of the physical. Genius may flame for a time in a weak or even a deformed body, but it burns out quickly, as we have seen in the ill-starred, erratic and short-lived careers of so many men of brilliant mental parts.

Many of the greatest authors found their best writing-desk in bed, because they found it difficult, if not impossible, to continue writing while sitting or standing erect, because the great heart muscle was not strong enough or too undeveloped to pump the blood up to the brain with sufficient vigour, when standing in the erect position. The great specialist, Sir Lauder Brunton, declared that he often felt it impossible to do literary work after an exhausting day, unless by writing in a semi-recumbent position, so permitting a better flow of blood to the brain. How much more brilliantly might many great men have shone if they had been developed from boyhood in perfect physical and mental balance. The life tragedies of a Keats, a Coleridge, a De Quincey, and hundreds of other " intellectuals " of the past might have been averted, had their youthful bodies and brains been cultivated and developed in absolute balance, for in them the mental and physical were in such dissonance as to compel mental instability and morbidity.

Their minds were delicate and susceptible exotics which flourished luxuriantly and brilliantly for a brief period but in an unnatural and quickly degenerative environment and atmosphere. Such unbalanced genius is almost inevitably neurasthenic, often neurotic, and in most cases where the mental so predominates over the physical, it is, indeed, too often true that " great wits to madness nearly are allied."

Indeed, it may be said that most representatives of what a French writer has well called the real enfants terribles of the world— these flashing meteors and " shooting stars " of the intellectual firmament—have been neuropathic to an extreme degree, because some cells have been over-developed and others under-nourished, through the neglected balanced movement of that physical body which is the commissariat of the brain. It may be said of many of them that they only accomplished their great work in spite of their weak bodies, their ill-nourished nervous systems and their utter disproportion of mental and physical development by habitual resource to artificial aids and stimulants, which would explain the popular but erroneous idea that a disorderly or disordered life was essential to inspiration.

A " CONSTITUTION FULL OF HARMONY."

In many cases, too, their very work has actually reflected their morbid physical state Rousseau's dissipation of his vital energy in youth is freely admitted in his " Confessions." Musset and Baudelaire and Flaubert were only of " the better class " of degenerates, and their works were tinged with thoughts, fancies and forebodings that could only exist in a person whose mental powers were hyper-developed and out of balance with his physical powers.

Contrast such men with robuster types of genius like the elder, Dumas, who lived the open-air and enjoyed healthy physical exercise; of Balzaac, "who lived like a monk when at work," and had an athlete's constitution; of Victor Hugo, whose physical and psychical constitution was " full of strength and harmony." Dumas père lived to 67, Victor Hugo to 82, and Michelet, the historian, who, in spite of a delicate constitution, kept his health " very even " by regulating his physical life, reached the age of 74.

These men had a high courage because they did not neglect or despise the physical body supporting their mighty brains. They had bodies, as it were, attuned to their brains, with a high tonicity of muscles, a strong blood circulation, a more abundant power of assimilation, secretion and elimination, immense reserves of vitality, and, consequently, superior functional activity that made them feel capable of overcoming almost any obstacle. So developed and proportioned a body will not tolerate disease, for, like the hardy and high-spirited Norman warrior of old, it will refuse to entertain even the thought of non-existence, will shut its portals against Disease and even defy Death itself.

BODIES WITH PAMPERED BRAINS.

The utter lack of self-control and self-mastery displayed by many men of genius and by the insane in some abnormality or eccentricity, is the result of the lack of physical balance, or, at least, of harmonious balance between body and brain, and is due most frequently to the excessive concentration of thought on one fixed idea or in one particular direction, with the result that certain cerebral cells are nourished, developed and strengthened at the expense of even more vital physical cells. In other words, the brain becomes in them the pampered and spoiled child of the body. Certain cells of the brain not being employed or kept actively in use become weaker and weaker until they are a ready prey for disease, while the cells of the body itself, upon the labours of which the brain is dependent for nourishment, air and all the essentials of life, are themselves deprived of these vital supplies through lack of use and movement, and so we find a brain altogether too strong and active for the physical body is not equally developed in balance.

Cells that are starved or poorly nourished sooner or later " down tools," and the blood itself becomes thin and pale. This impoverished blood, too, lacking even the necessary supplies to feed and support the cells of the brain, is not pumped vigorously enough to distribute even these diminished supplies fairly to every brain cell equally, because the heart muscle, through lack of sufficient movement, becomes too weak to do its work efficiently, causing cerebral anaemia, and so the physical and mental man is still further unbalanced. The frailty of so many men of genius, physical, moral, and spiritual, can often be traced to the too exclusive schooling and developing of certain mental and nervous cells out of-all proportion to the other cellular inhabitants of the body.

Gifted with such a powerful mental machine as man is, it was, perhaps, not unnatural in a comparatively unscientific age, that every care should be lavished by man upon that organ, which has justly been called " the real incarnation of the soul," until its cells waxed and grew prosperous at the expense of what have long and wrongly been regarded as the " lower orders " of the bodily cell population, those very cells, unfortunately, upon the health, strength, number and efficiency of which depends entirely bodily and mental well-being, just as Society in the last analysis depends upon its individual workers. In these circumstances, it is not to be wondered at that the mental " sceptre and throne often come tumbling down " after a brief and often riotous existence.

THE BAROMETER OF THE BRAIN.

The age-long mistake of attempting to split the human, body into mental, moral, spiritual, and physical chambers, and the foolish belief that the culture of the spiritual and the moral in man demand the mortification and the humiliation of the body they inhabit, are false conceptions, that have been exploded by comparatively recent progress in the science of mind. When we know, as we now do, that a man's conscious actions (for every conscious human act, right or wrong, good or evil, is only the translation and manifestation of a thought previously existent in the material cells of the brain) are determined and directed largely by the mere pressure of the blood in the cerebral arteries, that the force of this blood pressure, to a great extent, regulates all his thoughts, ideas, passions, impulses and emotions (as Professor Maurice de Fleury has demonstrated), and through them his acts and through repetition of these thoughts and acts his habits, that the force of the cerebral blood pressure, again, can be modified by physical movement, and that all human physical movement is performed by the muscular system, is it not at once over-whelmingly apparent that through the muscular man we can direct, regulate and control the mental, the moral and the spiritual man.

A system of scientific bodily reconstruction such as I am attempting to define and describe, must begin by recognising the unification of the body (also the unification of disease), and the absolute dependence of mental health and moral rectitude upon physical causes and activities. In science, truth alone can reign supreme, and science to-day boldly admits and proclaims that much of all that is moral or immoral in man, including passion and its control, is the result of measurable and discernible physical conditions.

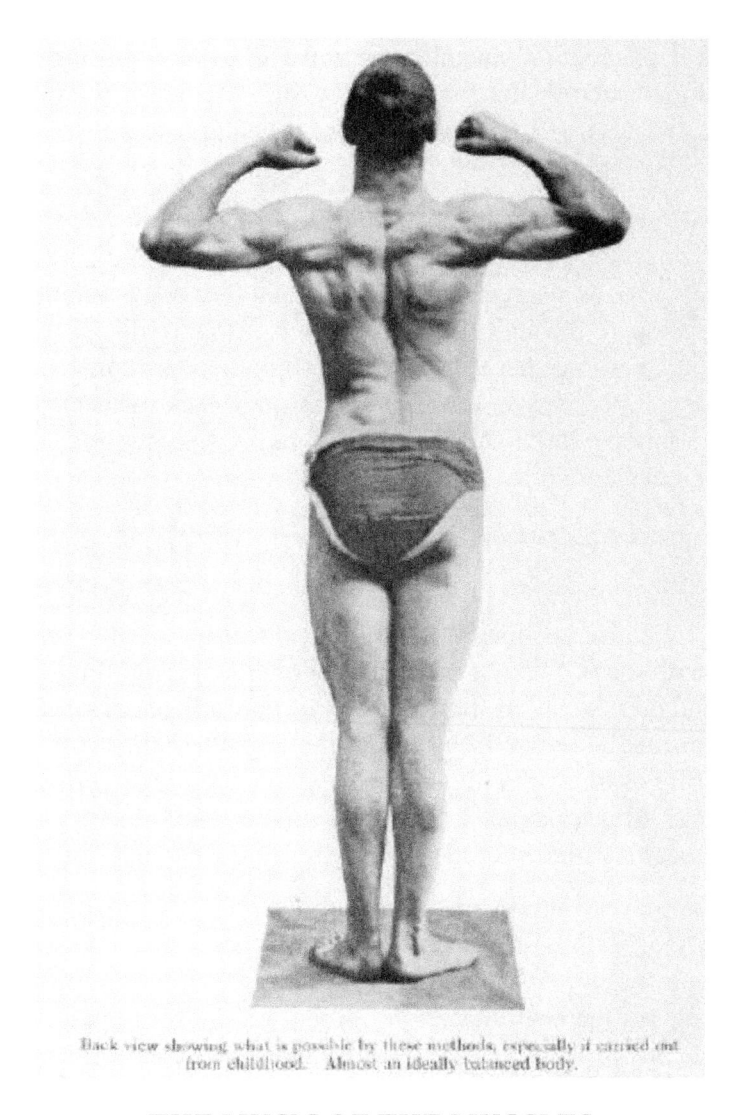

Back view showing what is possible by these methods, especially if carried out from childhood. Almost an ideally balanced body.

THE MUSIC OF THE MUSCLES.

The active carrying out of certain specific and harmonised physical movements, moderately and progressively, can be so guided and directed as to develop all the natural resources of energy in the individual, and undoubtedly influence the moral as well as the mental constitution of an individual and of the people as a whole in process of time. The rhythmic bodily harmony of health which evidences the smooth and perfect co-ordination of mind and muscle, of organ and function, of sense and nerve, is but the sweet music of the muscles brought forth by the touch of a master hand, exquisitely sensitive and in sympathetic affinity with the divine instrument at its disposal in the wonderful fabric of the body.

Where there is no actual organic disease or lesion of the brain, a diseased or degenerate mental tendency or condition may be corrected, prevented and cured by scientific physical training that restores balance to the joint mental and physical relationship. This scan be achieved, as I have personally proved in the treatment and cure of mentally defectives, by educating the neurotic and the neurasthenic to acquire gradual control over each and all of the voluntary muscles by carefully selected, rightly directed, balanced and progressive physical movements.

By this means the power of mental concentration and will-power, with greater self-mastery and control, are both developed, two of the faculties in which the neurasthenic, the neuropathic and the insane are lacking, because of their want of mental equipoise and physical and mental co-ordination.

The majority of mental and nervous troubles—with the exceptions already indicated—have a history of overwork (consciously or unconsciously) of mal-nutrition, and over-expenditure of nervous energy. Certain cells, as 1 have shown, are forced to work at over pressure, while others are starved and undeveloped through lack of movement and disuse (because supplies are unevenly consumed, and there is, therefore, over-development of some cells, while other cells "are neglected and undeveloped or become so weak through lack of use and movement that they become simply paupers in a badly balanced body and brain. Inevitably such an unbalanced state must end in bodily and mental anarchy.

STRENGTH COMES FROM WITHIN.

Until some such a system of scientific physical education and reconstruction as that indicated in this book is adopted by those responsible for the education of the rising generation, other methods of grappling with the problem of rescuing child-life and building up healthy and disease immune adolescents and adults can, at the best, be but partially successful. All must begin with the physical education of the body itself, through it making the brain stronger and more receptive. Well-intended and helpful as all such valuable movements are they overlook the radical and real source of evil, a weak, ill-developed body and stunted brain lacking the balance and co-ordination of vigorous health which should make it the conqueror and not the victim of Disease.

To-day it is recognised on every hand that to prevent disease rather than cure it is the duty of our doctors, but the majority of medical men are seeking for preventives of disease without the body that are only to be found within. A balanced and developed human body will thrive even in an unhygienic environment, but the healthiest environment will never make the weak child strong if its body is robbed of the physical and mental balance that is necessary for the vigorous functional activity which is the only guarantee of robust life and constitution. Strength of mind and body can only come from within by self-knowledge, self-respect, self-development and self-control.

It is evident, therefore, that such scientific physical education from childhood, as I advocate, must make one feel better, think better, work better, look better and be better in every way, because life is movement, and balanced strength through balanced movement alone will enable the body and brain to defy weakness and disease within and the deadly microbes ever ready to attack us from without. With the theory of the microbe—that " unseen, small, million-murdering " enemy—I propose to deal in my next chapter.

CHAPTER XVI.
Man's Most Deadly Foe.

THE microbe or bacillus of disease may well be called man's most deadly foe. It lurks for him everywhere, in the air he breathes, in the food he eats, in the beverages he drinks, in the clothes he wears, and subtly steals its way even into the most innermost parts of his body.

To recognise and know the enemy, however, to be able to trace his history, his habits, his methods and tactics, to discover his weak points and to attack him there, is to defeat him, always provided the body is strong enough within itself in every part. It was not until the bacillus of tuberculosis was discovered and identified that we could grapple with that disease even so successfully as we have done. The discovery of the tubercle bacillus, however, has not prevented and will not prevent consumption, for to prevent consumption we must make the human body itself physically too strong and resistant to the tubercle bacillus for the latter to overcome it, and not rest content even with the destruction of the bacillus of consumption.

DISEASE SHUNS THE STRONG.

Now, I have shown that the body is only as strong as its weakest individual cell, and that the only way to have a sufficient and an efficient army of healthy and resistant cells—the body's first and last line of defence—is to keep every individual living cell of the body fit and all in perfectly balanced strength in all its parts and systems. Such a body is not only more likely to resist and repel disease in cases of attack, but is, indeed, much less liable to attack, for just as the thief is more likely to select the weak, the infirm and the old for his predatory prowess rather than the prize-fighter or athlete, so disease prefers to attack the weak or the unfit.

Whilst admitting the wonderful triumphs of laboratory work and bacteriology in modern times, I sometimes am inclined to think that even to-day our medical and scientific men are almost as prone to a species of " germ mania" as they were in the 17th century, when the Dutch investigator Leeuwenhoek first discovered by means of his somewhat primitive microscope the existence of what he called "animalcules," but what we know to-day as microbes.

The greatest triumphs of bacteriology have been in the realm of infectious and contagious disease, and admittedly science has done much here to secure humanity's comparative immunity from various forms of disease that once were rife to the extreme of epidemics. In this way science has already done a great deal to help mankind to advance in its onward march towards that diseaseless world which, I contend, is no Utopian dream, but a by no means very remote possibility. Just as leprosy, dysentery and Asiatic cholera are now, to all intents and purposes, non-existent in civilised communities, so I hope to see every modern form of serious and deadly disease disappear from the earth, as it must assuredly do sooner or later if we apply scientific methods to the breeding and perfecting of the human being as thoroughly and as persistently as we do in other directions to-day.

ROUNDING UP HEALTH CRIMINALS.

And just here let me explain that when I use the expression " a diseaseless world," I mean that it is possible to have a world in which the conditions both within and without the body will not permit, tolerate or foster disease, and that our immunity from disease shall depend upon our approximation to these conditions. Christianity supplies us with the laws necessary to prevent or, repress crime and vice, but though Christianity has done a great deal to reduce the criminality and viciousness of the world it has never quite suppressed or eliminated them, because there are .still those who ignore and violate those laws. So though, as I contend, a national system of health education and bodily reconstruction as outlined here, supported by medical science and medical research, can and must ultimately give us these conditions, within and without the human body, necessary to rid the world of disease, it is possible to suppose that there will always exist a species of health-criminal and irresponsible that will ignore or challenge those conditions.

Even these, however, in course of time will gradually diminish and probably disappear, for the new environment and the stringent application of the law of "the survival of the fittest" will cause Nature to condemn them as unfit to survive, while those who continue to defy the laws of life and health will be treated as pariahs and outcasts. In other words, the sick man will rightly be regarded and treated much as we would treat a leper in our midst to-day, with mingled pity, horror and aversion.

However, this is a digression.

MICROBES AS YET UNDISCOVERED.

Though the bacteriologists have done a great service to mankind in tracing the bacilli of many diseases to their lair, so long as man must live under the artificial conditions of modern civilisation such bacilli will still continue to live, increase and flourish, and new microbes reveal themselves, just as other vermin still defy all the efforts of man to stamp them out under certain conditions, so that if we are to achieve the 'prevention rather than the cure of disease we must seek to make the body itself strong enough within to defy and conquer the most disease-inviting environment and every microbe of disease.

The most that bacteriology, with all its admitted triumphs, has so far been able to achieve for the sick and the diseased is to kill or sterilise disease germs or to counteract the poisons and ravages of these bacilli in the body. That, however, does not and cannot increase the bodily resistant power in the least. As I cannot state too often, the body itself must be made and kept so healthy and strong and so perfectly balanced in all its cells from childhood to the grave that it will be able to defy and defeat every microbe of every form of microbic disease—even microbes as yet undiscovered or unrecognised—and so prevent microbic disease altogether.

The introduction of sera and anti-toxins into an infected or susceptible body often fails even to sterilise the bacilli of disease, but only increases the immunity of the body from their evil influence by increasing its tolerance to them just as the body can be made tolerant to opium or morphia. Thus, in the case of small-pox, the vaccinationists endeavour to prevent that fearful disease by " acclimatising," as it were, the body to it, introducing what is, after all, only a milder form of the disease. In other words, their only hope and prospect of success lies in educating the body to withstand small-pox by inoculating it with cow-pox, just as the body can be habituated to large doses of the same poison by taking smaller doses. Moreover, vaccination often introduces other microbic diseases by blood poisoning, including syphilis.

80,000 NEW CASES OF SYPHILIS ANNUALLY.

It is worthy of notice that, notwithstanding the most heralded discoveries of Professor Ehrlich and his disciples in recent years, the terrible white scourge, syphilis, is increasing at an alarming rate, and that there are something like 80,000 new cases every year in the British Isles alone.

I may add, too, that it is now freely admitted that the much- advertised 606 treatment for the plague of syphilis is only palliative, and is itself accompanied by grave dangers to health. A famous French medical expert, M. Hallopean, says: " Salversan is not without serious drawbacks. In the first place, its efficacy is far from being absolute. In the second place, the remedy is not harmless when administered, for one has seen, up to the present, a large number of cases of death admittedly due to its action!"

" This remedy," says Dr Marshall, of the British Skin Hospital, " appears to be liable to cause severe toxic effects, sometimes ending fatally. No doubt many of the deaths after Salversan were due to faulty technique and like causes, but a certain number are difficult to explain except by arsenical poisoning."

It is, again, here evident that the best that this much-boomed " remedy " for syphilis can accomplish is only to introduce another poison into the system. It has not been established that it even makes a victim of syphilis immune from further attacks, even if it does succeed in effecting what is called a cure. Yet, it is stated on high authority that among the causes of death syphilis comes next to tuberculosis, while it is also a powerful and predisposing cause to consumption. The progress of syphilis depends entirely on the patient's own resistant power, and doctors know one person may have a very severe attack, another a milder form, and yet another escape altogether after contact with the same diseased person.

I am not going to be drawn into any controversy as to the moral aspect of the question, although my sympathies are entirely with those who advocate the most stringent laws to suppress all conditions that tend to foster venereal disease in any community, but I wish to show that from a purely physiological point of view the upbuilding of a body strong and balanced in every part is the surest and best preventive measure that society can take in this direction for the ultimate eradication of this terrible disease.

Physically, however, I contend that it is the strength within— the life-blood in the body itself, and the innate muscular strength and fitness of each individual cell (which has, in the majority of people to-day, been greatly diminished through lack of balanced- physical activity, and this inborn in most of us through generations of ancestors), that is the best security against the entrance into the system and the progress of this mind-and-body-destroying disease.

The lack of a liberal hygienic education among the people is no doubt, to some extent, also partly responsible for the awful and increasing ravages of syphilis, and I hope the time will soon arrive when the essential knowledge to the protection of each person's own body against the seeds of this and other microbic diseases will be as general as is our present common familiarity with the letters of the alphabet or the rudiments of simple arithmetic. The object should be to prevent syphilis altogether rather than to await its presence and development before grappling with it.

The killing and sterilising of the bacilli of parasitic disease— that is, disease caused by bacteria which only thrive on a living host —is, I repeat, only possible in a body where the life movement or vitality is already sufficient, and the fighting cells and working cells present in sufficient number and balanced strength to ensure victory. This is why the doctors say that even in the last great fight between life and death " everything depends on the patient's vitality."

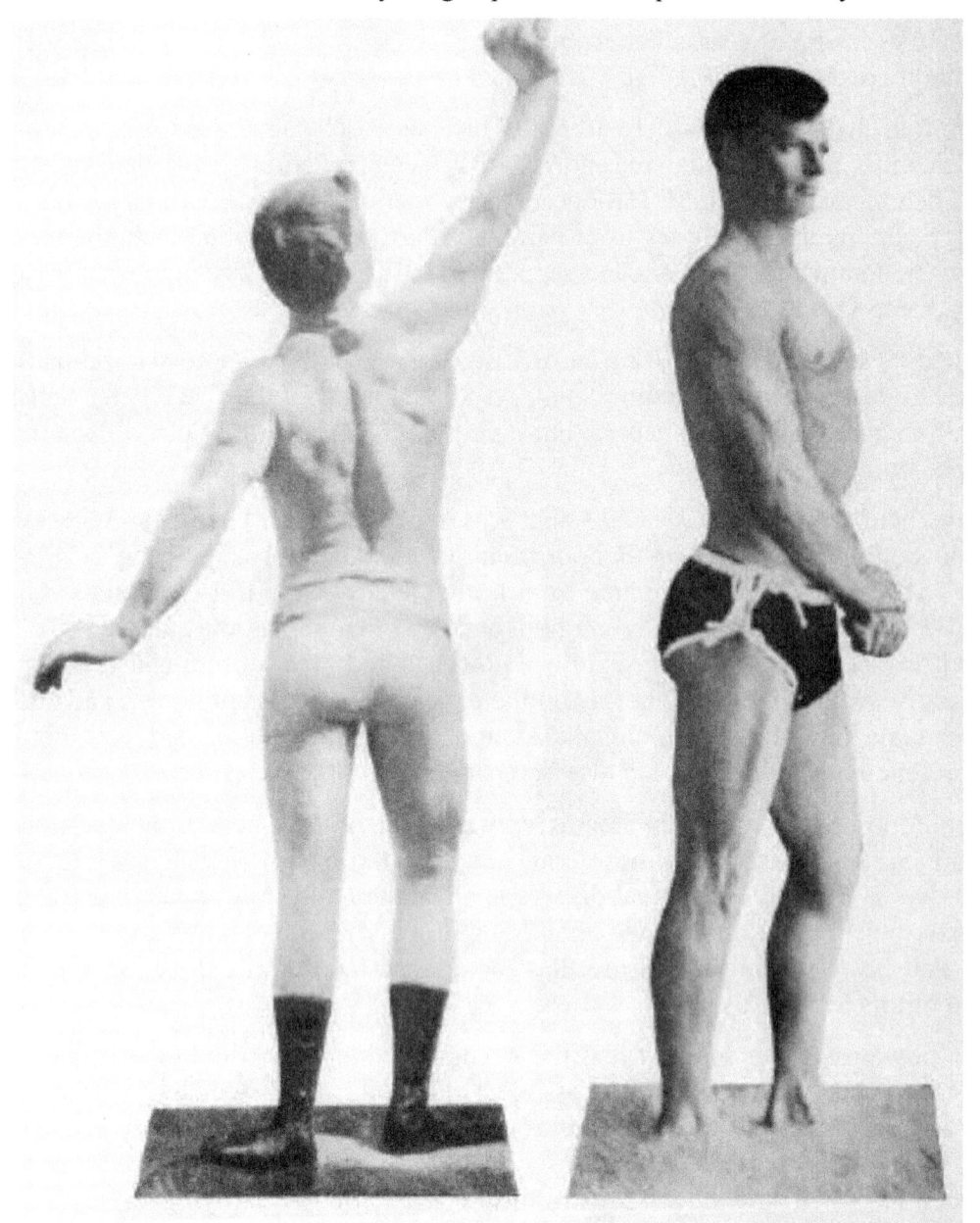

Two youths who would find little difficulty in passing the most severe army medical tests after following out the methods of physical teaching here laid down.

MUSCLES OF RESPIRATION, CIRCULATION, AND DIGESTION.

Now the first great source of vitality is air, and movement—the circulation of the blood—is essential to bring the life-giving oxygen of the air to every individual cell of the body, because this oxygen is carried on and distributed by the blood-stream which is kept moving continuously only by muscular movement; the beating of the heart and the contraction of the arteries. In the same way, nutrition, the other great source of vitality, is largely dependent on muscular movement—the movement of the muscular walls of the stomach— and the more vigorous and active every little living cell of the body is the better the body is oxygenated and nourished, and the greater, therefore, must be its store of vitality. So also the elimination of waste and poisonous matter that depletes a body of its vitality is accelerated by physical movement and greater circulation.

This brings me back to my first argument that if less attention were devoted to the germs that attack man and more first to the fundamental factor, the living cell, we should be travelling on a safer, speedier, and more reliable route towards the eradication and elimination of human disease.

After all the learned explanations of the way of the microbe and the best methods of encompassing its extermination, why, may we not ask, does the bacillus of disease successfully attack one man and not another? Why is it able to successfully attack anyone at all? The answer is that one patient succumbs to the disease because the life in the blood is not sufficient—i.e., all the fighting cells in the blood have not sufficient muscular health and vigour—to resist and conquer the enemy. One man dies because his bodily fighting cells or some of them are too weak to fight the bacilli of disease, or unable, at least, to fight them successfully. Another lives, but only after a terrific struggle between his very weak army of cell-soldiers and the invading disease germs, which have temporarily vanquished him because the fighting cells of the bodily army were unable to defeat them at the first onset.

The man whose vitality is strong to overflowing, whose cells are all equally strong and developed in perfect balance, is not attacked, or, if attacked, may not even feel the least symptom or discomfort. Why? Because, the cell-army of the blood and the fighting capacity of the bodily cells are sufficient to ward off the disease germs or kill them as soon as they enter the body.

THE "LIFE GUARDS" OF THE BODY.

The resistant power which, as Dr Sir George Newman says, is " the first line of defence " in the body, depends upon the number and well-being both of the fighting cells in the blood and of all the cells of the body upon which they are dependent. The fighting cells are roused into movement and activity in two ways (1) through the movement of the voluntary muscles by one's own will and direction, as I have explained, and (2) involuntarily, when disease attacks the body. In the latter case, all the fighting cells rush immediately to the spot or spots attacked with continuous reinforcements to resist and kill the enemy, and it is this mobilisation and combat of the fighting cells that causes such discomforts of disease as the rise of temperature, the quickening of the heart's action and, sometime^, local inflammations. The doctor can see how the battle is going as the temperature rises or falls or the pulse goes faster or slower, according to what we call the " vitality," or resistant power of the patient.

There is also another way in which the cells are sometimes aroused, viz., by some strong emotion, sudden shock, violent passion, etc., but this is psychical rather than physical. The great point I wish to impress upon the reader is the fact that the better balanced the body, the greater the number of bodily cells and the stronger and more developed they are in relationship to one another—for the fighting cells are dependent on the working cells for the continuation and transport of their supplies—the greater the resistant power to any and every form of disease. The fighting cells, in short, are the "lifeguards" of the body, with a great army of workers to support them, and upon the fitness individually and collectively of all these cells the safety of the body against disease microbes and disease of every kind depends.

Among my followers and patients in the East, where yellow fever, sleeping sickness, cholera, small-pox and infectious or contagious diseases are rife, there have been many whose balanced physical fitness, due to the natural methods as I am now advocating, has kept them immune in the midst of the most fearful epidemics, and many more who have " won through " only after a spirited fight with these awful enemies of man. Had they been weak, physically unfit, and lacking in vitality they would undoubtedly have succumbed. This splendid immunity from, or triumphant victory over, disease shows the value of scientific physical education, even in a comparatively late period of life. How much more valuable will it be when it becomes a compulsory and essential feature of our elementary educational system for the young.

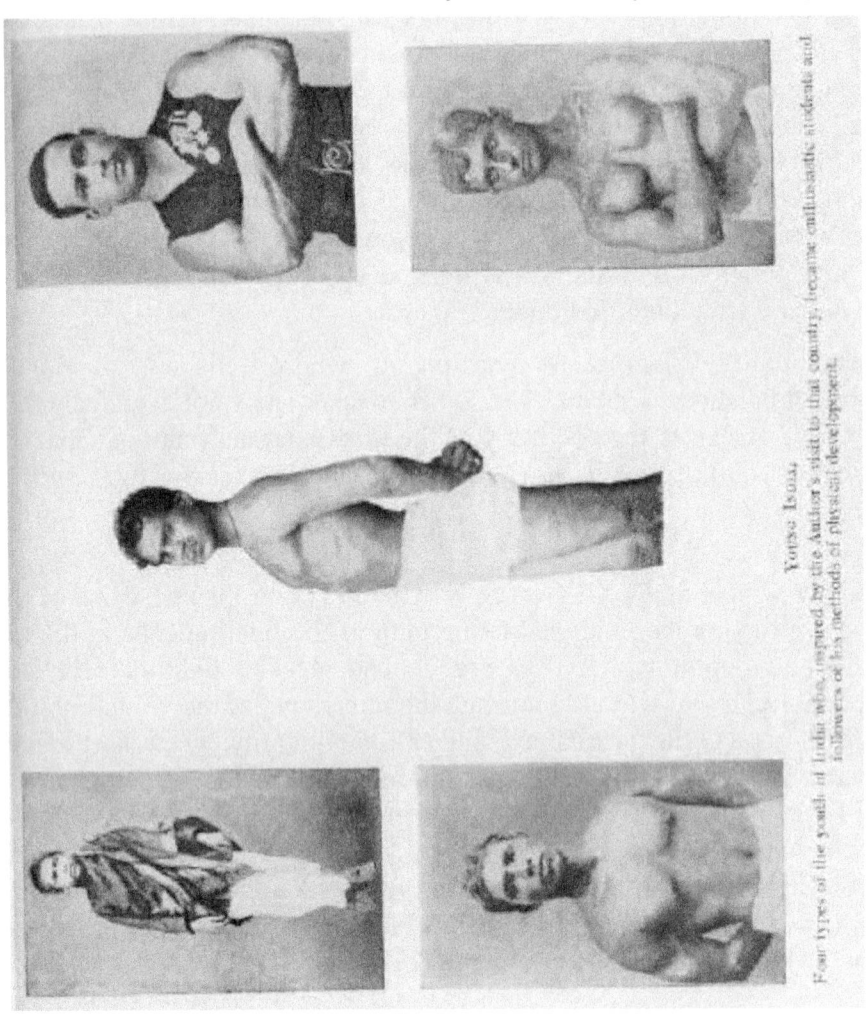

Four types of the youth of India who, inspired by the Author's visit to that country, became enthusiastic students and followers of his methods of physical development.

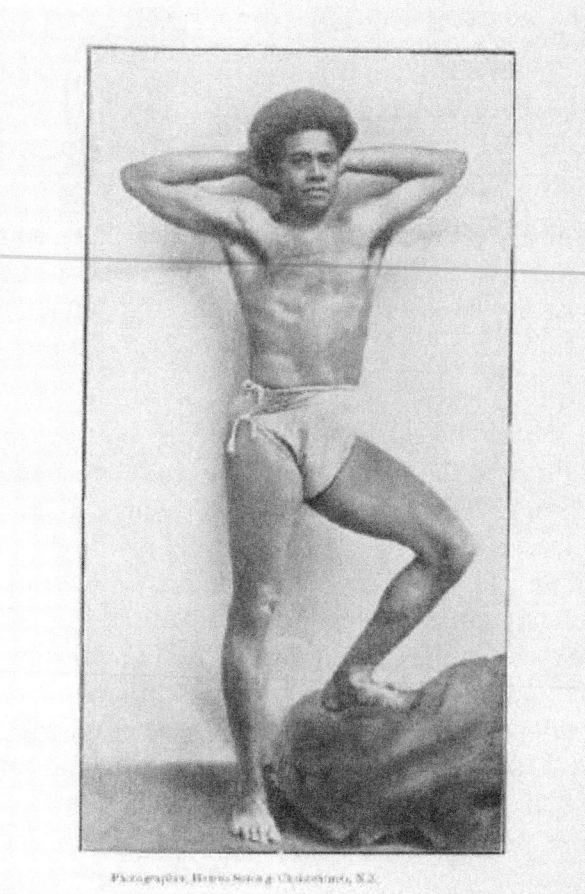

Young Fijian who takes a pride in his physical body, and who has brought it to a high state of physical excellence by these methods.

HOW TO PREVENT MICROBIC DISEASE.

It is because the natural methods advocated here replace and keep on replacing weak and feeble and disease-inviting cells by more and better cells which, in turn, breed still better and stronger cells, with greater muscular activity and greater resistant power, that the germs of disease cannot successfully attack and conquer a body so disciplined, and so full of fighting and resistant power with which to oppose the enemy. Microbic disease in man can only be prevented by developing this great cell-community of the body, encouraging the multiplication of the cells, and bringing to each and every cell within the body copious supplies of vitalising oxygen and nutriment, while, at the same time helping the skin, the lungs, the liver, the kidneys and the intestines to eject from the system all waste and poisonous products, whether of bacterial origin or self-generated by daily bodily wear and tear. Only such a body as this, supported by all the protective measures of modern medical science and by the most drastic legislation, will be able to win the victory over these venereal and microbic diseases which bequeath such a morbid heritage to humanity to-day.

" Surely, Mr Sandow, though, you do not contend that any method or methods of bodily reconstruction and body-culture can hope to eliminate such highly infectious and inherited disease as tuberculosis, syphilis, cancer, etc? " That statement, put to me recently by a well-known public man, brought from me this reply:—

THE BOGEY OF HEREDITY.

" In the first place, I am doubtful if there is any such thing as inherited disease. A child may, of course, be born with a weakness tending towards disease, because weakness of the frame and constitution has been inherited, and the conditions of modern civilisation and education at present only tend to tolerate and even aggravate that weakness.

" If both parents and child were placed and kept under State and medical supervision and guidance from the first, much of the so-called hereditary disease of to-day would be prevented from developing. As it is, the child grows up weakly, for neither parents nor child have the knowledge necessary to safeguard it, until, at last disease strikes the weakest spot and only then is the doctor tailed in."

Heredity has been made a bogey to affright many people, but it is the transmission of physical weakness that is the real threat to the children, and the children's children. A scientific system of physical reconstruction through balanced physical movement will gradually tend to the reduction and elimination of this inherited weakness in children by giving them parents with well-formed, well- organised, and well-developed bodies. A child cannot choose its ancestry, so we must 'help to choose for it. We can help, too, by taking the child early in life and arresting any tendency to disease that physical weakness implies. For instance, by strengthening the spinal muscles and the muscles of the shoulders and all trunk muscles in a child, one or both of whose parents were consumptive, and by developing its chest and lungs and increasing its lung capacity, we would be able to check and arrest the progress of that disease in the lung cells of the child. So, too, by preventing the development of phthisis in the child, itself a sexual being and capable of reproduction at a later age, we would do much to prevent the tendency to a similar weakness in its offspring, and thus gradually eliminate consumption from the family and finally from the human race.

My contention is that every mother should be under State medical supervision and guidance, and be instructed by the doctor, with the family history to guide him, as to the best steps to take to safeguard her child's life. Later, at school, the child itself should be kept under constant medical supervision, as I have fully described elsewhere, and have its whole body evenly developed and perfectly balanced to make it strongly resistant to disease, especially in its weaker parts which have less power of resistance, and which are, therefore, most likely to succumb. If this were done, very much of the so-called hereditary disease too familiar to-day would cease to be.

INTERNAL CLEANLINESS NECESSARY.

To save the children, it will be necessary to inculcate a sense of reverence for that body of which to-day most people, even in adulthood, know so little, and to teach them to keep it clean, both within and without. Cleanliness of the outward body is already made obligatory in many schools, colleges, and educational institutions, but it is even more important to teach the children—the man and woman of the future—to keep the inside of their bodies also clean by that healthy and scientific physical movement which is the first law of life, a law which, unfortunately, is too often forgotten, neglected or evaded in these days because there is no authority to enforce it.

When once the necessity of this interior cleanliness and sanitation of the bodily dwelling is firmly implanted in the youthful mind, and the occupant learns to take as great a pride in it as the good housewife does in the brightness and sweetness of the home in which she reigns, a great step forward will have been taken towards the prevention and elimination of all disease, infectious or otherwise.

Habits ingrained in early youth grow stronger with the years, and it is just as easy to implant good habits as to allow bad ones to be formed. Most forms of vice arise from evil habits that have become in time almost an obsession. Habits of health and virtue can also be sown early if proper steps be taken, and these, too, will partake in later life of the nature of an obsession too strong to be easily supplanted by other habits of an ill or evil tendency. A body schooled, trained and disciplined to a daily habit, of health-care will not lightly entertain, much less tolerate thoughts or actions to its own undoing.

OUR HERITAGE OF HEALTH.

Just as we can see the effects of a soldier's drill even in old age —it is generally easy to distinguish the trained soldier from others of about similar age by his erect carriage and bearing even in later years—so the building up of a strongly resistant body in youth will remain apparent even in later life, and such a man will certainly be less liable to disease then, even if he discontinues exercise, than a person whose body has never been so disciplined. The early scientific physical re-education and reconstruction of which I speak would build up a body too strong to be overcome by any germs of disease, which, after all, can only hope to triumph in a body that has already been made too weak or unbalanced through ignorance, neglect or ill-treatment, to resist it successfully.

Apart from the fact that a body well-developed, with a mind well-cultured in proportion, is little likely to fall a prey to infectious disease germs of any kind, it is also better able, if the disease does gain a footing therein, to repel it and to conquer it more quickly than a body not so developed. Thus one man will recover in a few days, another may take months or even years, and another, weaker still, will never recover but die a sudden or a lingering death.

EQUALITY OF HEALTH OPPORTUNITY.

I do not, for one instant, mean to argue that such methods as I advocate will give us a sort of health-socialism, in which there will be no rich or poor and no grades or ranks, for there will, at least for some time yet, be some with a heritage of health from birth greater than that of others not so happily circumstanced. Physical re-education, which means the reconstruction of the whole organism, however, in so far as it does tend to a levelling of the national health, will be a levelling-up rather than a levelling-down process, and in time we must obtain if not a physical equality an approximation to physical and health equality. At least, we can give all equal opportunities for health after birth.

To an almost incredible degree, it is true that microbic disease of every kind can be prevented by scrupulous internal and external cleanliness, and the upbuilding of clean, strong and healthy cellular tissue. Such methods of health education and culture as I advocate will, as I have already said, teach people from childhood to cleanse and purify the interior of the body as well as the exterior. Scientific physical movement will improve the circulation of the blood, and increase the ejection of the waste and refuse matter from the system. By inducing perspiration and opening every pore of the system it also leads to the greater purification and aeration of the blood (for each pore of the body is also a little lung taking in oxygen as well as discharging bodily waste matter), and also reduces the eliminatory work thrown upon the intestines, kidneys, liver and lungs.

All this means internal cleanliness as well as external, for many a man and woman to-day who prides himself or herself on his or her personal cleanliness, carries an unclean interior beneath a well- cleansed and pleasing exterior. The free opening of the pores would lead to the greater aeration of the blood, and its consequent purification, a fact which cannot be too clearly borne in mind when we remember that " the blood is the life," and that through the blood health or disease manifests itself. This, in turn, means that every living cell of the body receives greater supplies of oxygen and is, consequently, made stronger, more productive, more strong and healthy within itself to resist disease and all the conditions that are favourable to disease, either from within the body itself or from without.

The body that is scientifically trained and physically balanced has an ever-vigilant army of attendants to protect it. and promptly administer the coup de grace, or the " knock-out blow," to all these minute emissaries of disease called microbes or germs. Weaker bodies similarly attacked are often only " beaten on points," to use another boxing phrase, after a long and trying fight, while there are bodies so weak and run down and so conscious of the fact, that they lose their courage and are beaten without even a show of defence. Microbic diseases only win their showy victories over the weak and the physically unbalanced, as all medical men of prominence now know and admit. To be strong to resist and conquer one form of disease, is to resist and conquer all, and if we can conquer disease we can prevent it, as I show in my next chapter which, I hope, will especially appeal to medical men.

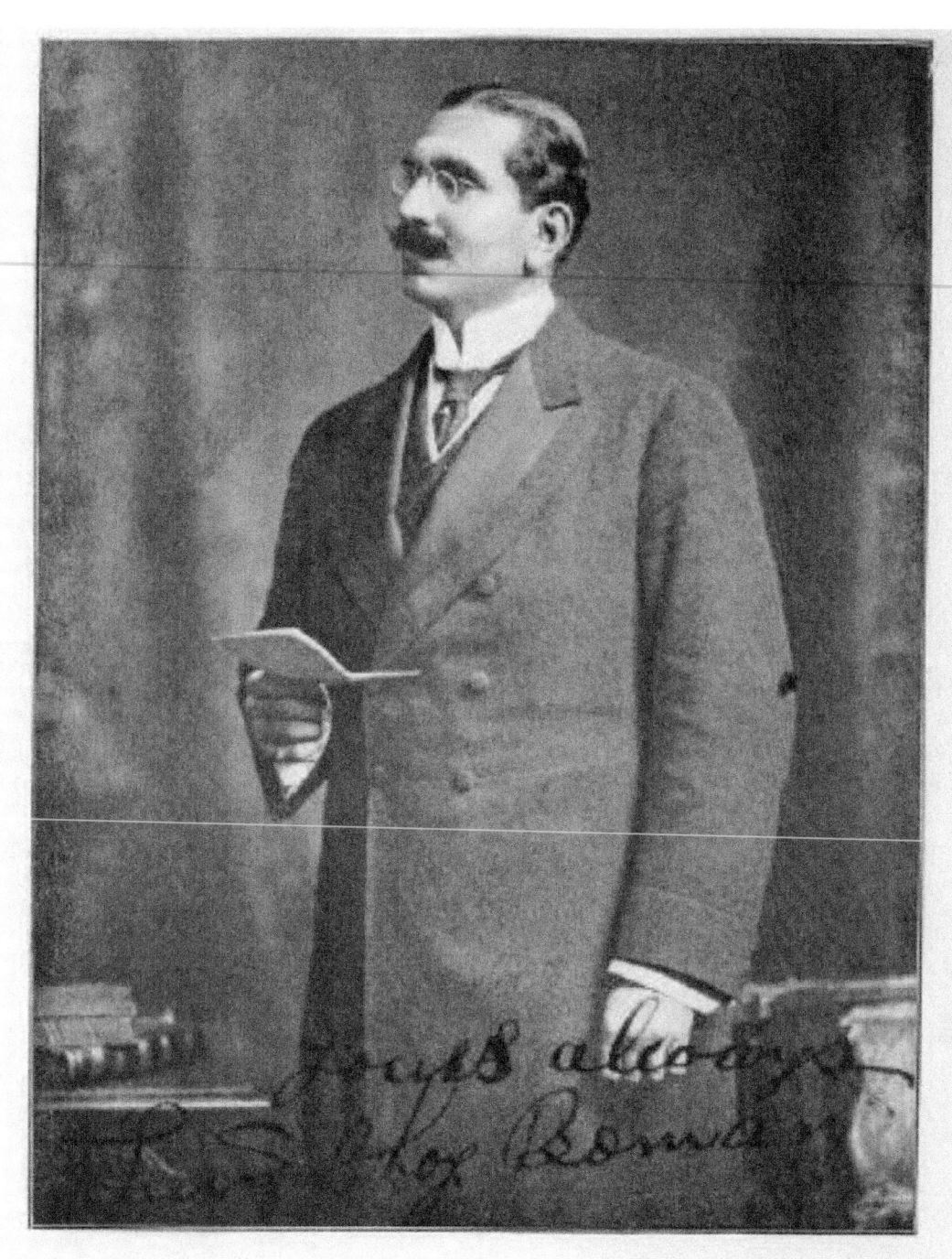

Photographers, Lafayette, London.

M. DHUNJIBHOY BOMANJI, OF BOMBAY.

This gentleman suffered severely from the terrible disease of elephantiasis, but to-day, thanks to the methods of physical reconstruction and cellular evolution described by the Author, he is one of the heartiest, strongest and most perfect of men, physically, in the whole of India. Of high birth and ancient lineage, it would be impossible anywhere to find one more worthy of both those fine and oft misused terms, man and gentleman. A son of the Empire whom it is proud to claim, and who honours it by his unwavering loyalty and distinguished services.

CHAPTER XVII.

Medical Facts for Medical Men about Medicine and Disease.

MEDICAL men now agree that much disease is preventable and that what they designate "preventive medicine" is the medical study of the future, though, as I point out later, the word prevention is scarcely the right word to use, as we cannot prevent the existence of disease germs or the weakness from birth that may be within tending towards disease. All we can do is to prevent disease from being victorious in its war against humanity by making man superior both to disease germs and to innate weakness.

PREVENTION BETTER THAN CURE.

The preventive aspect of such a scheme of physical reconstruction and regeneration as I now advocate must, in the present attitude of medical science, be its most attractive feature to medical men and medical students. But, in the meantime, there is a great work being accomplished by very similar methods for the relief and cure of existent disease both in the children and in adults—what I may call physical therapeutics or curative physical culture, though, after all, it matters little what name we employ so long as we employ the right methods.

The medical student of the future must thoroughly understand three things before he is qualified and certified to practise as a real Minister of Health. Firstly, he must understand the nature of disease, its history, occasions and causes. Secondly, Jie must understand the diagnosis, treatment, relief and cure of disease. Thirdly —and this will be the most important of all branches of medical knowledge and practice in the very near future—he must know the best, and indeed, the only method of prevention against disease, viz., the development of a body perfectly balanced in every part and itself too resistant to become diseased in its own cells or to succumb to disease from without.

Until he understands all about disease, and what we call " diseases," he cannot naturally be expected to cure them. To know how to cure them should teach him ultimately how to prevent them. After a little while, he will be able to do without the second of these qualifications, for through knowing all about disease, its treatment and cure, he will know the steps to take to prevent it, and what can be prevented should never need to be cured.

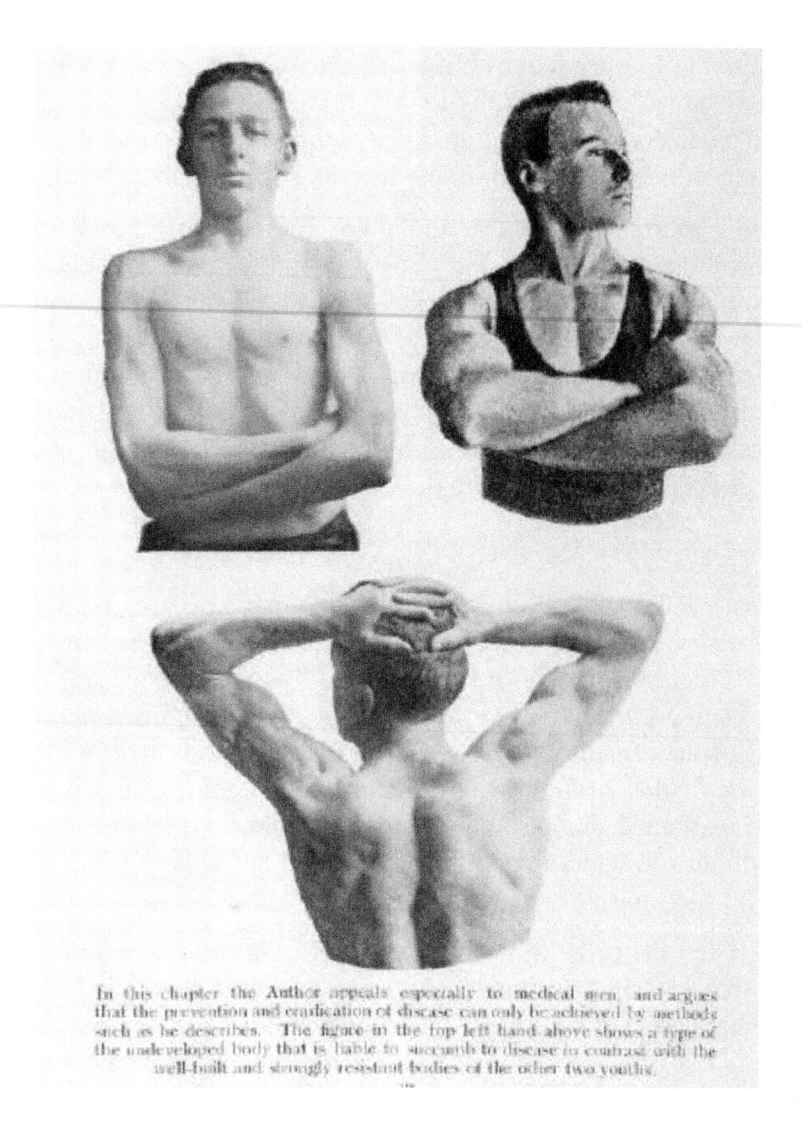

In this chapter the Author appeals especially to medical men, and argues that the prevention and eradication of disease can only be achieved by methods such as he describes. The figure in the top left hand above shows a type of the undeveloped body that is liable to succumb to disease in contrast with the well-built and strongly resistant bodies of the other two youths.

THE SCIENCE AND ART OF LIFE.

Medical men and medical students will be familiar with the wonderful report on "Medical Education," presented by Sir George Newman in 1918, to which I have already made reference. Commenting upon this report, a writer in The Times Educational Supplement said:—" From the summary of these views which we publish to-day it will be seen that his main object is to establish the harmony existing between all the branches of medical work, more especially between preventive and curative medicine. Preventive medicine is based upon a knowledge of the origins of disease: disease is most curable when it begins to manifest itself.

" The student must, therefore, be a man of wide general culture with the ability to grasp the relation of his future calling to the body politic, and also the bearing of each branch of his calling on the other branches. He must see medicine whole and must frame his mind to regard it, as a process, an evolution, a sequence. Loss of function rather than departure from standard form is the modern definition of disease; disease thus assumes a secondary place in the doctor's mind giving way to the primary idea of health. Medicine is no longer an occult art, it has become the science of the art of life."

However, before we attain to our ideal of a diseaseless world much existent disease will have to be combated or, as we say, " cured," though why should we " cure " disease? It is our place to kill disease by making the body so strong in every part that no ceil or cells will be so weak as to become diseased itself or to be the victim of any microbic disease from without.

This applies alike to children and adults, and the knowledge of the means that will cure or prevent disease in the children will be equally effective in the adult. The best method of " curing " disease, therefore, in both cases will be to employ the best means, and I contend that the method described in these pages, which will make the body in every part so strong as to defeat disease is the only real and permanent method of " curing " disease, because life is movement and it is through lack of balanced movement that we have physically fallen from grace. Only by literally re-creating a new body or part of a body in such a manner as I have described, can we eliminate and prevent disease altogether in an individual.

THE RE-CREATION OF THE BODY.

Drugs only cause destruction without construction. They have no creative or constructive power in themselves. No drug can have any effect on a body incapable itself of movement. The rational and scientific physical methods which I advocate not only assist the natural metabolistic changes in the body, improving both destructive and constructive metabolism, but they ensure that continually new and better cells are being born in a diseased body taking the place of the weak, the old and the diseased cells, so that the sufferer in time becomes, as it were, a new being free from disease. I have explained this elsewhere in greater detail. It has been said that the body is thus like a knife with an old handle supplied with new blades as the older ones wear thin and frail and too infirm for their purpose.

Will any medical man tell me if he knows of a single drug or medicine or of any combination of drugs or medicines that will increase healthy muscular flesh in this way? Can he tell me of any drugs or medicines that can give an added fraction of vitality to a sick person? Is there anything that will make a weak cell strong but movement? Will even the best of food do it if there is not physical movement to transform it into a suitable condition to be absorbed by the various parts of the body?

Medicine is simply a blackmailer in the body of a sick man levying toll on such little vitality as is left. It will irritate an organ or even a muscle into action by poisoning the nerve centres just as a galvanic battery can make the muscles of a dead frog twitch through stimulation. It will soothe or benumb a nerve, or, in some cases, supply the chemicals that diseased cells cannot themselves obtain. If anything, indeed, it retards nutrition and provokes malnutrition by increasing the toxins already existent in a weak and diseased body. Besides, the basis of many medicines, and especially patent medicines (which are taken indiscriminately and without medical prescription), are poisonous drugs of a most deleterious character in themselves and would suffice to cause death if given or taken in larger quantities. Medicine is not merely innocuous, it may even be injurious, and I hope will soon be as obsolete as the old-fashioned practice of cupping.

Doctors themselves—at least the more advanced thinkers among them—know and admit that, with very few exceptions, medicine, like the x in algebra, largely symbolises an unknown quantity, and that its administration is mainly for its psychical rather than for its physiological value. I could quote hundreds of professors and distinguished doctors who support me in this view, but I only give a few.

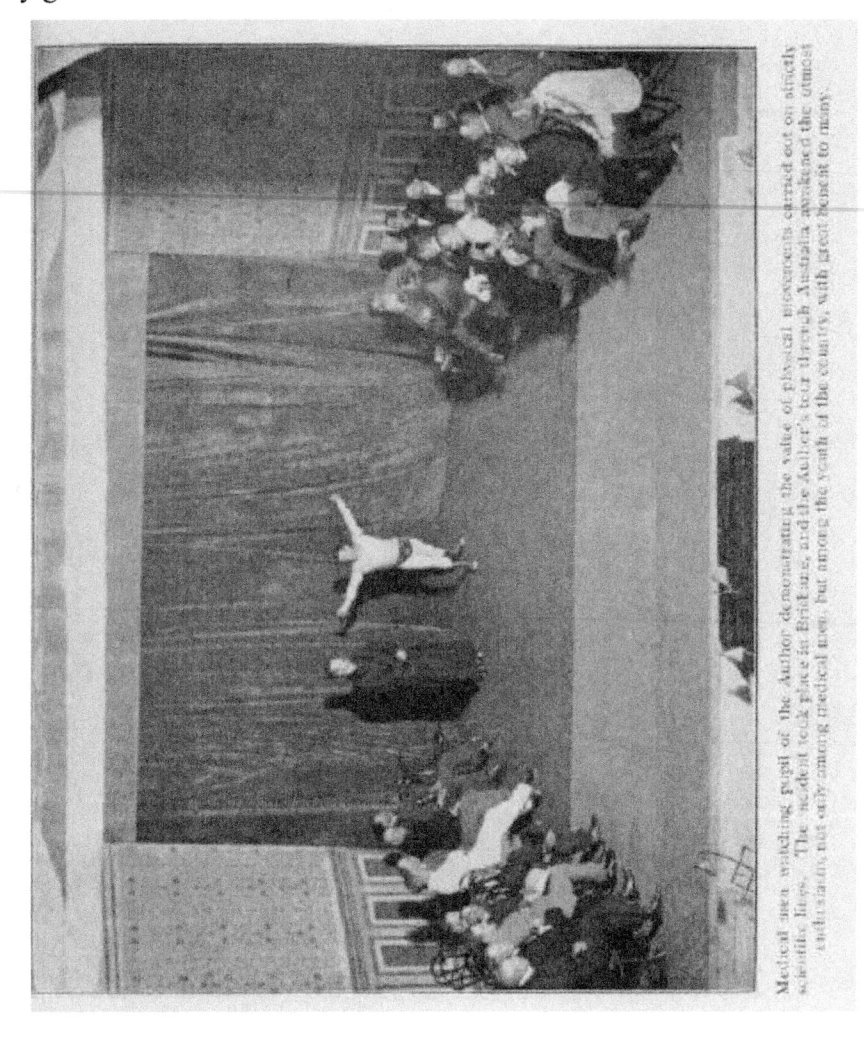

Medical men watching pupil of the Author demonstrating the value of physical movements carried out on strictly scientific lines. The incident took place in Brisbane, and the Author's tour through Australia awakened the utmost enthusiasm, not only among medical men, but among the youth of the country, with great honest to many.

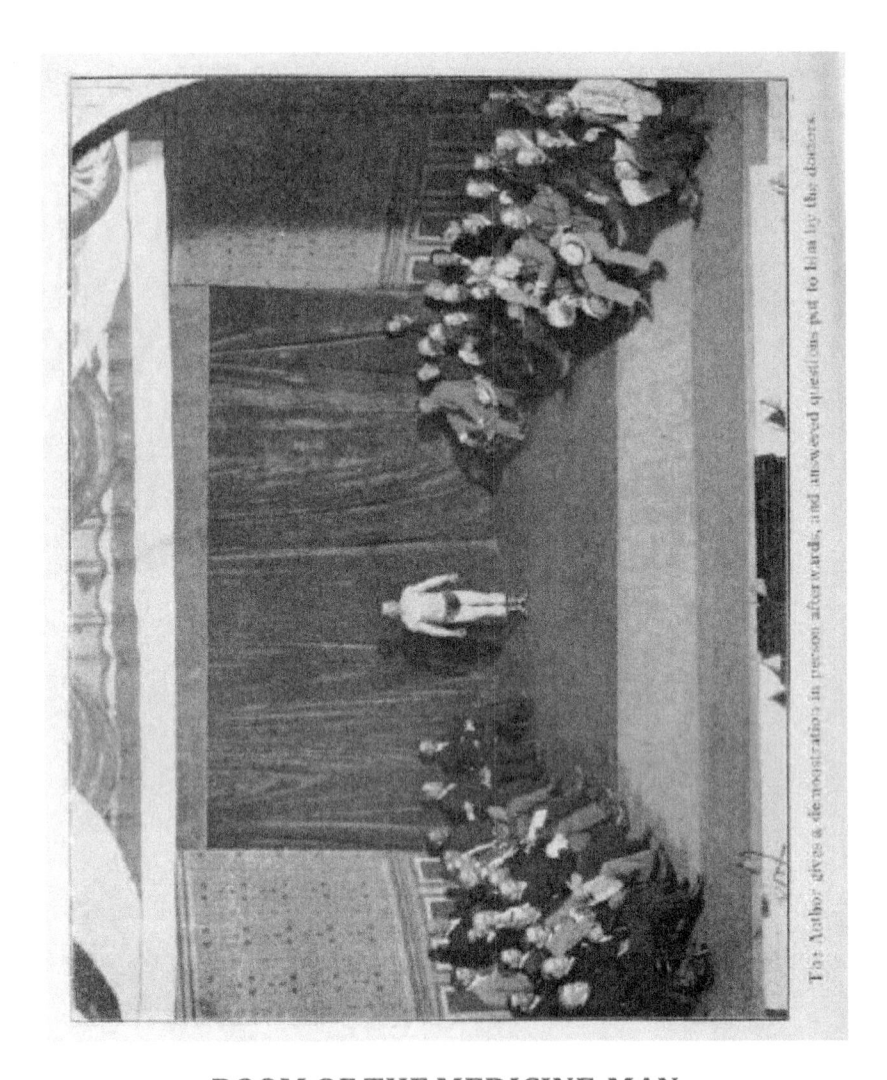

DOOM OF THE MEDICINE-MAN.

The famous French physiologist, Majendie, speaking before his medical class, said:—

" Gentlemen, I will tell you what I did when I was head physician at the Hotel Dieu. Some three or four thousand patients passed through my hands every week. I divided the patients into two classes. To one I gave the usual medicine without having the least idea why or wherefore. To the others I gave bread pills and coloured water, and occasionally, gentlemen, I created a third division to whom I gave nothing whatever. All the third class got well. There was but little mortality amongst those who received the bread pills and coloured water, but the mortality was greatest among those who were carefully drugged according to the dispensary."

Our own distinguished Sir James Paget declared that " every dose of medicine given to a patient is a blind experiment," and this also to an audience of young medical gentlemen.

Sir James Johnson, the brilliant editor of the Medico Chirurgical Review, said I—" I firmly believe that if there were not an apothecary, druggist, or drug on the face of the earth, there would be less sickness and less mortality than now prevail."

It is not " medical men " but " medicine men " who stand in the way of reform and progress.

From the great Sydenham and even before down to Osier, similar utterances have come from famous physicians themselves. The remedy for disease, as every doctor recognises, is in the body itself and not in any medicine or drug. As one medical man put it, " Nature cures and the doctor takes the fee," but even Nature cannot cure unless the most favourable conditions are supplied for the operation of Nature's healing power, and those conditions can only be supplied by the restoration of that balanced movement the lack of which has led to the present prevalence of disease.

The testimony I have just quoted is not the testimony of the ignorant or the prejudiced, and speaks louder than any words of mine.

What I may call balanced or harmonised movement or physical therapeutics is, as I have said, just as effective in the case of adults as it is in children, except, of course, that it may achieve its results more easily and more quickly in children than in grown-ups, because the older one gets the slower the cells are to increase and multiply. The principle, however, holds good at all ages, and, indeed, I contend that the old need physical movement applied scientifically even more than the young, so as to keep the cells of the body more young, more muscular and more reproductive.

To cite only one case, an old gentleman of 82 made the following improvement: chest 4 inches, upper arm 3 inches, forearm 2 inches, thigh 3 inches, calf 2 inches, with an increased chest expansion of 3 inches. The increase of bulk measurement was, of course, entirely due to the fact that more cells and better cells, with increasing muscular power and reproductiveness, were built up by harmonised physical movement applied, as they always ought to be, in a strictly scientific way, and this increase could only be obtained by getting perfect internal balance at the same time. The value of this in the final elimination and prevention of disease (which, after all, only means diseased cells, or cells weak towards disease), and their replacement by more and better cells, will be at once apparent to any medical man or student, and even to a lay reader of ordinary intelligence.

SELF-EXERCISING AND SELF-DRUGGING.

I venture to prophesy that in the very near future the doctor will require to know less of medicine as he learns more of the meaning and value of physical balance and still more of the human body itself. He will be a doctor of exercise rather than a doctor of medicine. He will prescribe necessary exercises as carefully as he prescribes medicine to-day.

What medicine man would turn to a sick man and tell him vaguely to take medicine—to go into a druggist's shop and take any or every medicine there. Yet thousands upon thousands of doctors to-day still tell their patients to take exercise in this off-hand way. A man might just as easily kill or injure himself in this way as by taking medicine when and how as he himself felt disposed.

For instance, fancy telling a neurasthenic vaguely to " take exercise," or " have a round on the golf links " as is, unfortunately, still done too often by medical men. Here is a man suffering from a physical condition induced by the continued over-expenditure of nervous energy and who, acting on medical advice, is quite likely to spend prodigally still more and more energy on golf or some other form of outdoor sport, instead of trying to save and bank new nervous energy every day. That way he will overdraw his account at the Bank of Health too heavily possibly with a fatal result. (See chapter on Neurasthenia later in this book.)

You might as well send him to a chemist for nux vomica without indicating the dose and times of taking. So with physical movement. If it is to be prescribed, administered and applied in a satisfactory way it must be given even more carefully and just as scientifically as medicine. The exact movements and number of movements must be prescribed after the most painstaking and accurate diagnosis of the patient's age and all individual conditions and requirements.

To assure this, it would, of course, be best for every student to be compelled to take up a course of practical physical therapeutics in his own person first, to qualify physically himself, before prescribing physical movements for others. It would, indeed, seem strange for a narrow-chested, physically undeveloped doctor to prescribe a " medicine " to others that he so visibly needed himself, and it only shows how credulous must be the sick public of to-day when it expects health from a bottle prescribed by a man, weak-looking and probably diseased himself, who has not even learnt, with all his knowledge of medicine, how to make and keep his own body healthy.

As Dr Hubert Higgins, M.R.C.S., says in his book on " Humani-culture," "As long as physicians are not conspicuous in attaining and maintaining more than average health themselves, it is legitimate to say that among the blind the one-eyed man is king, and to hope that the day is not far distant when none must necessarily be blind or even one-eyed." The spectacle of a medical man, bearing in his own person unmistakable evidence of weakness and disease, as we often see to-day, prescribing medicine to another well seems to me as ridiculous as the tipster one so often meets on a racecourse with wonderful " information " regarding " a certain winner " that one would think he would naturally seek first to benefit by himself.

Under the new system nothing of this paradoxical nature would be possible, for the doctor would have gone through a course of physical education in his own body:—would have "taken his own medicine " as the saying is—and would himself be the best and most convincing evidence of what he preached. His own body would be well developed and perfectly balanced physically. It would symbolise in its external appearance his very profession,' the power to confer health and strength on others. How much more confidence would any suffering man or woman put in a medical adviser of this stamp than in a physician who himself looked weak or ill, or even in a serious state of disease as we so often see to-day.

EXERCISE SHOULD BE PRESCRIBED LIKE MEDICINE.

Every student should be taught the prescription of what I call balanced physical movement. The muscles within voluntary control and their movements are known, and the student should learn to know the therapeutic effect of each movement or set of movements, the scientific and best method of carrying them out, how to diagnose and to prescribe physical movement with accuracy to any part of the body according to a patient's age, sex, condition and other individual considerations, how the movements should be blended, varied, and graduated to meet the patient's changing condition—everything, in fact, about the scientific prescription and application of harmonised physical movements for the treatment, cure and future prevention of disease both in children and adults.

All that I have written here may seem strange and startling to the medical man steeped in tradition, but is a fact, an absolute and proved fact. For disease and all weakness towards disease can be cured and even prevented by the upbuilding of a balanced and strongly resistant body. This is no mere and unsupported ipse dixit on my part, nor mere theorising or speculation.

Indeed there is surely sufficient evidence of its truth to convince the most sceptical in the splendid array of photographs that accompany this book. Some of them are real " living pictures," and one could not imagine these people easily succumbing to any disease. Many of the originals were weakly and undeveloped when they first commenced treatment, and their photographs show what wonderful improvement was wrought in them.

WONDERFUL RESULTS ACHIEVED.

Just here, I might say that I do not say it would be impossible for any of these to become diseased again if they persistently neglected the balanced physical movement always essential to healthy life, although muscle, once made, remains to some extent. But under all circumstances I do argue that they would be less liable to disease than those who have neglected physical movement all their lives, and never at any time possessed a well-balanced organism and constitution. It is always possible even for the strongest, by neglect or carelessness, to get diseased or in that physical condition which makes them liable to disease. Those, however, who have acquired bodily balance by such methods as I describe, seldom discontinue the practice, but come to regard it as essential to health and comfort as the washing of their face or their daily bath.

Some of these were guided by post, some by my books, and some personally. Some required only enough daily physical movement to keep them in normal health and resistant to disease. Some required a better physique and general physical development, and naturally derived also a considerable accession of robust health at the same time. Some had physical defects or deformities that made life unhappy or threatened serious disease, and had their physical deformities smoothed away. A great many had some Illness or disease that needed specific physical treatment, and many were sent to me by well-known medical men.

The worst cases were, of course, those who only came to me after they had been chasing a will-o'-the-wisp of health through all the swamps and marshes of chemistry until they had nearly wrought their own destruction; they were all ages and-both sexes, from children of two years to old men and women of 80 and over. They represented every grade of society and every type of humanity. Nothing but methods such as I am now advocating here as a national system of physical reconstruction for all was employed, and the remarkable record of success which has been achieved has been vouched for by no less critical and conscientious a periodical as Mr Labouchere's world-famous organ of exposure, Truth.

The result of a Special Commissioner's investigations caused a tremendous sensation at the time, not only in England, but all over the world. It was one of the most amazing health reports ever issued by any newspaper. Here are a few extracts from it:—

> " So far as actual disease is concerned, the Sandow system of curative physical culture is employed at the Institute in four principal groups of illnesses. They are:—
>
>> " (1) Weakness and diseases of the chest, and lungs.
>>
>> " (2) Digestive and kidney troubles.
>>
>> " (3) Illnesses arising from failure in some function of the nervous system.
>>
>> " (4) Skeletal deformities, as, for instance, curvature of the spine.
>
> " Taking (the figures) for one day I find the cases may be grouped under the following heads:—

	Per cent.
" Cases of Dyspepsia in its many forms	44
" Nervous disorders, insomnia, etc.	16
" Gout, rheumatism	4
" Cases of Paralysis	3
" Heart affections	5
" Chest and lung complaints	10
" Various and other complaints	5
" No special illness, but treated for reduction of obesity or for general physical improvement	13

" Such figures go to show that the Sandow treatment is applicable and applied to a large number of serious cases.

" I learned that ultimately, of all the cases treated over the latest period for which figures were available, the treatment had only failed entirely in less than on£ per cent, of cases. Satisfactory improvement, therefore, was produced in over 99 per cent, of cases, and the treatment had completely achieved the object for which it was undertaken in no fewer than 94 per cent, of cases."

NATURAL LAWS OF MATHEMATICAL EXACTITUDE.

If I have been more successful than others it is simply because of the unique knowledge I have acquired during thirty odd years of devoted study to this subject exclusively, of my experiments on my own body, and of my experience in this natural treatment of thousands of others. The movements that I employ are as old as Adam himself, and as natural, except that they are now consciously carried on with a distinct object. My " system " is based on an accurate diagnosis of each individual case—perhaps the most difficult matter of all—enabling me to select and apply the correct movements to suit that case only, first to the particular part or parts immediately affected and simultaneously or consecutively in the building up and balancing of every organ, muscle, nerve, bone, system and every individual cell of the body, movements varied and gradually increased as the patient progresses.

This is a result that can never be achieved without special study, experience and by well-balanced physical movements applied not in any half-hearted or haphazard way, but in a scientific manner as mathematically exact as to quantity and quality as if subject to a mechanical or mathematical law.

The great aim of the doctor should always be to obtain both external and internal physical balance, the balancing of the mental and muscular, especially in the child, the balancing of organ and muscle and function, and the ideal is, of course, the establishment of a perfect cellular balance in every part of the body of each part with every other part, and the nice adjustment of the body to its environment.

But the greatest care must, above everything else, be exercised to regulate the selection and prescription of all physical movement according to the condition of the heart, and always to make certain that the movements will strengthen the pupil or patient's heart action. Even persons with weak and functionally defective hearts can have their hearts made strong by scientific physical movement if this precaution is observed, and I even contend that except where there is serious structural disease it is possible to rebuild a new and stronger heart by accelerating and improving cellular change as you can the rest of the body, so that heart troubles would practically cease to exist, especially if we began, as I suggest, with the children.

CO-PARTNERSHIP OF DOCTOR AND PATIENT.

Doctors will, of course, understand that much depends upon the hearty co-partnership of the patient, for if this is lacking nothing can prove successful. At the same time it is not to be expected that if a patient waits until heart disease or consumption or any deadly disease has become so far advanced that death may occur at any moment, a cure is possible, though it is really wonderful what can be achieved with patience on the part of patient and doctor. Unfortunately, many patients do not know that they have heart trouble and will not be made to realise that the treatment can only be employed gradually and slowly as the heart permits. Hence they grow discontented, and perhaps may give up in consequence and feel that it is no good simply because it does not produce some speedy and magical effect upon them. When sufferers learn to understand this, much better results will be obtained.

Both curatively and preventively, there is a great field for future medical study in this department of physical therapeutics. By beginning early with the children and teaching them to live healthfully, the curative aspect of the question will gradually grow of less and less importance until no disease remains to be cured. Coroner's inquests and post-mortem examinations will only be necessary after accidents or self-inflicted injuries, for knifeless anti- mortems will have taught us how to live, to live healthfully and to live happily.

It will naturally be somewhat difficult for conservative physicians of the old school to adjust themselves readily to this tremendous change in the whole medical outlook, although the younger generation will most certainly welcome it, for already there is a healthy and ever-increasing resentment in the new medical school against pharmacology, the more advanced thinkers agreeing that medicine and drugs, if not actually innocuous, have at least very circumscribed limitations.

NATION LOOKING TO THE DOCTORS.

It is to the rising generation of medical men, therefore, and the medical students present and future, to whom we must look chiefly for support in such a system as I propose, although I have no doubt that many of the great leaders of the profession to-day will be entirely with me in this matter. Should there, however, be evidence of any concerted movement against such a system of physical education and reconstruction for the children of the nation, I would still persist in my own unrelaxed advocacy of it.

It is my sincere and earnest hope, however, that the medical profession will see the wisdom of these measures against disease and of thus ensuring the health, happiness and efficiency of the people, measures, indeed, that will depend mainly for their success upon the generous and unanimous support of the medical men of the world

The great number and wonderful variety of diseases, even of an obstinate character that have defied medical, or rather, medicinal treatment and which have proved readily amenable to treatment by scientific physical movements will surprise everyone who has not had an opportunity of studying the subject, or whose experience has been confined altogether to orthodox treatment which must, under such a regime as I suggest, in a few years from now have become obsolete and unnecessary.

Indeed, all that I say here will be new to doctors whose study has been devoted to the influence and effect of medicine on the body and not the effect and possibilities of physical movement both as a preventive and a cure for disease, especially its power to improve cellular structure and function and through it organic function, which is Nature's way of curing and preventing disease.

This is a subject of the utmost interest, not only to medical men but to every man and woman, and I have dealt with it more fully in a later chapter of this book where anyone specially interested in the curative aspect of the question will find a mass of useful and helpful information, especially with regard to the natural treatment of nervous and functional disorders, by methods and means which bring new life and vigour to every cell in equal and harmonious proportion.

Under the new system it will be the individual patient who requires treatment rather than the disease. An engineer carefully ascertains just what strain materials and constructions meant to bear weights can stand, and never imposes tasks to the point of breaking strain. So we should do with the individual before prescribing physical movement.

By the methods I advocate we can not only replace, but even improve upon, the natural movements that kept man healthy in primitive life, and bring about the regeneration—at least in a physical sense—of the whole people.

PHYSICAL AND MENTAL EVOLUTION.

I was talking this over with a friend recently when he remarked, " But, Mr Sandow, you know we can't all be Sandows." Certainly, as men are to-day, the physical deterioration being greater in some than in others through ancestry, one will be able to develop greater muscular power and all-round organic strength and balance than another, because he starts, as it were, less severely handicapped by the condition of the body he already possesses and, by the physical family and medical history of his forebears.

When, however, we adopt a national and rational system of physical education and training on really scientific lines, and educate the children almost from the dawn of their life to habits of balanced physical movement, healthy living, and self-respect for the bodies they possess, each generation will become stronger and healthier, so that in a few generations the handicaps at present dividing humanity will not be so severe, the physical differences in children and adults not so great and, starting with equal opportunities, all will be able to attain at least to their maximum standard of physical perfection, and that complete bodily balance, internally and externally, that prevents the invasion or intrusion of disease or cells becoming diseased in themselves.

There is, of course, a limit to physical perfection and development, and those who make the greatest progress in the shortest time will then stand still while others make up the leeway, though there will never be absolute equality among all. The men and women of the future under such a system as I advocate may be so physically perfect that even I myself, recognised as the strongest of men in modern times, might be regarded almost as a weak man in comparison with the greatly improved type of the future.

While for a time the doctor will, of course, have to exercise the utmost care in diagnosis and prescription according to the individual needs of each child, it must be evident that after such a system has been in vogue for any length of time, the physical standard of the race and condition of the people from birth will be so much improved that this may no longer be absolutely necessary though it will always, perhaps, be advisable as a precautionary measure.

FLOUTED BY A MICROBE.

In our present physical condition, however, no physical movements should ever be prescribed for remedial or curative purposes except after careful diagnosis by a qualified medical man, and to suit the individual child or adult. Physical movements from books or charts of a general character are only for those who are physically and organically sound.

To the doctor more and more in the future the State and the people must look for the health of the nation. Even while I am writing this chapter the worst epidemic in influenza the world has ever known is raging, doctors are being kept busy night and day, and the public press is clamouring for more and more medical men and a Board of Health. It is evident, therefore, that the physician must play a still more prominent part in the whole national life than he has ever done in the past, but I ask medical men candidly if it is flattering to their profession in the twentieth century to find disease still flourishing more vigorously than ever even after all their studies, all their research, all their experimentation and all their experience.

Does it not argue something wrong radically in the system of grappling with an enemy that seems to grow more powerful after each reported defeat! The triumph of Lister, of Koch, of Pasteur, of Ehrlich, and of dozens of other great bacteriologists, surgeons and physicians shrink into small measures when a grinning microbe of influenza prostrates the people of the world, kills its millions, and defies the united efforts of the world's physicians to stamp it out.

The world has stood too long on the defensive against disease. The time has now arrived for a great offensive. We must no longer leave the initiative to disease and be content to parry its blows. We must fight it with a new weapon. Imagination must be added to the medical armoury, and the doctor must seek to anticipate, to circumvent and to prevent its onslaughts, or to render them abortive if attempted. Disease must be killed in the womb of humanity. It must be a still-born child.

Humanity must never give birth to such an offspring alive with all its vicious possibilities. To prevent the birth of disease in the human body is infinitely better, safer and cheaper than to seek to destroy it afterwards. Fortunately, the whole medical profession is fast awakening to this fact, and is devoting itself more and more to preventive measures, none of which, however, I contend, can succeed until we begin by making the human body itself too powerful everywhere and too resistant to be vanquished by disease in any shape or form.

In my next chapter I bring before my readers some remarkable statements by distinguished members of the medical profession as to the present and future medical attitude towards disease, and its prevention rather than its cure. Many of them I have collected from out of the way sources and will come as a surprise both to medical men and students, and even more so to my lay readers. All of them are indicative of a complete revolution in the new medical attitude towards disease. In many directions it is evident that medical science is looking for something that will really prevent disease, but looking in wrong quarters. When they turn their attention and study, as I have done, to the power and possibilities of physical reconstruction by natural methods, to build up a body in balanced strength, they will find what they are looking for everywhere else in vain

CHAPTER XVIII.

The "No-Medicine" Medical Man of the Future.

I HOPE my readers will excuse me for beginning this chapter on an unavoidably personal note, but I assure them I only intrude my personal experience in the hope that it may help to enforce my argument and consolidate my position, and I am confident that medical men not only in England but throughout the world will be interested in what I have to say here.

I think I may claim, without undue egotism, to be a fairly strong man—indeed, of more than average strength. Also I do claim, whether egotistically or not, to be a very healthy one. Indeed, according to my own argument, I could not be the former unless I were the latter. How did I make myself so healthy and so strong, for I was of delicate constitution in early youth. Simply in the manner I am now advocating in the public interest,, by developing my whole bodily organism in perfect balance by the simple methods I have already described. What I could do personally there is no reason why others cannot do also.

REFUTING A POPULAR DELUSION.

Some time ago I was desirous, for the sake of my wife and family, of insuring my life. Now, there was the common but erroneous impression that because I was " a strong man," as the phrase goes, I could not be healthy and sound. I must, some argued, have an overstrained heart and other infirmities caused by performing my feats of strength.

Well, I was medically examined by the Norwich Union Insurance Co.'s medical representative, and what was the result? Not only was I medically passed and accepted by the Company as a first-class life, and insured for £20,000, but I was accepted at a reduced rate of premium, because, as a letter I received from the general manager said, " my directors have decided to act upon the very exceptionally excellent medical examination you have passed."

Now my sole reason for bringing in this incident here is because it points a moral which I desire to emphasise. If I may say it without offence, the tradition of the medical profession has been to pay too much attention to the study of the body diseased and too little to ascertaining how to make and keep it healthy and free from disease, though I am glad to see a great trend at present towards the more desirable goal of preventing disease rather than curing it when once established. I have travelled all over the world in response to invitations to show my own physique and to lecture on physical culture, yet no doctor has ever voluntarily asked to examine me, because 'probably his traditional education and training had schooled him to exhibit curiosity only towards a diseased body, and not towards the discovery of my secret of developing and maintaining for more than half a century a perfectly healthy one.

And, remember, I have not only made myself healthy and strong, after having been born of weak constitution, but i have made thousands of others healthy and strong also. Had I complained of a cough, or of a pain in the region of my heart, I have no doubt that any of the many medical men whom I have met in many parts of the world would have gladly produced his stethoscope and examined my lungs or heart and given me the most excellent advice.

SECRET OF A DISEASE-FREE BODY.

I mention this to show that even a more than usually strong man with no sign of disease of any kind did not arouse sufficient curiosity in any of these medical men to make them anxious to ascertain the cause of that health and strength or how I maintained it through life. Yet I had travelled in many countries and had lived in climates very sympathetic to disease of the most infectious and most virulent character. If I could do this and have done this, surely the medical profession might well have sought to know the why and the wherefore of my immunity, and to understand why others could not be made similarly immune by similar methods.

It has all along been my contention that the causation of disease is lack of balance in the body or between the body and its environment, and though we may help the body by ameliorating the conditions of its environment, the more logical method is surely to adapt or adjust the body to its environment, or rather, to make it not the creature and slave of its environment but, as it should be, its conqueror and master.

If, as is now generally admitted, lack of balance between the individual and his environment is the chief factor in degeneration and disease, then, surely, if we can make man the master of his environment—as I have myself proved we can do—we are nearer the solution of this problem than we can ever attain by laboratory research (valuable as it undoubtedly is to this end), clinical studies and reports, and all the other methods now devoted to the study of existent disease, rather than to the study of its prevention in a structure so perfect in form, substance and organism as the human body, and its ultimate elimination and eradication of disease from the human race.

WEAKNESS OF MEDICAL METHODS.

The average practitioner only sees his patient when disease has actually triumphed over the patient's body. His " clinical notes " are made when the patient is already in a state of disease, and made from information supplied by a patient not only unskilled in the keen observation necessary to be of value, but even ignorant of the everyday working processes of his own body. Can the unskilled observations of such a man, already in the abnormal condition of disease, enable the doctor to be accurate in his deductions and conclusions as to the true cause and origin of the ailment.

Is a man stretched on the rack of disease and ignorant, even in health, of what is going on within his own body from day to day, to be able to give information that would explain the true reason why he had been defeated in the battle of life, or to help the doctor in making an accurate diagnosis. This has been too long the modern method, and shows how weak is our defensive armour against the intrusion of disease even now after centuries of medical research and experiment.

Indeed, as an American writer had put it in a typically quaint and humorous way, " the patient is too probably just sufficiently ' cured ' to enable him to have another ' round ' with his environment, to be defeated again and again, to be patched up, till finally he dies and gives up the struggle, the end of which was assured from the start."

My scheme of things, on the other hand, would be to have every individual consult his doctor periodically, just as a business man calls in an accountant to check and examine his books from time to time, thus taking steps to safeguard himself against failure, rather than looking round for advice when failure has come to him. Every individual from childhood should be taught to obtain and maintain a health-balance, to study his health expenditure, balance or overdraft, as the case may be, and to have his health accounts " audited " at least annually by a qualified medical man. The doctor of the future might, indeed, more aptly be called a Physical or Health Auditor, and people will consult him as business men to-day consult their accountants to avoid financial disaster.

POPULARISING HEALTH KNOWLEDGE.

Even the most humble individual should be watched over as constantly and as carefully as Royalty is to-day. For, as every doctor knows, Royalty is wonderfully free from disease, and usually lives to a ripe old age because of this constant medical vigilance and supervision. For children at school, indeed, I would have such a health-audit by skilled medical men made compulsory, so that health-care and health-culture would become a habit with them in later life, while the doctor in future, would be paid for the prevention of disease than for its cure.

The record of the medical profession is a noble one and it has achieved marvels of good, considering its limitations and handicaps, its lack of State support, its opportunities of securing sufficient data, and the disinclination of the older type of medical men for what one of the medical profession's most distinguished representatives called " the vulgarisation of knowledge." Just as medical men themselves in earlier ages were thwarted by the religious orders who sought to restrict the healing art, as it was known in those days, to their own priestly craft, and who even accused Hippocrates of robbing the temples of their prescriptions, so to-day the average layman is permitted to know little or nothing of his own body, and anatomy, physiology and hygiene are too often regarded by medical men as subjects to be dealt with only in " chained books " exclusively reserved and preserved for the benefits of something like a monastic order of medicine.

The attitude of too many medical men to-day is, indeed, not at all unlike that of the clergy who, in other days, sought to keep the people ignorant lest they should lose their own power and influence over the people. The spread of education, however, has not jeopardised ministers of the Church in the least, and we have at the same time a world better enlightened, more truly religious and more intelligent: In the old days, merchants had to entrust the clergy with all their business transactions, and so the layman was never entirely master of his own worldly affairs, just as in health matters to-day, he is not master of his own health capital owing to lack of health knowledge, that ought to be in his possession from youth.

HEALTH A SOCIAL DUTY.

The medical profession would itself benefit in many ways if it were so, and much disease would be prevented that now flourishes through ignorance and tardiness on the part of the individual. A patient with some knowledge of his own body and its myriad activities would, naturally, consult his doctor earlier and oftener, for he would observe early departures from health more quickly, and in this way would materially assist in preventing disease. Lawyers say that they are more often consulted by clients who know a little law than by those ignorant or suspicious of the law. The same would hold good between medical men and their patients, with the popularisation cf knowledge essential to the health of the people.

The schoolmaster, however, is abroad and the walls of what may be called medical monasticism or occultism, like the walls of the city of Jericho, will soon crumble and fall before the uplifted voice of the people, unless medical men themselves perceive the trend of the times, and open the gates of their own free will. That they will choose the latter course I feel confident, for after all, the co-operation of an intelligent subject is far more likely to lead to successful results and greater rewards than the present empiricism that robs the physician of most valuable information, and too often degrades the noblest of all professions in the eyes of an educated and observant public.

Besides, health and disease are matters that do not merely affect the individual and the doctor, but are matters affecting the whole community. If the individual, whose body and brain are often his only capital in life, is reduced in economic value by disease, the loss is not only his but falls directly or indirectly upon society. It is, then, the business and the duty of society to see that all disease is prevented, cured or alleviated, and, if possible (as I contend it is) eliminated altogether.

As showing the changing view of medical opinion——the result mainly of the appalling reports of the physical condition of the people in war-time and of the medical examination of school children—I may here refer to a leading article that appeared some little time ago in The Lancet, describing what was truly called "a new orientation of outlook with regard to existing medical teaching." A distinguished physician and professor were quoted as expressing the views of the General Medical Council that " the whole conduct of life from the point of view of national efficiency must be the objective of a new system of medical education on preventive lines." That in itself is a noteworthy utterance coming from such a quarter. It was a statement endorsed, too, by no less an authority than Professor G. Elliott Smith, while the same prominent journal of medical opinion quotes an equally remarkable statement of a similar nature by Dr J. S. Haldane.

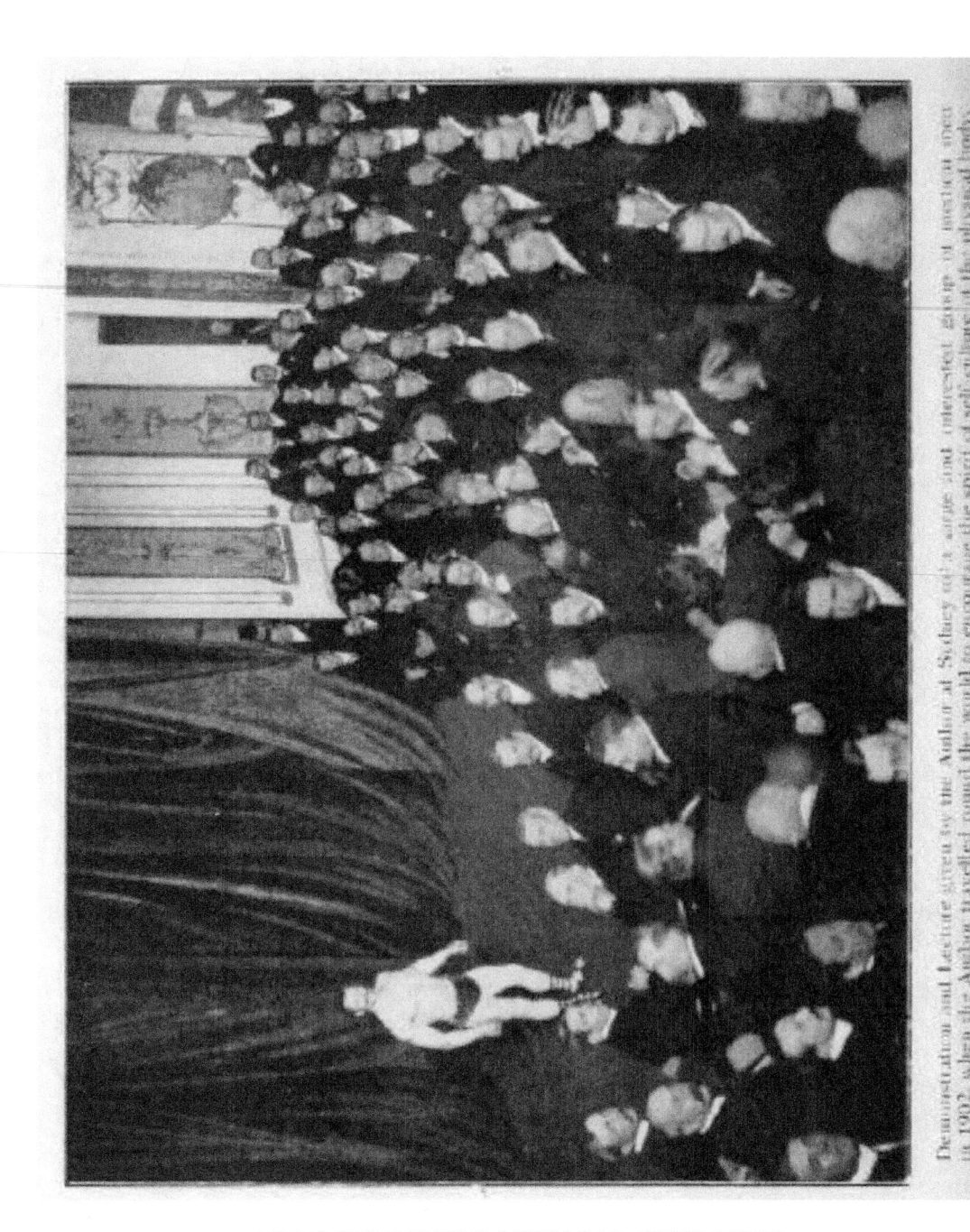

Demonstration and Lecture given by the Author at Sidney [?] of a large and interested group of medical men in 1902, when the Author travelled round the world to encourage the spirit of self-reliance of the physical body, and to combat the physical deterioration which was even then menacing the people everywhere.

NEW STUDY FOR MEDICAL STUDENTS.

The medical man of the future is the medical student of to-day, and I am most anxious that the present and future medical student will fully realise his relationship to the public in the new era when we shall prevent disease altogether and not permit it to exist in individuals made and kept too healthy to become diseased. To quote from a Times review of Sir George Newman's now famous Report on " Medical Education," already referred to, " the view that the general practitioner must be ready to discharge the work of a preventer of disease admits of no question. The general practitioner is the man who sees disease in its beginnings, he it is who makes the early diagnosis, he it is who can apply treatment at a moment when treatment is likely to be of value.

" His position grows more, not less, important to the whole State; his education is a vital matter. He must be taught that there is no cult in preventive medicine any more than in curative medicine. He is the foundation upon which both prevention and cure are builded. As a student he must, therefore, be taught that the least of 'his functions is the attempt to cure established, disease, the greatest policy of preventing the onset and establishment of disease

Speaking before the Edinburgh Pathological Club, Dr Haldane drew a striking picture of what he called the vis directrix of the healthy body as opposed to the vis medicatrix of the sick one, and this physician pointed out that " disease is but the breakdown of regulation at one point or another," or, as I call it, lack of balance. If we can prevent this " breakdown of regulation " we can prevent disease, and it is my contention that only through the voluntary muscles over which we have been given control we can do so. And it is towards the prevention of disease that all medical teaching is now trending, for we are at least beginning to realise that health, after all, is cheaper than disease.

This is one of the points that I have sought and am seeking to emphasise, and I contend that health can only be secured for all by developing the body in balanced cellular strength everywhere.

THE VIEWS OF SOME MEDICAL MEN.

Opinions, of course, still differ as to how disease can be prevented, and I have gathered together here some varied suggestions from distinguished medical men and Officers of Health. In a most interesting paper which was reported in the Edinburgh Medical Journal, Dr John Robertson, Medical Officer of Health for Birmingham, opened a striking debate on Preventive Medicine—a conjunction of words somewhat opposed to one another and indicative of the traditional medical mind. In that paper he said:—" There is no group of men who have the opportunities of the general medical practitioner for dealing with individuals who require advice on the methods of prevention of the spread of disease."

"As a matter of fact, there are very few diseases in regard to which preventive measures cannot effectively be taken. In my opinion, there is at present a vast field of work almost untouched in the domain of the prevention of disease. It cannot be too often impressed upon the profession that the 'prevention of disease is more important than the cure of it, and this ought to be impressed also on the medical student." Professor Stockman, in reply, said, " the relative use of drugs and other agencies does not, I think, come into this discussion. Personally, I teach physical therapeutics."

Even more remarkable in the expressions of opinion it elicited was the debate on a paper by Professor Hunter Stewart, of the University of Edinburgh. Dr Leslie Mackenzie, a distinguished Scottish physician, said that " the normal attitude of the medical man is primarily clinical. Not only that, his clinical insight is limited to cases of gross disease. The medical inspection of school children has helped the practitioner into a greater insight into preventive medicine." And under such a system as I advocate this insight and experience will be greatly increased and extended. I may quote other medical men in brief to save space:—

> Dr Guy—" They should get the idea fairly implanted in their mind that their highest aim ought to be the prevention of disease."

"The prominent ideas should be the prevention of disease, the maintenance of the adult in good health, and the important 'position that the student, as the future practitioner, will be called to occupy in relation to these ideals."

Dr Leslie Mackenzie—" In view of the development in the Army, one cannot forget that during the next four or five years the importance of the question of physical education and remedial massage and gymnastics—in fact, the whole of physical methods as applied to health—will be vastly enhanced."

In fact, the medical man of the future will be, or I hope will be, as far advanced from the practitioner of to-day as the present-day physician is ahead of the medicine man or witch-doctor of the .savage.

Professor Lorrain Smith—" There are very few diseases in regard to which preventive measures cannot effectively be taken."

Dr Robertson—" The question of physical culture is emphasised by the conditions in the Army. This also might well be taught as a part of preventive medicine. In America, it is considered such an important subject that several Universities have appointed professors of physical culture, who are doing magnificent work in this direction." Again he said: " If chairs of preventive medicine were established, duodenal ulcer, gastric ulcer, colitis and many other diseases could be tackled with advantage."

If old methods of physical culture came in for such commendation, what may we not expect from a scientific method such as I describe here.

Dr Traquair—" The loss of time and wages due to preventive affections of the eve is enormous. If the general practitioner regarded prevention seriously the public would in time do so also. In connection with diseases of the eye. I suppose there are about 30,000 blind people in the United Kingdom, half of whom owe their blindness to preventable causes."

Dr Gibbs—" It is a clinical fact that we can, if we wish, prevent dental diseases, and it could be taught to the student in one lecture. Dental caries and pyorrhoea alveolaris are the two commonest diseases of western civilised life, and the most easily prevented. The child can grow up with no dental caries; the adult can keep his teeth to old age. I have been preaching this for the last fifteen years, but the ignorance of the general practitioner undoes practically everything that many of us keenly interested in preventive medicine in this direction are trying to do."

These are only a few of some hundreds of similar medical opinions which have been expressed of late, and show only too plainly that the future medical practitioner will stand in a very different relationship to his patient than the old. It is evident, however, that the great objective of the medical profession will be that complete prevention of disease which is proverbially better than cure, and that physical methods of reconstructing the body and scientific physical education will be vital factors in helping medical men to reach that objective.

HOW CAN DISEASE BE PREVENTED?

While it is very satisfactory to note this changed attitude of the medical profession of recent years and to find a representative professional journal like The Medical Press declaring that " it is but yesterday that we were all for finding cures, to-day we seek above all things to cultivate prevention," yet I am still inclined to wonder if medical men even yet are approaching this tremendous problem in a really scientific and radical way.

What is this " preventive medicine " of which they speak? How can we "prevent" disease? Medicine that, after thousands of years, has failed to cure disease can scarcely be expected ever to prevent it. The only real preventive measure, I repeat, that can ever achieve success is to make man himself so strong within that his body contains not a single weak cell that can become diseased itself, and is strong enough to conquer and crush every microbe of disease that attacks it, and to obtain perfect cellular balance everywhere and equilibrium between the body and its environment.

You cannot do this by throwing out " fenders " around a weak and disease-tempting body. You cannot do it by giving such a body " escorts " and " body guards " in the form of drugs and medicines, for the moment these are taken away from it, it is an easier victim than ever before to disease. You can only defy and conquer disease by making the body innately so strong and so impregnably protected in its own muscular armour-plate that disease will always and ever attack it in vain.

RESEARCH WITHIN THE BODY ITSELF.

The new curriculum of the medical student will have more to do with the study of strength and health rather than the study of medicine and disease, and will save the money that is at present being spent on research in laboratories and foreign lands instead of within the body itself. Even after over 30 years of practically exclusive study in this subject I can say truly that, as the great Newton said modestly of his new discoveries, " I have merely picked a few pebbles on the sea-shore of knowledge," and long after I am gone, this great work of investigation will, I hope, be continued by others, with the facts that I have set down in this book as nuclei. We must, to again quote Dr Haldane's words, " seek to discover the vis directrix of the healthy body rather than the vis medicatrix or self-healing power of a diseased one," the power, that is, to assist Nature in regulating and directing at every moment the activity of the healthy body.

There is much yet to be studied and learnt in the direction of balancing the living, human engine and making it so healthy, strong and stable that it will be made practically immune from disease from childhood to old age. This is a great vision surely, and one the realisation of which would compensate for every sacrifice and all the cost. If " disease," to again quote the distinguished physician above mentioned, " is the breakdown of regulation at one point or another," it ought surely to be possible for medical men, with all our modern scientific knowledge and experience, to secure the restoration of that regulation to all the functions and activities of the body.

This will not, however, be attained in a day. It means more and more concentrated study of the living body, of the relation of cell to structure and function, of harmonious balance between organ and function and muscle, of mental and muscular co-ordination, of the nature and relationship of the various species of bodily cells, in fact, all forms of study and scientific thought which can help us to produce a perfectly balanced, healthy, harmonious and strong human engine. When we have solved the problem of balancing every organ, muscle, nerve, bone, yes, even every tiny drop of blood, both as to quality and distribution, and every microscopic cell, we shall have found the true and only secret of health and strength for all from childhood to the grave.

Surgery has done more, perhaps, to defeat disease than medicine, yet even surgery can never avail to eradicate disease from humanity or to prevent it. Surgeons may, of course, prevent an organ from becoming diseased, just as they may " cure " a diseased organ by cutting it out of the body, for disease cannot either attack or defeat the non-existent. If the organ is healthy there is no reason for its excision. If it is diseased, would it not be far better to re-create and reconstruct a new and healthy organ in its place, as I maintain we can do, by supplying it with younger, stronger and more vigorous cells, or improving its cellular constituents in health and strength rather than by removing an organ altogether or depriving the system of its services.

NOTHING IN THE BODY WITHOUT A PURPOSE.

We do not uproot and destroy a garden because it contains weeds, and there should be no need for the destruction and removal even of a diseased organ if it were dealt with in time as, of course, it would be under such a system as I advocate. In fact, the condition, even in a minor degree, could never arise. It is nothing but flat blasphemy to say that there is a single useless organ in the body, or that any organ is present there without a distinct purpose and duty, though surgeons sometimes speak of dispensable organs. The human body was not built with hands, and whatever even constructive surgery or medicine has accomplished, no doctor or surgeon has ever been able to make by hand a living man. As I have shown in another chapter, however, it is possible by assisting great natural laws to reconstruct a new and better body in whole or in any part, and that can only be done by the use, as I have explained, of the muscles under our own direction to rebuild progressively improving and stronger cells free of any weakness that tends to disease, and powerful enough to kill any microbes of disease that attack them.

To be able thus to prescribe muscular movement, in perfect balance, either for the cure or prevention of disease, is a study really worthy of a great profession, for it implies, above everything else, the study of man—a far greater study than either the study of medicines or disease. Doctors should even now be preparing themselves for the great work of national physical reconstruction that lies before them by studying this vast subject with all its ramifications and possibilities, present or remote, and by availing themselves of such knowledge and experience as we already possess. Their great object should be to learn bow to train the body to health and strength from, early childhood and not to wait until the body becomes diseased as it present, for as a great Scottish physician has said, "the student of to-day when he becomes physician is too often called upon to deal with an altogether new physiology from that which he studied." To know and understand the laws that keep the body so healthy and strong as to be literally disease-proof and to apply them will accomplish even greater miracles than helping a sick man to rise from his bed and walk.

All disease really begins in the body itself, and is not so much to be attributable to microbes, unhygienic environment and external conditions generally as to a physique and constitution impaired, as the inevitable result of our modern and enervating civilisation and lack of balanced movement, until its power of resistance to disease has been greatly diminished and, in some case, has disappeared altogether. Health, too, like disease, comes from within and never from without the body itself.

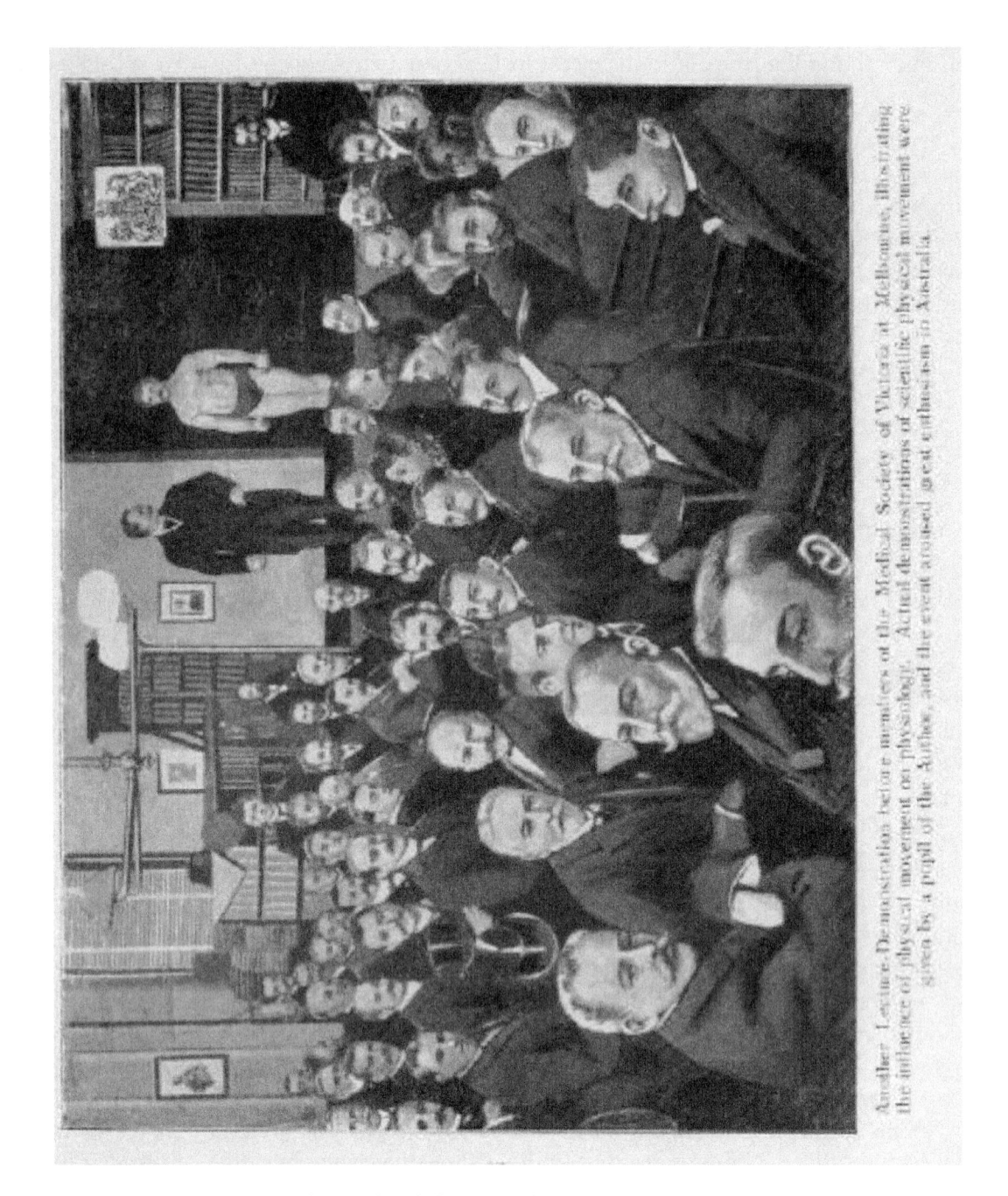

Another Lecture-Demonstration before members of the Medical Society of Victoria at Melbourne, illustrating the influence of physical movement on physiology. Actual demonstrations of scientific physical movement were given by a pupil of the Author, and the event aroused great enthusiasm in Australia.

MILLIONS SPENT ON MICROBES.

The microbe hunters of to-day can run their quarry to earth and kill microbes until they are tired, but they will never eradicate disease in this way any more than we could hope to exterminate a nest of wasps by killing stray specimens here and there. The weak body attracts the microbe while the strong one repels it, and even if it does find a lodgment in the latter the body will not tolerate is presence long, but will quickly kill or sterilise it. Our main object, then, should be to prevent the physical and especially the muscular and organic deterioration which alone enables disease to exist and flourish in the body, or healthy cells to deteriorate and become diseased, rather than to waste more millions of money and the best professional brains on tracking microbes to their lair. For, even if we keep on killing microbes, there will always be new and as yet unknown microbes of other sorts to take their place so long as we neglect the physical defences of the body itself or leave any " weak spots " in the bodily lines of defence at which enemy germs can break through.

The real enemy is not disease or disease germs but the physical deterioration that permits disease. This deterioration, through centuries of ever-diminishing balanced physical activity, is bad enough already, but it is and will continue to be progressive if some such method of individual physical re-education and reconstruction as I advocate is not begun immediately—NOW. As Dr J. Wallace Clarke says:—" Preventive measures to be effective must be conducted on individual lines and cannot begin too soon. Inoculation cannot transform a weakling and turn him into a robust citizen; there is no magical power which can transform the feeble, whose vital energy has been impregnated at its inception."

As we grow weaker and weaker still, which we are doing and will continue to do so long as we neglect the balanced physical movement of the human body that Nature intended us to maintain, old diseases will take a more virulent form and new diseases will appear and develop. On the other hand, as Sir George Newman says:— " Hygiene is the great medical subject of the future. As it advances the importance of the clinical subjects will decline; as it increases they must decrease."

BODIES THAT WELCOME MICROBES.

Influenza seemed never so virulent or so deadly as in war-time, say the medical men. Why? Because, owing to the fearful strain of war conditions, vitality, physique, constitution and innate resistant power to disease were lower than ever before. The disease of to-day is not, as some medical men proclaim, a new type or a more severe and deadly type, but possibly, as one doctor asserts, the old microbe accompanied by a more vicious companion. It will, however, most likely be established yet that it is but the same microbe meeting a weaker human opposition and more favourable reception that was responsible for its greater ravages. The shock was greater in proportion to the greater physical deterioration and weakness of the attacked, and if we allow this physical deterioration to continue increasing at even the same rate of progress as during the last fifty years, we shall find still newer and as yet unrecognised diseases triumphing over man, while even diseases like influenza will wreck as much human havoc as did cholera, typhus; or small-pox in other days, because of the further lowered resistant power of the individual. On the other hand, if through the voluntary muscles we make the individual stronger in himself with a perfectly balanced physique and organism, even the most virulent diseases will be little more deadly than influenza in its mildest form.

Writing on the ravages of influenza in war-time, the Weekly Dispatch had a very sensible leader at the time which I cannot refrain from quoting in part:—

" What," asks the writer, " after the experience of the past few weeks, are we to expect if other and perhaps more deadly infectious diseases invade this country? Medical science and organisation may have successfully kept from our shores the deadly enteric and typhus fevers, the cholera, and the plague, which are the usual heritage of war; we may hug ourselves with the belief that these diseases will be none of ours, and that for once history will fail to repeat itself, but medical science is not yet able to close every avenue through which the germs of infectious disease can reach us.

" Besides, however good may be our supplies of food, four years of war strain of anxiety, and of strenuous effort, often for seven days of the week of striving in hundreds of thousands of cases to do two or three persons' work, have undermined the power of resistance to disease, and the sooner the State public health recognise these facts the better.

I It should remember that the pick of the physical strength of the nation is in the Army or Navy, that the work of the nation outside munition and other factories producing war material is being carried on by 'crocks,' by old men and by young boys, girls and women, all of whom are forcing their nerve power in the effort to carry on.

" The next autumn and winter will be the most trying we have ever known, even if the war ends this year. (This article appeared in 1918.) The drain of man-power goes on steadily—it must go on, if we are to win the war. And if the civilian population is to stand the strain it must be as physically fit as war conditions allow it to be. The physical fitness of the people is a matter of supreme importance of the State at all times, and never more So than now. It is the business of the Health Department of the Government to watch over and protect that fitness.

" The grip of influenza which laid millions low and caused the deaths of thousands—indeed the medical correspondent of 'The Times' estimated the mortality alone from influenza in 12 weeks to be at least 6,000,000 —was, it may be safely said, due to impaired physical strength; but the lesson it taught seems to have gone unheeded."

It must not continue to be unheeded, however, for those who neglect to profit must go under.

Man at the beginning of things was created and intended to be master of his environment and master of himself. He was, however, a physical rather than a mental being, and his education was of necessity physical rather than mental. To-day, we have changed all that and we are paying the full penalty. It is our bounden duty to get back to first principles, and to make the child, to use Spencer's famous phrase, " a healthy animal " before all things else.

WANTED, HEALTHY CHILDREN.

When we have given the children a sound physical foundation and taught them how to keep the body in health and free from disease, it will be time enough to attend to the cultivation of the higher regions of the brain and soul. Health before all must be our motto for the future, for again to quote Spencer, it is true that even yet " there are few who seem to understand that there exists in the world what may be called physical morality." He was right, for morality, just like health, is mainly dependent upon and determined by physical condition. After securing this basic physical fitness, all the hygienic and preventive measures modern science can devise may be called into requisition as auxiliary services for the maintenance and preservation of bodily efficiency against disease, vice and crime in all their forms. Even in the present generation we can do much in the way I have indicated to banish disease and prevent its recurrence, while, after a single generation, half the auxiliary movements now put forward for the prevention and removal of disease will be quite unnecessary for the reasons I have fully put forward.

I might suggest that healthy children will constitute the best insurance policy that any nation can have. "Wanted, healthy children," should be the watchword of the medical profession and nothing should be left undone to see that every child, rich and poor alike, is watched over most vigilantly until it reaches years of discretion, so that it may not be handicapped by disease or infirmity that is unavoidable, and should be given an early insight into the laws that govern its own bodily architecture and construction, not likely to be easily lost or forgotten in adult life. The children of to-day are the parents of the future, and when we ensure that the children of the future will have healthy parents, and make every child's prospect of success in life equally hopeful, which must be the result of such physical education as I suggest, we can rely upon it that the world will soon learn to be so jealous of Hygiea, as to prevent Disease from even wooing her.

And we shall not, in the biting irony of Mr John Galsworthy, be in the position of an owner who enters a donkey for the Derby and expects it to hold its own against racehorses bred and trained to the highest standard of equine perfection, from a long line of equally high-bred and physically perfected ancestors. The child of the poorest must start with a body and mind as fit for the struggle as the child of the plutocrat.

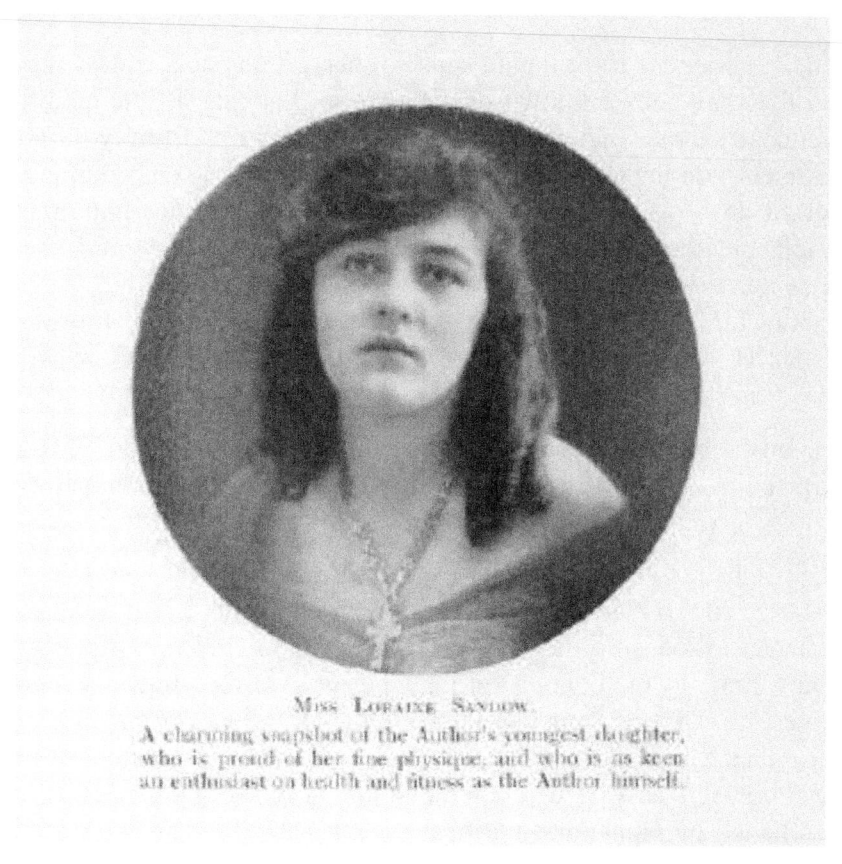

MISS LORAINE SANDOW.
A charming snapshot of the Author's youngest daughter, who is proud of her fine physique, and who is as keen an enthusiast on health and fitness as the Author himself.

CHAPTER XIX.

The Joy of a Healthy Life.

LIFE without health is merely, at best, human vegetation. Only the healthy know what it is to live.

Health, like wealth, is an expression of comparison. What would be but a servant's tip to one man would seem undreamt-of wealth to a pauper, and between the pauper and the millionaire there are many degrees of richness and poverty. There are health millionaires and health paupers also, with many gradations between.

Not to be ill does not imply the possession of perfect health. Health is positive, not negative. Civilisation has so " acclimatised " many people to weakness and deviations from the health maximum that they only think they are well and healthy because they are not actually ailing or ill. They have acquired, after centuries of civilisation, an acquiescence with or tolerance to certain conditions which blinds them to their real position. Many, indeed, have been so long familiar with sickness, suffering and disease as to take a morbid pride in its companionship. It is this false spirit of contentment that robs them of the ambition towards that perfect physical and mental health which alone can bring to them the real fullness of what the French joi de vivre, the sheer joy in living that thrills the bird upon the wing or the young colt that frolics in the field.

THE "STRAPHANGERS" OF LIFE.

Never once having experienced the exultant sense of perfect physical fitness they can scarcely be said to miss what they have never known or understood. Lacking all the qualities that make the healthy man advance to success and enable him to seize every opportunity for advancement, they are only " straphangers " on the journey of life, while others fill the cosy corners and comfortable seats. They never sit down at the banquet-table of Health, but, Dives-like, are content with the crumbs that are left, or, like the tame pigeons of large cities, flutter round the corn-bag of the feeding horse to snatch the few oats that it carelessly scatters around out of its own superfluity. Such existence is not Life, and the streets of every large city to-day are full of such people, that class which Dr Sir B. W. Richardson described as the " morituri," or which is popularly described as being " more dead than alive."

I was reading recently some reminiscences of the prize-fighter, " Charlie " Mitchell, and I could not fail to be attracted by one of his appositely shrewd remarks on the monetary value of fitness and health.

" Nearly all the millionaires I had met," he says, describing his New York experiences, " and I met many, had started life on a nickel, and had won wealth there in quick order by their brain force. I at once began to measure those successful men and find out wherein lay the secret of their success, and I came to the conclusion that the two words ' industry ' and ' enterprise ' covered the whole bill. They were workers, though, who always kept themselves fit for any opening that came their way, and when their chances came they jumped in and won. It didn't matter what their ' graft ' was, it was all the same—mining men, railway magnates, horse-owners, stock exchange manipulators, political bosses—the fit man won and the others went under. It was the tactics of the ring carried into the hives of industry."

RICHER THAN MIDAS.

True, the accumulation of Wealth is not the real mission of Health—indeed, many of these very rich men have sacrificed their health in attaining that very objective—but health brings far greater wealth than money, and purchases what the gold of Midas could not buy. It means good digestion and every good that good digestion brings. It sets the blood swinging and surging through every blood- channel of the body. It brings the colour to the cheeks and lips and the sparkle to the eye. It gives the erect carriage, the firm yet elastic tread, and the courage that only springs from confidence.

It ensures sound sleep better than all the bromides and sleeping draughts known to doctor or pharmacist. The healthy man awakes with a song in his lips and goes whistling to his day's work, for he feels himself the master of his fate and not its slave. Courage, confidence, nerve, cheeriness are stamped on his every act of life. Before such a man, fear, melancholy, despair and disease shrink timorously away. Such a man may well " bestride the world like a Colossus," while the poor in health and even the bourgeois of health feel abashed and humiliated in his presence.

Nor is it, as so many may imagine, any drudging or " hard labour " for such a man to take care of his body any more than it is a drudgery say, for the drunkard to get drunk. Each schools himself by repeated thought and act to one fixed idea of happiness, and only in thus thinking and acting finds the form of pleasure which satisfies him.

SOULS IN SLUM TENEMENTS.

But what a difference in the mental, moral and physical state of the two. The drunkard lives in a false, fleeting and delusive happiness which is followed by a very real and increasing depression and remorse, until the unnatural appetite is appeased once more. He is the victim of an obsession, a moral pervert, and finds happiness nowhere but in the dramshop. The man who has made the physical upkeep of his body his daily habit would miss the physical exercising of his body, which he regards as essential to his pleasure and comfort as the daily washing of his face, just as much as the drunkard would miss his favourite tipple.

He has, as reward, a thousand happinesses that the other has not. His eyes are wide open to the joys of life and living that ever unfold like a panorama before him. His mental and moral senses are keen-edged and unblunted. He sees things clearly and sees them whole. His pleasures are followed by no reaction or remorse. He is in harmony with Nature, in attunement with the Divine. He is not fear-haunted, worried, depressed or downcast, for he is one who truly lives as God meant man to live. His food tastes better, the air seems lighter, the flowers smell sweeter, his brain works quicker, he knows and feels the joy, the zest, and " the wild glad lust " of living as no one else can.

Such a man works better, and is better in every way than a person with a body as uncared for as a slum tenement. The slum body will have the slum mind, and we should always especially remember this when the children are under consideration.

Lack of physical activity will turn even a bodily palace into a slum dwelling for mind and soul. Through lack of movement the muscles become feeble and flabby, the body suffers in various organs and functions, the brain is insufficiently nourished through lack of air and exercise, waste and poisonous products are uneliminated from the system and cause what is called auto-toxication, a species of intoxication little different from that provided by alcohol. These waste products accumulate and ferment because there is a lack of balance between the processes of waste and repair that are ever going on in the body.

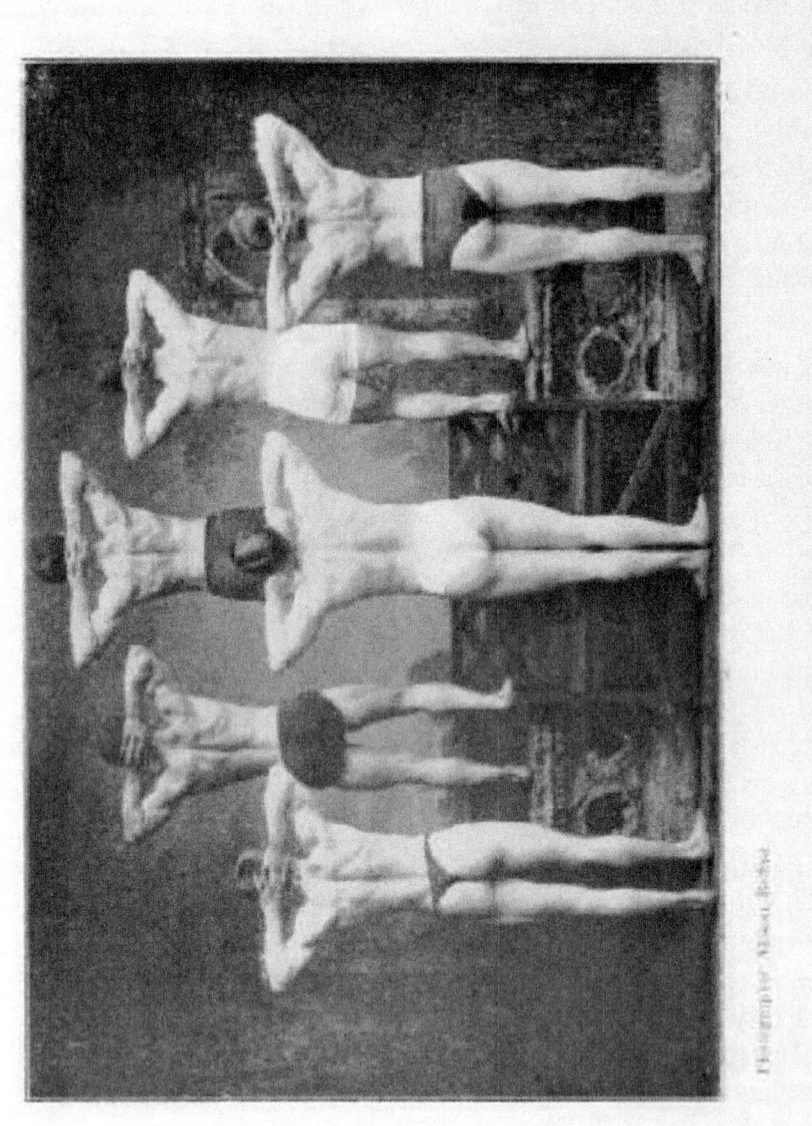

SELF-KNOWLEDGE, SELF-REVERENCE, SELF-CONTROL.

The cells that should do the work of elimination become weak or too few in number through lack of that balanced movement of the voluntary muscles which means life and health to every cell of the body. Some become diseased and die through lack of nutrition and sufficient physical movement, others, in the same way, become feeble and unfit, many continue to live in that state of existence in which the tide of life never reaches its flood but is ever on the ebb.

People of this type, unfortunately, are too common, because the conveniences and comforts of civilisation have made so many mere lotus-eaters in a world that demands physical activity and effort as the price of Health. So long as children are allowed to grow up into men and women without that self-knowledge which alone leads life to self-reverence and self-control, so long as their minds are developed at the expense of their bodies, so long as they are taught to conform to an unhygienic environment rather than to adjust the body into balance with its environment, or by education to make, as it were, their own environment, just so long will we have the weak, the degenerate and the diseased.

We want men and women who have the strength and the courage to be nonconformists to conditions and circumstances that rob them of their most valuable asset in life, physical health and fitness. A system of education for the people that justifies itself by its results is demanded, an education that will not point to the way to physical deterioration, degeneracy and disease. That is the true, natural, and only way to breed healthy and happy men in every sense of those often abused words. It will do more to raise the standard of humanity than all the other creeds, 'ologies and doctrines ever inculcated into the young.

Just as the body is only the multiplication of the individual cell, so the State is only the multiplication of the individual, and the State that does not do everything to improve the physical as well as the mental efficiency of every individual child must and will fall in the battles of brain and body that will take place for commercial supremacy, long after the guns have ceased to thunder and the bayonets and the sword have been beaten into ploughshares and pruning hooks.

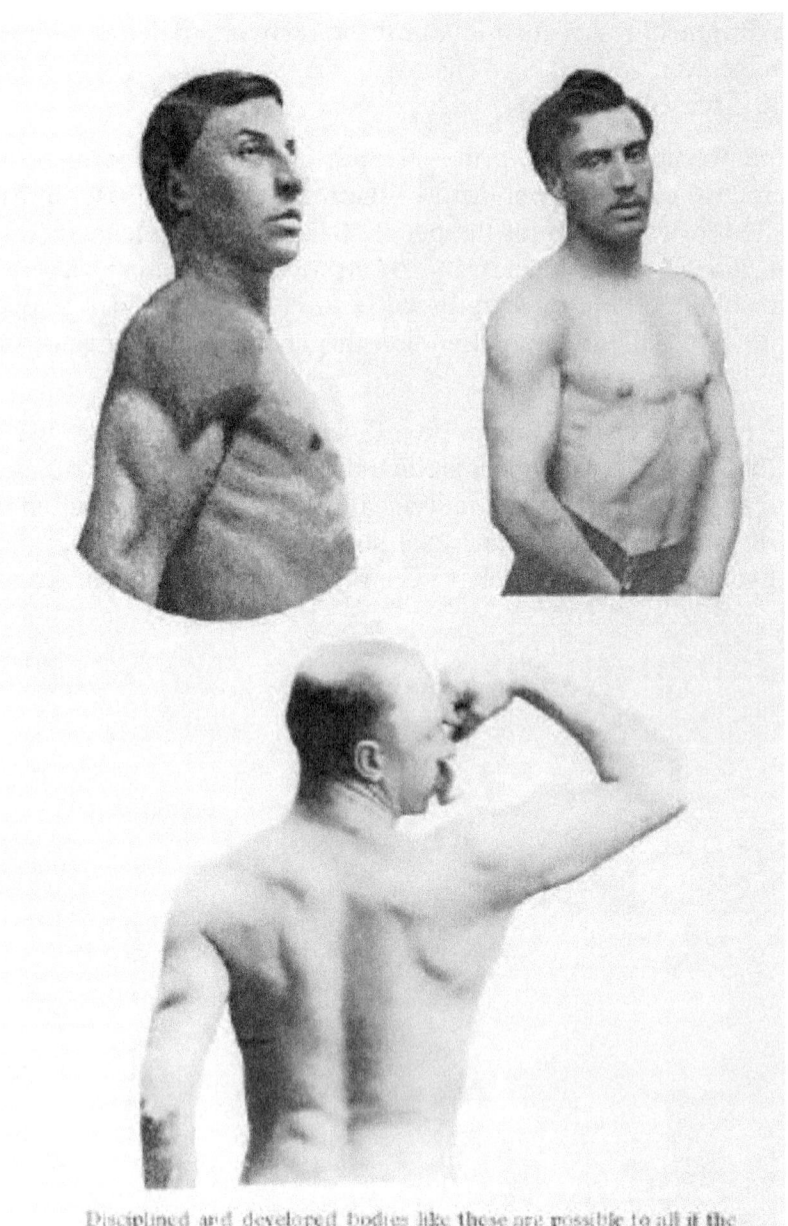

Disciplined and developed bodies like those are possible to all if the advice given in this book is put into practice. There is no reason why every man should not possess such a body, strong healthy, and disease-defying.

FEEBLE BODIES AND DEFECTIVE BRAINS.

Every individual—the children above all—must learn to know and appreciate what the joy of life is, how to attain it and the best methods of attaining it. When perfect health becomes the normal in our individual and natural life, no one will be content with less, just as to-day no one really cares to be poor. There will and must, of course, always be degrees of health as of wealth, but each individual will be able to attain to his highest possible standard or, if necessary, will be compelled by law to do so after reaching an age of personal responsibility. Those, however, who once experience the full joy of a balanced and healthy life will be little likely to become spendthrifts of it afterwards, if only for the sake of preserving to themselves the many pleasures it brings.

Adults, after all, are " but children of a larger growth," and what applies to the child equally applies to the " grown-up," so far, at least, as the application of the first Law of Life to the body goes. And it is not only the body that benefits, but the mind also reaps the harvest of Health. Mind, after all, is largely the mirror of the body, and one cannot expect even the best mental machine to work perfectly and easily on an ill-balanced physical structure. Faulty elimination of waste products that rise up to cloud, depress and irritate the mind are responsible for much of the bad temper, the vicious impulses, the immoral tendencies, and even the crime which exists in the world to-day.

That a feeble body is also an inevitable cause of a feeble mind is now recognised by all the great alienists and specialists on mental diseases, and I hope to see the day when the State will take as much care of the physically defective as they do at present of the feeble-minded and the mentally defective. Were there no feeble-bodied in our midst there would probably be no feeble-minded, for I contend that mental failure in the great majority of instances may be ultimately traced to the condition of the physical body.

KEEPING THE BODY YOUNG.

The mind is but " the upper storey " of the bodily building, and it can only be made secure by strengthening and establishing the physical " storeys " below on a strong, deep and sure foundation. As the well-known authority on mental and nervous diseases, Dr

David F. Lincoln, truly says, " the first storey of the educational fabric is built of and by muscular activities."

Tissue is the material of which every part of the body is made, and tissue, as I have explained already, is composed of cells that live, die and have their being just as you or I must do. Scientific physical movement makes these living cells of the bodily tissue more fertile, and as each old and decayed cell dies off, newer, younger, and livelier cells in abundance take their place. The cellular birth-rate, in fact, is greater than the cellular death-rate, and just as a good birth-rate is a nation's best guarantee of prosperity for the future, so this improving birth-rate of the cells ensures a healthy, strong; and happy corporeal body.

These recruits to the cell-population of the body being young and active themselves communicate their own feeling of youthfulness to the body they habit. This explains why harmonised physical movement makes a person possess that bubbling sense of youth which reveals itself in brighter spirits, increased mental activity, a light-ness and a gaiety that soar above all those clouds of depression and dejection that harass the weak, the ill and the unfit. It makes you feel as if new life had been infused into your body, as, indeed, it literally has been, by the introduction of new and youthful cells, better oxygenated and nourished than the old because more active. It gives you a sense of oneness with all Nature, a feeling of goodness, of happiness, of benignant toleration to everything alive, because it puts you in touch with the Infinite and leads you sub-consciously through Nature up to Nature's God.

PERFECT HEALTH CASTETH OUT FEAR.

There is an old saying that " the nearer you get to Nature the nearer you get to God," and if you put your faith in the Creator Who made and meant you to be healthy and happy, and obey Him by living the life of movement which He intended you to live, you will experience a sheer joy in being that nothing on earth can surpass, for you will, as it were, enter a little Heaven of your own on earth. To be healthy is to be happy, for health is the pivot upon which practically every moment of your life turns. Well may such sing:

> " How good is man's life, the mere living! how fit to employ,
>
> All for the head and the soul and the senses for ever in joy."

Knowing no fear—for perfect health like perfect love casteth out fear—the healthy and the strong remain free from illness and disease where others succumb. For fear—in itself the subconscious recognition of physical weakness and incapacity—is a prolific parent of many diseases. Where Disease kills its thousands, Fear kills its tens of thousands. The weak in body are weak in the will that endures to victory, and fear will kill a host of the weak-willed, while a strong and stubborn will " endureth to the end," and defies not only Disease but even Death itself.

THE REAL " ELIXIR OF LIFE."

It is my life-long ambition to see all men and women revelling in the luxury of perfect health, to enable them to look through its rosy lenses rather than through the green and sickly glasses of physical weakness and poor health. It has been my pleasure to see thousands transformed into new beings through the application of the methods I advocate. If this can be done in the already diseased, in the weak, the obese, the emaciated, even the deformed, what hopes can we not hold out to the many who are not so grievously afflicted but who are just "below par," or temporarily "run-down" through living lives lacking in the right kind of physical activity.

No fabled " elixir of life " so regenerates and so rejuvenates as this natural method of developing and extracting the wonderful powers within the body itself to enable it to tower over all the disease- inviting, disease-propagating and disease-engendering conditions and environment of modern life.

Is it to be wondered at that I write and speak with enthusiasm in such a cause! I know what scientific bodily culture and reconstruction have done for thousands and thousands of fully-grown men and women. And what it can do and has done for those of set habit, often with well-established defects of organisation, surely it can and will do with even greater success when the body is young, pliant and plastic in youth and childhood, as, indeed, I have proved in my own and in thousands of other cases.

HEALTH ON THE THRONE.

When we ourselves and those in authority realise that our very conception of what elementary education means will have to be revolutionised, and that the physical establishment of the children should be the prelude to all mental education, when mind and nerve and muscle come to be regarded as one compound organ, when body and brain are recognised to be a mutual co-partnership, the sceptre shall be knocked from the hand of Disease, and Health will take its right and legitimate place on the throne of Humanity.

So long as we neglect the physical needs and demands of a body that was made to live by movement, as we have too long done, we must lay ourselves open to weakness and disease and to all the miseries that inevitably accompany them. There are thousands upon thousands of men and women to-day whose whole lives have been shadowed by disease through a lack of balanced physical movement. There are millions who, though they have never been ill, have never known the real joy and zest of life through the same cause. Very few, indeed, to-day, live out their full span of life, or die what can really and truly be called a natural death. Such a death would be as gradual and calm a progress as was growth in childhood. It would be a peaceful decline towards the earth from which we sprang, a graded declension of the physical body and mental faculties, a mere falling asleep after the long and arduous journey of life.

Those who wish to know the real happiness that health alone can bring, the sheer joy and lust of living that makes every minute of your life dance with gladness, the vim, the vigour, and the flexibility of mind and body that alone command success in a world of strife, must live, as Nature and as the Creator intended them to live, a life of natural and healthy and balanced physical movement.

CHAPTER XX.

Temporary Aids and Auxiliaries.

SUCH a system as that which I have just outlined would be sufficient in itself to give us the highest possible type of men and women, both physically and mentally, either for times of peace or war, if we were not unfortunately handicapped at the very beginning through our present-day civilised and unhygienic conditions and environment, lack of popular knowledge on health matters, and long years of the neglect of bodily culture.

We have at present, however, to deal with children as they are, and also with the parents of these children, who have not themselves had the advantage of such an education as I advocate. One does not expect flowers to bloom and thrive in mud or sand, and the child's environment must, for the present, also be improved as far as possible by wise schemes to better the existing conditions of most children and that of their parents also. For the time being, too, the education of both parents and children must also be attended to, and it will probably be necessary for some time yet to enforce certain conditions and introduce additional statutory measures that will bridge over the gap until our higher and healthier type arrives. This is, I am afraid, inevitable, under present conditions, to hasten the speedier advent of that better time. But the necessity for these auxiliaries to our scheme will automatically pass away with the upbuilding of healthier and hygienically better educated people, and, indeed, the methods of early health and physical education, which I now propose, will, if adapted, not very long tolerate conditions that are prejudicial to the health and happiness of the commonweal.

DENTAL DECAYS AND MALNUTRITION.

For instance, the teeth of most civilised nations to-day have most seriously deteriorated through lack of physical condition (inborn through generations), and a similar want of knowledge of the laws of bodily hygiene, without a full realisation of the dangers accruing. At present, the teeth are not only too often diseased themselves but are also a prolific cause of disease. Statistics show that half the school children to-day need dental treatment, and about 600,000 are suffering from malnutrition, chiefly because of this. To prevent this in the future, each school should have attached to it a dentist or dental staff according to the number of pupils, or each district should have a dental institute in a central position for the children to attend, especially in a country where the teeth of the people are much more neglected than in, say, America, a country where, by comparison with the British Isles, very few persons, rich or poor, are compelled to have recourse to false teeth in adult life through the care taken of their own from childhood, although even in America statistics also show a large percentage of cases of malnutrition in children are due to faulty and diseased teeth.

Among the better classes in England the same thing holds good to some extent, and it is evident that the poorer people suffer terribly from this neglect of or indifference to, the teeth in infancy and youth. Hence the prevalence of caries (decay), the decalcification of the teeth by lactic acid, periostitis (inflammation of the membrane which covers the roots of the teeth and lines their sockets), often followed by alveolar abscesses and pyorrhoea (with a most pernicious influence upon digestion and the nervous system), and the necessity later for the removal of the teeth and their replacement by false ones.

Under such a system as I suggest it would be the duty of the dentist to examine every child's teeth whenever necessary, and he should make a dental examination of all the children's teeth at least once in every three months. It would, of course, be the teacher's duty every morning to see that the children's teeth were cleaned as well as their hands and faces before they began their lessons, and it is needless to say that these precautionary measures would do much to prevent many diseases of the digestive and the nervous system, for the teeth, it has truly been said, dig more graves than spades.

INTERNAL AND EXTERNAL CLEANLINESS.

Equally necessary for some time is it to instil in the children the lesson of strict cleanliness both of the internal body by means of scientific physical movement and of the external body by other means. Public baths should be centrally erected or attached to every school, with fumigation arrangements to kill disease germs and vermin, and the children should attend these baths at least once a week. Afterwards, it should be the duty of the teachers to examine them most carefully.

The parents should be notified of filth or vermin, and on repetition of the offence, should be held liable to the law. This would not only help the child of careless or neglectful parents, but would often save the children of others from contamination by infection and the spreading of vermin. The homes of the children should also be liable to legal inspection from time to time, and every landlord should be compelled by law to provide each home with at least one bath-room, while its sanitary arrangements should be most scrupulously examined by competent sanitary officers.

All these measures would be steps towards the establishment and maintenance of health, and they constitute a debt that every State owes to its children, a debt that would be repaid with interest by the raising of a sound national human stock, healthy, happy, strong and practically free from the degeneracy that precedes, is associated with, or follows disease.

It may be argued that if the poor are taught to be so careful over bodily cleanliness, the Government or authorities or landlords will have to add bath-rooms to the working-man's dwellings. And why should they not? But I predict that if vim and self-respect are once implanted in the people from their earliest years there will be no need for the Government to do this. In time, I repeat, a people so educated and trained will not only be able to pay for their own bath-rooms, but their own homes, and will see to it that they have them.

REGULATION OF MATRIMONY AND PARENTHOOD.

Marriage is the threshold of parenthood, and marriage being something more than a mere civil contract between two persons should be more strictly regulated. Though we cannot breed men and women as we do horses and dogs, we can at least do much to ensure healthy parents and healthy offspring by making it impossible, as they already do in certain States of America, for the insane, the degenerate and habitual criminals to propagate their species. Many doctors, indeed, urge the introduction of a medical marriage certificate, but the establishment of really scientific physical education and body culture in the schools would, I am sure, in a few generations, make all such enactments unnecessary, for such a system would lead to the certain elimination of these classes and these carriers or spreaders of disease.

In Connecticut marriage is forbidden between a woman under 45 years of age and a man, either of whom is epileptic, imbecile or feeble-minded. The penalty for infraction is three years' penal servitude. In Pennsylvania a fine of six months' imprisonment or £100 fine, or both, can be inflicted on persons beknowingly celebrating, procuring or abetting the marriage of the insane or feeble-minded, or even of one who has been insane in the past, except from accidental as distinguished from natural causes, and a similar penalty for the principals in such a marriage. I would like to see, for some time at least, the propagation of disease by marriage made as sternly prohibitive as the propagation of insanity or imbecility.

And, in fairness to the married, I would make divorce legal and possible to all where one of the parties has concealed vital facts such as the pre-existence of insanity, syphilis or epilepsy. Even chronic alcoholism amounting to inebriety, and a prolific source of mental and bodily degeneracy, should be a bar to marriage or a just cause for the annulment of marriage. But in time, as I say, health education and the rebuilding of better physical bodies will, I hope and believe, practically eliminate these forms of disease altogether, and also many forms of vice arising from physical degeneracy.

THE MORBID BIRTHRIGHT OF THE POOR.

When the marriage ceremony has been performed the parents at once enter into a new civic responsibility, and it should be the object of the State to lighten that responsibility to the very utmost of its power by education, for by so doing it would at least lessen the morbid inheritance which is the only birthright of so many poor children to-day. Every wife and potential mother should receive, as she receives her marriage certificate, a book issued as a sort of Government Blue Book, containing all that the future mother ought to know concerning the sexual relationship, bodily hygiene, pregnancy, nursing, and other vital matters.

So, too, when a child is registered, every mother should, at the same time, receive a guide-book to motherhood, containing all the information that can be gathered together that will help her in the upbringing of her child or children, and warn her against all the dangers that threaten child life to-day. Such a book should contain full information as to the nature and symptoms of infantile diseases, so that she could call in the doctor at the earliest possible moment when necessary, and should deal most thoroughly with the whole subject of infant feeding. (The subject of food and diet is more fully dealt with in my chapter on " The Fuel of the Human Engine.") In this way alone, thousands of children's lives that are now needlessly sacrificed through ignorance would be saved and conserved to the State.

At a time when children are so precious to the country, and when the birth-rate has fallen to a startlingly low ebb, when even the children who survive are often of the poorest physical quality, everything that can encourage men and women to have larger families should be done, and everything possible to improve the physical quality of the children when they are born. For, to again quote Sir George Newman, " it seems futile to attempt to reform education apart from the physical condition of the child. It seems unreasonable to expect healthy citizenship if we continue to neglect the remedy of the physical disabilities of childhood, and the prevention of their cause."

One hears of Malthusianism and much condemnation from those with " money in their purses " of married women who refuse to bear children, or from bachelor divines who forget apparently that more than ever money has strictly limited purchasing powers, and that the domestic chancellor of the working-man's exchequer may well ponder before adding even a single unit to the family. A higher standard of wages will do more to stimulate population, at least among the masses, than pulpit philippics to penurious parents, which only irritate o people already too heavily taxed.

TAXING THE PROLIFIC MOTHER.

As each additional child is added to a family, with the father's income remaining stationary or practically stationary, a severe tax is placed on motherhood. With equal wages coming in, the woman with only one child has an immense advantage over her neighbour with three, or, perhaps five, and each addition to the latter handicaps the more fertile mother and her child still further. It will be quite easily seen that with five children in a family the same amount of food will not go so far to nourish each of the five as where there is only one child in a family. If a sixth be added, it means that either it must go short of the rations or the food of the others reduced.

But the new child's food should not be an added burden to the parents, or even mean short rations for the others, as both or either of these are equally bad for the State, and the State should, therefore, support and encourage motherhood by securing to each child at least one good nourishing meal a day, while small State pensions might even be given for the encouragement of motherhood, and for every child over the number of three a mother should be allowed a grant. Many women at present prefer to sacrifice their own maternal instincts rather than allow the living children they already have to run the risk of going short to help the unborn and unlikely-to-be-born' children which the State so badly needs.

In the future there should be no excuse for either parental ignorance, neglect, or ill-treatment of the children that are born, and such should be made a statutory offence with stringent punitive laws to support it.

A GOOD START IN LIFE.

To safeguard itself, the State should hold the parents responsible for the health, the maintenance and the morals of their offspring, until a certain age has been reached, and the people, in turn, should hold the State responsible for the commonweal of the nation. Public sentiment can do much in this direction, and I appeal with confidence to all right thinking men and women to take their part in what is literally a great crusade on behalf of the children, born, and as yet unborn.

Thus even before its birth a child would be, to some extent at least, ensured on its entrance into the world of a reasonable chance of life and a sound constitution, and during its pre-school days of favourable prospects of growing up healthy and strong. Every child, in short, would have a really good and fair start in life.

THE SAVING OF CHILD-LIFE.

When, too, we begin by educating the little girls to understand, respect and develop their bodies to the highest possible degree, the prospect of being a mother will no longer be looked forward to with something akin to terror as it is to-day, and child-birth in the future will be robbed of many of its present-day dangers, pain and subsequent exhaustion due mainly to muscular deterioration brought about •gradually by the diminished necessity for physical activity and muscular strength

To-day, child-birth is fraught with intense suffering because of this muscular deterioration in women, and naturally many women shirk the ordeal, much against the natural instinct of every woman but against the best interests and greater necessities of the State. The birth-rate has shrunk and is still shrinking more and more at the very moment when the demand for children is more insistent than ever, not only here, but in every country of the world. Even when children are brought into the world, it is with such risk to the life both of mother and child that something must be done to stop the appalling and altogether unnecessary sacrifice of these precious lives.

Women in a natural state did not suffer as the women of to-day in child-labour, because their abdominal and groin muscles and ail the internal muscles associated with the bearing and expulsion of the child were naturally stronger through their physically active daily life, and even the women of to-day who live in countries less civilised do not suffer as women of our cities and towns do. Nor is the birth of children accompanied with so much risk to both mother and child.

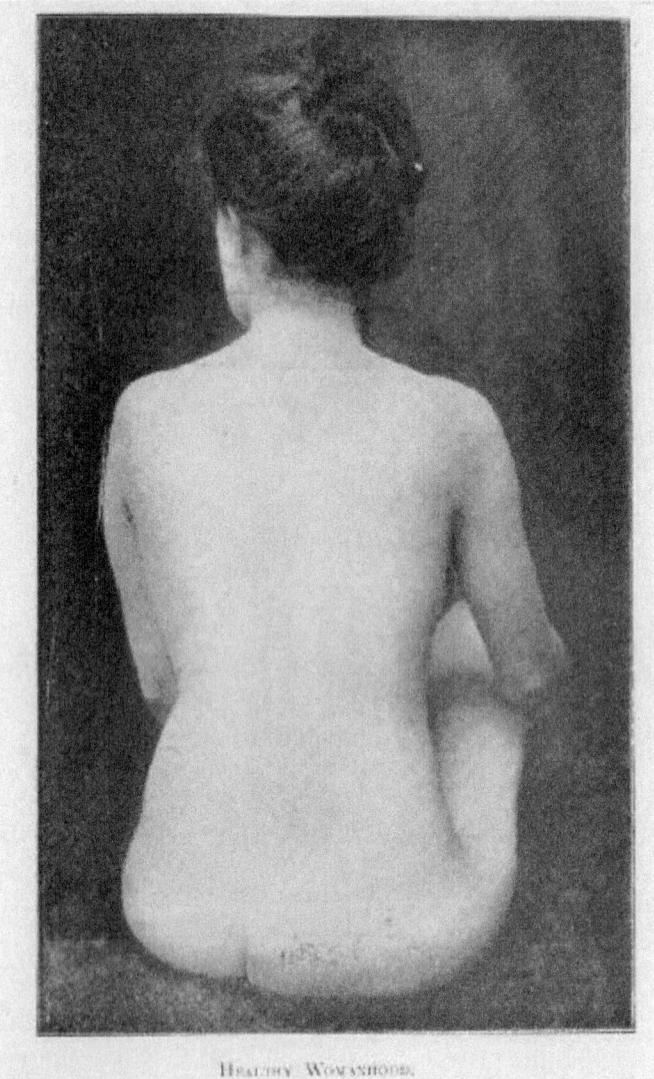

HEALTHY WOMANHOOD.
The best guarantee for the future of our national life. A naturally good figure developed in symmetry by these methods to the betterment of health and beauty.

A Study in Contrasts.

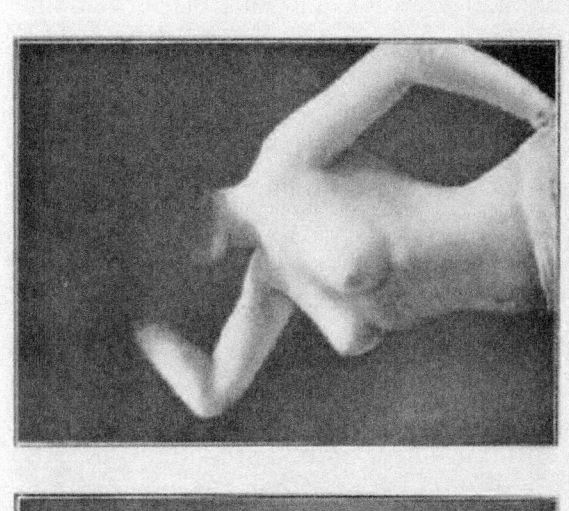

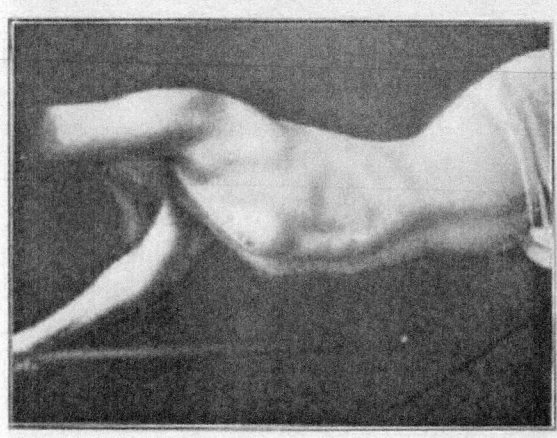

The female form divine as it should and as it should not be. The picture to the left shows the body lacking in development and contrasts very unfavourably with that to the right, which is the result of body culture, which is here described. Woman holds the key of the future in her hands, for her health and physical capacity largely determines the future of the nation's children.

WANTED, MORE MUSCULAR MOTHERS.

The woman of the past did not have to remain in bed for weeks after the birth of her child through sheer physical weakness and exhaustion, nor was she incapacitated from her duties for weeks before. Birth was with her a natural function naturally performed, because all the muscles engaged or affected were strong enough to perform the function quickly and easily without overstrain or tearing. Midwives and all the accompaniments of modern child-birth were unnecessary and unknown. Often, indeed, the child was born while the mother was at work in the fields, with only a slight disturbance of her labours.

In those days they knew nothing of " twilight sleep," for women were muscularly strong naturally through their healthy and active physical life, with bodies well developed and balanced, and the result was that not only was child-birth easy and natural but healthier and sturdier babies were born. Besides, the period of child-birth was not so terrifying as to make her look forward with fear and anxiety towards a recurrence of similar anguish. In fact, the event quickly faded from her memory, and the dread of the pains of previous child-birth did not then menace the birth-rate as it does to-day.

So that once again we see the importance of muscle and muscular development even in this vital matter of child-birth to every nation. To-day, women are so weak muscularly that they naturally shirk an ordeal not only accompanied by the most fearful suffering, but which leaves them for weeks sometimes for months, in a state of indescribable exhaustion, hovering often for days, between life and death just as if they had passed through what surgeons call a major operation. Little wonder then, that statesmen, sociologists and divines alike call in vain upon the women of the country for children and yet more children. They will never get them either in the quantity or quality the country so much needs until women are educated in the matter and physically re-educated in the scientific way I describe from early girlhood, and also assisted in the other ways I have suggested when and where necessary.

ADVICE TO PROSPECTIVE MOTHERS.

In the meantime, however, for the encouragement of motherhood it is essential that we should do all we can to lighten the lot of the mother-to-be. to assuage her pain, and to diminish, as far as humanly possible, the strain, the pain and the exhaustion usually associated with child-birth to-day, undoubtedly the result mainly of physical and organic deterioration, together with lunder-feeding, large families, and often starvation for the mother herself which might also mean starvation to the child in the womb.

Many ladies who were pupils of mine before their marriage, and whose whole muscular and organic systems had been developed by physical training to the highest degree and in the most admirable balance, have since written to me telling me that they passed through their confinement with comparatively little pain, and that their babe was safely delivered with little exhaustion and no injury. Others who had not this physical preparation before marriage, and whose first child was delivered with much suffering and exhaustion subsequently found, after a course of physical education and body culture that the next child was delivered with much less suffering or exhaustion.

I have even found that it has made delivery less painful, dangerous and exhausting, when special physical movements have been carried out by women during, say, the first six months of pregnancy, to develop and strengthen the groin and abdominal muscles and all the muscles associated with the bearing of children, and the act of repulsion. Even this temporary and partial physical and muscular development has led to a great diminution of suffering and made child-birth less exhausting and less dangerous to the life of both mother and child.

Besides, children so brought into the world cannot fail to have a better physical foundation from the very beginning of their little lives than children born in intense maternal agony and overstrain after months of pre-natal anxiety, which also must be most injurious to the child when born. Every woman, indeed, who wishes to make her delivery of a child less painful and less exhausting would benefit by such physical preparation, and should consult her medical man as to this the moment she realises she is pregnant.

If even a temporary and partial physical training of the adult such as this will afford so much relief, it is easy to realise that when from girlhood all women are educated physically and have bodies strong in perfectly balanced strength, through such educational methods as I suggest, it will be as easy and natural for them to be delivered of children as for women of primitive times. It will also be apparent that one of the greatest obstacles to motherhood will have been removed, and that the dread of child-birth, especially after the birth of the first child, will no longer cause potential mothers to cheat the country by illicit methods of its most precious possession, the children who are the life-blood of a nation.

REAL TEMPERANCE REFORM.

The war has proved the greatest temperance reform crusade ever known. Weaker alcoholic beverages, restriction of hours, and the " no treating " order have undoubtedly weaned many a sot from the public-house altogether. He has learnt not only to do without but also the pleasure of doing without.

The old-style public-house, with its ever-open door and standing counter, its " confessional box " partition behind whose swivel windows unseen barmaids sold vicious decoctions at so much a glass often to unseen customers, its free-and-easy atmosphere that made intrusion from strangers no impertinence but rather invited it, and the inevitable " let's have another one " among friends and acquaintances that often induced a man to take half-a-dozen drinks where he would have taken but one alone, could not but lead to excessive drinking if not to drunkenness.

The dipsomaniac would take a furtive look round, dash in and swallow a drink hastily, and the operation would be repeated many times a day. Secret " nipping " went on all day, the very worst form of alcoholism known to medical men and the most difficult to combat was encouraged. Parents got drunk, or at least, slightly inebriated inside, while children took occasional and furtive peeps into the mysterious parental heaven whose portals they dare not cross. One can easily imagine how indignantly many a high-spirited boy resented this ostracism and how eagerly he awaited the time when he, too, could follow in his father's footsteps. Such a law, it seems to me, is but an agent provocateur to any high-spirited boy.

The war, of course, improved matters considerably. The reduction of alcoholic strength in all beverages, the curtailment of the drinking hours, and the order against " treating " have all helped to dissipate this atmosphere; but its restrictions have not been welcome, because they savour of compulsion and prejudice the liberty of the subject.

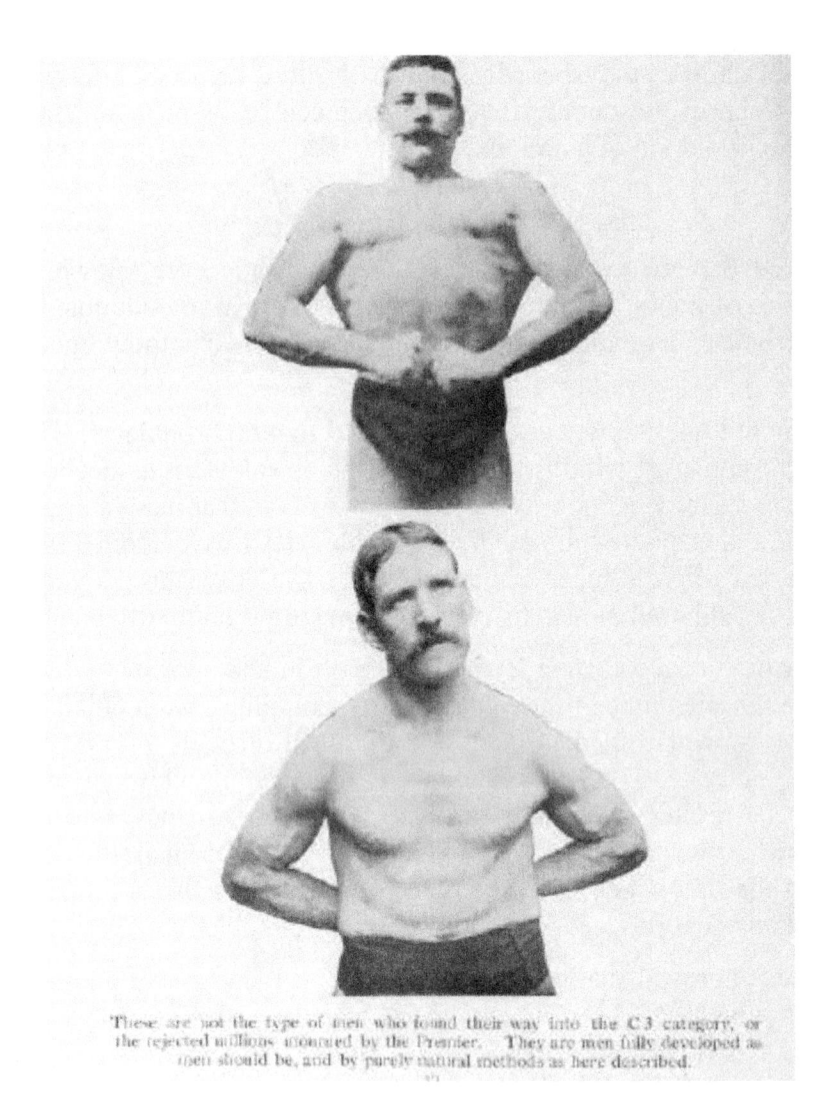

These are not the type of men who found their way into the C3 category, or the rejected millions mourned by the Premier. They are men fully developed as men should be, and by purely natural methods as here described.

THE HOUSE OF THE PUBLIC.

There is room now for a new and better type of public-house, or, rather, house of the public, in which we shall be able to have all the benefits of curtailed hours and " no treating " orders without such compulsion. The new public-house should have its bar out of sight of the customer, with no young ladies acting as attractive magnets. Instead of standing at a counter, each party would sit down at cosy little tables in a semi-private state, into which the most pachydermatous strangers would not dare to intrude without invitation or permission.

A busy man or woman would hesitate before entering such an establishment, and to sit down and call for refreshment unless he or she really needed it or had leisure time to spare, and the furtive visitors and secret drink snatchers would receive their quietus. Children, too, would be able to remain with their parents, for the new public-house would have plenty of good food and tea, coffee, cocoa, and cake for either the little ones or for those who did not desire alcoholic beverages.

The place need no longer be hidden from the view of onlookers from outside, indeed, it would be all the better to have big, wide windows admitting plenty of light, and enabling those inside to see the passing world outside, and those outside to glance at the happy folk within. In such a public-house it would easily be possible to obtain all the benefits which war-time restrictions and curtailment of hours have admittedly brought with them, but without offence or any infringement of individual liberty. In the larger houses an orchestra would dispense good music, and instead of the present vicious and demoralising atmosphere the crowd would consist of happy, smiling and healthy people seeking and obtaining rational, innocent, and recreating refreshment and enjoyment.

THE NEW ERA OF INDUSTRY.

In the great upward movement that the new methods of physical education and bodily culture will inaugurate, we must look to employers of labour to play a prominent part. Children, so well-nurtured and educated on leaving the school behind, will have been taught habits of life and conduct too precious to be ruthlessly sacrificed to greed or selfishness on the part of unscrupulous or even thoughtless employers.

One hears too often the expression that there is no sentiment in business. That is false and a false principle. There is a well of sentiment in business relationships, and successful businesses are built on sentiment. There is no motive 'power in the world, no method of scientific efficiency, no "speeding up" process that has the driving force of sentiment, and it is the employer who enlists not merely the service of his workpeople but their affection and loyalty whose business will wax fat and prosper.

MORE MODEL EMPLOYERS NEEDED.

We know to-day how welfare work in large industrial and commercial establishments, both in America and in this country, has rewarded employers with healthier, happier, more loyal and more efficient work people, and indeed, many children have been heart- glad to leave the old-fashioned school for the model factory, workshop or business establishment with its medical care, its splendid canteens, its magnificent playing centres, its baths, athletic arenas and organisations, and all the accessories of the model modern place of business.

Men like Lord Leverhulme and George Cadbury may well call their great industrial centres at Port Sunlight and Bourneville by the euphonious terms of " a model village " and " a factory in a garden." The heart of John Ruskin or William Morris would have pulsed with joy had they lived to see those ideal business and industrial colonies of modern life, and I am glad to say that the example set by these employers is being copied all over England to-day.

We know how splendidly and carefully the health and other vital interests of the munition workers were looked after during the war, and the splendid results. Industrial poisoning was almost completely erased from workshop risks, and this in one of the most dangerous trades imaginable. The report of the Health of Munition Workers' Committee ought to be made the Bible of Business, and the basis for the conduct of every large and industrial and commercial establishment.

It is certainly an illuminating document dealing with almost every phase of the industrial problem, and shows what might be accomplished by really scientific organisation under a real Ministry of Health. It touches the subject of industrial efficiency and worker's welfare from nearly every point of view, and the only fault I have to find with it is that the importance of physical training in the sense I mean had not at that time been brought to the notice of the medical authorities responsible, as then even better results would have been undoubtedly attained.

PHYSICAL AND INDUSTRIAL EFFICIENCY.

To some extent the business establishment ought to be a physical " continuation school," so as to prevent pupils who have left schools for the workshop or office from forgetting all they had learnt and to keep themselves in the best physical condition. It is, indeed, the interest as well as the duty of employers to secure the highest physical efficiency of the workers, and in many American houses an instructor in physical culture is an important member of the staff, while, of course, a doctor and nursing staff are always in attendance.

Employers must realise, if only for their own sake, that the condition of the worker is reflected in his work, especially the. physical condition. Every house of business should devote at least one hour a day to real 'physical education and culture on a scientific basis—not mere recreation—for which time the workers would be paid at their ordinary rate of remuneration. American employers who have done so say it pays, and American employers are too shrewd to pay workers merely for enjoying themselves. Baths and washhouses should be erected, fitted, as the house advertisements say, with every modern convenience so that an employee could leave off work as clean and tidy as when he entered.

To save the worker's clothes, also to keep them clean during work, overalls or special suits should be provided. Thus we would no longer see grimy and stained workmen leaving off work and entering public conveyances often to the inconvenience of others and to their own distress. There is no reason why any workman should not quit work, and emerge from the premises as clean and immaculate as the average City clerk.

THE WORKER MIRRORED IN HIS WORK.

This would all help the workers to maintain their self-respect, and all this would also be reflected in their work. The workers would naturally feel new ambitions stirred within them, and though higher wages would naturally be demanded, the workers would be found to be far more sober, regular in attendance and efficient in their work, so that the balance at the end of the year would be to the credit of the employer.

Apart altogether from profits, however, it is to our benefit to evolve a higher and ever higher type of worker in the great commercial and industrial struggle that confronts us. And physical health is the basis of good workmanship, the corner-stone of national industrial efficiency.

As the British Medical Journal said in its review of the Report to which I have referred 1—" Physical health is the basis, and its physiological justification must be a correct understanding of the part played by nutrition, by rest, by fatigue and general conditions affecting health. This, because physical health is necessary to mental well-being and is at the basis of moral and social development.

" The matters dealt with in the Munition Workers' Report concern the future as well as the present, and are among the root problems of preventive medicine which has as its object the removal of the occasion of disease and physical inefficiency, combined with the husbanding of the physical resources of the worker, in such a way and to such a degree that he can exert his free power unhampered with benefit to himself and his countrymen." In this great work the employers can do the State some service and help us forward to the diseaseless era. The money lost to employers and to workers annually by sickness and disease must represent millions annually, and this huge deficit can be reduced to an imperceptible minimum, if the whole community united in the great forward movement, which, it is hoped, is now about to begin, and to inspire which this book has been written. To live healthfully is to do work more easily, do more and do it better, increase efficiency and earning power, and to enjoy life as only those who are fit and healthy can.

CHAPTER XXI.
The True Position of Sports and Pastimes.

WHEREVER you find English-speaking people in any part of the world you find a colony of sportsmen. The playing fields of Eton have done more than won a Waterloo. They have set a fashion to the world, and games and sports essentially British in their origin are not only played and participated in to-day by Britishers everywhere, but by people of every nationality and country. Sport has become the real international language of the world, and sportsmen form a cosmopolis of their own.

A very great poet once had the rashness to speak disparagingly of " muddied oafs and flannelled fools," and had to eat his words in sackcloth and ashes. I must not follow in his footsteps even if I would. Let me, therefore, at the outset, declare my unbounded admiration for sports and games of every kind, and for those who find in them the most natural and rational enjoyment offered to man. Sport is the perpetuation of the eternal child in man, the adolescent and adult expression of the instinct implanted in every healthy child to evidence its health and vitality in physical and muscular activity of some kind.

Unfortunately, to-day, it is only the select few who are either physically fit or have time and means at their command, to revel in this natural and physically active life as they ought to do. Civilisation, with its unceasing demands upon the vitality of the people, intervenes. We all live the strenuous life to-day, but it is not the strenuous physical life of our forefathers, the hardworking, hard- playing physical strenuousness that kept the blood quickly coursing in their veins, braced their nerves and hardened their frames. Today, it is the mentally strenuous life that the majority live, working at office desks and in huge business establishments, where the physical man is treated with indifference or even contempt until he rebels and advertises his presence in well-known pains and discomforts.

This, of course, is the inevitable result of an early system of education that has led most men and women into a sort of mental cul-de-sac, from which there has seemed so far but little hope of escape. So we go on breeding a people more and more physically decrepit and less and less fitted for indulgence in the vigorous and muscle-testing sports, games and pastimes of our ancestors. The antagonism of civilisation and muscular movement have wrought unspeakable harm, and faulty educational methods have helped to carry on the evil work that civilisation began.

To-day, our educationalists are trying to atone for the defects and shortcomings of the past, and physical education of some sort is now a part of the scholastic system in most of our schools, while games, sports, pastimes and dancing are also receiving more time and attention than ever they did before. But there is a lack of scientific method even in the most modern schemes for the physical education of children that will, I am afraid, produce results very little better than before. The sense of proportion is absent. The perspective is false. There is a disposition to place last things first that betrays what Burns calls the "prentice hand."

Correct theory is the essential to successful practice, and it is incorrect theory that permits a child to plunge into games and sports that are usually of a severely testing character, as children are constituted in modern life, before they have had, as it were, the faults of long generations of ancestors and civilisation safeguarded against in their own little bodies. Physical education that will really upbuild or rebuild the body of the average child as he or she is born to-day ought to take precedence of all games and sports, and such education and physical reconstruction is not to be effectively carried out by the scanty or haphazard provision of a useless kind of physical movements admingled with games, sports, dancing and pastimes of various kinds. In fact, such methods are likely not only to perpetuate but even aggravate the conditions existent to-day in which we find millions of spectators for hundreds of contestants in all our games or sports.

Great athletes, like great poets, are made not born, but that is no reason why the athletic potentialities within every child should not be given every opportunity of development and expansion by providing it with a sound physique and organism from the very threshold of life— that is, by a system of physical education and reconstruction on truly scientific lines from its earliest days. Such methods as I have outlined in this book would, I contend, give us men and women in later life who would not be content to play the role of mere spectators in all our athletic games, but would be fit and fitted from childhood to be active participants in them if they desired to do so.

Such children would grow up with bodies having within them the basic element that makes for success in every game, sport and pastime, in which the determining factors are muscular power and vital force. This is why I strive so eagerly to define the true position of sports, games and pastimes in any system of physical education that has the least claim to be called scientific. The scientific physical culture of the body should be the first step in the preparation of the physical body for the athletic sports and pastimes which, in adolescent and adult life to-day, are, after all, the recreation only of the fittest and strongest of the nation. In fact, it is the result of that lack of such early physical preparatory work in the past that provides us with the spectacle of thronged galleries watching others at play instead of themselves being actual players and competitors, because they are physically unfit just as so many also could only be onlookers during the war instead of being able to defend home and country for the same reason.

In the athletic, as well as in the military sense, the body must be schooled patiently for feats that demand muscular power and ability as their prime factor to success, because civilisation and long- ingrained habits of physical inactivity have left the people with bodies that cannot immediately be taxed in this way. The average young man, for instance, who wishes to take up pedestrianism or football must first have special muscles prepared for those feats by weeks or even months of training, and even then it is only the strongest who can stand this training or who are able to take it up safely. Many, on the other hand, damage and ruin their health for life by attempting feats that would have been quite within their power if they had been physically prepared for them from childhood in the manner I am now advocating. As it is, probably not one man in every hundred is able to participate in such strenuous field sports to-day with safety and success or to stand the training necessary for victory in them.

Even, however, if all were so physically sound that it would be quite safe for them medically to join in these strenuous contests, a man or woman would have to devote his or her life to them— to make them their sole profession in life and devote ail their time to a great variety of them—to build up a body in anything approaching that balanced strength which is essential to the successful warfare that the body must wage war against disease. This, of course, is impossible in modern times when there are so many other more pressing demands upon the average person's time, and besides, none, even then, would have either the strength of constitution or the money and time to spare to participate in the great number and variety of sports and games that would build up such a body. For this great mass of the people, therefore, the natural methods of body-building, scientifically applied, which are indicated here, provide a most admirable substitute, for with such methods at hand, these men and women are able to carry out simple exercises that will be as beneficial to their bodily health in ten minutes as would games or sports and pastimes, in hours of sub-conscious physical activity. After all, the main essential of all physical exercise is to build up a body healthy, strong and disease-free, and if that is the criterion, then I say that games and sports alone cannot do it under modern conditions of existence. Only such natural methods of scientific physical reconstruction as are described in this book can provide the exercise which is one of the essential elements of health and strength in a convenient, compressed and concentrated form compatible with modern circumstances of life.

By all means let us have plenty of games and sports, but let us have them in their true position from their physical and health value as compared with methods of physical upbuilding from schooldays that lay down a physical foundation for life, and build up muscle and tissue and a healthy organism not for the mere performance of any particular game or sport or athletic feat, but as the finest insurance policy in the world against physical deterioration and disease. The training of the body for competitive sports and severely testing games must of necessity be spasmodic and unbalanced in character, and is something very different from a continuous and consistent physical upbuilding of a body that is meant to keep it always and under all conditions in the highest and most balanced strength, not in one or more parts, but in each and every part, erecting, as it were, a physical building with foundations sunk deep and each part or parts in perfectly balanced strength to the whole, presenting rather to all the forces that may strive to overthrow it a single front, with no weak points anywhere and illimitable reserves and reinforcements of muscular power and vital energy to resist and defeat them.

The very schooling that will build up a body in perfectly balanced strength, with correct adjustment between contraction and relaxation, between flexors and extensors and between mind and muscle will make a man better fitted for boxing or cricketing or any other sport or pastime than the spasmodic and unscientific training of to-day, in which, by specialised training of certain muscles, the bodily balance is apt to be more disturbed. Perfect mental and muscular co-ordination is the secret of rapidity in action, and the more muscular strength within balance to support it the greater prospect of success or victory, all other things being equal.

The fact is that methods of physical training that make a man slow are not scientific but the very reverse, because through not exercising and developing opposing muscles in absolute balance they do tend to make a man muscle-bound. Slowness in movement comes from this lack of balance, because the extensors have not been trained in equal balance with the flexors, relaxation is inferior to contraction, and there is apt to be a consequent shortening and stiffening of the tendons of one muscle or sets of muscles that destroys speed of action.

Photographer, G. H. Cassell, Boxer.

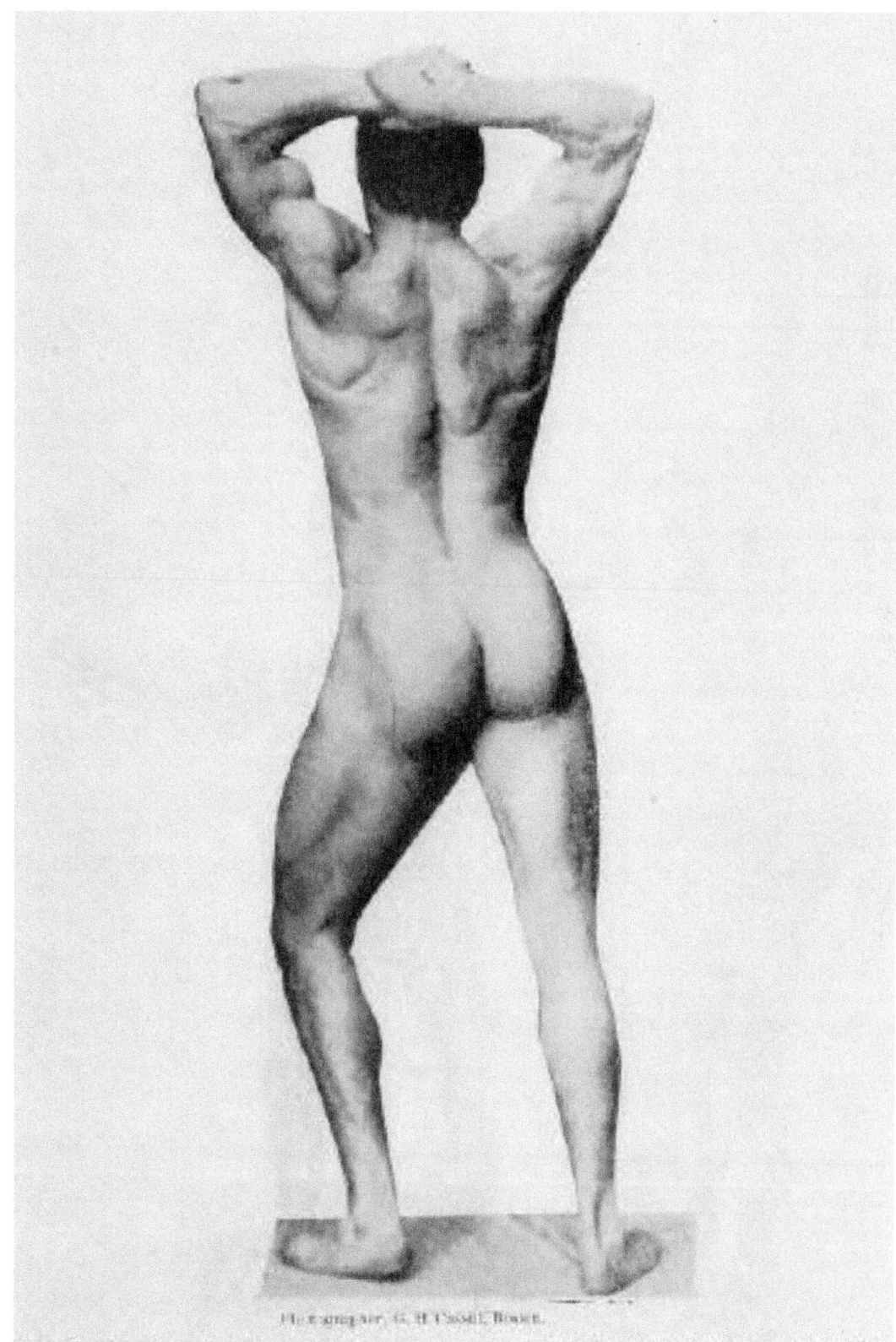

This is the type of athlete built all over in perfectly balanced muscular strength which the methods of scientific physical reconstruction described here would give us as models and examples for the encouragement of the whole nation.

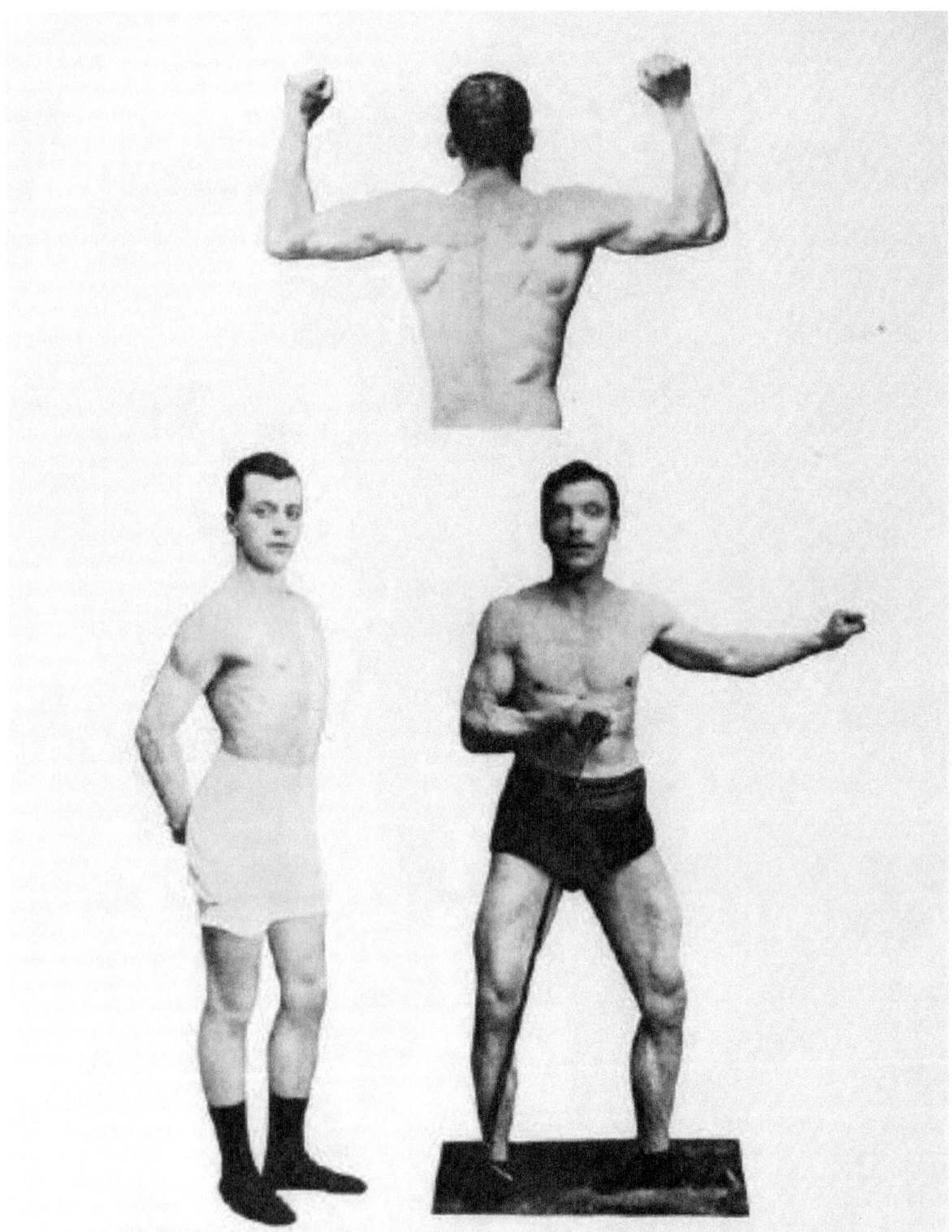

The Youth of the Nation as it should and would be if framed and developed along the lines indicated.

Take boxing, for instance, I have shown how, by scientific tests, my own blow was more rapid than that of even a professional boxer. And it was not only more rapidly delivered, but the force behind it was infinitely greater, because the cells of the muscles and brain employed in act of striking were far superior in their development and power to those of my friendly antagonist who was a trained boxer, while there was better mental and muscular co-ordination. Speed in action admittedly comes from the brain, or rather, from perfect mental and muscular co-ordination, but even mental effort is primarily dependent on physical conditions and upon the relation-ship of mental and physical cells. In other words, you cannot develop the physical side by truly scientific means without increasing mental aptness and efficiency and mental and muscular co-ordination, for scientific exercise of the muscles always means also the exercising and developing of brain and nerve cells.

The boxer so trained Will not only have muscles able to hit at their highest possible power, but will also possess the mental capacity necessary to send out his blows with lightning-like rapidity, an elasticity of brain, if I might so describe it, equal and proportionate to the contractile and relaxing power of his muscular system. Such a man would not only strike more rapidly and more powerfully than another, but might very easily break an opponent's arm, or seriously injure some part of his body, because there would be infinitely more and better-balanced muscular power and nerve-force behind his blows.

But naturally such physical preparation would never teach him the rules and craft of the game. That he must learn by practice and to know all the rules and tricks and how to use them to the best advantage. For, of course, in all games and sports, mental skill, craft and cunning count perhaps as much as muscle, and what is called generalship wins as often as much as muscular strength, speed

and stamina. Natural aptitude is often also a determining factor,, for no matter how well we might qualify a man physically and organically, by early and scientific physical education, he might never become a first-class cricketer through lack of natural aptitude for the game and for many other reasons. So, in pedestrianism, more races, after all, are won by the brain than by the muscles of the limbs engaged, for one man will be quicker to judge pace, to estimate and seize chances, and to invent and use a thousand tricks and wiles that may win where a really superior runner in point of speed or stamina would lose. Physical and muscular strength and stamina, however, are the basic factors in all such contests, and I contend that the man whose body has been steadily upbuilt from childhood by really scientific methods will always have a better physical groundwork to build upon for success in all games, sports and pastimes. Given two men with equal knowledge of the craft of the game, and the strongest in balance must always prove the winner.

Too many to-day plunge into games and sports for which they are physically unfit, and a few weeks or even months' spasmodic and partial training of the body is a poor substitute for scientific physical culture of the body from childhood, when a youth or man will better be prepared for the sterner training necessary for any particular athletic feat or sport.

Just think what magnificent athletes any country will have when its children are thus scientifically educated and physically prepared for later life by Nature's own methods. I say that by these means we can breed athletes yet of a higher standard in every way than any the world has yet seen. Our playing fields and athletic arenas will then see gladiators greater than those of ancient Rome and athletes superior even to those of once peerless Greece. Not one man (or even woman) but everyone would have a body training and built up scientifically to a degree of physical perfection and beauty never known in history, and we would have nations scientifically prepared and fitted from childhood for the athletic arena just as Germany has scientifically schooled its people even from their school days to worship and wield the arms of warfare.

But what is, after all, far more important is the upbuilding of a people sane in mind and sound in body, a people at least equal if not superior to the splendid men and women of Greece's palmiest days, men and women healthy, happy, strong and free from disease, men and women so educated from childhood that the culture, development and care of their physical bodies would come as natural to them as the matutinal wash or their daily meals, a people taught to delight and take a pride in physical power and prowess just as to-day they bow down before mental strength and success at however costly a physical price it may be temporarily obtained.

In bringing about such a consummation, games, sports and pastimes can truly play a foremost part when seen in their true perspective and relegated to their proper position in the physical life of the people. In fact, the encouragement of these on a far greater scale than ever before would be the best propaganda work on behalf of the physical renaissance which is coming, and which is necessary if, as a people, we are to avoid the physical deterioration that has already enslaved us to disease and has brought us nearly to the very verge of destruction.

As I have said elsewhere, children instinctively admire physical strength and skill. Let that instinct be encouraged in every way, not by turning them recklessly into the playing fields and athletic grounds until their bodies are ripe and ready for such efforts, but by instilling in the childish mind a sense of reverence for the physical body, a knowledge of its needs and requirements, and the best physical and hygienic education that human ingenuity can devise and money can obtain.

Let us have athletic games and sports of every kind on the greatest scale the world has ever seen, with rewards for the victors such as were never offered before. The whole thought of the nation would then be turned into new channels, and every child at school would have a far higher physical ideal set before it than had even the children of ancient Greece. Our athletes and leaders in every branch of outdoor sport would become national heroes in a far higher sense than they are to-day. Even professionalism would lose what of stigma is associated with to-day. On the other hand, a man would have to be a professor of each branch of sport to be able to achieve victory, and his profession would become an honoured one as it really ought to be.

Nothing that could help in every way to stimulate in the youthful mind the idea of physical health and beauty and of body culture should be left undone. Olympic games ought to be held annually, under the patronage of the King, on an unprecedented scale at which the finest physical types of the nation would compete in every form of outdoor and manly sport. These would form the great annual struggles between the giants of the various sports from every part of the country, who had previously won their right to appear in county or local Olympics on a smaller scale, and it would be a good idea if special free seats were allocated for those children who could not afford payment for admission to witness these games and contests.

The great value of all this would be to arouse and encourage and foster ambition in the young, and even in adolescents and adults, towards the development of their own physical bodies in strength and beauty. It would divert the stream of popular favour and admiration away from pursuits and studies that have proved subversive of the best interests of the nation. An ideal would be implanted of a far loftier type than the mammon and mental worship which has usurped its place in modern life.

Not everyone, of course, could hope to win the honours and rewards of the athletic arena or in the realms of sport, but all would be set a physical standard to strive upwards to from youth, and the ambition to possess a body as beautiful and strong as the bodies of these physical paragons could not fail to result in a general upraising of the physical standard of the people.

This is just the goal to which the State, the educationalists and the people themselves must turn their eyes, if the people are to be rescued from the physical slough of despond into which they have fallen, and re-established in the physical beauty and strength and freedom from disease that they have sacrificed to the blind worship of civilisation, ease, luxury and a mental education that has outrun their physical capacity, based, too, on an insecure physical foundation. By these natural methods of physical movement, every man, woman and child, even though he or she may not secure the laurels of an Olympic hero, can, at least—and this without interference with the daily life or the progress of our civilisation or serious encroachment upon their time—possess a body beautiful in its balanced strength, as vigorous and disease-free as that of man in his pristine prime, because in a few minutes they will be able to obtain a sufficiency of physical movement to compensate for the havoc wrought by habits and methods of life through long ages of civilisation that have slowly but surely deprived modern mankind of the prime essential of life and health, the balanced physical movement which alone will enable the human body to tower above the miasma of physical deterioration and disease that is still creeping over our heads. Back to Nature we cannot go as things are to-day, but we can profit by her example, lessons and warnings, and this is the only way to do so, for these are the methods by which Nature maintained primitive man in his very prime of physical strength, health, and beauty.

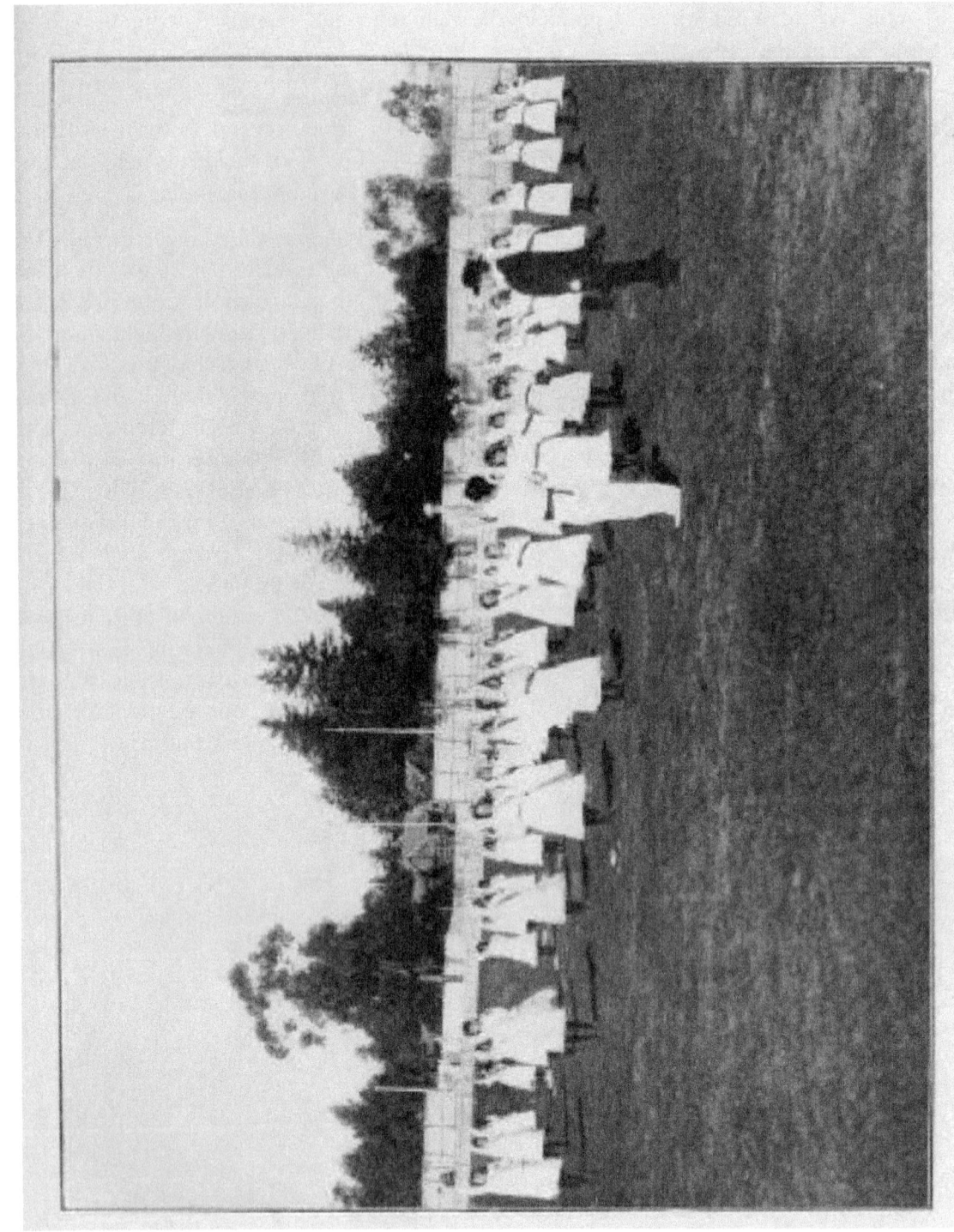

The Author inspecting a charming and graceful display by little girls, who are being schooled in a way that is likely to make them healthy, happy, and graceful women in later years.

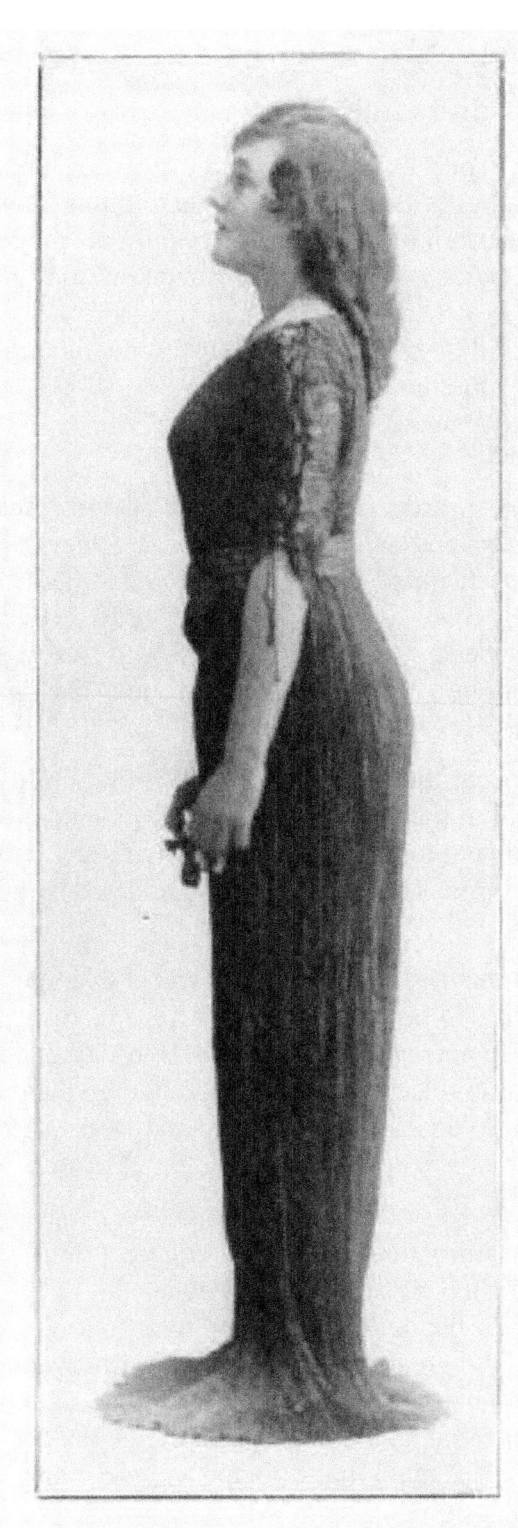

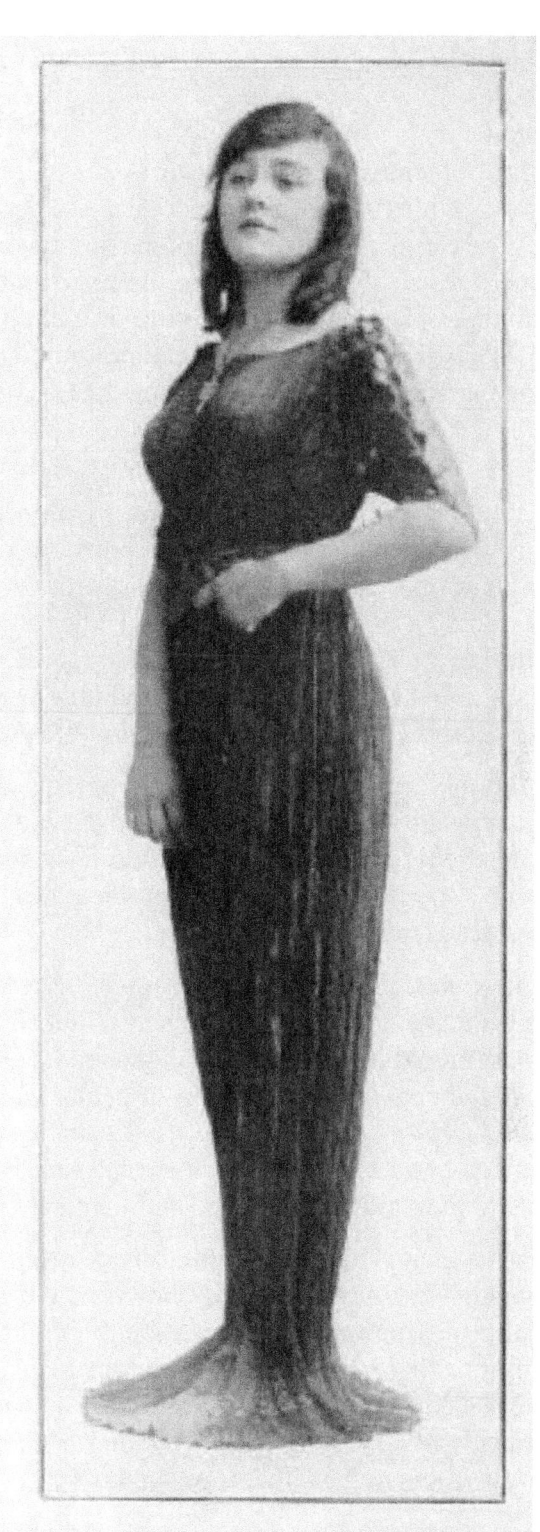

"*Standing with reluctant feet
Where the brook and river meet.*" —LONGFELLOW.

Miss Lorraine Sandow, the younger daughter of the Author, photographed at 15, an almost perfect study in pose, poise and grace. An enthusiastic follower of the methods described, with resulting grace of figure and healthy physical development.

CHAPTER XXII.

A Word to Parents and Guardians.

THE most precious thing in the world is a child, especially in the loving eyes of a parent. What father and mother do not but experience the ecstatic thrill of creation in their children as keenly as does the true artist, musician and poet in the children of their creative brain. This perpetuation of themselves in their children is the only idol before which civilised mankind may prostrate itself without blasphemy. For the life of a child is something sacred to every parent, something that awakens the instincts of true religion implanted in every human breast, something that links weak and erring man with the kingdom of Heaven and the angels.

THE GREAT PILGRIMAGE OF LIFE.

Every child is in the eyes of a parent more or less a dream-child. It touches the imagination as nothing else can. It conjures up visions by days and wonderful dreams by night. It is an inspiration to inspire poetry in the most prosaic of men and women, a beacon that flares up with the illumination of a thousand hopes. Father and mother live again in their children, and look to them to live after they are gone. In this respect, indeed, man is truly eternal, and lives again and yet again in his children and their children's children to be until the end of time. The death of a child is not the death of an individual, but the sacrifice of future generations.

From the moment a child is born the parents accept the burden of a new responsibility to the child, to society and to themselves—but above all to the little ones whose tiny foot are about to begin the great pilgrimage of life, whose eyes look out unseeing into the misty future, and whose bodies and brains will yet be called upon to bear strains heavier than any shouldered by humanity in times dead and dying.

The " new world " into which we are about to enter will not be a better world than the old one unless we make it better. In many ways, indeed, it will be a harder one, and the men and women who must mould its destinies are in the cradles, the nurseries and the schools to-day. Parents and guardians, themselves the victims of centuries of civilised and disease-producing habits of life and of educational methods that have sought to divorce brain and body and treat them as two single parts of a human being, cannot but face the prospect with anxiety and trepidation, and it is to come to their aid and guidance that I am penning this chapter.

In their hands it is at once a power and a responsibility that might well stagger a timid soul and overwhelm it with awe. I have shown in the earlier part of my book what the State and the medical profession may do to prepare the child for the battle of life and to accoutre it with the only armour that carry it to victory over mankind's greatest enemy, disease. But whatever the State or the educational authorities may or may not do—and I know from painful past experience how quickly waves of enthusiasm arising from national danger subside when the danger appears to be past— it is to the fathers and mothers themselves that I make my most powerful appeal.

OVER-DEVELOPED BRAINS ON UNFIT BODIES.

I know how truly anxious is every parent to send their children out into the stern fray of life fully armed and accoutred at all points and with every prospect of success. But I know also the handicap that their own lack of knowledge and experience of vital points impose on them, a handicap which has been often forced upon them by wrong educational methods in their own youth or by the restriction and limitation of that knowledge of the human body and its needs for health and strength, both mental and physical, which is vital and essential to the successful conduct of life, and which will be still more necessary for the children of to-day and the future in the strenuous days that lie before them.

How can parents, who are themselves deficient in their knowledge of laws and principles without which no life, however zealously guarded, is ever safe from the intrusion of disease, be expected to school their children until such knowledge is brought within their ken. How can the children of such parents be expected to thrive under conditions of existence demanding higher standards of physical and mental efficiency than ever, if they are not initiated into things that are at present mysteries even to their parents.

I solemnly warn every parent to-day that their children will be assuredly done grievous injury in either health of body or mind and not improbably in both if methods of education are persisted in that neglect the physical body, or, at least, will not develop it to its fullest power and capacity, while the brain is being " forced " in a sort of educational greenhouse. Their very first step to ensure the safety, mentally and physically, of the children they love is to see that the physical child is attended to in every way before its mind is artificially hurried forward, like some delicate exotic, to fade and wither at the first chill blast from a sterner clime.

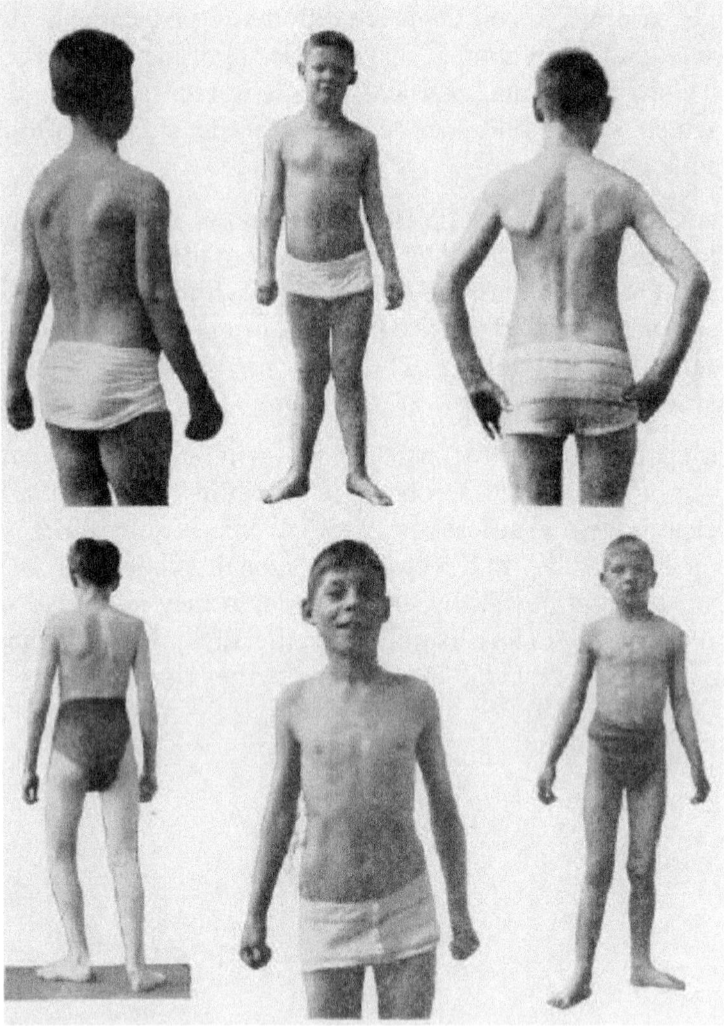

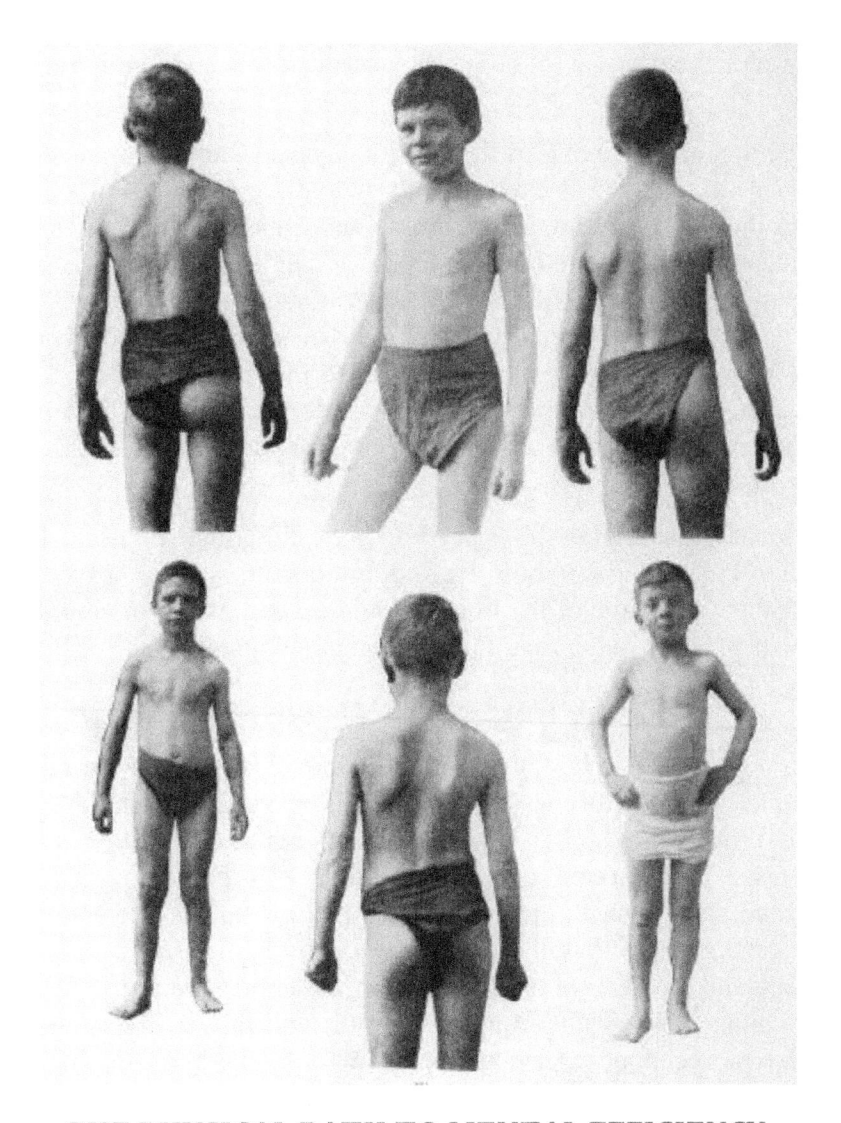

THE PHYSICAL PATH TO MENTAL EFFICIENCY.

Here lies the danger—the same danger that I have thundered against for years, the danger that can but still further perpetuate weakness and disease in our midst, and rob millions of children from the very threshold of life of that very outfit for the journey which all parents are so anxious to provide. If they continue to believe that they are doing their best for the children by developing unnaturally and unhealthfully an abnormal brain—whether for making money, winning fame, or attaining some other high ambition —upon a physical foundation not first prepared and built up to sustain it, they are sending these little pilgrims along a lion- infested path without the armour of defence necessary to protect them. The way to health and strength from childhood, and even to the highest mental efficiency, leads along the straight and narrow path of physical fitness and strength, and not by tortuous mental mazes and quagmires that may encompass the pilgrim's destruction ere he has rod far upon his journey.

Let every parent take that warning to heart as he or she prizes his or her children. Misguided enthusiasm and love misapplied may do as much harm as indifference or cold neglect. To the parent who is seeking he very best that can be done to serve his or her child, I emphasise and reiterate my warning for them to see to the physical wants of its body and brain on the only deep and safe foundation.

How can this best be done I The laying of the child's physical foundation must begin in the home. There are difficulties, of course, at present, but with the spreading of education as I have suggested earlier in this book, among both parents and children, these difficulties will quickly pass away. In the meantime, there are certain steps that can be taken at once, and which, indeed, must be taken, if parents are to shield their children from risks and dangers that may very greatly be avoided. Indeed, these are essential steps if disease is really to be prevented, and I feel confident that parents who read this book will not need much impressment from me when they realise how much better will be the prospects and outlook of their children by observing and studying what I say here in the light of a long and very embracing experience.

A great advance will be made when every parent begins to teach the child from the earliest possible moment to be proud of its physical body, to delight in physical beauty, to turn its childish thoughts into channels that would lead its mind in the direction of physical health and well-being. The whole atmosphere of the home should be one of health, and the child should be encouraged to grow physically rather than to display a precocious mental skill and ability.

HEALTH EDUCATION IN THE HOME.

In its most impressionable period of life, it would be easy to give its habit of thought an orientation that would imperceptibly instil in it hygienic desires and ambitions which would go far in later life to protect it against weakening thoughts and tendencies that lead towards unfitness and disease. To surround it with picture books containing coloured pictures of handsome women and brave, strong men, to inspire it from statues and photographs of ancient and modern Heroes and athletes, to tell it stories of the noble men and women who inspired the great epics of Greece and Rome, and to fix firmly in the child's mind the fact that health is the beginning of all wealth, that the sane mind is the fruit and flower of the sound body, that the brain that will endure and conquer in every sphere of life is the brain that naturally followed in its rise and development the upbuilding of a body physically prepared to support and sustain it.

Children should be taught from early days to take a pride in the whiteness and soundness of their teeth, to love cleanliness and practice it both in their persons and surroundings, to shun everything calculated to antagonise the health and efficiency of body or brain, to be proud of their muscles and healthy firm flesh, the colour of their cheeks, their straight backs and erect carriage, their gait and deportment, everything, in short, that bears evidence to a physical body well-cared for, well-nourished and consciously cultured in every possible way. Think how valuable would all this he in preparing children for a life that will test them physically and mentally in the future to the utmost.

The little ones should be encouraged to romp and play and exercise their muscles in every way that Nature prompts. Their growth and development should be watched and noted by the family physician, who would be able to advise parents and guardians, and to see that the children were receiving a physical education and upbringing at home that would fit and prepare them for the sterner phase of life they would soon enter upon. At least once a year, too, the family doctor should be invited to make a most careful physical examination of the child and to report upon its progress, while he should most certainly be consulted regularly from the very moment its mental education begins.

HOW PARENTS MAY SAVE CHILDREN.

Parents themselves should never permit a false modesty, or more pressing claims upon their time to prevent them from making a personal examination of their 'children's bodies, at least until a certain age has been reached, nor to withhold from any child information that might be necessary for preserving it in the path of health and happiness. The most vigilant watch and ward over the physical body of the child in its early home life may often save a father or mother after years of remorse, for slight defects and deviations from the normal may be observed in time to prevent them from developing into serious physical deformities or disease.

I write of this feelingly and with sympathy, for time and again parents have come to me with tears in their eyes, horrified almost beyond words to find some loved child afflicted with spinal curvature or rounded shoulders or rickety limbs or some other physical defect that might have been easily checked and never even have been allowed to appear at all, if the parents had only done as I am now suggesting. Many children, too, are often punished or wrongly blamed for some mental deficiency that is really attributable to a physical cause, and especially to the enforcement of mental education upon a brain that is kept in a state of anaemia and ill-nutrition because the physical body is not able to provide it with the supplies that are necessary for its healthy functioning, and, indeed, the lack of which threaten its integrity and diminish its receptive power.

Parents should always keep in mind the fact that the basis of all education is the establishment of a sound, healthy and well-functioned body, and that without it the brain of the most intelligent child is simply " a castle in the air," deficient in support or sustaining power and liable to collapse even if the undeveloped body itself does not first give way. To give any child a strong, stable and receptive mind, to make its way easy for the assimilation of knowledge, and to give it the prospect of winning wealth and prosperity in life the surest and, indeed, the only method, is to begin with the education and upbuilding of its physical body and the securing of the physiological foundation essentially for the highest product of mind as well as body.

As long as possible the home influence should make its presence felt, because so far as I can see, the educational authorities of to-day find it difficult; if not impossible, to grasp the stern fact that the physical education and progress of a child is of far greater importance than its mental, and that, at least, it must be conducted by as scientific methods as mental education is to-day. I have read the latest Annual Report issued by the Board of Education, and I must confess I am not favourably impressed with the ideas of the authorities as to what they call " physical education." The mere provision of physical exercises to be carried out in a haphazard way, of dancing, and games, swimming and play centres is not only insufficient, as has been proved in the past, but may even do a child irretrievable injury, especially if there is a latent tendency towards the disease of a parent or ancestor.

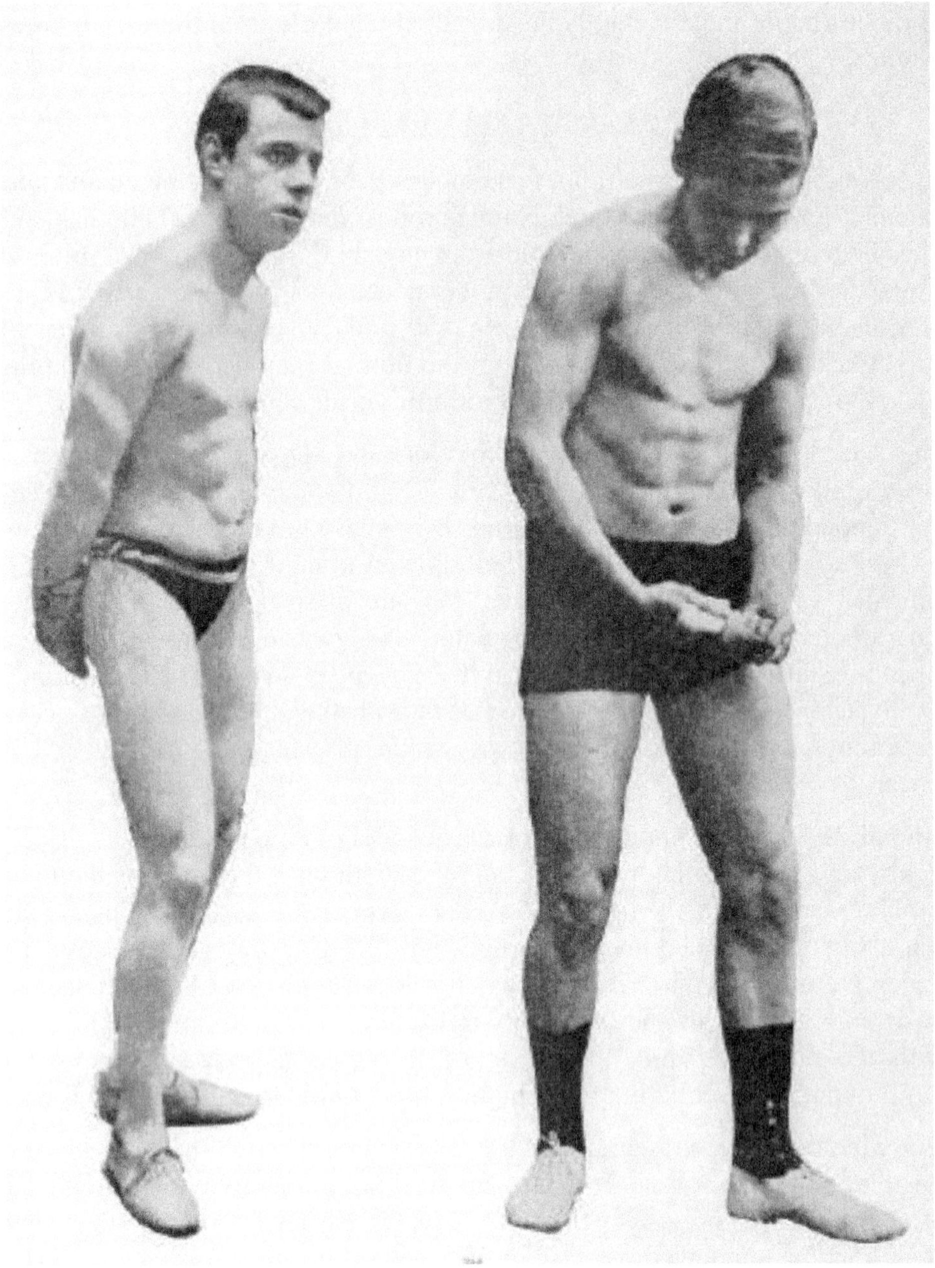

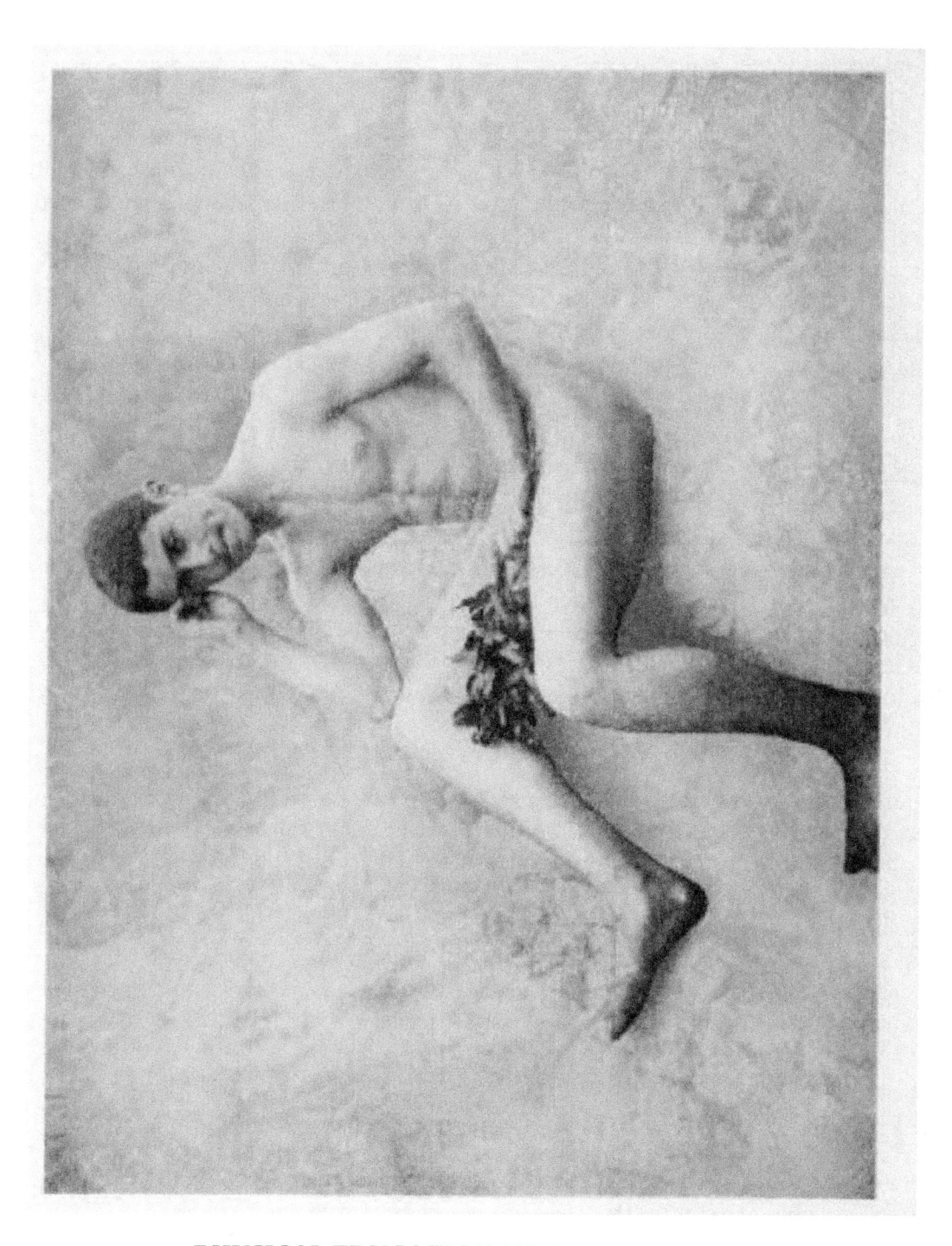

PHYSICAL EDUCATION MUST COME FIRST.

The physical education of a child is too serious a matter to be treated as a mere addendum or appendix to mental education, but, on the other hand, ought to be the very basis of all education and culture. It is a matter calling for a far deeper appreciation of the part that physical movement plays in the making and perfecting of the body as a physiological machine or engine than even the medical profession yet seems to possess. It is a matter upon which, indeed, the medical profession is even vague and indistinct, because it has never given to the subject the long and detailed study it deserves.

I cannot warn parents and guardians too solemnly to exercise their individual parental authority whenever necessary in this matter, and not always to leave the matter in the hands entirely of educational authorities who do not educate, and who may even destroy the career of the most promising child at the most susceptible period of its life by forcing its mental growth beyond its physical capacity. The school doctors are admittedly anxious to do their best, but they have neither sufficient experience nor authority yet to devise and carry out a really scientific system of physical education and bodily reconstruction. In the case of children especially, games and sports and dancing may work injury for life unless the child's physical condition is such as to warrant these, for all these should be the reward of physical fitness rather than means to that end.

Even at the moment of writing I see nothing that bids me hope for better things until there is a radical change in the ordinary medical conception of what constitutes a really scientific method of building up the human body by natural physical movements alone that will ensure the very highest standard of physical and mental power and balance in the children. It is because of this that I want all parents and child lovers to study the methods I describe in these pages, and that I am most anxious to win over medical men to a fuller understanding of them, for I know that such evidence as I adduce cannot fail to carry conviction to the inquiring minds of men used to scientific thought and logical deduction, but which have been kept operating too long in a groove or trench deeply dug through long years of tradition and conservation.

CORRECTING AND PREVENTING PAST ERRORS.

Parents anxious about the health and future well-being of their children will, I hope, support me in this matter not only for the sake of their own little ones but for the sake of all those children who, perhaps, from circumstances of fortune, are less happily placed I am glad to say that already the more advanced school of medical thinkers are rallying to my side because time is ever proving that physical education is a subject which embodies the solution of both the suppression and prevention of disease, and the provision of those natural essentials of a healthy mind in a strong and healthy body. The reproach that disease is not only not being prevented but that it is actually increasing is, I think, the best evidence that during all these years our medical men have sought too long for a preventive of disease where it was not to be found. In a really scientific system of physical education from childhood, with body culture carried out from early days on the lines indicated here, may I express the hope and belief that they will find the real corrective for and prevention of physical conditions and disease that are but the product of over-civilisation and a lop-sided system of education. Until such methods are taught and practised in our schools I strongly advise all parents and guardians to give their personal attention to what may be a matter of health or disease, success or failure, even, indeed of life or death to those they love even more than life itself.

The care of the children is, indeed, a labour of love that can never be in vain, and their health-education and culture will bring their own reward to the fathers and mothers of the country. The way that I point out is the only way to provide a real education that will make the acquisition of knowledge a pleasure and not a drudge for the little ones, and that will place mental training on a still more stable and valuable basis. Mind is, after all, the functioning of a material brain, and that material brain is primarily dependent for all its needs upon the too-long and too-often despised physical body. This attitude of depreciation and disparagement of the corporeal body is one that parents should take the van in changing, for muscle and blood and bone and nerve and sinew have all a part to play in the upbuilding as well as in the maintenance of the efficient mind.

A LEAGUE OF HEALTH.

Whatever may be the outcome of my advocacy of this cause, I am personally determined to carry on my own mission work to the last, for I have no doubt as to its final success so long as all lovers of children rally round me. It will not be my fault if a future Premier of England mourns in lamentations deep and loud over the physical unfitness and deterioration of the people. But it is to the children and to the parents and guardians and all child-lovers that I must look for encouragement and support. I want to see in every city, town and village at least one organisation devoted to the teaching and practice of natural physical reconstruction on scientific lines. Every home might well be a nursery of a finer, healthier, and stronger race of men and women. The watchword of the people to-day might well be All-for-Health, and the time was never better adapted for the beginning of a great physical renaissance movement throughout the British Empire than it is to-day.

Under its banner all might be proud to march towards that glorious goal and summit of human ambition—the sane, sound mind in the strong and healthy body. In a later chapter, I make an announcement which I feel certain will meet with a warm response from every right-thinking man and woman, especially from those who are the guerdons of the future, and who wish to save the children from that physical decline which almost encompassed our national destruction in the awful and recent past. I propose to form an All-for-Health League, not only at home but in that even greater Britain beyond the seas, for the purpose of a great national health propaganda, and to use it as the fulcrum of a lever that may yet move the world.

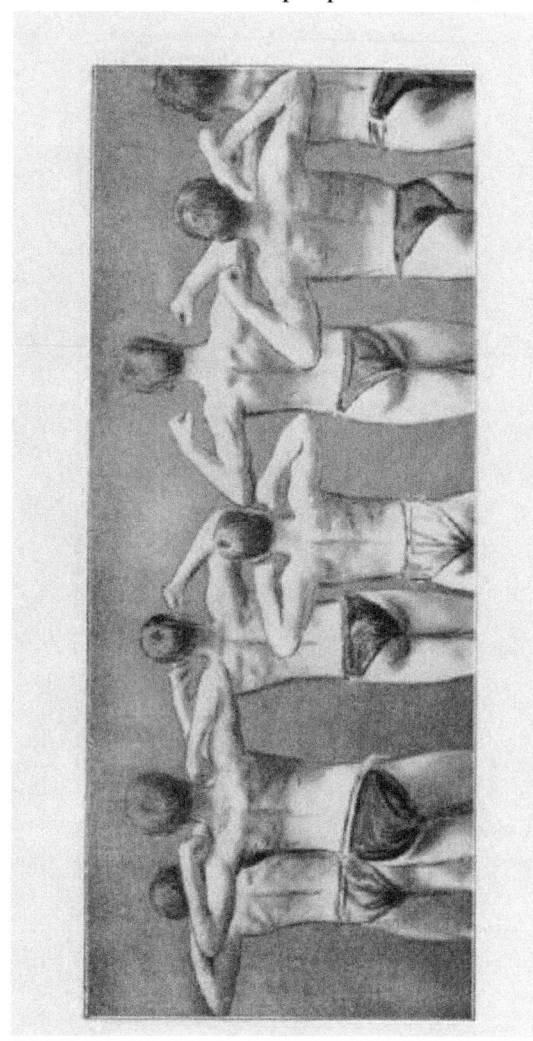

JOHN PETERS

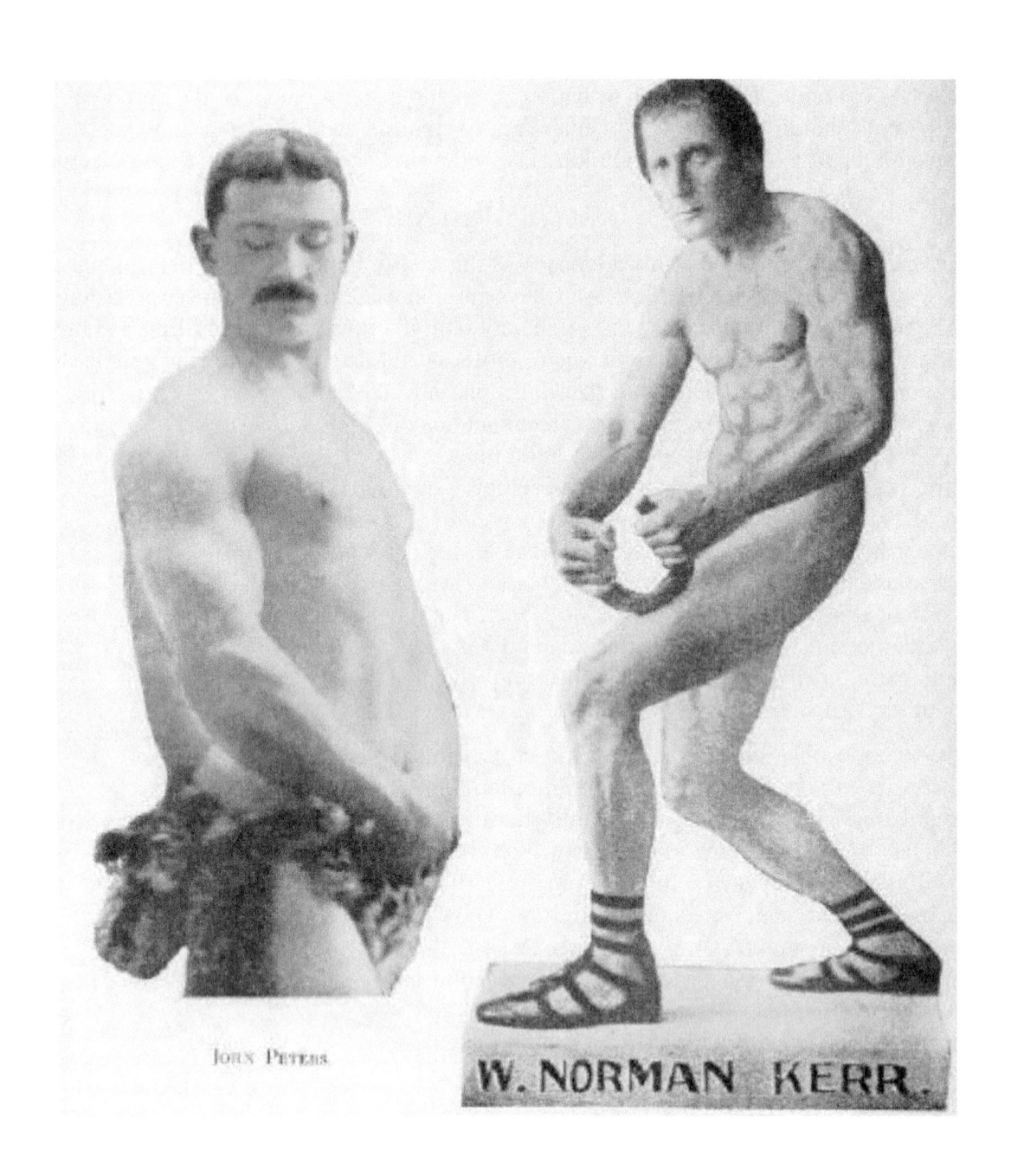

W. NORMAN KERR.

CHAPTER XXIII.
NEURASTHENIA—A NEW CONCEPTION.

What it is, How it Arises, Symptoms of its Presence, and how it can be Prevented or Overcome.

FOREWORD.

This chapter has been specially prepared for neurasthenics and all those who are interested in one of the most puzzling of modern ailments. I give my opinions and inferences not as mere theory, but as the actually proved and provable results of personal experience—an experience that, I think, I may say with all modesty is unique. As it has been my especial province occurred to me that the result of observations, as presented here for to study the best method of attaining and maintaining physical fitness, strength and health, and as a natural corollary, the best method of husbanding and economising it when once secured, it has the first time, will not be without interest to all who are afflicted with this condition, the more so at a time like the present when, despite all efforts to check or arrest it, neurasthenia is revealing itself more and in worse forms than ever.

No other book on this subject that I have seen has probed to the root-cause of this condition, and no author, medical or otherwise, has seemed to realise that it is entirely the result of a diminished and diminishing nervous income with an increased and increasing expenditure, and that to obtain and maintain balance between them, and still better, to increase income far beyond expenditure, is the only way to overcome this condition and that permanently. This we can only do by the natural methods hereafter described. That it can be done by scientific and balanced physical movement I know and have proved to demonstration, and I wish others, and especially sufferers from it, to know the how and the why of it. Hence this chapter.

"The Disease with 150 Symptoms."

Neurasthenia has been called "the disease with 150 symptoms," but as new symptoms are continually making their appearance from time to time, it is probable that they now number even more. As, however, many of these symptoms converge so closely to one another in nature and character, and as the differences are sometimes so fine as to be scarcely perceptible, I have endeavoured here to enumerate only the distinct and characteristic mental and physical symptoms that betray the neurasthenic condition, sometimes embracing many under one generic appellation. Some of these symptoms are invariably present in true neurasthenia, and all of them are indicative of some weakness, disorder or irritation of the nervous system.

Fear in many forms.
Pressure on top of head.
Stiffness at back of neck.
Pain on top of head.
Pain at back of neck.
Shooting pains.
Pain over eyebrows.
Pain at temples.
Head noises and dizziness.
Nervous irritability.
Acute sensitiveness of skin.
Feelings of "pins and needles."
Sensation of insects on skin.
Numbness in limbs.
Tenderness of scalp.
Loss of power in limbs.
Dizziness, especially when eyes are closed.
Palpitation and breathlessness.
Nervous headaches.
Dread of insanity.
Suicidal impulse and fears.
Failure of memory.
Self-consciousness.
Loss of self-confidence.
Loss of self-control.
Irresolution and doubt.

Irresistible impulses.
Sense of impending disaster.
Dread of heart failure.
Fits of depression.
Loss of interest in work or play.
Trembling of limbs.
Twitching of muscles.
Sleeplessness.
Vague anxieties.
Flushing and blushing.
Alternate feelings of hot and cold.
Loss of appetite.
Capricious appetite.
Sense of confusion.
Feeling of oppression.
Magnifying of trifles.
Dragging pains in small of back.
Inability to maintain erect position.
Lack of vigour.
Restlessness.
Vacillation and want of decision.
Nervous dyspepsia.
Craving for drugs or stimulant.
Palpitation and breathlessness.

Dread of company or crowds.
Dread of being alone.
Afraid of crossing open spaces.
Afraid of being closed up in carriages or closed places.
Dread of jumping from windows or high places.
Craving for excitement and change.
Intense excitability.
Unaccountable dislikes and aversions.
Fretfulness and moodiness.
Concentration of thoughts on self.
Suspicion of friends.
Inability to adhere to plans and resolutions.
Stuttering and stammering in presence of others.
Difficulty in writing in presence of others.
Susceptibility to sound.
Hearing imaginary voices.
Sense of failing mental power.
Delusions and hallucinations.

I HAVE now pointed out how everyone can possess a body built up in such perfectly balanced strength as to be disease-free, and, if so kept, even disease-immune. I now wish to show every reader how to regain the priceless treasure of health once it has been won and secured.

The possession and retention of health, like that of wealth, is contingent and dependent upon its intelligent and wise use, the relationship of income and expenditure, and the avoidance of any infringement on capital or reserve. An expenditure within income, ample capital, and a reserve fund sufficient to meet unforeseen and unexpected emergencies, are all necessary to ensure the successful conduct of any business, and to safeguard its financial position.

To maintain these vital principles, the services of auditors and accountants are retained, whose duty it is to check the firm's books and accounts, to study fluctuations of income and expenditure, to ascertain the exact relationship of profit and loss, to balance assets against liabilities, to safeguard the firm in every way against insolvency and bankruptcy, and to keep the directors always apprised of the true financial position of the house.

THE DOCTOR AS HEALTH ACCOUNTANT.

Something very much like that should, I argue, be the relationship between patient and physician. The doctor of the future will be very much in the position of a Health Accountant, performing somewhat similar duties to his patient in the matter of his health possessions, and helping him to avoid those health crises and disasters which we call disease rather than, as at present, waiting until they occur before the patient requires his services.

Just as the soundest and oldest of business houses can be brought to disaster by mismanagement, so the strongest and healthiest body may succumb to neurasthenia by some misconduct or misdirection of its affairs, or for want of that close supervision over income and outgo which is necessary to the successful conduct of every business enterprise. Though I can give you the wealth of health, as I have described in the earlier section of my book, anyone may afterwards, by over-expenditure of health-capital or income, drift into the distressing condition of nervous exhaustion called neurasthenia.

Neurasthenia is of all health troubles the one most self-incurred. It is a morbid condition rather than a disease, although it is a condition most favourable to other diseases, as I will show later. It does not arise from any germ or microbe that attacks the body from without, nor from diseased cells within. It is brought about, in the first place, through one's own mismanagement of one's vital affairs, mainly through lack of knowledge and experience, and for want of a proper system of what I may call health-accountancy.

I want now, in this chapter, to show every sufferer from neurasthenia that the knowledge and expert application of natural laws in the scientific manner I describe in the earlier part of this book, is the one and only way by which this most distressing condition can be mastered, and by so doing, to show also the absolute necessity for that health education and bodily culture which I say each and everyone should have from the earliest days of childhood. With such education and knowledge, and a really scientific system of physical reconstruction from childhood, millions will, in the future, be saved from its mental anguish and physical agony.

RUNNING THE BODY AS A BUSINESS.

To-day, the majority of men and women embark in the business of life not only with no suitable education and training, but handicapped from birth by ancestry and inheritance through generations of civilised life. In the majority of cases, it is needless to say that the result is failure—just as it would be in any other business in which a human being engaged without knowledge of the requirements and the conditions for success, or without the experience necessary to ensure its successful conduct.

Of their own bodies and its operations most people have little or no knowledge until disaster occurs, and only then is the doctor called in.

What would we think of any business man, who embarked in a business he did not understand, who took no note of his income and expenditure, and who only called in an auditor and accountant to attempt to put him right again when he had utterly failed in a business where he could never justly have expected to succeed.

So the average man or woman to-day lives through the daily business of life in haphazard fashion, unfamiliar with its details, unable to keep any check on his incomings and outgoings, never thinks of treating the doctor as a health auditor and accountant to assist him in the management of his affairs, and is generally surprised when disaster overtakes him.

RUINOUS EDUCATIONAL METHODS.

Many suffer even from childhood through what a famous continental specialist calls " an anomaly of constitution," and even from their youthful days they are apt to spend nervous energy beyond their capital and income. Even, however, where this is not so', our modern educational methods, by cramming the brain, with little care of the physical body as compensation, and by inculcating and fostering the competitive spirit early in life, lay the foundation of neurasthenia while children are at school.

Children are taught to worship the brain, and to pay every attention to it with the object of making money or a career, and to regard the body as its humble servant, and an inferior part of the individual. Indeed, in England, as the Dean of St. Paul's has tersely put it, " even learning is estimated by what it will bring in." While this remains so one cannot expect anything better. For, as I have pointed out in the earlier part of my book, the mental and nervous system depends for its supplies mainly on the digestion and the blood, and both the preparation of these supplies and their distribution, like every other bodily function, are performed partly by muscular movement.

Stating out in adolescent and continuing in adult life with the idea that the brain and nerves are better money-earners than the body, and with the competitive spirit firmly installed and implanted, these two persistent ideas continue to flog along a starved, weakened and finally irritated nervous system to the point of exhaustion, because the physical body itself at last becomes too weak through lack of movement to meet its insatiable demands. The ambition to defeat a rival, to make more money, to gain some honour or win some success, whips many people along unceasingly no matter how steep the hill they have to climb or how hard the road they must traverse.

MAN MUST LEARN TO LIVE.

Man, in short, is the only animal that has to be taught everything he must know for healthy life. Yet he is usually left untaught in the most vital essentials. Other animals have been given the knowledge they require in that which we call instinct. The bird knows instinctively how to obtain its food and rear its young. It can fly for miles over sea and land to some warmer clime in autumn, and find its way back again in the spring to the tree in the branches of which it first peeped out upon the world.

The bee knows how to gather wax and honey, and how to construct its hygienic cells and keep them sanitary. The salmon needs no chart or compass to come back to its own river after miles of journeying through many seas. Man alone must be taught how to live, what food to eat, what to drink and what to avoid, how to economise and how to expend his life force.

PHYSICAL AND MENTAL OVERWORK.

Neurasthenia is essentially the outcome of this ignorance as to the correct conduct of the business of life. It is the result of spending nervous energy faster than it can be made, or replenished, and is almost invariably the result of mental or nervous overstrain, shock and worry. It is, indeed, a state that cannot be produced by purely physical conditions, because the body cannot continue to perform physical work after the point of exhaustion, but sinks to sleep, during which time there is no further expenditure of nervous energy for during sound and dreamless sleep even the machinery of life runs more slowly, while Nature is helping one to heap up new supplies of nervous energy for the morrow. The heart beats more slowly, breathing is lighter and easier, for the time being the whole body exists only in a state of suspended or diminished animation, so that the sleeper awakes all the richer in nervous energy however much tired muscles still may ache.

Where there is intense mental or nervous strain it is very different. The over-tensed or long-tensed brain and nerve-cells refuse to relax and cause insomnia or, remaining over-tensed even in sleep, continue to operate sub-consciously and beyond the domination or direction of the will, causing restlessness, dreams, and nightmares, and thus the victim is literally consuming nervous energy continuously day and night. I have explained very fully what I mean by this sub-conscious over-tension of the brain and nerve-cells in my chapter on " Muscle, Mind and Nerve." in the earlier part of this book, and I will return to the subject of sleeplessness later on in the present chapter.

To revert to my statement that it is the mental and not the physical over-strain that causes neurasthenia, although it is just the same energy that is spent in both, it will be evident then that temperament plays no small part in this dread condition, and it is not surprising that neurasthenia chooses as its favourite victims those with the most delicate, hyper-sensitive and refined nerve-texture, whilst it rarely attacks manual workers except where there is also some great mental or nervous pressure. It is the brain worker and those of the artistic temperament who are naturally the most predisposed to neurasthenia, those in the higher professions and all those who live T)y their brains and nerves rather than by their muscles.

THE OCCASIONS OF NEURASTHENIA.

Sedentary workers and those engaged in the more responsible commercial positions come next, while to these must be added that vast army of men and women in every sphere of life upon whom " the daily round, the common task " "fall with merciless severity and monotony, literally crushing and squeezing mind and nerve with a relentless and increasing pressure. The war, needless to say, has stretched millions on the rack of neurasthenia, for it was a war of nerves as well as a war of munitions and strategy, a war, too, in which the millions who never saw the trenches suffered through tense strain, poignant sorrow, and overwhelming anxiety or grief, just as acutely as many of those shell-shocked and nerve-wracked by the noise, horror, and sufferings of battle waged under the most awful conditions in history. Palpitation is nearly always an early symptom, the heart fluttering, racing, and not infrequently appearing to miss a beat. This is very different from the increased action following exercise, being of purely nervous origin. It means expenditure of energy with no return, whereas in the former case income is increased. It also arouses fear, which still further consumes vital force in this way.

To enumerate all the occasions that give rise to neurasthenia, is, of course, impossible in the space at my disposal here. Prolonged mental work, business worry, professional ambition and aspiration, worry, shock, grief, fear, shame and, indeed, any deep emotion or passion or even feeling, will cause the expenditure of nervous energy at a rate which not even a millionaire of health could long withstand.

The lover, plunged in grief at the loss of one to him more than all else in the world, spends his energy in vain regrets and repinings until the point of exhaustion. The soldier, through shock or fear, amid the wild frenzy of war and dazed by the roar of guns, loses all control over himself, and is drained quickly of his last reserves of nervous force. The merchant with forebodings of failure, the doctor anxious over some most critical case, the stockbroker fearing the disgrace of " hammering," the student burning at once the midnight oil and his own life-force, these and hundreds of similarly situated men and women all help to swell the already huge army of the neurasthenic, for all are incurring the most prodigal expenditure of nerve-force.

FIRST SYMPTOMS OF NEURASTHENIA.

The first symptom of the loss of power in brain and nerve-cells is almost invariably pain or stiffness at the back of the neck or pressure on the top of the head, just as your arm would feel stiff and painful if the muscles were kept firmly contracted for a long time. There may be also sharp darting pains of a neuralgic type through the head or over or around the eyes, or, perhaps, an alarming sense of constriction as if the brain were being held firmly in a vice, while sometimes the nerves seem almost to jump and dance on the skin at the top or back of the head.

If a person can, at such a time, throw over all claims of business, there is no better plan to arrest the almost inevitable progress of this condition than to seek immediate change of scene, company and air, preferably in some foreign country, where foreign scenery and language will help to distract his thoughts and relieve cells in the brain and nervous system that have become strained and painful through severe or prolonged tension, conscious and sub-conscious, as I have already explained in the chapter on " Muscle, Mind and Nerve."

Unfortunately, few can afford to go to the enormous expense that this entails, fewer still are disposed to break the chain of everyday habit even if they could, and far fewer neurasthenics have sufficient will-power left to do so. So they continue madly on a career as devastating in its own way as the ride of Mazeppa. There is often to be observed in such cases a pathetic heroism, because the victim receives little sympathy from others, the symptoms of his condition being subjective rather than objective, and not often apparent to others, except in a form that alienates rather than arouses sympathy. So he feels shunned by a world that lacks sympathy and understanding, and he feels more and more that he must fight his battle alone and unbefriended.

DOGGED BY DESPONDENCY AND DESPAIR.

At first there is the conscious recognition that something, he knows not what, is wrong with his health, although he may possibly be told he is organically sound and is really the victim of no actual disease. This only intensifies his sufferings, and he includes the doctor among his enemies. Suspicions give birth to fear and lack of faith in everyone around him. A business man devoted to his business, for instance, begins to doubt his ability to carry it on successfully and to doubt those who work for or with him.

As a result, he causes more and more work to devolve upon himself at the very time when he should be saving his own nervous energy in every possible way. He imagines that everything depends upon his own efforts alone, and that if anything does cause him to break down, the business or pursuit will have to be sacrificed. It is the same with the artist, the author, the doctor and others who see the shadow of Failure stalking them everywhere, and whose every minute seems dogged by Despondency and Despair.

DISLIKE FOR WORK OR PLAY.

Added to all this is an increasing sense of difficulty in performing any task or duty, or even of engaging in or enjoying any pleasure or recreation. Intense depression supervenes, and the victim is borne down by a vague but ever-haunting sense of impending disaster. Headaches become frequent, and the sufferer becomes irritable, restless, and sometimes possessed of a morbid craving for excitement and novelty. Even the most microscopic difficulties are magnified into insurmountable obstacles. There gradually develops a growing dislike even for work that was formerly the chief object in life, and a loss of interest in all his surroundings. It becomes more and more difficult to concentrate the mind on one's daily labour; the mind gives way to strange and irresistible impulses; there is lack of continuity and even reading or talking cohesively on any subject becomes difficult if not impossible.

All this fear, lack of faith, and lack of self-confidence and self-control work together and form a vicious circle, the one perpetuating the other, and all together devouring and consuming nervous energy at a most destructive rate, putting extra work upon the digestive organs and the cells in the blood that act as food carriers and distributors, which, as a result of this prodigal consumption of vital force, make frantic endeavours to supply the additional nutrition now demanded by the brain and nerve cells through their increased expenditure, although all these cells in neurasthenia are already overworked. As a result malnutrition supervenes, to be quickly followed by many functional disorders, for it has been truly said that " neurasthenia is the parent of a whole family of functional diseases."

WHAT MALNUTRITION MEANS.

In the first place, food now often passes unassimilated through the system, because the digestive cells themselves do not receive sufficient supplies of nerve-force to convert the food that is eaten into nutrient material, while supplies, too, are diverted to brain and nerve cells that through their use and movement demand an unfair proportion of food that should be more equally distributed and consumed among other cells, with the result that the other cells at last " down tools," as it were, and refuse the supplies demanded by the ravenous and clamorous brain and nerve cells.

The result is that the neurasthenic's already heavy burden is now added to, this increased expenditure of nervous energy is aggravated still further by the cutting down of income, and while more nerve-force is being spent as the condition becomes more acute, less and less is coming in through the lack of supplies, or, rather, through lack of the power to convert food into nutritive material or its unfair and unequal distribution and consumption even if so converted. In short, the neurasthenic now begins to spend capital and reserve rather than income, so hastening his own destruction.

Malnutrition is a condition which may be accompanied by gastric pains or not, but which, in either case, means simply that food is not fulfilling its proper function in the body, viz., nutrition, because only a small percentage of the food eaten is converted into assimilable form and the various tissues of the body are not, therefore, nourished and sustained by it. On the other hand, much food not only passes through the body in an absolutely undigested and unassimilable form, and is of no value to feed the hungry and starving nervous system, but much also remains in the system to putrefy, ferment, and generate poisonous gases and acids, causing derangements in various systems, and often leading to acute nervous dyspepsia, neuritis, sciatica, neuralgia, and other painful complaints. Sometimes the food supplies are perverted into excessive fatty tissue that infiltrates various muscles and organs, and may again lead to serious forms of disease.

When there is malnutrition, there is rapid deterioration of tissue, with pronounced functional derangement and disturbance, especially of the nervous system, through which any or every other system of the body may be injuriously affected. In this condition, even so-called " nerve-foods," though they contain the essential elements in an inorganic form, of which nerve-tissue is made, are useless, because they cannot be assimilated by the enfeebled digestive cells, and generally pass through and out of the body unchanged or remain and cause constipation.

IS IT A MALADE IMAGINAIRE?

In this condition it is not difficult to imagine how rapid now becomes the deterioration of the nervous system, and how quickly new symptoms develop as the condition progresses. The brain itself becomes more and more affected through the functional disturbance of the various organs associated with digestion, assimilation and elimination. Sleeplessness and the most acute depression become more marked and more frequent. A sort of physical miasma arises in the body to ascend and float over the sufferer's brain, a cloud through which no sun of hope peers. The victim reflects the gloom within him, and becomes something of an Ishmaelite even among his friends. Important affairs are neglected or treated with difference. He becomes morbidly introspective and self-centred. His conversation becomes one " never-ending tale of morbid maladies." He becomes obsessed with himself and his symptoms and can think or talk of little else.

To his best friends even he often becomes a bore if not a butt, and people of more robust and cruder nerve-texture despise him. They look upon him as a hypochrondriac, the victim solely of a malade imaginaire. Unfortunately, for the victim, neurasthenia, while it may, to some extent, be called a disease of the imagination, is no mere imaginary disease, but a condition distressing in the extreme and deserving of the utmost consideration and sympathy.

In his own imagination he creates a hideous monster, a mental Frankenstein to devour him. He is now drawing deeply and more deeply upon his reserves of vital energy and begins to lose weight rapidly. Probably he consults a physician, or friends, who, in a well- meaning way, advise him to take more exercise, for in some vague, undefined sort of way, everyone instinctively recognises the benefits to be derived from physical exercise, although few, even among the medical profession, yet fully realise the fact that physical exercise, like medicine, may be a valuable friend or a dangerous enemy.

Perhaps they tell him lightly to "try a game of golf," or to " get a bicycle," or to " try mountain climbing," or to " take long walks," all of which may simply add to the sufferer's expenditure of nervous energy by anything from 25 to 50 per cent, at a time when new energy should be being placed to his credit. Not unlikely, the neurasthenic, acting on such advice, will give up what was meant to be a day of rest in every seven to the competitive or physical effort involved in some game or form of sport. The fact that the Creator allotted one day in every seven for the purpose of rest, and such rest is absolutely essential for recuperation, is too often forgotten or ignored in these days. At first, the excitement and novelty may give him a transient sense of improvement in health and spirits acting as does a " cocktail " on a jaded palate or appetite, but such " cocktails " often repeated can only have a disastrous termination for one suffering from neurasthenia. In his condition, physical exercise should be most carefully indulged, according to his condition, peculiar circumstances and in balance with the time he allows or can allow for rest and recuperation and other individual considerations.

BRAINS THAT NEVER REST.

Every form of material has its " breaking strain." Engineers know that and avoid it whenever possible. But the wonderful material that comprises the human body and brain is too often taxed to the very verge of breaking point by overwork, worry and the stress of modern life. Even steel and iron, we know, gets " tired " and overworked, and required a " rest " to enable it to recuperate.

Yet human flesh and blood and brain and nerve are often asked to work on untiringly, and even to continue " working " in the form of recreation and play, beyond the point of breaking strain, when it is really rest they require. A man, in short, is often more considerate to his razor, which he puts by at times for a much-needed rest, than to himself. For the neurasthenic to indulge in vigorous and strenuous physical effort to the point of exhaustion is like keeping the engine of a motor-car running while in the garage and not in actual use.

The result in such cases is almost invariably total collapse sooner or later, or when the nervous system breaks down completely, as in true neurasthenia, it affects the whole human body in all its departments of life very much as a great railway disaster at an important junction like Crewe, in which both the railway and the telegraph systems were disordered, would affect the life of the whole country. The direct and indirect results are scarcely calculable.

In the first place the neurasthenia increases malnutrition, and this, in turn, causes internal functional disturbances that provoke insomnia, with sleepless, restless, or dream-infested nights, when the sufferer begins to feel the more acute ravages of neurasthenia, and is tormented with the fear of insanity or the dread thought that he is about to commit suicide, perhaps the most agonising mental distress associated with this condition. The lot of the neurasthenic now, often passing night after night with " no oasis of sweet slumber," is, indeed, a pathetic one. To be robbed of sound and dreamless sleep, often after weary and tiring days, is like spending money with both hands. Nervous energy is now being wasted almost continuously, and the brain and nervous system has no opportunity to replenish stores.

HOW TO WOO SOUND SLEEP.

Sleep, next to nutrition, must be restored if neurasthenia is to be overcome, because it is during healthy and natural sleep—the deep dreamless sleep of a healthy child—that Nature is most bountiful in furnishing the body with new funds of energy. Expenditure by conscious effort is then compulsorily prohibited and our subconscious expenditure of nervous energy is cut down to the very minimum. The great workshop of the body is almost still, except for the operations and activities absolutely essential to its maintenance. The heart continues to beat but more slowly, the breathing is slower, only such functions as are necessary for repair and the replenishing of supplies are carried out, so that the healthy person wakes up much richer in nervous energy than when he lay down. Not so the neurasthenic.

He wakes up poorer in his vital force than when he lay down, and so he has to face another day with less reserve than ever to fall back upon. His bodily workshop is going on at full speed day and night, and, indeed, working faster than ever during nights of sleeplessness or broken sleep. Even when he sleeps the expenditure continues in dreams. So again income is reduced while expenditure increases, and he is losing in a double sense.

Now everything in Nature is the result of immutable and unchangeable laws. There is a law that regulates the sound and dreamless sleep of the child, and the broken sleep or sleeplessness of the neurasthenic is the result of a transgression of that law. The neurasthenic cannot change the law and cannot transgress it with impunity. When he obeys the law, Nature will again reward him with the precious gift of sleep.

Let him woo sleep by conforming to the law in every way. He must eschew everything that tends to interfere with sleep. He should avoid the late and heavy supper. He should see that his surroundings are congenial and tranquillising. He should occupy a bedroom that is at a proper temperature and well ventilated. Above all, he should school and discipline his mind and nerves by repeated efforts to sleep. He should practise dismissing every thought from his mind on retiring, and, in the popular phrase, endeavour to make his mind a blank.

He will find this difficult and even impossible at first, but in time he will be able to master his thoughts and feelings. Remember that a habit which has become fixed cannot be broken down in a moment. It may take days, even weeks, perhaps months, to secure even a few minutes' sleep at will in this way; but the effort, at first difficult, will Gradually become easier and more and more successful, until the new habit of sleep is acquired, and sleep comes automatically as soon almost as his head is on the pillow.

Practice proverbially makes perfect. " Practice, practice, practice," answered a famous pianist, when asked what was the secret of his unique musical skill, and the neurasthenic who is afflicted with insomnia should profit by the hint. Man is, after all, largely a creature of habit, and can by steady and persistent effort and constant practice, school himself to the habit of sleep just as the pianist learnt the mastery of his instrument by regular and conscientious practice. At first it will, no doubt, be very difficult, just as difficult and as tedious as learning to play the piano well. Persistence and patience, however, will meet their reward as by the practice at first of one- finger and then five-finger musical exercises the child can ultimately learn to be a skilled pianist.

THE AFTERMATH OF INSOMNIA.

Remember that all this effort will mean a much smaller expenditure of nervous energy than hours spent in sleepless fretting and worrying and thinking of self, so that even if you do not win sleep at first you are still cutting down your nervous expenditure, for your mind is being diverted, at least partially, from its usual course, and less energy is spent in this way in the same time than in thinking of your fears and worries during the same period. Every hour so spent you are thus saving energy that would otherwise be wasted, and if at first you only obtain a few moments sleep, you are further saving the energy you would have spent in that time had you remained sleepless. With patience, the minutes will become an hour, the hour becomes two hours, until you will at last be able to enjoy your normal amount of healthy, dream-free sleep. Besides, all this time you will be disciplining mind and nerves, and steadily acquiring that self- mastery over the brain and nervous system which will enable you the better to regulate your income and expenditure of nervous energy in the future.

There is no surer evidence of supreme self-control over the mental and nervous system than the power to sleep at will, as was possessed by great commanders of the past like Napoleon and Wellington, and which was the great nerve-sustainer of men like Foch and Haig in the immensely testing struggle that has just ended in their great victory. This is not a gift, though some possess it in greater degree than others, but like everything else can be cultivated by practice, and is worth more from the health point of view than all the drugs ever compounded.

The aftermath of the insomnia of neurasthenia is one of the most terrible penalties associated with that condition, for one is now reduced to a state of nervous trepidation in which faith and hope in everything departs. The loss of faith in oneself, in one's friends, even in God too often follows, and the sufferer becomes melancholic to a degree that menaces even mental sanity unless prompt steps be taken to check this condition. Even the atheist, though he denies the existence of God, feels a sense of dependence, in the last resort, upon something unknown, beyond and above him, as, in the other extreme, the Pantheist worships God as revealed in all things.

The neurasthenic of religious mind feels that the Almighty has withdrawn His favour from him, a sense that something has departed from him and he is left helpless and alone, and that fear develops as he grows weaker. The man who has lived a careless or irreligious life feels that, perhaps, God is punishing him for his neglect or worship. The atheist is worse still, for he feels that there is nothing to which he can cling and becomes even more despondent.

FEARS OF MANY KINDS.

All feel their utter helplessness alone, and through this loss of faith, and the fact that the world offers them either little sympathy or consolation, they are driven more and more within themselves, while their fear often engenders a hundred other fears. In this mental attitude, deprived even of man's last and only hope in his hour of greatest distress, their whole mental attitude is one that lowers bodily resistant power and makes the path easier for disease.

The fear of failure in a thousand directions is present in practically every case, taking some form generally traceable to concentrated thought on one object or in one direction. There are few neurasthenics who escape entirely one or more of these fears, the fear of insanity (a fear, happily, that is more alarming in itself than in the possibility of its actual occurrence), the fear of a suicide's ending, the fear of being alone, the dread of company or crowds, the fear of open or closed spaces, the fear of high places, the fear of disease, the fear of Divine disfavour, the fear of something they know not what, the fear of showing cowardice, the fear of being thought afraid, the fear of monetary loss and poverty, the fear of disappointment—these and a thousand other fears and forebodings place a tremendous tax and tension upon nerve-centres, already ill-nourished and irritated through lack of nutrition and overwork, until the nervous system is at last insidiously and utterly undermined and exhausted.

Even were one as rich as a Carnegie or a Rockefeller in this more-precious-than-gold vital force, the combination of neurasthenia, with its inseparable allies, insomnia and malnutrition, will bring him to health bankruptcy, indeed, more likely so, for the richer one is in nervous energy the less will he feel disposed to conserve and economise it. On the other hand, he will be tempted to expend it still more freely because he possesses it in such abundance. Nothing will cause this extravagance more freely than enthusiasm, the whip and spur which one drives himself when he consecrates himself to some labour of love. Then, indeed, is it that " vaulting ambition o'erleaps itself " in a way very different to that suggested by the poet.

HOW I, MYSELF, BROKE DOWN.

The artist, the musician, the author, the actor, the doctor, the clergyman, the statesman, immersing their own individuality in a cause to which they are devoted, do not count the cost and may easily fail to note the signs that foretell the declination of nervous power until suddenly faced with the wreckage of their former selves.

It is always possible in any walk of life that the spirit of even the strongest man will drive his brain and nervous system to the point of exhaustion and cause them to break down suddenly under too severe a strain. No one can be so strong physically that the power of a driving mind may not sometimes lead to disastrous over-expenditure and inevitable collapse.

Strong and robust as I was not so very many years ago, and in the very prime of my vigour, I was impelled, under the driving spirit of a great enthusiasm in the very cause I am now advocating, to spend nervous energy faster—much faster—than I could make it, although I lived a stern and disciplined life otherwise, and was always, to some degree, in good physical condition, while my accumulated reserves of health and vitality, through years of such living, gave me undoubted advantages over the average man and woman. On this occasion, however, my enthusiasm took wings that outsped even my physical strength, and though I never had a day's illness or suffered from any disease in my life, I had at last a very serious nervous collapse.

My weight sank from 15st. to 8st. My muscles seemed almost to fade away. My skin simply covered my bones. Indeed, those who see me to-day at 52, as fit as, if not better than, I ever was in my life (as my most recent photos reproduced in this book will prove), and again turning the scale at about 15st., can scarcely credit this, when I tell them the facts. Yet by my own methods, and exactly on the lines I am now advocating, I made myself as strong and healthy again in every way as I was in my youthful prime, just as I transformed myself in earlier life from a delicate youth into a strong and healthy young man, and I mention this incident for the encouragement of others and to give them the assurance that I have a sympathetic understanding in similar cases. I restored myself entirely by increasing my income of nervous energy and restricting my expenditure in the exact way I am describing in this book.

MENTAL AND NERVOUS EARTHQUAKES.

There is a breaking strain with the toughest physical material, mental and physical, beyond which even the most perfectly developed and balanced man or woman may fail. Any tremendous and unexpected crisis may cause the best physical structure to collapse, just as a violent earthquake will bring down the strongest building and uproot the deepest and most firmly-laid foundation. But as in an earthquake, the strongest built building upon the deepest and surest foundation will be the most likely to resist the unwonted shock while weaker and less securely established buildings fall, so the mental and nervous system that has its physical foundation the better and more securely established will the more readily withstand even the most terrific mental upheaval.

There are, however, as the greatest of all poets has truly said; more things in heaven and earth than- are dreamt of in our philosophy, and over and beyond all human calculations there may come at times abnormal mental storms, tempests, cyclones and earthquakes, that will shake even the strongest in their very foundation.

Here, again, however, those who have made man the chief object of their study rather than disease or medicine, who have added a deep knowledge of psychology to a comprehensive knowledge of human physiology, who have learned to study man not as a mere material product of dust but as a reflection of the Divine essence that permeates and animates this tenement of clay, will be able to grapple with and overcome neurasthenia most successfully.

The most sympathetic understanding, an almost superhuman insight into the mental processes of the human mind, a most intimate acquaintance with the inter-relationship of body and brain and nerve, and a just recognition of the importance of physical, mental and nervous balance, will be demanded from those who, in the future, aspire to the highest of human titles, physician and healer.

THE LATH AND PLASTER OF DRUGS.

The human construction that has been devastated by one of these mental and nervous upheavals is not to be stuck together again in jerry-built fashion with the lath and plaster of medicine or drugs. It must be re-erected from the very foundation upwards, and rebuilt stouter and stronger than ever, braced with unbreakable girders of human muscle, buttressed and fortified by a mental and nervous system as flexible and yet as enduring as finest tempered steel, underpinned and strutted for the future so that the fiercest tornado of mental or physical disease will sweep against it in vain.

The fear of any recurrence of similar mental " earthquakes " must be overcome if neurasthenia is to be successfully treated, and the study of the neurasthenic tells us that not only does this fear precipitate disaster, but it often hinders or prevents recovery and hinders reconstruction. Eear-thoughts will even bring about the very disaster which they have long morbidly anticipated, and cause the very wreckage which they so anxiously have sought to avoid, for there was true psychology in St. Paul's utterance, 1 the thing I feared has come upon me."

A business man, for instance, in a state of neurasthenia may strive so assiduously to avert financial disaster that his very anxiety will drive him to overwork and so to precipitate the disaster he so dreads. He is afraid, say, of bankruptcy. Such a person must be schooled to realise that fear is itself an infirmity of the mind, and that the surest way to conquer fear is not to shrink from it but to challenge that which he fears. To suggest to a person that there is nothing despicable in failure, financial or otherwise, to encourage hope by pointing out that he himself can will fear away, to help him to regain his self-confidence and courage, and to be positive not negative in character, methods of mental therapeutics may well be associated with the physical therapeutics I so strongly advocate.

WHAT LOSS OF NERVE-FORCE MEANS.

The great aim in the treatment of this condition must always be to prevent over-expenditure of nerve-force, to economise it in every way and to increase its replenishment. Over-expenditure is the chief enemy, and the sufferer must be saved from himself or, rather, be taught how to save himself from himself in this matter.

Treatment, then, must be partly physical and physiological and partly psychical, Mentally much help may be given to a sufferer by teaching him to practise self-suggestion, especially if the neurasthenic feels that there is a bond of sympathy between, and the neurasthenic has an almost uncanny power of divining the presence or absence of sympathy in another. He is usually exquisitely sensitive in this direction, and for that reason all successful treatment must be based on a perfect and sympathetic understanding between patient and healer.

In no other form of illness does psychology play so important a part in treatment, and for that reason one who can, from personal experience, cross, as it were, the threshold of the sufferer's mind, is likely to be successful where stereotyped and traditional methods will completely fail. Indeed, many of those who have found relief and cure in the methods I advocate have told me, without being aware of the fact which I have divulged here for the first time, they felt that I must have myself suffered at some time from neurasthenia to understand their feelings and needs so perfectly.

Hypnotic treatment has a certain logical basis, but personally I think it much the better plan for a sufferer from neurasthenia to acquire the habit of self-suggestion rather than to submit his own will to the subjection of another, for the former method helps to build up will-power, whereas the other tends rather to weaken it and to still further undermine the self-confidence and self-reliance of the neurasthenic. A very good plan, indeed, is for neurasthenics to commence each day with a code of affirmations that will help them to fight against the many habits, tendencies and inclinations that are responsible for an enormous wastage of nerve-force, and especially against any one or more of which they are especially the victim. For instance, the timorous should suggest to themselves to face boldly any difficulty, the bashful to be bold, the indecisive to be decisive, and the restless to cultivate repose and stolidity.

It is not a bad principle, indeed, for the sufferer to discipline himself to do those things he dislikes to do, and to resist the things he feels tempted to do where circumstances admit and no moral or other law should restrain. A few such exercises as the following will do much to strengthen and discipline the will. Let the neurasthenic repeat to himself these or some similar phrases to suit his own personal needs every morning.

LESSONS IN SELF-SUGGESTION

1. I will have faith in God, in my friends and in myself;
2. I will not worry under any circumstances;
3. I will not talk of myself or my symptoms;
4. I will do my duty fearlessly and have faith in God;
5. I will control all my thoughts and actions;
6. I will keep cool, calm and cheerful;
7. I will cultivate repose and serenity;
8. I will be good-tempered and not irritable;
9. I will not be jealous or greedy;
10. I will be patient;
11. I will think good of everyone;
12. I will cultivate good and pleasant thoughts;
13. I will be slow to suspect and quick to forgive;
14. I will economise my energy in every way;
15. I will defeat depression and despair.

Neurasthenics will be surprised, indeed, if they strive to model their daily life on some such lines as this, to find in how many directions they will be able to economise energy that is otherwise wasted in life's daily round of thoughts, deeds, and innumerable annoyances and worries, great or small.

I have shown now that neurasthenia is simply the result of (1) excessive expenditure of nervous energy, and (2) to the decrease of vital income, and that in both these, malnutrition and insomnia play a predominant part. Logically, therefore, it will be evident that whatever decreases expenditure and increases income will help to restore the balance that that has been disturbed in the nervous system and to pay off all overdrafts on the Bank of Health, and finally to possess an ample reserve fund for future contingencies. How can we best achieve that object and reach that goal? My contention is that we can only do so permanently and legitimately by the employment of Nature's own methods, used and applied scientifically as I describe, because all other methods must interfere with great natural laws and curative forces already existent in the body itself, and can, at best, be but transient in their effect, because artificial and unnatural.

NATURE AND NATURE'S LAW.

I have said that everything in Nature is ruled by law. The law is fixed and unchangeable. Unfortunately, many to-day live in ignorance of the law, and, in consequence, transgress it. It is to prevent this state of things in the future that I advocate a system of health education and bodily culture in every school, supported by the State, because, unfortunately, ignorance of the law is no excuse, and Nature is inexorable. To obey the law without knowledge of it is not easy, so if we wish to prevent the sins either of omission or commission that lead to neurasthenia, or, indeed, any diseased condition in the people, it is only fair that the people should be instructed in the law and instructed from childhood. Indeed, part of the school duty in such a scheme as I suggest should be to instruct the children on this most vital subject of the economy and expenditure of nervous energy.

Even this knowledge, however, will not prevent many from still expending nervous energy, as it were, " beyond their means," for competition, ambition, enthusiasm and even desperation will always tempt many to take risks in this matter in the hope that the attainment of their goal and object will compensate them later. It is for these and other reasons that this condition is likely to continue some time yet, even when every other form of disease has been eradicated, and this is why I have particularly chosen to deal with it here as distinct entirely from other diseases, and to show just how and why the methods I indicate can prevent it, if the sufferer adheres to the law, or overcome it if, for any reason, over-expenditure of energy causes its occurrence.

This book, indeed, would not be complete if I did not give this knowledge, for knowledge on the part of the patient is essential to an intelligent co-partnership between patient and healer, and every sufferer, therefore, from neurasthenia should not only study the advice given in this chapter most carefully, but should also read and grasp fully the lessons conveyed in the earlier chapters.

The fundamental law of life, as I think I have proved conclusively in the previous pages of this book, is movement, which in all animal life is muscular movement. Now all muscular movement comprises contraction and relaxation, and I have explained in the chapter on 1 What is Scientific Physical Movement " how the voluntary muscles, by their contraction and relaxation, can be used to bring into play all the involuntary muscles of the body and through them reach every cell and influence every function of the body, including the cells of the brain and nervous system. I have also pointed out in another chapter, " The Machinery of Natural Physical Training," the importance alike of mental concentration and equivalent relaxation in carrying out physical movements to the very best advantage not merely for the physical body but to strengthen brain and nerve.

THE PARASITIC BRAIN.

In real and acute neurasthenia the brain and nerve-cells are and have been kept in an almost perpetual state of over-tension, sometimes consciously and sometimes sub-consciously, the sufferer being unable to relax them by any effort of will. This continuous conscious or sub-conscious over-tension of brain and nerve cells means that the great central nervous system is drawing to itself greater supplies of blood and consuming more supplies than the amount to which it is entitled in an equitable arrangement of the bodily affairs.

The brain, indeed, becomes, for a time, a sort of parasite in the body, but as these exorbitant demands continue, the digestive cells at last grow too weak and exhausted to meet them, through weakness and lack of movement, and they themselves collapse. So with all the other cells in the bodily community, the cells that should act in the body as chemists, stokers, distributors, scavengers, etc., ail of whom are brought in time to the point of exhaustion, and cannot even sustain themselves, much less the rebellious cells of the mental and nervous system.

VALUE OF RELAXATION.

Now it must be evident that the first necessity of a body and brain in this condition is the relaxation of the over-tensed cells. But it is only possible in this state to relax the nerve-cells through the relaxation of the voluntary muscles. Primitive man doing purely physical work had no such necessity thrust upon him, for physical overwork, alone, unaccompanied by mental overstrain, could never cause such a condition as neurasthenia. It is only mental overwork or overstrain that can do it, or mental work super-added to physical work. Physical exhaustion compels sleep during which time the brain and nerve centres relax and recuperate. Mental or nervous exhaustion banishes or diminishes sleep. Nature intervenes when physical effort is made to exhaustion.

For instance, the soldiers in the retreat from Mons, physically worn out, wounded, bleeding and exhausted, sank down at last into sound sleep the moment they reached a place of safety and could scarcely be awakened. Indeed, some slept or dosed while on their horses, others even while marching on foot, their legs moving automatically without any effort of the mind. Their muscles then relaxed naturally and spontaneously when the limit of muscular effort had been reached, just as the muscles of a weight-lifter, after being exerted to their utmost power in some feat, relax, and cannot repeat that feat until they are allowed to rest and recuperate. The active brain, however, is not controlled or checked by nature in this way, but will go on thinking and worrying both night and day beyond its normal power if means are not taken to arrest or suspend its operation.

Here, I think, is the reason why it is the man or woman of high mentality, the brain-worker, the highly-strung, the person of artistic temperament, the refined, the hypersensitive, those in positions of authority and those of every class who live mentally rather than muscularly, that constitute the pathetic legion of the neurasthenic, those, that is, whose daily duties demand mental and nervous strain rather than physical and muscular. Indeed, few who do severe and prolonged mental work having little time for recuperation, escape neurasthenia altogether, and probably none escape malnutrition in some degree.

This is because the brain and nerve cells overtax the cells of the digestive system far beyond their normal powers, without supplying that compensation which balanced physical movement gives, and which is as necessary for their nourishment and fitness as for the cells of a muscle.

In other words, the digestive cells become too weak to extract the utmost amount of nourishment out of food, and so, in time, all the other cells of the body must suffer similarly, because each and all are interdependent and all actually dependent on the digestive cells for nutrition.

This, no doubt, explains why the hustling American, with brain and nerves ever on the alert, is so great a victim of neurasthenia and nervous dyspepsia, and why, indeed, neurasthenia has been called " the American disease." indeed, the name neurasthenia was first given to this condition by a famous American neurologist, Dr A. M. Beard, a name, I regret to say, that in itself is inclined to alarm the victim of it, or, at least, to aggravate the state of fear ever present, and especially in a people who have not been educated from childhood in the language of anatomy, physiology and pathology, or, indeed, in scarcely anything attaching to the human form, shape, substance, organisation, and the manifold operations ever going on in the body.

WHY A HEALTHY CHILD SLEEPS SOUNDLY.

Now it will be quite evident that to increase income and curtail expenditure of nervous energy it is necessary (1) to learn how to relax the severely contracted brain and nerve cells, and (2) to improve digestion and nutrition and increase the revenue of the nervous system. I have shown in an earlier chapter that relaxation of the muscles is, and can only be, equal to contraction, and that by learning how to completely relax the muscles within our control we will learn also how to relax the brain and nerve cells.

Let me explain this a little more fully. The healthy child (an example I am fond of using you will note) retires to bed and drops instantly into sound and restful sleep. Why? Because at that age it has no mental worries and completely relaxes muscle, mind and nerves on lying down. Later in life, it has to provide itself with food, shelter and clothing, and has other worries and troubles to contend against. So the mind intervenes between its body and sleep. The grown-up person too often takes his work and his troubles to bed with him, and the sound sleep of childhood gives place to disturbed, broken and dream-haunted sleep, and probably banishes sleep altogether. Very few to-day can enjoy the dreamless sleep of a healthy child because they cannot relax either their muscles or nerves fully.

The sufferer from neurasthenia must practise relaxation both of the muscles and of the mind and nerves as a first lesson in the economy of his nervous energy. To begin with, he should practise relaxing first one pair or set of muscles only at a time, as far as is possible, say, those of the arm. Raise one arm above the head to its utmost limit of extension, and then let it fall as limply by the side and as helpless as if you had no power of mental control over it in any way.

When relaxed thus, the muscles of the arm should be quite soft and flabby, the very antithesis of a muscle is a state of full contraction. Repeat the movement five or six times, and then do the same with the other arm, afterwards carrying out the same movements of full and complete relaxation with both arms simultaneously.

Then do similar movements with the legs whilst sitting or reclining. Finally, practise equally complete relaxation of every muscle in the body while sitting in a chair. Sit up straight, with muscles firmly braced and shoulders squared, every muscle engaged as tense as those of a mounted trooper on parade. Then allow all of them to relax as limply as if you had suddenly swooned, offering no resistance and letting the body sink helpless into the chair with the arms drooping and apparently powerless.

EQUAL CONTRACTION AND RELAXATION.

When you retire to bed, endeavour to relax every muscle of the body in the same way. Try to imagine that your body is a heavy weight which you are utterly exhausted carrying about—and which is, after all, really to some extent the case—and, with a sigh of relief, let it drop as heavily on the bed as if it weighed a ton. All this will be most valuable in acquiring both the habit of complete relaxation, and also in schooling the mind and nervous system as I have explained in " Muscle, Mind and Nerve."

To give a popular illustration of what is meant by complete relaxation of all the muscles of the body, I know no better example than that of a man, in the condition which is familiarly described as 1 helplessly drunk," without the slightest mental control or direction of the muscles of his body, and who, when he falls, sinks down " all of a heap," as the saying is, without the least effort of resistance. It is because of this utter lack of resistance that the drunken man escapes the injuries that would result from such a fall in a condition of sobriety, where resistance would be made automatically in falling.

In carrying out contraction movements, on the other hand, the mind must be intensely concentrated on the muscles moved during the whole effort of contraction, and these contractions should be made vigorously and slow, not quick and jerkily. The mental concentration draws the blood in greater quantities to the part to which it is directed, causing greater oxidation and an increased demand for oxygen, and the vigour and slowness of the contraction means that the poisonous waste and worn materials are more thoroughly squeezed out, making more room for new blood to take its place with fresh supplies of nutrient material in greater quantity.

It is the force of the contraction that counts, not the speed, for fast and jerky muscular movements increase the strain upon the heart and tend to exhaust nervous vitality instead of strengthening the one and economising the other. All contraction movements, therefore, should be performed slowly but with the very maximum of physical and mental effort, but they must never be carried to the point of fatigue, or, on the other hand, allowed to degenerate into monotonous and only semi-conscious effort.

This contraction and relaxation of the voluntary muscles, with mental concentration on the parts or muscles moved, has both a psychical and a physiological value in neurasthenia. The fact that thinking of a part determines the flow of blood to that part gives the mental concentration a high physiological value and also disciplines the mind and schools one in the culture of that self-control which is so essential to the regulation of one's nervous income and expenditure. Physiologically, we know the value of this determination of the blood to any part in the digestion of a meal.

When the mind is active in other directions, the whole function of digestion is disturbed and the gastric juices cease to flow freely. But when a person is thinking only of his stomach and the enjoyment of a good meal gives, the blood is drawn to the stomach in greater quantities, the secretions are stimulated, and the food better digested. This is why so many feel sleepy after enjoying a good dinner.

EQUAL HEALTH FOR EVERY CELL.

It is the same with the cells of the muscles when moved with the mind thinking on the muscles moved, and not of other matters. The living cells of the muscles themselves are, of course, better nourished, because the blood brings them better supplies. But when this movement of the voluntary muscles is made in balance, all the cells of the body are benefited in turn, as the blood is pumped more vigorously everywhere in the body afterwards, and supplies are better distributed and more fairly consumed.

The balanced movement of all the voluntary muscles, as I explain in the previous part of this book, automatically sets cells of all kinds in every part of the body in action. It is, in short, as if you gave exercise to every cell of the body and brain, and this increases their appetite, leads to their better nutrition, oxygenation and purification, and develops them all in equally balanced strength. There you have the whole secret of how and why such methods as I advocate will secure, maintain or regain nervous stability. Every brain and nerve cell is " drilled " into health and strength by movement.

Those who carry out this treatment by means of balanced physical movements must never forget how important a part the mind plays in all treatment. When they have learnt how to contract and ' relax the muscles perfectly they should also practise that relaxation , of the mind which is essential to complete relaxation.

HOW TO CULTIVATE SERENITY.

Habits of repose should be cultivated except when the movements are actually being carried out, and all fidgetiness and restlessness fought against so as to economise energy to the utmost. The exact prescription of exercise in relationship to work and rest differentiates such treatment as I advocate from ordinary physical work or from games, sports and pastimes, which are too often indulged in at the cost of a terrific expenditure of nerve-force. As the great object in the treatment of neurasthenia is to save and bank nervous energy, not to still further dissipate it, only such physical movements as are specified should be carried out, and all other physical and mental activity reduced to a minimum. Sufferers should school themselves into the habit of serenity, and try as far as possible to give the mind an occasional holiday.

The three necessary steps in treatment are (1) to cut down expenditure in the ways I have described and increase income and (2) to make good the overdrafts on the Bank of Health, and (3) to place a good supply of nervous energy as a Reserve Fund for future emergencies. The question, then, for the physician or healer (or, as I prefer to call him in this case, the Health Accountant) is to first determine, by painstaking diagnosis in each individual case, to what particular causes the over-expenditure and decrease of income may be due, and to prescribe treatment in each individual case accordingly.

In one the cause may be worry, in another shock, great grief in another, and so on; and, of course, treatment must be regulated according to the state of each patient's health account, and such physical movement as is prescribed must be administered and regulated in such a way as just to compensate the sufferer and not to still further deplete his energy. All exercise should only be carried out directly according to prescription, and though gentle walks may be recommended, the time and distance even of these should be distinctly stated by the person in charge of each case.

TWIN DESTROYERS OF ENERGY.

As in practically every case of neurasthenia there is malnutrition, it will also be the duty of those prescribing treatment to be able to estimate from the sufferer's condition just the nature and amount of exercising that will strengthen the exhausted nervous system and make good the energy lost by malnutrition (the perversion or diversion of food). In insomnia, where there is an almost continuous leakage of energy, physical movement will have to be prescribed in very careful doses according to the stage of the disease, the amount of loss of sleep and consequent dissipation of energy and the movement that will just suffice to woo " Nature's tired restorer," and slowly replenish the exhausted nervous system by providing that sound sleep which economises the patient's expenditure of nerve-force.

The quantity and quality of sleep, the amount of brain work, the appetite and a great many other vital matters must be taken into consideration, so it will be seen that in the prescription of physical movement so as to restore and rebuild an exhausted nervous system, a physician will have a much more delicate work to perform than he has in the prescription of medicine.

RE-BUILDING THE NERVOUS SYSTEM.

Rest and physical movement must be kept within exact balance, and this alone is a work requiring the most exact diagnosis and a keen and sympathetic insight into human nature, a perfect knowledge of the physiological effect of each and every muscular movement, the power to adjust movement to recruit the exhausted nervous system in specific cases by better digestion and better sleep, the ability to ensure balance between income and outgo of nervous energy, and all those rare gifts of health accountancy which can raise a body and nervous system from a state of liquidation to solvency and the possession of a handsome Reserve Fund in the Bank of Health.

To summarise, then, let me present the case briefly to the reader as follows:—

THE HOW AND WHY OF NEURASTHENIA.

1. Neurasthenia, strictly speaking, is not a disease, but a nervous condition brought about by the over-expenditure of nervous energy with a diminished income, until the condition of physical bankruptcy has been reached.

2. The nervous system being the regulator of all the bodily functions, its failure has an evil effect on every other function of the body. It starts the body on a sort of " rake's progress," in which every system, organ and function is involved. It impairs digestion (and so decreases income still more), it provokes insomnia (and so swells nervous expenditure), it causes a lowering of all the vital functions of life and so sets up a vicious circle in the body reacting again injuriously on the central nervous system and brain.

3. It almost invariably arises from mental work or overstrain, intense emotion, passion or feeling, or sudden shock. It is characterised by many symptoms, the chief of which are lack of faith, fear, depression, doubt, loss of confidence and loss of self-control.

4. The brain and nervous system, kept in a continual state of over-tension, conscious or sub-conscious, with a perpetual leakage of nervous energy by overwork, consumes supplies to such an extent that the digestive cells become exhausted and are unable to feed themselves, much less supply the hungry and starving brain and nerve-cells. The brain and nervous system becomes a parasite, and (slowly robs other 'systems of their vitality. Other cells of other systems then begin to suffer and deteriorate through malnutrition, and at last the whole physical organism becomes bankrupt. There has been a " run " on the Bank of Health until it stops payment altogether. The sufferer is like a person who has been living on borrowed money and who has pledged everything he possesses and borrowed from every source until the crisis comes, and he is unable to satisfy his creditors.

5.	Through ignorance of the laws of health and its management his body has gone into liquidation, and only now is the doctor usually called in to set matters right if he can. It is just as if a business firm refused to call in an auditor and accountant until it became insolvent. The real duty of the doctor should be to make periodical examinations of the state of the patient's health affairs, to ascertain his health assets and his liabilities, and to avoid or avert bankruptcy by keeping a strict record of the health income and expenditure of the patient.

6.	What is now to be done? The first thing is to cut down expenditure. The next to increase income, pay off all debts, and place a plentiful supply of nervous energy as a Reserve Fund in the Bank of Health. How can this be done? Drugs alone cannot do it. Food alone will not do it. Only balanced physical movement will replenish the system with new stores of nervous energy.

HOW IT CAN BE CONQUERED.

7.	Everything that lives manifests its life by movement. The nerve-cells and the cells of the brain are living things. They live by movement, their own movement and the movement also of all these cells in the body upon which they are dependent for their supplies of new energy.

8.	Food and air are the two chief sources of vitality or nervous energy. But food without movement is dead, and the oxygen in the air can only be taken into the body in sufficient quantities through movement.

9.	The movement of the voluntary muscles brings into step every cell of the body, as already shown. By increasing respiration it means the intake of more oxygen. It also increases the muscular movement of the cells of the involuntary muscles associated with digestion, circulation and elimination. Thus, physical movement means more oxygen to vitalise the nerve centres and every nerve-cell, and more nutrition because the food is more thoroughly digested and more nourishment extracted from it.

10.	But the movement of all the voluntary muscles in balance means more than this. It also means the freer elimination of waste matter and self-generated poison caused by the many vital activities of the body, so that the blood—through which the nerve-cells are supplied—is both purified and enriched, for the cells of the eliminatory system are also automatically set moving by the movement of all the voluntary muscles in proper relationship.

11.	All this movement, then, means the better aeration, nutrition and purification of the whole nervous system from the beginning. The nerve-cells live, as it were, in a healthier environment, are better nourished and made stronger in every way. Thus the income of nervous energy is greatly increased.

12.	Further, a more equable circulation of the blood is established by this all-round physical movement with a fairer rationing system to every cell of the body and brain, which relieves the cerebral congestion and over-tension of the brain cells, dispels morbid mental and nervous symptoms due to circulatory disturbance, and so promotes healthy, natural sleep.

13. Venous and abdominal congestion is also relieved, still further assisting in the removal of waste and poisonous refuse that otherwise would remain to irritate and inflame the nerves.

14. Physical movements, carried out with mental concentration on the parts moved, school the will and give one the power of self-control, the lack of which is one of the chief symptoms of neurasthenia. This means power to restrain or suppress superfluous and unnecessary muscular movements, restlessness, and mental aberrations that cause a vast and extravagant expenditure to the neurasthenic. So the expenditure of nervous energy is cut down to an irreducible minimum.

This natural method of treating neurasthenia, in short, cultivates and increases all the resources of the body that will add to the depleted nervous income of the neurasthenic, enforce a fairer distribution both of labour and supplies in body and brain, and prevent extravagance and waste in the expenditure of nervous energy, thus enriching not only the nervous system but the whole body, and infusing the whole organism with new life and energy. The tension on brain and nerve cells is reduced to normal, and the cells multiply more fruitfully, younger and better cells take their place, healthier, stronger and more vigorous, so that in time the sufferer may be said literally to have a new and better brain and nervous system as well as a new and better body.

For long, neurasthenia has been regarded as a sort of mystery disease, the no-man's-land of medical science, because it is a condition entirely beyond the domain of medicine, and to give a neurasthenic medicines or drugs is at best only like giving a temporary dole to one who really needs new sources of income. Here are the means at hand by which the exhausted nervous system can be firmly and permanently re-established by methods which, I am confident every serious medical student will agree, are based on a sound physiological foundation. I have no desire to usurp the rightful place of the medical man nor to arrogate to myself an authority I do not possess. All I am anxious to do is to present facts, proved facts, that I have gleaned in a field of therapeutics which I have made peculiarly my own after nearly 30 years of personal study, observation and experience, to the medical profession, and I offer them both to physician and patient for serious consideration in the belief and faith that they will be of service in the alleviation of human suffering and the physical reconstruction of humanity. The methods are Nature's not mine, and all that I have done is to enlist and employ them, as I hope the medical profession soon also will do,—will, indeed, be compelled yet to do,—in the service of all who suffer and are in pain.

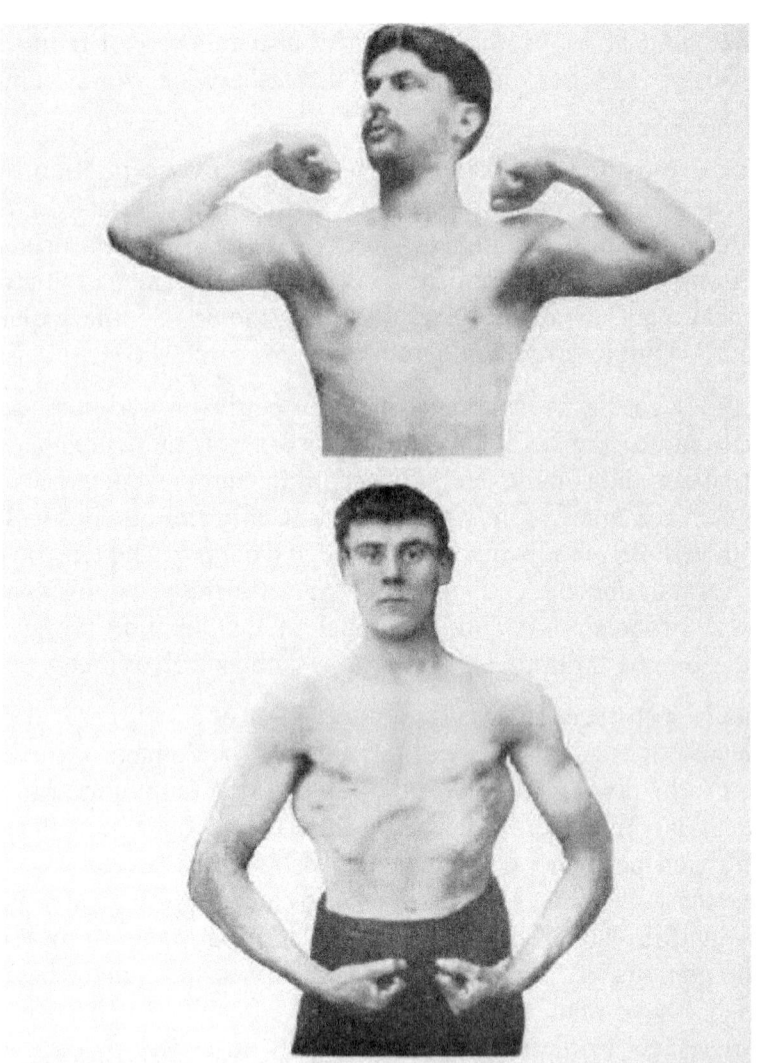

Two young men whose bodies were built up scientifically by the methods described in this book. The lower one shows remarkable chest development and expansion, and is a fine example to encourage the youth of the country.

The attention of those who are ailing or diseased, and of medical men and medical students, is particularly directed to the Appendix to this chapter, dealing with a most interesting article and letter on Physical Treatment that appeared in The Lancet, the leading medical journal, after this chapter had been written.—Author.

CHAPTER XXIV.

How and Why Scientific Physical Movement is Nature's Cure for Disease.

ALTHOUGH this book has been written primarily with the object of showing how the State can, by a rational and national system of compulsory physical education and reconstruction in our schools, go very far on the road to the complete prevention and elimination of disease, there is nothing in this book that does not apply with equal, or almost equal, force to the adult who is to-day suffering for the mistakes of faulty educational methods and the disease-tending habits of modern civilised life.

In other words, the methods I have described will be found equally as valuable in the cure of existent disease (with very few exceptions) as for its ultimate prevention in the individual and final elimination from a world in which it should have no place. For this reason, therefore, I would like everyone, whether of normal condition seeking to prevent weakness and disease or who is suffering from that physical weakness which assuredly leads to disease, or who is actually already in a state of disease, to read most carefully the earlier part of this book, to study and understand the basic principles of the methods there more fully explained, and to realise that there is scarcely any form of physical weakness or disease with which we are familiar to-day that is not amenable to successful treatment by this simple and quite natural method.

THE DECLINE AND FALL OF MAN.

Disease, as I have shown, is largely the product of that lack of all-round physical movement which was absolutely a necessity of mere existence in those far-off days when disease was unknown to man. It has taken centuries upon centuries for man to fall from his former high physical estate, and the process has been so slow and insidious that its progress has scarcely been observed until man has become an easy prey to forms of disease that were unheard of even a century or two ago. Just as man rose by slow degrees to his erect physical position and the vertebrate brain, so he has fallen from health by a kind of inverted geometrical progression until his body has lost its pristine vigour and resistant power to disease.

The first step, therefore, in the successful treatment and cure of disease, as in its prevention, must be to restore to the human body that individual strength to resist which alone can overcome disease. We must return, so far as is possible to-day, to the path marked out for us by Nature, and intended for us by Nature's God. The law of movement, which is the law of life, has been violated, and disease is humanity's punishment. That law is as exact and as unvarying as the law that holds the sun in its course and guides the seasons in their coming and going.

Elsewhere in this book I have said that all disease may be attributed ultimately to defective metabolism, that is, to loss of balance between the waste and repair that is ever going on in the body, but I might reduce this definition even to simpler terms by saying that all disease is really the evidence of some disturbance of the circulation of the blood, or the apparatus of circulation, including the heart, arteries, veins, and capillaries, and in the consequent lowering effect on the resistant power of the bodily cells. Feeble, congested, impaired, or arrested circulation from some cause or other can be said to be the most prolific cause of all disease, because it interferes with and arrests nutrition, growth, and development in some part or parts of the body and prevents the free elimination of waste and poisonous matter.

When the blood travels slowly and sluggishly in its channels, or is impeded in any way, it means that supplies are held up or brought slowly, and, consequently, in insufficient quantities to every part of the body, and also that the waste which is produced daily by the vital operations of the body and its cells is imperfectly eliminated. In fact, a sort of bodily blockade is established, transport and distribution are interrupted, and the cellular community of the body is not only ill-nourished, but is left to live in an insanitary state because the sewerage system of the body is unflushed by the slowly moving blood, and foetid matter accumulates. Starvation and stagnation unite to produce, encourage and foster disease just as the slimy and stagnant pool is provocative of deadly disease and fatal to every form of life.

Now, as I have explained, through the voluntary muscular system, we can reach every cell in every part, organ, and system of the body. The blood-circulation is the connecting-rod, and the various muscles may be described as so many keys that wind up the engine of the whole system, the heart, and set the connecting-rod moving more fastly. In this way the heart, like a powerful force pump, sets the blood circulating rapidly and vigorously in all its myriad channels, carrying copious supplies of food, air, and vitality to every cell even in the remotest part of the body, and sweeping out all refuse and waste matter just as a powerful hose cleans out a sewer.

This means that every cell is well fed, well nourished, and kept living in the most hygienic environment. Consequently the cells are built up strong, healthy, and free from any weakness or disease by the natural movement of the voluntary muscles in balance, until the whole body presents an invincible front to disease, while the cells multiply more rapidly, and continue constantly to develop in strength and resistant power until they attain to their highest standard and limit of fitness and efficiency. To prevent disease, therefore, seems so natural that one wonders why civilisation has been allowed to deprive humanity so long of the chief and basic essential of healthy life, the natural and balanced movement of the voluntary muscular system in a scientific way to suit present-day demands of life and to help rather than hinder the onward march of civilisation.

The elements of health—the essentials as distinct from the non- essentials—are so simple and easy to obtain that one wonders why humanity has not been better shielded from disease through the ages than it has, and why it has been necessary for the expenditure of such enormous sums of money to combat it.

" I die," said the great Sydenham, " but I leave behind me three greater physicians—-Air, Exercise, and Water;" and travelling far down the corridors of Time, we find such a distinguished modern as Professor Osier, Regius Professor of Cambridge University, supporting me in this, for he declares that " modern treatment relies greatly upon the natural methods, in other words, giving the natural forces the fullest scope by easy and thorough nutrition, increased flow of blood, and removal of obstructions to the excretory system or the circulation in the tissues."

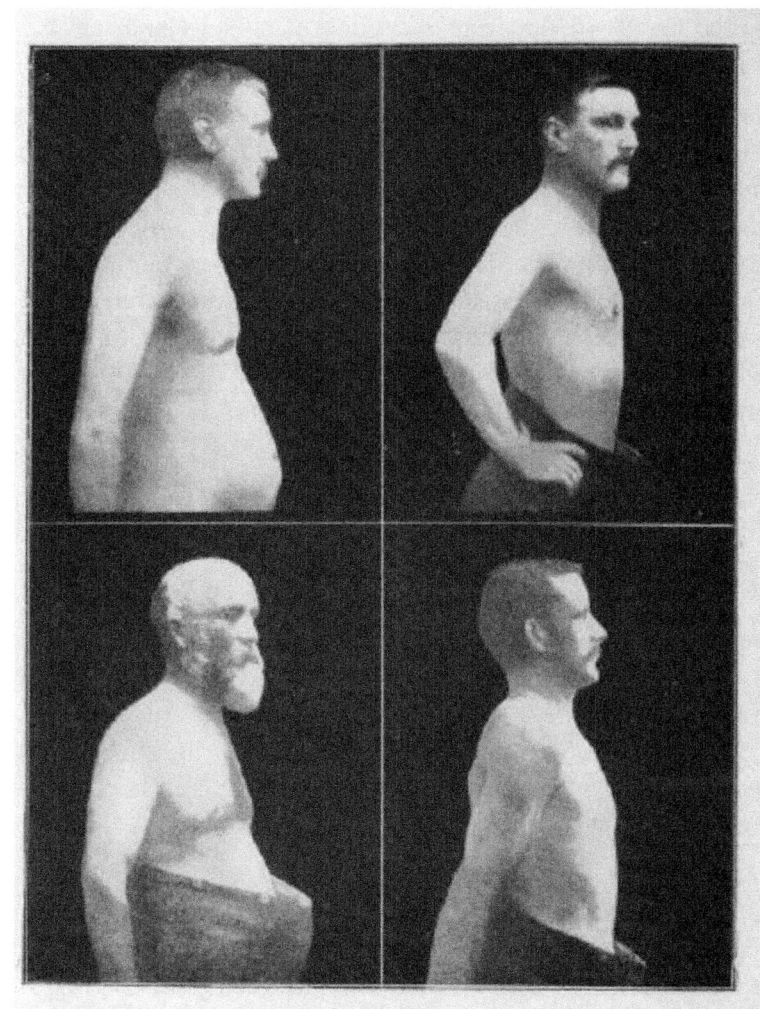

Before and after photos of cases of abdominal obesity successfully treated by these methods, without any restrictions on diet or the use of drugs. These, of course, are only a few out of thousands who have equally benefited in various forms of obesity. This is Nature's method of reducing superfluous flesh without risk of injury to the general health.

RELATION OF FUNCTION TO MUSCLE.

What does this mean? It means that the successful treatment and cure of disease depend mainly on improving the functions of respiration, nutrition, circulation, secretion and excretion. The most serious diseases may be traced ultimately to some minute departure from the normal in the functioning of the body, and anything that will improve and stimulate function must, therefore, strike at the very root and source of disease. In other words, impaired or arrested functioning, especially of circulation, lowers bodily resistant power to disease in any or all of its forms, and, conversely, the restoration of functional activity everywhere, and of a free-flowing circulation of the blood in the body must increase bodily resistant power and enable it to conquer disease.

But I have proved in my chapter on " The Physiology of Bodily Reconstruction " that function is dependent upon muscular power, assisted by the nervous system, although so great a physiologist as Professor Schiff has shown that muscular tissue has a contractile power independent of that supplied to it by the nerves. Whether, however, the motive power comes from the nervous system or is latent in muscular tissue is not to the point here, because we know that the muscles are the agents of function; indeed, that muscle is, after all,, only " crystallised function."

Thus, by natural and easy stages we are led to the logical conclusion that muscle plays a predominant part in function, and that through the muscular system over which we have direct control we can reach, develop and improve every bodily function, and thus, at one blow, reach and remove the most fruitful cause of disease, viz., impaired, diminished, or arrested function. Now is it not equally logical to deduce from this, the now proved fact, that if we use and develop all the voluntary muscles in balance, thus, as I have shown, automatically bringing into play all the involuntary muscles, we are also increasing and improving the functional activity of every organ and of every cell of every organ, and in this way also developing in strength every organ by its own use and movement.

NO SYSTEM DISEASED ALONE.

The medical profession has undoubtedly made a very great mistake in the specialised treatment of disease—and by that I mean not treatment by special methods but the consideration and treatment only of special organs and systems—as it has done by its classification and multiplication of so-called diseases. As I have said, all disease is one, and what are called diseases are merely various expressions and evidences of a single cause. In one, it takes the form of indigestion; in another, rheumatism; in another, say, tubercular disease. How much even of the latter most deadly disease may be traced ultimately to faulty digestion and elimination causing malnutrition and loss of vital resistant power it would not be easy to say, but the percentage must certainly be very high.

If there is disease anywhere in the body there must be disease everywhere, just as the derangement of one wheel in a machine will interfere with and upset the working of every part of the machine. True, certain organs and systems are more closely inter-related and inter-dependent than others, but all are affected in degree by each and all of the others. For anyone to attempt to overcome nervous troubles, for instance, by treating the nervous system only, is, as Euclid says, absurd.

The digestive system and the respiratory system must be affected injuriously by any breakdown of the nervous system, and, on the other hand, the nervous breakdown cannot but interfere with the healthy functioning of the digestive system, and in a minor degree also of the respiratory system. The circulatory and eliminatory systems, the beating of the heart, the passage of supplies to every part of the body, and the elimination of waste and poisonous matter from the entire organism are all dependent of the nervous system. How then can a man propose to specialise in nervous disorders, when so many other systems and organs are malignly affected by them.

CURING ONE DISEASE OFTEN PREVENTS ANOTHER.

Again, on the same principle, what cures one disease should cure all, for the same basic principles must underlie all successful treatment, or, at least, all treatment that is really radical and not palliative, or what I have heard described as " medical patchwork." To heal and cure a diseased body is not merely to put, as it were, a patch on here or there, but to build up, or rebuild, a body so strong and healthy in unison that it will tower invincible not over any particular form of disease in any particular bodily locality, but over disease in every form and in every system.

Furthermore, it must always be borne in mind that to build up the body in such balanced strength in any and every part is not only to cure some actual form of disease, but to prevent others of a more gross and deadly character. To cure dyspepsia may appear no very great triumph in itself, but it must be remembered that by banishing the dyspepsia, and consequent malnutrition, we are also preventing all the more deadly diseases that are contingent upon the dyspeptic condition. To cure—or, rather, to radically overcome—any form of disease may he, indeed, also to prevent others, because any form of disease diminishes vitality and resistant power not only in the actual seat of the ailment but everywhere else in the body.

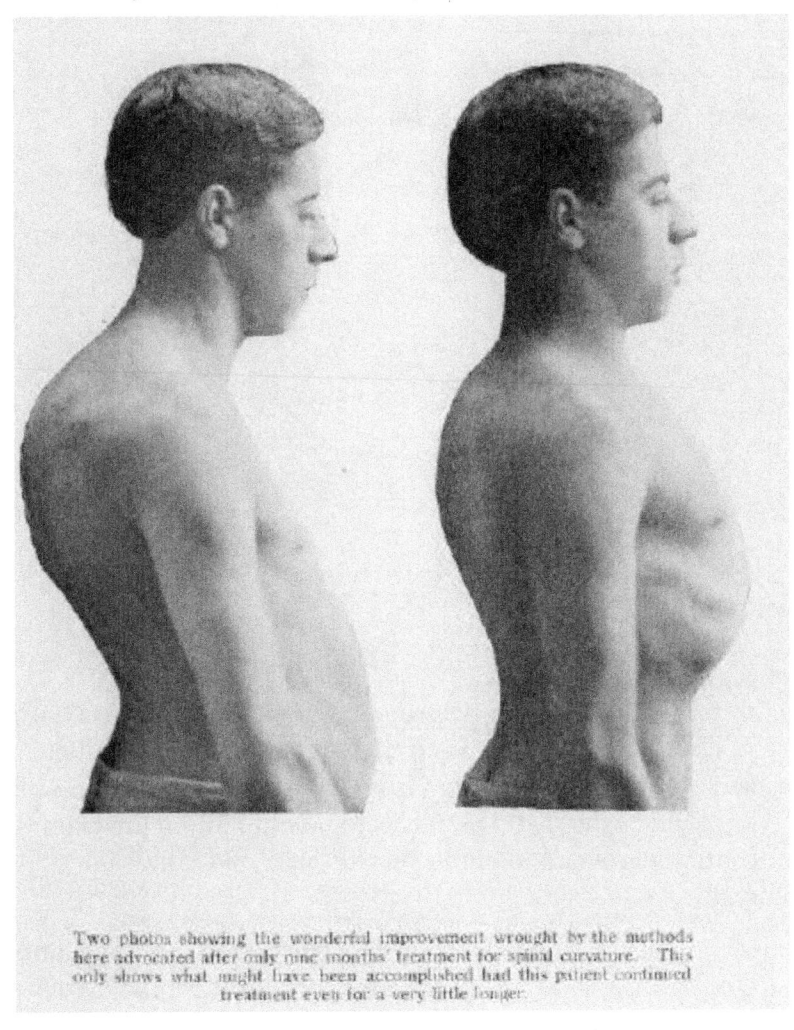

Two photos showing the wonderful improvement wrought by the methods here advocated after only nine months' treatment for spinal curvature. This only shows what might have been accomplished had this patient continued treatment even for a very little longer.

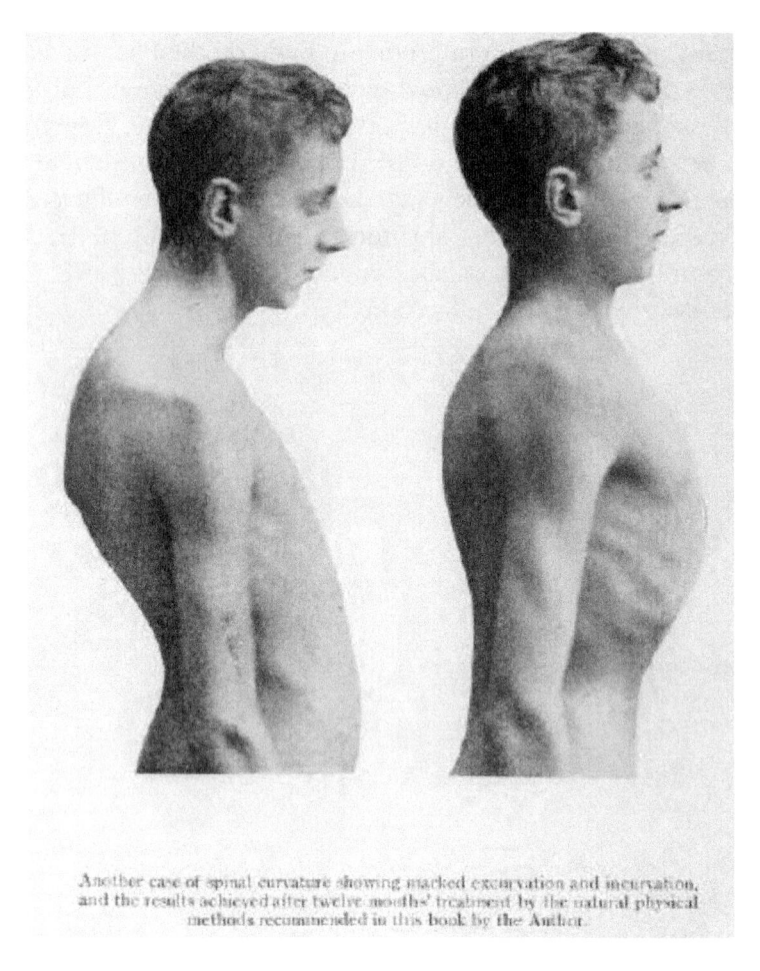

Another case of spinal curvature showing marked excurvation and incurvation, and the results achieved after twelve months' treatment by the natural physical methods recommended in this book by the Author.

DISEASE HAS A SINGLE CAUSE.

It will be evident, therefore, that the only real cure for disease— just as it is the only real preventive of it—is to develop the body in such perfect and balanced strength everywhere that it will offer an impregnable front to disease. That is to say, nothing really cures any form of disease that will not cure every form of disease. There was logic after all, in the claim of the charlatan or quack who sold a nostrum warranted to cure every disease under the sun. If it could cure one it should be able to cure all.

The curative physical therapeutics described here, being but the application of natural and fundamental laws to the diseased body, with the provision of the most favourable conditions for Nature to minister to it, have been so successful in a vast and varied number of nearly every form of human disease, that their very success has, to some extent, caused them to be regarded with doubt and suspicion by those who have too long regarded disease as separate and distinct morbid entities rather than as effects all arising from a single and similar cause.

That cause is the diminished, resistant power of the body itself, and especially in some particular part or parts where the weakness most manifests itself, for disease invariably attacks at the weakest spot, and too often, also, breaks through the bodily line of resistance. Reinforcements must be rushed to that part if the situation is to be saved, and the whole bodily chain must be secure in equal strength in each and every link.

The body is only as strong as its weakest cell, and only through the voluntary muscles within our control and the circulatory system, can we bring the balanced movement to each and every cell of the body that is essential to make and keep it in the highest state of physical efficiency to supply the body in every part, with that capital and reserve of vitality to make and keep it strong enough to resist disease and to make and keep all the cells in harmonious strength and relationship to each other, so that the body presents in each and every part an insuperable barrier to every form of disease.

CELLS GROW WEAK THROUGH LACK OF MOVEMENT.

Let us take, for example, an everyday case of indigestion or dyspepsia, a condition, by the way, that is too often lightly regarded as a necessary evil of modern life, whereas, it is really responsible for many of the most serious and deadly diseases that develop through its presence and neglect. Now what are the usual and traditional measures taken in the effort to relieve and cure this condition. Certain foods are debarred. Diet is cut down. Pepsin and other so-called digestives are prescribed. In other words, instead of seeking to make the cells of the stomach and digestive system stronger, everything possible is done to make them weaker.

The fact is quite overlooked that all these cells are living muscular entities and that their muscular power is not to be developed by diminishing their use and movement but by increasing it gradually, just as we build up the muscles of an arm or a leg. By the usual methods adapted, these cells of the whole digestive tract that are directly responsible for the nutrition of the body can never be made stronger, but must become weaker through lack of movement, so that the patient grows weaker through lack of nutrition. The appetite fails through lack of the movement necessary to make the cells hungry. The cells require then but little food, or food eaten is of little or no value to them, and even injurious, through lack of the necessary motive-power to digest and assimilate it, because the voluntary muscle-cells do not receive sufficient movement to keep all the voluntary cells active, and so create appetite and digestive power.

But the trouble does not end here. When the digestive cells fail, strike or mutiny either through unemployment and consequent innutrition, a series of what might be called sympathetic strikes begin to take place in other systems of the body. All the other cells suffer through innutrition and may cry out in pain because they are irritated, inflamed and injured by the accumulation of waste in the system through lack of sufficient movement in some part or parts' to ensure its removal. The cells of the bodily sanitary system become too weak to carry out their important function of elimination. All the bodily cells, in fact, suffer in unison with the suffering digestive cells. Their muscular power decreases just as the muscles of the arm would shrink, through lack of use and movement.

ASSISTING THE NATURAL CHANCES IN THE BODY.

Digestion and the assimilation of nutriment with the free elimination of waste and poisonous matter—the two main factors in the establishment of sound bodily health—are mainly carried out by muscles that can be strengthened and developed by natural physical movements. The churning movement by which the food is tossed about in the stomach, and by which it is more thoroughly submitted to the digestive action of the gastric juice, is increased by such movement, and the cells of the muscles of digestion are all made stronger and more efficient in the performance of their functions. So, too, the cells that are responsible for the elimination of waste and poisonous matter can only be kept in the highest state of efficiency and capable of working to their full capacity through the movement of the voluntary muscular system in the way I have described. The cells of both these systems are not only made stronger and more vigorous, but they multiply more quickly, and each generation of new cells is better in every way than the preceding ones. Thus these two systems responsible for nutrition and elimination are practically rebuilt by improved and accelerated metabolism, that is, more rapid repair of the waste that is continually going on in the body, and more perfect elimination of that waste from the system, through the better and faster circulation of the blood.

When all the voluntary muscles of the body are brought into play in balance, it is very much like winding up a clock with a key, and by such an act every organ and system is set moving and kept moving. The cells of the muscles moved need more supplies to repair the force spent by the movement. The digestive cells are thus called up to do their work more thoroughly to meet this demand, and so themselves become stronger and fitter by this movement. The cell chemists of the body are also made to move about their duties smartly and efficiently, and are maintained at their highest capacity. And the " little vessels " in the blood that carry nourishment and air to each and every part of the body travel faster and further as a result of the movement. Every cell of every system, in short, is, as it were, exercised and developed when all the voluntary muscles are moved in balance, and all these cells are better nourished, more thoroughly oxygenated, and provided with the hygienic bodily environment that enables them to thrive vigorously and multiply rapidly, with a continually improving progeny.

Thus the movement of all the voluntary muscles in balance is the only possible way by which we can literally rebuild a new and better body in every part, or strengthen and make disease-free any part that is weak or diseased by bringing the whole organism into perfect balance. This was Nature's method from the beginning of things, by which man was given and enabled to maintain a body in such perfect balance as to be supreme over weakness or disease, because he was compelled to live a life of all-round physical activity in those days. It is still Nature's way of maintaining the body in health and preventing disease, and it is the only way in which Nature will cure and overcome disease, but we must to-day obtain the same balanced physical activity in a concentrated form, because of the conditions and demands of modern life.

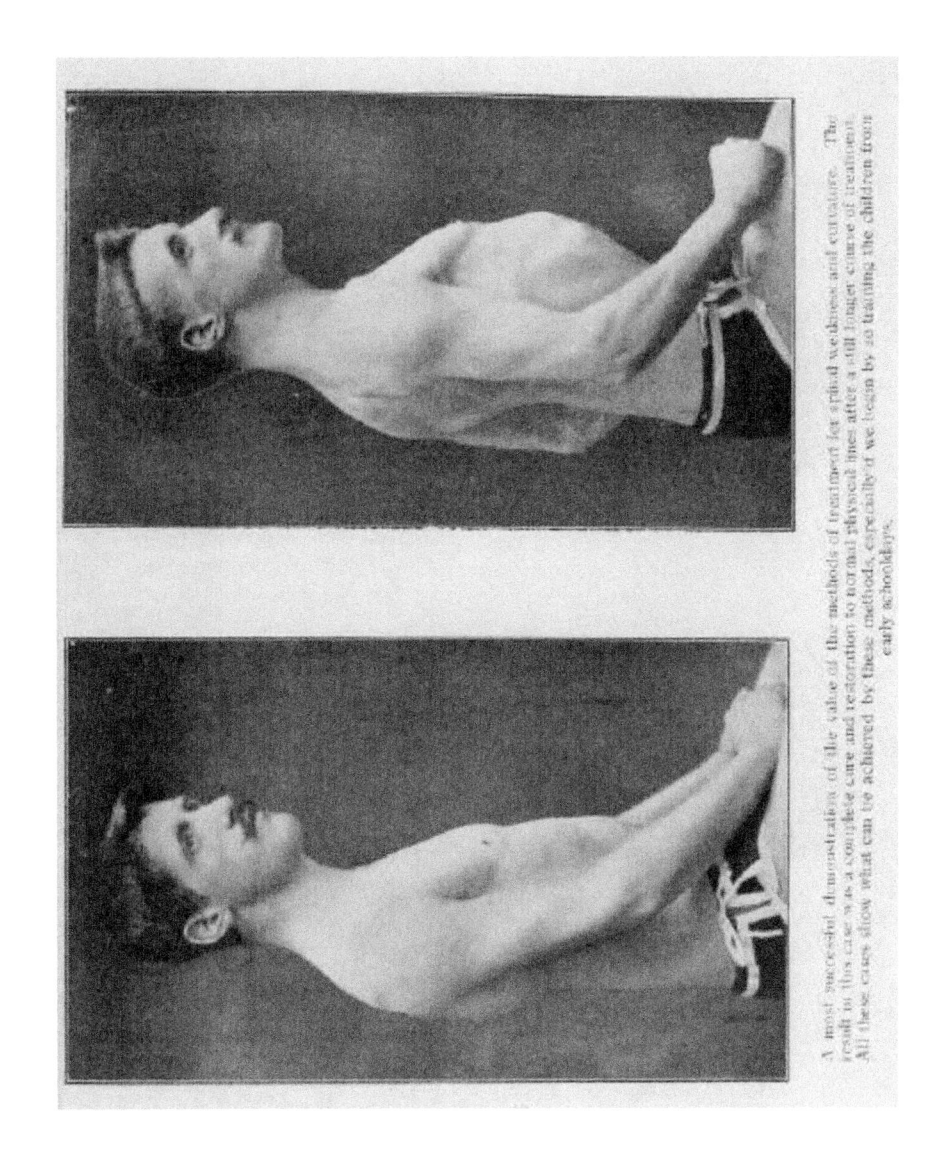

A most successful demonstration of the value of the methods of treatment set forth we discuss and curvature. The result in this case was a complete cure and restoration to normal physical lines after a still longer course of treatment. All these cases show what can be achieved by these methods, especially if we begin by so training the children from early schooldays.

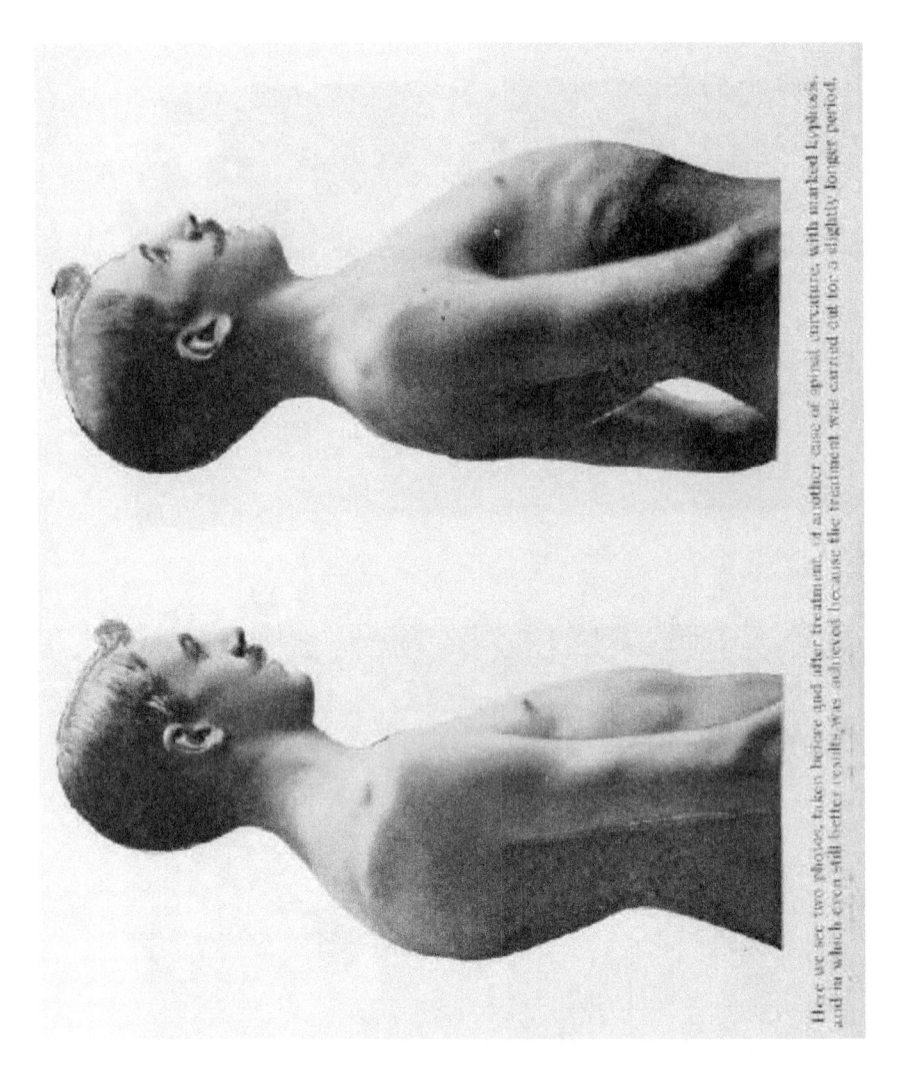

Here we see two photos, taken before and after treatment, of another case of spinal curvature, with marked kyphosis, and in which even still better results was achieved because the treatment was carried out for a slightly longer period.

NATURE'S GREATEST HEALING AGENT.

Muscular movement is Nature's greatest therapeutic agent, and the scientific application of natural physical movement to a weak, diseased or deformed body in any part does not give a mere artificial and transient sense of increased strength and betterment in that part, but actually rebuilds any organ or system of better material and enables all the cell-workers and fighters of the body to carry out their functional duties better and more easily. In short, organic function is developed by the improvement of cellular function, while in actual organic disease an organ can itself be rebuilt by the increased movement and multiplication of its cells, and by permitting only the survival of the fittest and strongest.

To impress upon medical men the almost incredible possibilities of what may be achieved by the process of cellular evolution, I am reproducing here photographs of a remarkable case in which there was not only very marked spinal curvature but actual tubercular disease of the spine and pulmonary consumption, so serious, indeed, that it had been given up as incurable by medical men. The patient was a Mr Harold Robinson, of Oldham, and the lateral curvature was originally to the extent of quite 7\ inches from the normal. In addition to his other afflictions, Mr Robinson also suffered from a dislocation of the hip. He was informed that it would be impossible for him to live any length of time, and that he would never be able to walk again.

The patient is to-day a well-known man in Oldham, and his case naturally aroused something like a local sensation, for he is now not only living and well, but has an exceptionally well-developed physique, and his spine is almost straight again. In addition to this, he is something of an athlete, and, apart from the fact that he has been able to discard crutches altogether, he is a cyclist and a swimmer.

This remarkable cure and transformation was brought about entirely by the natural methods that I am describing and advocating, and accomplished in a grown-up person. I select it for illustration because it is one that can best be understood from photographic and ocular evidence, and because it is easier to illustrate deformities than disease for obvious reasons, but these same natural methods are equally successful in the cure of disease. I could, of course, present many photographs of persons who have been freed from lordosis and scoliosis, but feel confident that the photographs of Mr Robinson and a few others will be sufficient to satisfy and convince the most sceptical.

The facts in Mr Robinson's case particularly are so remarkable that many well-known Oldham people have had pleasure in subscribing their names to the following form: —

" We, the undersigned, have pleasure in stating that Mr Harold Robinson, of 100, Chadderton Road, Oldham, who a few years ago was only able to walk with crutches, is able to dispense with crutches entirely, and he can now walk for miles without them.

For many years Mr Robinson suffered with very marked curvature of the spine, the spine being quite 7½ inches out of line. There was also dislocation of the hip. Mr Robinson was informed that it would be impossible for him to live any length of time, and that he would never be able to walk again. His spine is now almost straight. He enjoys perfect health, and has a remarkably good physique, the muscular development being wonderfully marked, and it is unquestionable he is far above the average man in physical strength. In addition to now being able to walk without crutches, he can ride a bicycle and swim. We have asked Mr Robinson to what he attributes these splendid results, and he states emphatically that his marvellous improvement is entirely due to the careful and regular following out of Mr Sandow's treatment."

The names attached to this memorandum include some of Oldham's best known people, and the following are only a few of the signatures:—

(Signed) W. ANDREW, J.P.

(Signed) COUNCILLOR H. KEMPE, O.M.

(Signed) W. H. PIGOTT, Superintendent of Police.

(Signed) REV. STANLEY BUCKLEY.

(Signed) SQUIRE DUNKERLEY, Alderman.

(Signed) GEO. ROBERTS, Missionary.

(Signed) W. SCHOLES, Manager.

(Signed) H. RILEY, Salvation Army.

(Signed) E. J. CHAMPETT, Instructor of Physical Training to Oldham Schools.

(Signed) THOS. BEATTIE, General Superintendent.

etc., etc.

Now it will be conceded that if such a remarkable rebuilding of the human body can be accomplished in the case of a grown-up person much greater results may well be expected when the physical bodies of all receive this attention from early childhood.

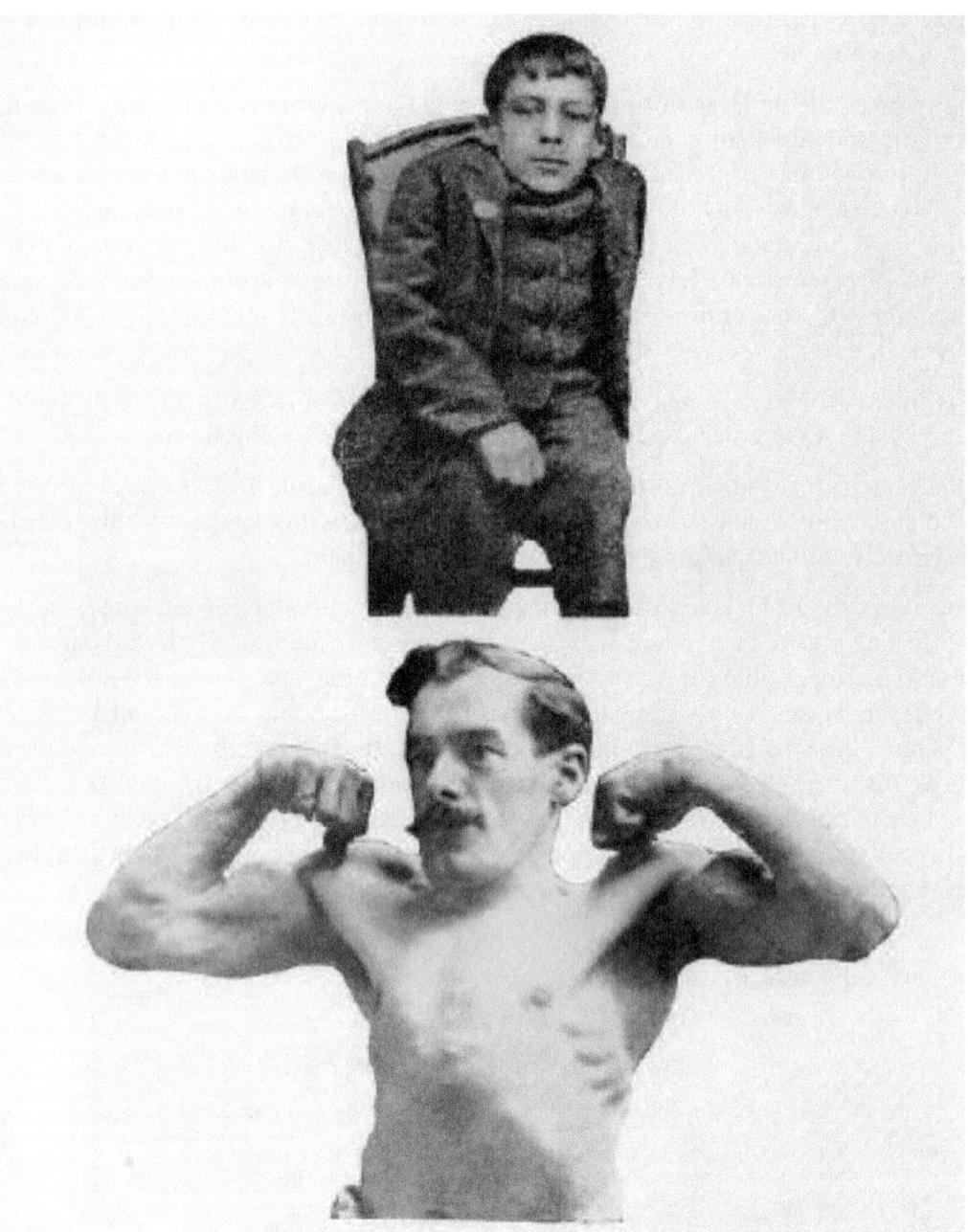

MR. HAROLD ROBINSON, of Oldham, Lancs.

These are two photos of the gentleman whose case is fully described in this chapter. Were it not for these photographs showing him as he was, a helpless cripple, and as he is to-day, a healthy and robust man; together with the contributory evidence supplied by local gentlemen, who have known his whole life-story, such a physical transformation might well tax anyone's credulity to breaking point. This was achieved solely by the methods described in these pages, and this is only one of thousands of cases of curvature and deformities overcome by such natural methods of treatment applied in a scientific way. The photos opposite show

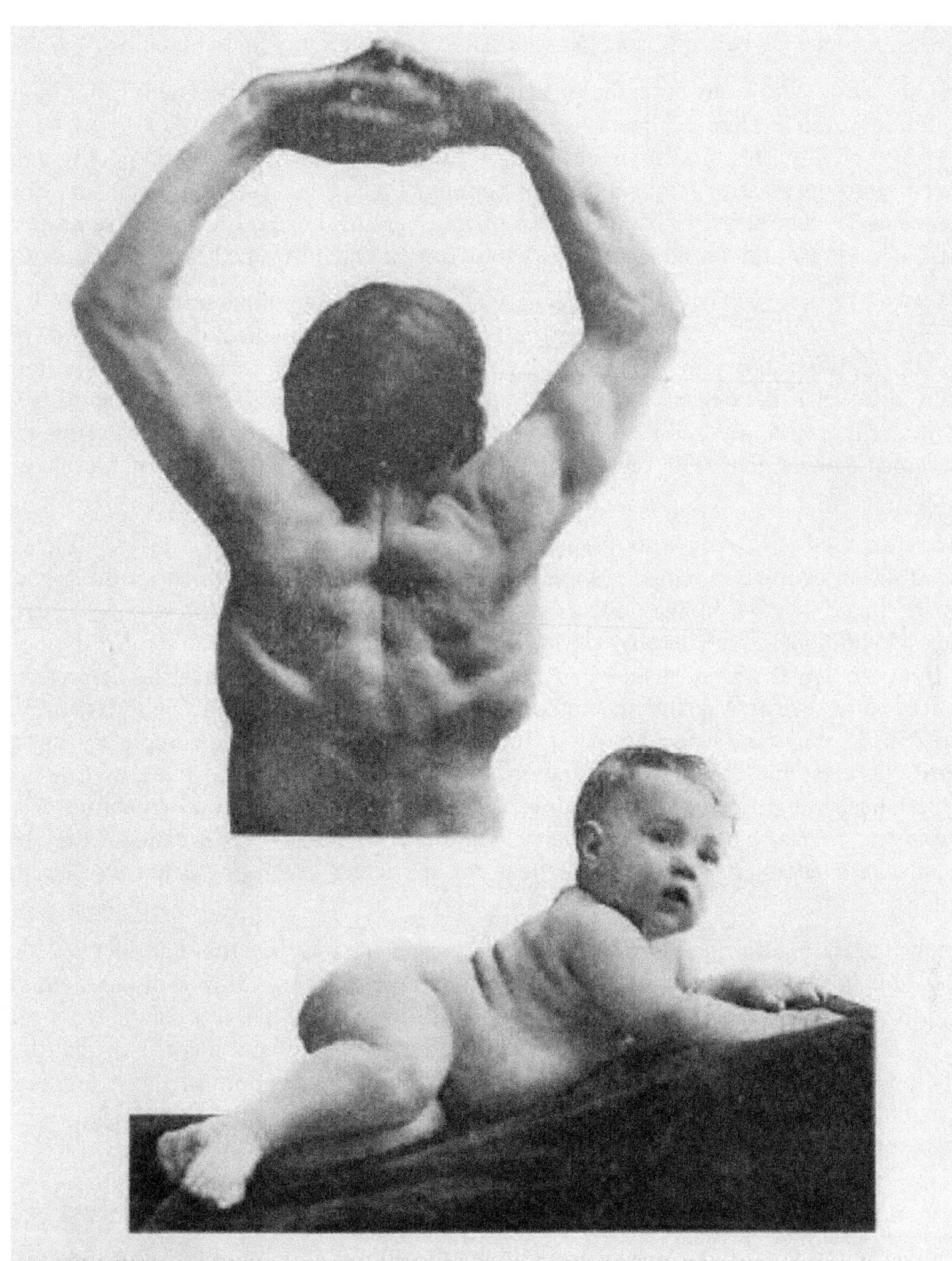

(1) a back view showing the now straightened spine—the spine was no less than 7½ inches from the perpendicular—and fine muscular back and shoulders, with (2) a photo of Mr. Robinson's healthy, chubby and well-formed child. Sensitive as to his own physical defects, Mr. Robinson hesitated long before marrying lest the children who might follow would be similarly afflicted. His cure, however, was so complete that he hesitated no longer, and this sturdy child is the fruit of his marriage. How important, therefore, from the national point of view, are methods of physical reconstruction in their influence through parentage alone upon the children of the future.

WALKING IN NATURE'S FOOTSTEPS.

It is not only the effect of this upon the present generation but upon subsequent generations that must be borne in mind. Here is a man given up by physicians as a hopeless case, yet he is now the father of a child perfect and symmetrical in form, as will be seen from the photograph here reproduced, with no trace of its parental shortcomings. When one sees and considers the vista thus opened up for the release of Nature's own magnificent healing and recuperative properties it will, I am sure, attract and fascinate all those whose duty it is to alleviate human sufferings.

In fact, I go so far as to say that in this discovery of the application of natural physical movement so as to reach and influence each and every cell of the body, the medical profession will be able to solve the greatest problem of life to-day, the one and only method of overcoming or preventing disease. It is Nature's way, and I am certain that the medical men themselves will agree with me that it is impossible to improve upon Nature, which contains and carries the one and only medicament that will rebuild and reconstruct the cellular body of which man is composed.

This natural method of dealing with diseases and even deformities does not deal so much with a diseased stomach or liver or lungs or spine as with a unified body in which all the organs and systems are linked together by the nervous system as a single and indivisible whole. A disturbed and diseased condition of any organ or system may have its origin in some part of the body far remote from the actual seat of disturbance. The whole nervous system may be deranged when there is gastric or digestive disturbance, and may express it in parts of the body far away from the stomach. In the same way, a very trifling nervous disorder will completely upset and temporarily paralyse the function of digestion. A diseased or disordered liver, as most people have experienced some time or other, will cause acute mental depression, irritability or severe head pains and mental confusion. The value, therefore, of methods of treatment that seek to restore balance everywhere rather than to treat any particular organ or system will be at once apparent.

It is because these natural methods regulate cellular and organic function and increase organic strength and balance everywhere that they are so successful in every form of disease. No system or part of the body is allowed to jeopardise the other nor is allowed to live a parasitic existence in the body at the expense of others. Balance is obtained everywhere, and this means that the cells of all the bodily systems are rebuilt and maintained in their due proportion and relationship for the provisioning of the whole organism, its sanitation, and security against disease.

ACCURACY OF DIAGNOSIS AND PRESCRIPTION.

Although I have had to emphasise the importance of exact and correct diagnosis and prescriptions elsewhere, I am reluctantly compelled, owing to its vital importance to success, to refer to this matter again here, especially its necessity in the treatment of actual and existent disease. In ascertaining a true diagnosis nothing is too trifling to be omitted. The patient's age, constitution, organic condition, complaint and existing muscular power must first be ascertained, the conditions that have brought about deterioration and disease fully understood, the true seat of the loss of balance located, the exact nature, quality and amount of movement to suit the patient must be estimated with the utmost exactitude, temperament, family history, habits of life and other purely personal considerations must be noted, and in the selection of movements every care must be taken to prescribe all movements to strict subjection to the state of the heart. Changes of exercises must be prescribed by easy gradations according to a patient's improvement, and no time or labour spared to strengthen particular weak spots until the body, as a complete and organised whole, is made so powerful everywhere in balanced strength as to resist and conquer disease in any form. Needless to add, it is also most essential that the movements are carried out by the patient with his mind wholly concentrated on the muscles being moved.

I am convinced that doctors must and will yet be forced to adopt them, however long they may hesitate and procrastinate. It may be that my grandchildren or great-grandchildren will see what I myself may not live to see, viz., the decision of the whole medical profession to employ natural therapeutics only in the prevention, treatment and cure of disease. But I am confident that, sooner or later, and, if for no other reason, the increasing prevalence of disease will force them to look away from their present methods, and seek their own physical salvation and that of their patients in the true and only way. Already, I know, there are those who will continue my work when I am gone, but I am especially anxious that medical men will give these methods the unanimous support of their profession and at least devote more study and attention to this subject.

So long as the medical profession neglects or fails to give a more just recognition to the part played by the muscular .system in its effect and influence on physiology, so long will disease continue to persist despite their most strenuous efforts towards either its prevention or cure. This is the essential point which I wish to impress upon physician and patient alike. The " bottle-of-medicine-man," to use Sir George Newman's own phrase, is already passing, and doctors everywhere are coming to appreciate the fact that nothing of an artificial character can be introduced into the body that can equal in its beneficent action the power that is ever present in Nature itself. To minister to Nature and to permit the most favourable conditions for the manifestation of that inherent healing power is the best ser v ice that the physician can render to the ailing and diseased body. This can only be done by an approach to those natural conditions under which man was intended to live, viz., a life of balanced physical activity which gave to each and every cell of the body that movement which, in turn, is essential to its living and well-being.

THE CELL THE UNIT OF HEALTH OR DISEASE.

I have shown, and I hope proved, conclusively in this book how we can nearest approximate to that natural healthy life. I have shown how, with our present-day amassed and organised knowledge, we can supply this necessary movement through the voluntary muscular system to every cell of the body, and do so conveniently to suit modern conditions of life. I have shown how it is only through the cellular body that we can re-educate the nerve-centres and reestablish the healthy functioning of every organ and system. This is the way and the only way by which we can either prevent or cure disease. It is in the cell, that microscopic living entity which represents us in miniature, that we will find the true method of emancipating the human body from disease. The prospect is such a fascinating one that it should impel every medical man to turn his thoughts in this direction. Movement is the fundamental phenomenon of life, and when medical men have studied and mastered its influence on cellular function and through it on organic structure and function, they will have gone far towards the solution of a problem that has long baffled, and, indeed, is still baffling, the acutest minds of medical professors throughout the world. I say this with all modesty, and not in any spirit of arrogance, but simply as an honest expression of opinion based on a life of specialised study and personal experience in a subject to which the medical profession has scarcely yet paid sufficient attention. If disease can be cured and prevented, as I most emphatically believe it can, no methods of preventing it or treating it should be considered beneath the dignity of a profession to which the very existence of disease must be a reproach.

The physiological effect of curative physical movement, such as is described in these pages, may be briefly summarised as follows:

1. The body must be regarded as the most perfect automatic machine in the world, not as a number of separate and distinct machines each operating independently of one another.

2. Disease, therefore, must be considered as a unit, for what upsets or hinders the effective operations of any one wheel or even cog in this human automatic machine must interfere with the operations of the machine as a whole.

3. The circulatory system is the connecting-rod through which power is brought from the voluntary muscular system, through the digestive and respiratory system to maintain all the human cogs and wheels in a state of efficiency.

4. Now, to keep the whole machine in perfect working order, each and every part must do its fair and proportionate share of the work, operating at its fullest capacity easily and efficiently. All this work of the body is done by the living cells, which can only be kept fit and strong and able to reproduce better cells of their own species by movement and use.

5. Life is movement, and unless kept moving, any part and, in time, every part of the body will weaken and become diseased, or, if deprived of movement long enough, must die, just as machinery will rust and rot if not kept constantly in use.

6. In health, the living cells that carry on the work of the body constitute an ideal community of muscular workers and fighters. Each species of these millions of cells has its allotted task to perform. Some build tissue, some prepare the supplies for bodily maintenance, some are chemists, some soldiers, some look after distribution, and some are scavengers.

7. Every organ and system of the body is upbuilt and maintained by the movement of these cells, and every bodily function is performed by them. Over some of these cells we can exercise direct control, others are beyond our direct control or only partially subject to it. All can be reached and influenced, however, through the voluntary muscles and the cells of which they are composed. Nourishment and air are supplied to them from the digestive and respiratory systems by the circulatory blood, and the distribution is improved by this movement of the voluntary muscles. So, too, is the elimination of all waste and poisonous matter.

8. The cells of the voluntary muscles are the only cells we can move directly at will, and by so moving them we increase their capacity, efficiency and output, improve them in quality and increase them in number, old and feeble cells succumbing, leaving only the youthful and strongest. Thus we make a voluntary muscle bigger and better by moving it at will, and this movement, bringing the blood to it more vigorously, all the cells,

including the nerve-cells it contains, are better nourished and their waste matter more freely carried away. These nerve cells, it is important to remember, keep that particular part of the body in communication with every part of the body, including the brain. All the cells in the muscles moved are rejuvenated by the movement of the muscle, and if every voluntary muscle were moved in the same way in balance all would be similarly benefited.

9. Conversely, if the muscles or any of the muscles are kept without movement, the cells of those muscles, including the nerve-cells which link them up with other parts of the body, are deprived of their full share of supplies and the free elimination of their waste through the lack of movement, and so become weak and unfit, while many die. Thus the unmoved muscle or muscles diminish in size and substance, and the muscle, if kept long enough unmoved, atrophies. The nerve-cells in all such unmoved muscles also suffer in the same way, and this is immediately communicated to other parts of the body by the nervous telegraphic system, causing disease and disharmony, or lack of balance.

10. But. as I have shown in my chapter on " What is Scientific Physical Movement," the voluntary movement of even one muscle only or group of muscles immediately sets the involuntary cells of every other system of the body in motion to supply again the force that has-been consumed by its, or their own, movement, and to carry away the waste that has been caused by the contraction.

11. Now this simple muscular movement of any muscle of group of muscles not only strengthens and develops its own muscle-cells and nerve-cells by bringing them more and better nourishment, and by removing waste matter which would injure their health, through the better circulation of the blood, and by causing them to multiply their species more rapidly by division and sub-division, thus improving the " breed " continuously, but its demands also give all the involuntary cells—whose duty it is to supply all these demands—" employment," as it were, makes them move more, and so keeps them fit, weeds out unfit cells, and causes a higher and better birth-rate of new cells.

12. In other words, even the contraction of the biceps means an increased demand upon the services of the digestive cells to make good the waste, upon the eliminatory cells to remove it from the system, upon the cells in the blood to carry and distribute air and food, and to bear away refuse, and, indeed, upon all the involuntary cells of the body so that all the involuntary cells are proportionately strengthened and developed by their own movement, become more reproductive and are able to carry out their functions easily and vigorously through the initial movement of only one voluntary muscle or set of muscles.

13. But these involuntary cells will only move and work to the extent required to meet the demands of the one muscle or set of muscles moved. This means that they are working only up to restricted output, running below power, because they are not getting sufficient movement to keep them in the highest efficiency. To ensure this all or nearly all the voluntary muscles must be made to move. When only one muscle or set of muscles is used some cells in the unmoved parts will die off, some grow weak towards disease, and all will fail to reproduce younger and still more vigorous cells, propagating instead cells as inefficient or even weaker until disease attacks some part of the body

successfully, because the feeble cells are unable to resist and conquer it. This is what is meant by lowered resistant power to disease. The nerve-cells in the unmoved parts also suffer, and so the whole body is thrown out of balance.

14. From creation, man was given a great number of muscles to move and use, and by their united use and movement his body was maintained in health and strength as it was designed and created to be. The sufficient movement of all, or nearly all, his voluntary muscles was essential to existence in those days, and as a result he was disease-free, because these muscles, all being brought into play, brought all the involuntary cells of every bodily system also into movement as I have explained, and kept all these cells moving and functioning to their maximum capacity, in order to supply and keep pure the greater number of muscles that were then being used in everyday life. Not a weak spot of cell was to be found anywhere, and all the cells, organs, and systems were in absolutely balanced strength to resist all the encroachments of disease.

15. As time advanced and civilisation made it less and less necessary for man to use all his voluntary muscles, the cells of the involuntary muscles and systems were, consequently, also called upon less and less to move, for the diminution of voluntary muscular movement made less demands upon them in every way. Thus through this gradual loss of movement essential to their well-being they became poorly nourished, reduced in power and efficiency, contaminated by uneliminated waste and poisonous matter, while they are diminished in number, all this reducing resistant power to disease and still weaker cells often take their place instead of stronger.

16. Muscles that were unmoved and unused caused certain cells especially to weaken and become diseased because the cells in the unused parts suffered most, and that part or parts became so weak as to fall before disease, while the cells reproduced even more infirm descendants.

17. When that occurred, however, the nerve cells of that part or parts also suffered, and the cells of other systems suffered in sympathy, and thus disease was manifested in systems and parts of the body often far removed from the seat of actual disturbance, just as a defective drain will cause and spread disease afar off from the actual place of breakdown. That is what I mean when I say that as the nerve-cells are in communication in every part of the body, disease must be considered as a unit and the whole body also as a unit.

18. Only by bringing all—or nearly all—the voluntary muscles of the body into action within balance—which is what I mean by scientific physical movement taking the place of the everyday and all-round physical movement of primitive life in a concentrated form to suit modern life—and through them keeping every cell and all the cells of the body moving at their maximum of effort and efficiency to serve the needs of the body, can we again restore functional efficiency to these cells, and through them strengthen every organ and every function so as to overcome existent disease or the weakness that leads to disease, or to prevent it in the modern human body as Nature compelled man to do in primitive days. This is a new study for medical men, which will give them better results than the present methods of grappling with disease, and is Nature's own method of prevention and cure.

19. In this way we can even build up an entirely new and better body in any or every part, and make the body so strong in balance in all its cells, as either to prevent or cure any and every form of disease, and by what I call cellular evolution in the earlier part of my book, rebuild a body even better and more resistant to disease than it was at birth. The greater nutrition, oxygenation and purification of the cells of every system is secured by balanced physical movement. Old and feeble cells die off through incapacity and only the younger and more vigorous cells are left to continually reproduce still stronger and healthier cells of their species.

20. I think it will be evident from all this (a) that if there is disease of disorder in one part of the body there is disease in all parts of the body, (b) that to cure the part or parts that is or are affected is to cure every part, (c) that to remove the common cause of disease, viz., lack of resistant power in certain cells or in all the cells by making each and all of them so strong in balance is to either cure disease or to prevent it by making all the cells of the body equally strong and disease- immune. This, I say, we can only do in Nature's way by restoring to the body that balanced movement of the voluntary muscles which was its right and prerogative in the days of our splendid prime, and which alone can give it that 'strong, tenacious and conquering resistant power which is its first and greatest line of defence against disease.

Note.—It may be objected that most of the photos reproduced in the book are of young or comparatively young men showing an external muscular development above the average to-day, but only normal as men were intended to be. This is so, but it- must be remembered that many of these were weak and even suffering from some ailment when they first began to follow out the methods advocated here, and. were built up entirely in this way. Equally satisfactory results, from a curative point of view, are obtainable by men and women of all ages, though naturally the process must he slower in old age than in youth. In every case, however, and at all ages, these methods are valuable to build up organic and' vital reserve power and so to combat and conquer disease.

Important to Readers of this Chapter. Remarkable Article in "The Lancet," the Leading Medical Journal.

Readers of this chapter will be pleased to hear that the greatest medical journal in the world had a leading article and a letter in its issue of December 21st, 1918, in strong support of physical treatment, and admitting its great success in overcoming many forms of disease. The leading article contains, the most remarkable admissions as to the value of what Dr Radcliffe, the author of the letter, calls " Nature's remedies and I want every reader of this chapter to read this appendix to what I have just said, as it is of the greatest importance to sick and suffering mankind.

APPENDIX.

WHILST engaged on this my very last chapter, the current issue of The Lancet, under date of December 21st, 1918, lies on my desk. It contains a most interesting article on " Primitive Agents in Treatment," and an equally attractive letter on " The Value of Physical Treatment," from the pen of Dr Frank Radcliffe, medical officer in charge of a Manchester hospital for the physical treatment of soldier-victims of the war. The sanity of the views expressed in both of these is to me, indeed, a welcome sign of a new orientation of thought even in the very sanctum sanctorum of the medical profession, the editorial columns of the recognised official organ and probably the leading medical journal of the world. Both article and letter are welcomed by me as thin rays of sunlight peeping through a sky as yet somewhat cloudy and troubled. Yet there are points in both article and letter with which I venture to disagree, and upon which I would like to comment.

It is, for instance, distinctly gratifying to find that stern, unbending organ of medical tradition and authority not only lending itself to the support of natural physical methods of treatment, but even admitting that "the ordinary practitioner has, largely of his own free will, surrendered any say in these matters," and that the first step is for the profession to set its house in order and to make sure that physical treatment is placed on a satisfactory, scientific basis.

The admission here that those chiefly responsible for the healing of broken and suffering humanity have voluntarily allowed any proved methods of healing, but especially simple and natural methods coeval with Adam, to pass neglected, until others had accomplished cures almost miraculous by them, is by no means flattering to the sagacity of those responsible for high medical policy, and proved my contention that medical tradition has too long drugged and blinded those whose special mission it should always have been to seek for and employ methods of treatment of any and every kind likely to reduce the huge casualty lists of sickness and disease that have been increasing every year despite orthodox methods of medicinal treatment.

Instead of contemning or condemning others who refused to be handicapped by tradition, The Lancet might rather acknowledge, even in a modest way, all those whose efforts have at last forced the present recognition of natural, physical and primitive methods from such a staunch defender of medical tradition and orthodoxy, and whose work along natural lines have proved so beneficent to hundreds of thousands of suffering men and women, unreached by the orthodox methods of treatment—that great physically " submerged tenth," whose bodies could only be saved and regenerated by the very methods which doctors have for years, according to The Lancet itself, neglected, despised and " surrendered."

In the meantime, I would, with all modesty, suggest that medical men, who have for so long closed their eyes to methods which are, as I am proving in this book, Nature's own and only way of overcoming disease, and whose whole training has dealt with the effects of medicine on a diseased body rather than the application of natural physical movement scientifically to pathological conditions—the latter a subject, by the way, which has not even yet deigned to study and investigate fully—will have much to learn when they do turn their mind in this direction. It is for this very reason that I have advocated in this book special colleges for the exclusive study of this subject and special courses of physical therapeutics for doctors, and still more for the medical students of the future, included in all future medical education.

To deal now with Dr Radcliffe's letter, there is, after all, little in it that every medical man does not know since the days of Hippocrates. It gives concrete proof of the value of physical exercise, and natural therapeutics, even in an unscientific way, in releasing the healing force of Nature. It gives a long list of conditions in which these natural methods of physical treatment have proved successful. These include:—

    1.   Debility from any cause, e.g., pneumonia, typhoid, dysentery, all post-operative conditions, e.g., appendicitis, hernia, etc.

    2.   Rheumatism, including myositis, myalgia, fibrositis, rheumatoid arthritis, osteoarthritis, both in the earlier stages.

3. Neuritis, including neuralgias of all kinds, particularly headaches, which are often of rheumatic origin, due to fibrositis of the cervical muscles.

4. Nervous conditions, including neurasthenia, loss of nerve tone, general tremors and insomnia, associated at the present time with the overstrain of war and shell shock.

5. Heart conditions, particularly arrhythmia, tachycardia, bradycardia, loss of myocardial tone; dilatation, whether associated with valvular disease or not.

6. Post-operative conditions, such as adhesions following abdominal operations, contracted scars producing deformity by the trapping of nerves of tendons.

7. Fractures with only fibrous union; in other words, deficiency of callus.

8. Paralysis with paresis of any nerve, more particularly facial, ulnar, median, musculo-spiral, sciatic and branches.

9. Synovitis and fibrous ankylosis of large or small joints where breaking down of tissue and re-education of movement are necessary.

10. Circulatory conditions, such as trench feet, post-frost-bite and erythromelalgia.

For the benefit of the uninitiated reader, unfamiliar with the medical nomenclature of pathological conditions, I give the following explanation of such medical terms used above as may be puzzling in simpler English terms:—

Dysentery	Inflammation of the large intestine.
Pneumonia	Inflammation of the lungs.
Appendicitis	Inflammation of the appendix.
Hernia	Commonly called rupture.
Typhoid	A fever, usually attended with ulceration of bowels.
Myalgia	Pain in the muscles.
Myositis	Inflammation of the muscles.
Fibrositis	Inflammation of the fibrous tissue.
Rheumatoid arthritis	Inflammation of the joints from rheumatism.
Osteo-arthritis	Inflammation of the bony structure of a joint.
Neuritis	Inflammation of a nerve.
Neuralgia	Pain of a nerve or nerves.
Neurasthenia	Nerve weakness and exhaustion.
Arrhythmia	Irregular action of the heart.
Tachycardia	Rapid action of the heart.
Bradycardia	Slow action of the heart.
Myocardial tone	Tone of the muscular tissue of the heart.
Dilatation	Enlargement of an organ.
Post	After.
Adhesions	A matting together of tissues.
Callus	The new material that unites a broken bone.
Paresis	Slight form of paralysis.
Ulnar	Pertaining to the elbow and forearm near the inner bone.
Median	In the middle.
Musculo-spiral	A nerve of the arm.
Sciatica	Neuralgia of the large nerve of the hip and back of thigh.
Synovitis	Inflammation of the membrane of a joint, most common in the knee joint.
Ankylosis	Fixity of a joint.
Erythromelalgia	Redness of skin with pain in lower extremities.

This is a report on cases which came under Dr Radcliffe's own personal observations as medical officer in charge of an hospital near Manchester for the treatment of wounded soldiers and sailors whose health had suffered in the ways above mentioned as a result of war conditions, after a course of physical treatment as understood and practised there. For the information of Dr Radcliffe and his fellow practitioners, and also for the encouragement of such of the public as may be personally interested, I would like, however, to give here particulars of the still more remarkable results that have been achieved, not only in such cases as he reports, but in many other forms of disease and in orthopaedic cases of various kinds. I know that the medical profession having now had their attention professionally directed to the matter will be interested to know what can be and actually has been accomplished by natural physical movements alone, but applied and carried out in the most scientific way, and for that reason I add my own experience here to that of Dr Radcliffe.

Among the many and varied diseases and deformities treated with the utmost success by the natural methods here described by me may be mentioned the following:—

1. Indigestion and Dyspepsia, both in acute and chronic form, including acid dyspepsia, atonic dyspepsia, nervous dyspepsia, flatulent dyspepsia, biliousness, nausea, sick headache, gastric cattarrh, dilated stomach, heartburn, loss of appetite, pains in chest, shoulders and back, etc.

2. Constipation, a condition especially amenable to this treatment by bringing into use abdominal muscles rarely used in modern life, and employing them to act as a natural massage to the viscera; even in colitis these methods have proved successful.

3. Liver Troubles.—Exceptional results have been obtained in these conditions. Liver congestion, torpor and sluggishness have been completely overcome, and great relief has been obtained even in more obstinate forms of liver trouble such as jaundice and fatty degeneration, and cirrhosis of the liver in its early stages.

4. Neurasthenia and all Functional Nervous Disorders lend themselves more readily to these natural methods of treatment than to any other. Splendid results have been obtained in shellshock cases, cerebral neurasthenia, sexual neurasthenia, dyspeptic neurasthenia, spinal neurasthenia and cardiac neurasthenia, and in neuritis, hysteria, St. Vitus's Dance, epileptic fits, neuralgia and sciatica, while minor forms of paralysis have also been greatly benefited. Nervous disorders arising from feminine troubles and spinal weakness have been treated with results that have amazed the medical men in charge of the cases.

5. Obesity in Men and Women.—In the reduction of superfluous flesh and the amelioration of the dangerous conditions it induces, threatening vital organs, physical treatment is, of course, naturally indicated, and is not only far more successful but far safer than drugs, medicines, purgatives, violent sweating or " banting." The photographs reproduced will give a better idea of results that have actually been achieved by these methods to the health, benefit, and comfort of the persons so treated.

6. Heart Affections.—Hearts weak and irregular in their functions, especially if the functional disturbance is of nervous origin, have been made strong and normal in their functioning, and, in addition to the heart troubles mentioned by Dr Radcliffe, many more

serious cardiac disorders have, after medical advice, been most successfully treated. especially when taken in time. The heart itself has been improved organically, and the influence of the nervous system has been considerably modified, while the psychological effect has been most helpful in cases where there was often undue and even needless alarm.

7. Lung and Chest Complaints, it is scarcely necessary to say, are among the diseases that have lent themselves most readily to these methods of natural physical treatment, and, in many cases, phthisis, when not too far advanced, has been arrested and prevented. The improvement of the carriage, the deepening and broadening of the chest, and the toughening of the lung tissue are all contributory to this result. Bronchitis, asthma, emphysema, and other diseases of the respiratory system are also conditions in which these methods have conquered.

8. Rheumatism and Gout.—The improvement of circulation, the increased elimination of waste products and the dispersal of uric acid deposits and crystals have been easily and naturally accomplished by these methods, and rheumatism in all its forms, gout, lumbago, sciatica and uric acid disorders of various kinds have been quickly and permanently overcome.

9. Anaemia— In this condition, physical movements scientifically applied, have been uniformly successful, strengthening all the digestive organs and so improving digestion and nutrition, enriching and purifying the blood by increased oxygenation and elimination.

10. Kidney Disorders, functional and chronic, have all been successfully treated, and conditions leading to Bright's disease, dropsy, and stone have been overcome. The effect of physical movement, when applied scientifically, in promoting renal activity, is now well established and recognised by many medical men.

11. Lack of Vigour.—-In this state of diminished vitality, whether from sexual causes or otherwise, the benefits of the treatment have been placed beyond dispute. The whole nervous system regains tone, nutrition and elimination are increased, and such conditions as spermatorrhoea and impotence banished by purely natural means.

12. Physical Deformities and Defects.—A glance at the photographs reproduced elsewhere will convince the most sceptical of the value of these methods in cases of lateral spinal curvature and in kyphosis or lordosis. Other defects and deformities that have been overcome by the same means are knock-knees, bow legs, pigeon chest, etc.

13. Circulatory Disorders, including hyperaemias and congestions, local inflammations, varicose veins and other venous troubles, arterio-sclerosis, and other serious disturbances of the circulation have all been benefited and cured by methods that, promote the normal and equitable distribution of the blood through all its channels.

14. Skin Disorders, likewise, have also lent themselves most readily to this natural treatment, including erysipelas, acne, herpes, eczema and other distressing skin troubles.

15. Physical Development for Men.—A very large percentage of the physical troubles from which men suffer to-day may be traced to an imperfect and unbalanced physical development that injures or hampers organs and disturbs their functions. Many of the

men whose magnificent physical development may be seen in the photographs appearing in these pages were very poor in physique and sub-normal in their general condition, and their present superb physique and robust constitution may be attributed entirely to these natural methods of drawing out the best that is in a man at least in the physical sense.

16. Figure Culture for Women.—The same may be said to apply to the women depicted in a number of the illustrations who owe their splendid figures, physical beauty and perfect health to-day to this natural method of health and beauty culture.

17. Boys' and Girls' Ailments.—In cases of rickets, round shoulders, debility, anaemia, wasting, and many of the weaknesses and ailments to which the little folks are peculiarly liable, the results have been most gratifying, and many children have been saved from years of subsequent suffering and misery.

18. Insomnia, that terrible condition which has well been called " the vestibule of insanity," and which is especially the product of modern civilisation and mental rather than physical labour, has proved itself more tractable to natural treatment by physical movement than anything else.

The above statements have been verified by the most critical journal in the world, Truth, whose editor sent a special investigator to personally report upon the remarkable cures that were continually being reported by those who had tried these natural methods of regaining health and strength. The investigator ultimately bore public testimony to the fact that personal investigation compelled him to admit that actual "cures were achieved in no less than 94 cases out of every hundred and great relief given in 99," while, personally, I believe that these figures might have been still higher but for the impatience of many of those under treatment, who expected in a few weeks something approximating to the miraculous.

Indeed, 1 go so far as to assert that practically every form of deadly disease, especially if taken in its earlier stages, can be checked and overcome in its devastating progress by these natural methods of cellular reconstruction and evolution, and not merely some forms of disease as suggested in " The Lancet." No case, indeed, is beyond hope except if the sufferer is figuratively if not literally a dying man, or is prohibited by muscular atrophy or pain from carrying out these movements. If the voluntary muscles cannot be moved or only used with great pain, then such auxiliary methods of promoting what 1 may call artificial movement as massage, electricity or hydropathy will, no doubt, prove beneficial to re=establish the free and voluntary use of the patient's muscles, after which they no longer be necessary.

But; as I have said, in this subject doctors have yet a very great deal to learn, and I say this modestly as an unqualified man should to men who have chosen as their profession the science and art of healing sick and suffering humanity. As already observed, what I would like to see is physical treatment by means of natural physical movements alone made a special subject of study added to the present curriculum of every medical student, and, even colleges opened for •exclusive study and practice in this subject, for those who desire to specialise in it. For in this matter it is fusion not fissure that is needed.

I would like here to quote a short extract from a very interesting .article that I have just read in The World's Work from the pen of a Mr E. Wooton, in which he says truly:

> " A pure anatomist and physiologist has nothing experientially that may guide him in the matter of choosing exercises. Judging of the body's actions merely as a student of the normal and the natural, he is quite unfamiliar with the effects following that which is distinctly abnormal system of training."

For physical culture to become a really satisfactory science there must be an intimate acquaintance with the training itself, and this should be in harmony with the indications of physiological law. Quite obviously medico-physical culture affords a fair field for specialising to the qualified medical practitioner.

Prevention, of course, is the goal, and as the writer truly adds:—

> " If there is one subject on which human knowledge has arrived at certitude—although not finality—it is in relation to the influence on health of exercise, air, temperature, baths and foods. These are, so to speak, objective agencies working through physiological laws, and their application can, as a rule, be made far more rationally—that is, with a surer knowledge of need, and of result—than a doctor can treat a disease."

And Dr Radcliffe adds:

> " There are many other conditions which might be mentioned where physical treatment is indicated. It is the accurate and direct therapeutic application of exercise in its many forms which is absolutely necessary to ensure a scientific and well-balanced method of procedure. It will certainly replace many bottles of medicine, and benefit the patient by Nature's remedy."

But I fail, I am sorry to say, to see even yet a really true, deep and just appreciation in either The Lancet article or in Dr Radcliffe's letter of just how and why physical movement, scientifically applied, will both cure and prevent disease. In fact, the physiological effect of such physical movement on cellular structure and function has never yet been understood or even realised by medical men, whose studies have only led them to observe the action of medicine and other orthodox agents upon the body, and to judge rather by clinical observation and results than by processes from cause to effect. They see and admit the value of physical movement, but have not probed yet the reason why.

Even an advanced medical man, like Dr Radcliffe, cannot be expected to distinguish between the action and influence of scientific physical movement alone in stimulating cellular function, reproduction and evolution, as distinct entirely from ordinary physical exercise and methods of treatment that employ as aids and auxiliaries electricity, hydrology, and passive massage, for his studies and observations have been identified with methods of treatment embracing all these in combination. The value of scientific and balanced physical movement alone, as I mean it, has not so far been made clear to them.

It is because I have made the study of physical movement, applied in a scientific way for the cure and prevention of disease, the chief work of my life-time that, I think, the facts I am adducing in this book will come as a startling revelation to medical men, and will make clear to them, for the first time, just how and why such movement has achieved so great success and in such a variety of human diseases and physical defects.

Passive massage as recommended and employed by Dr Radcliffe, while valuable, and indeed, essential in some cases to improve circulation in the part to which it is applied or give artificial movement locally only to the cells in that part to break down adhesions, or to bring back lost power to an atrophied muscle by affording artificial movement to the cells without compensation, has no such deep-searching influence on the great involuntary and cellular man as has physical movement applied scientifically, because its effect is only local and affects only the voluntary cells and nerve cells in that part. Massage is valuable where a voluntary muscle has become so weak that it cannot be moved at the direction of a patient's will, but conscious physical movement alone will develop all his voluntary and involuntary muscles and cells as I explain in a previous chapter, and cause all the cells to multiply more rapidly and reproduce better and still better cells. In fact, in passive massage the masseur derives far more health benefit in every way than his patient, for the latter gets little or no compensation for the effort but the former does.

Electricity will, we know, cause the muscles of a dead frog to twitch, but it cannot stimulate the beating of the heart, or increase respiration, or beneficially influence the millions of involuntary cells in the body. This equally applies to massage. Conscious physical movement can and does.

So with wet packs and hydrotherapy in general. They are valuable for determining circulation to some local area of the body, to repair injured or inflamed tissue more rapidly, or for dispersing congestion, but they do not and cannot set all the cells of the body moving, multiplying and developing in vigour and power as does the physical movement of the voluntary muscles.

Natural methods of moving all the muscles by conscious and willed effort, except where there is too great pain or the muscle has become so atrophied as to be practically powerless, are the best, and, indeed, the only methods of developing not only the voluntary muscles themselves, but when carried out in perfect balance, movements can be applied so as to develop and increase both in number and vigour, the living cells of any or every system in the body, improve their functioning and actually rebuild the human body in whole or in part, as necessary, because it is the only way to supply that movement to all these cells which is essential to their healthy existence, to surround him with a hygienic environment, to eliminate all waste and poisonous matter, and to bring the whole into such balanced strength as to conquer and defy disease.

This is my conception of the only kind of movement that can truly be called scientific physical exercise, and it is just such movement that must be provided if doctors are to conquer, prevent and eradicate disease. It is movement of this kind, accurately and scientifically applied, that few doctors as yet understand or know how to apply successfully to a weak or diseased body, because they have not yet devoted sufficient and serious study to the subject. I am putting all the facts before them here so that they can see for themselves how great a study such a subject presents to them, and to explain to them the true reason why of what, I think, I may almost call its amazing and miraculous success over medicine and orthodox therapeutics. It is a more far-reaching study even than medicine, and it offers prospects of reward to medical men far greater than any they have yet had in their many admitted victories and triumphs over disease.

But all physical movement for the cure or prevention of disease must be carried out in an absolutely scientific way. For this reason I am quite in accord with the writer in The Lancet when he 'expresses the desire that it should not be left to those who might carry it out unscientifically, as, I am afraid, is too often the case at present. The prescription of remedial and curative movements is quite as serious a matter as the prescription of medicine, if not more so, and the gravest danger will be incurred to millions unless it is prescribed and applied in a strictly scientific way.

Under any circumstances to think that the best results can ever be obtained from these methods, whether prescribed by medical men or others, unless they are prescribed and employed by those who have long and seriously studied the subject in all its phases, and who have had experience of its wonderful possibilities, both in their own person and in theory and practice, and who are quite certain that they are really practising and prescribing scientific and curative or preventive physical movement as distinct from physical movement that is not scientific, as in ordinary everyday work or games or even commonly accepted ideas of physical training that are erroneous even in their conception and of little value for remedial or preventive purposes.

This, indeed, brings me back to the leading article in The Lancet already referred to. A portion of it deals with attempts that are being made and expected to have wonderful results in the treatment of disabled and debilitated soldiers by what is called " the agricultural cure." According to The Lancet, The agricultural colonies at Port Villez, Juvisy, Martillac, Milan, Poseia, and Palermo, have already proved what Professor Silvio Rolando, of Genoa, calls the veritable resurrection of the soldier during the agricultural cure. In agricultural work a great variety of exercises is possible all day long."

Now, all of us must admit that fresh country air and farm work, with the change from the excitement and allurements of town life or the frenzy of war conditions to pastoral conditions and healthy refreshing sleep must exercise a healthful influence, but to expect it to bring about what Professor Silvio Rolando, of Genoa, calls i the veritable resurrection of the soldier," is, I think, an exaggerated claim, for the physical effort expended in agricultural work is distinct from scientific physical exercise, as it gives no compensation, or, indeed, physical exercise, as distinct from work which is not intended to benefit the body but to accomplish a certain task. Between the two there is just as much difference as between food and medicine.

Here, again, is evidence that even in these quarters there is no exact conception of what is strictly scientific and curative exercise or what its great potentialities. Movements that are carried out in a sub-conscious way, as in agriculture, without the maximum of physical effort and mental concentration on the muscles or parts moved, can have no therapeutic value from an exercise point of view. The intense physical movement of only one set of muscles in the conscious and concentrated way I have described would be more beneficial than long hours in, say, guiding a plough with the mind engaged on the work being done instead of being concentrated entirely on the bodily parts being moved. This is no more effective for curative purposes than to quote The Lancet's own words, I physical treatment carelessly carried out, motions without aim repeated without energy, and soon forsaken as being without interest or, at all events, leaving a sense of boredom and insincerity."

Light, natural physical movements done solely for the purpose of exercise and carried out with full mental concentration on the muscles moved and with the maximum of physical power will always be found to be of a far higher curative value than sub-conscious, automatic, or semi-conscious physical movements as in agricultural or any other physical work, in which the mind may be directed altogether away from the movement being performed. Such movements applied in balance and due ratio as to many of the voluntary muscles as possible provides the life-movement essential to the very life of the millions of cells in the body to their nutrition, sanitation, propagation and evolution. Through the conscious direction and movement of the voluntary muscles of the body in balance we alone can build up the body in such balanced strength that it will be able to overcome existent disease or resist and prevent the first encroachments or the most violent assaults of disease from without or the weakness within that imperils the bodily citadel, and which, if neglected, betrays it to disease. To do this it is necessary first to locate exactly where there is loss of balance and to strengthen it.

For, as I have already said, loss of balance somewhere in the body, with resultant diminished resistant power, throws open the gateway of the human citadel to disease, and long generations of civilised life have caused most of us to-day to be afflicted through ancestry and birth, as well as by modern conditions of life, with some disturbance of balance. In some this imperfect balance is more marked than others, and such are, of course, more liable to disease.

Before this loss of balance can be restored, it is necessary to discover exactly where the loss of balance is. That implies the greatest accuracy of diagnosis and long study and experience in prescribing just the exact movement and in the exact way to the exact part or parts that will bring back the unfit or diseased body to a condition of perfectly balanced strength. For this reason, therefore, agricultural work or ordinary physical labour of any kind has, and can have, no actual curative value, because it does not and cannot restore balance to the unbalanced body as it does not apply to unbalanced part or parts, but is liable to disturb it still further. Physical labour is not physical exercise applied and carried out with a distinct and specific object, but is, as I have said, physical effort without compensation, and in the case of a sick person may be even worse than valueless and dangerous, just like medicine taken without medical prescription. Physical labour cannot cure or prevent disease, but often causes it. Were it not so, physical labourers, even agricultural workers, would not have to consult medical men so often.

There is just one other point in the letter to The Lancet under notice which I would like to refer, because, although it has no direct hearing on the subject under treatment in this chapter, it indirectly affects the great army of human sufferers whom it is the chief aim and end of all of us to assist and relieve. It is a matter, however, in which I can only venture my own honest opinion, but upon which I feel acutely, for it refers to another of the bonds of conservatism and traditional etiquette which hampers medical men from rendering still greater services to humanity, and is, I know, irksome and galling to many worthy and distinguished members of the profession.

If the object of the medical profession is, as it should be, to do the greatest good to the greatest number, it cannot continue to ignore the great possibilities of newspaper publicity and the ramifying network of postal communications that offer to every medical man new avenues to greater fields of service, and which would widen and extend his present parochial and limited horizon reminiscent of a feudal period and the parish pump. In The Lancet, Dr Radcliffe —still clinging to an etiquette that is altogether out of place in these democratic days—finishes up his letter with a sly dig at advertising, but, to-day, publicity has attained a dignity that robs it of much that was formerly adduced against it, and I see no reason whatever why British professors of medicine should not follow the example of their brethren in America and elsewhere, and so place their knowledge, experience and discoveries at the benefit of the whole world instead of restricting these, as at present, to a comparatively limited few in their own neighbourhood and district.

There should be nothing infra dig in a medical man enlisting the agency of the greatest power in the world in announcing any method of treatment or discovery for the alleviation or eradication of human suffering. On the other hand, it has everything in its favour, and it would provide an international consulting room for medical men that might bring new life and hope to thousands and in the defence of humanity against an enemy that recognises no frontiers.

In my own modest way, because untrammelled by professional etiquette, the press and the post have enabled me to do everlasting good to suffering men and women in every part of the globe, who might never have received relief otherwise from years of pain and suffering, and, instead of decrying the lay press, I and ailing humanity, to the contrary, must ever feel under an unpayable debt of gratitude to it, as thousands upon thousands who have been relieved and cured by the methods described alone, have gladly borne testimony to me in person or in correspondence by post. I see no reason whatever why qualified men should continue to curtail and restrict their good offices to humanity by refusing any longer to avail themselves of such an agency for doing public good as I have personally proved it to be.

However, to return to the subject of physical movement, in a scientific way, as distinct from the ideas of physical treatment held by medical men generally and The Lancet writer, which show how little the medical profession even yet understands this subject. To make myself quite clear I am compelled again to reiterate some of the salient points already referred to elsewhere, but this, I hope, will be excused, as I am very anxious to prevent any confusion or conflict of ideas. Let me endeavour then, briefly, and, I hope, quite clearly, to put my case for what I mean by the really scientific application of natural movements for the cure as well as for the prevention of disease in the proverbial nutshell as follows:—

1. Life is movement. Without muscular movement and the circulation of the blood, the living cells of the body would get neither nourishment nor air, and would be poisoned by deadly carbonic acid gas. They would die, like ourselves, whom they represent in miniature.

2. The slightest movement of a voluntary muscle brings an increased rush of blood to that muscle to carry away the waste and to bring supplies of nourishment and air to make good that waste. All physical movement achieves this object. It will be seen, therefore, how important a factor is the circulation of the blood in health or in disease.

3. This same movement also causes all the involuntary cells of the various organs and systems to move automatically, to prepare, transport and distribute this nourishment and air which are the prime necessities of life, and to eliminate the poisonous gas and waste matter which would be fatal to life if retained, as I have shown in my chapter " What is Physical Movement? "

4. Therefore, in some form, movement is the prime essential of life. The movement of one or more voluntary muscles in any part of the body immediately calls upon the heart to pump the blood faster to that part to carry away the waste and poisonous matter caused by this movement, and to replace the materials destroyed and repair the waste. The action of the heart is gradually strengthened by this natural movement, and it then is able to force the blood faster through the various channels of circulation to every part of the body, while this natural movement, also, by quickening or deepening respiration, increases the oxygenation of the blood, relieves it of the poisonous carbonic acid gas so injurious and even fatal to animal life. Massage, electricity or hydropathy does not improve the heart's action in this way, but only draws the blood locally to the spot where

it is applied in greater quantity for a time, without any increase of force either in that spot or in any other part of the body.

5. But movement may be performed by the conscious direction of the brain or performed automatically or sub-consciously. So long as it is performed consciously—that is, by a direct command from the brain through the nervous system to the muscles, the cells of body, nerve and brain are set and kept moving, and are developed and evolved continuously by this conscious movement. The moment a conscious act becomes a sub-conscious one, all these cells cease to develop and evolve further than required for the performance of that act.

6. Only so long as the mind is fixed on the muscles or parts moved do the particular cells employed in those parts, and the cells in the brain and nervous system also employed continue to develop, multiply and increase in number and efficiency on a continuously ascending plane. In other words, only conscious physical movement keeps on increasing the cells both in number and efficiency by continuously evolving better cells in all the parts brought into action by any physical movement.

7. This means that where the cells in the brain, the nerve cells and the muscle cells, involved in a movement that is carried out without the mind being concentrated and directed to the muscles or parts to be moved, cellular progress and development automatically ceases, as in ordinary work or play which has become automatic and sub-conscious by reiteration, and can even be accomplished while the mind is occupied on something else beside the work or feat to be performed. When all the cells directly and locally employed have arrived at that stage they remain stationary. This is what I mean when I say there is no compensation for sub-conscious physical effort.

8. But I have shown that the act of one muscle or group of muscles brings into play also millions of cells in all the other systems and parts of the body automatically, i.e., sets and keeps all these moving also, so that when a voluntary muscular movement is no longer performed with the mind on the muscles or parts moved, not only do the cells actually employed cease to receive compensation and suffer from arrested development, but all these millions of other associated cells also similarly suffer, and make no progress beyond the point necessary for the performance of the particular feat or task to be accomplished.

9. So that work or play performed automatically has no value in increasing cellular efficiency or breeding better cells in body and brain beyond the standard needed to accomplish some feat or do some allotted task. Neither physical labour, therefore, or sports and games go on improving cells by multiplication and evolution beyond a certain point. The benefit, too, to the voluntary muscles is only to those muscles and parts actually moved, while many of the involuntary cells everywhere in the body are only called upon to keep moving sufficiently to supply the demands of the directing cells of the brain, the nerve-cells and the muscle cells actually engaged, which usually represent only some of the more than 500 muscles of the body.

10. Now, on the other hand, what I call scientific physical movement is, in the first place, movement carried out with the mind exclusively engaged on the muscles and parts moved for the time being. Physical movement is not scientific if it is carried out sub-

consciously or automatically, whether in play or in work, or in what is by courtesy sometimes called physical training.

11.   Secondly, only simple and natural movements are employed—the movements that Nature instinctively implants in the healthy infant to keep it healthy. By combining and collating and regulating our present-day knowledge of the possibilities of these primitive and natural physical movements, and " Bovrilising " them into a compressed and " tabloid " form compatible with civilisation and modern methods of life, these methods are no mere man-invented system of physical therapeutics, but are rather my discovery of how to supply and apply these natural and ancient movements and agents which kept primitive man strong, healthy and disease- free, for the cure and prevention of disease in an easy, agreeable and highly concentrated form to-day. In other words, these methods are Nature's remedies applied scientifically for the first time, and all I claim is to have devised certain movements and combinations of movements that give in a few minutes the benefits from the all-day and all-round physical active life of primitive man.

12.   Now, when these movements are scientifically carried out, they must be done with the utmost vigour of contraction and full and equal relaxation, thus increasing (1) the nutrition of the muscle cells and nerve-cells of the voluntary muscles moved and the complete removal of all waste and poisonous matter that if uneliminated most freely would lead to unfitness and disease, and (2) equally of all the involuntary cells of every system and part of the body as I have shown. (There is no danger to the organically sound person and free from any physical weakness, such as a tendency to rupture, in putting this maximum effort into every movement, because he cannot put more into the effort than he possesses. But for the organically unsound or physically defective it is advisable that the effort exerted should be graduated by easy stages from the beginning.)

13.   Thirdly, when I speak of " conscious " physical movement I mean emphatically that the mind must be concentrated solely on the muscles and parts being moved at the moment, and not drawn away from it to anything else. This is why I do not believe in musical drills except as play, because the mind is diverted from the muscles and parts being moved. It is also why I say that physical work games, sports and pastimes are not scientific movement, because the mind is more centred on the work or the game or the feat to be performed than upon the muscles being employed. And in saying this I speak of that which I do know from long and varied experience and not from text-books.

14.   In other words, the importance of this conscious and concentrated effort upon the muscles moved means this. By putting in the maximum of effort into each contraction a continuous development and betterment of the cells is maintained, because the effort, of course, is increasing though imperceptibly, as the strength of the individual also increases and the effect upon the cells is cumulative. It is much as in the case of Milo's cells, which were continuously developed by lifting the growing calf from birth until he could lift a full-grown ox. The daily progress, though scarcely perceptible, was Cumulative, because a greater effort was being made daily, though also imperceptibly, and new and stronger cells were being evolved on an ever-ascending scale until the feat of lifting the ox was accomplished But the moment the ox ceased to increase in weight, and only the same effort was required to repeat the feat, the process of cellular evolution ceased. This is what happens in all sub-conscious physical movement where a task or a feat has to be

accomplished, and once accomplished, the cells cease to develop and improve further, and will even degenerate if the task or feat be discontinued for a time.

15. Conscious physical movement as I define it, viz., with the mind wholly centred on the muscles moved, and not on the feat or task being done, means the permanent and continuous evolution of the cells until the highest attainable maximum of efficiency is reached, and even then the cells, by this conscious effort, are maintained in this 100 per cent., efficiency, old and feeble cells being " weeded out " and only the youngest and strongest allowed to exist. Had Milo put his whole energy daily into the effort necessary to lift an imaginary and growing calf until it was a full- grown ox, the evolution of the cells would have continued even after the hypothetical ox had ceased to increase in weight, until the living cells had reached their very maximum of strength and efficiency, and so long as he continued to make his maximum physical effort with full concentration of the mind on the muscles the cells would have been maintained at their highest possible standard of efficiency, because his mind was not being diverted to the actual feat he was performing, and cellular evolution continued until the absolute maximum of efficiency was attained and maintained. In sub-conscious movement, as in work or flay, there is merely cellular evolution until the quality' of cells necessary to perform a certain work or feat is obtained, when they will become stationary and degenerate if the feat or work is not continued. Conscious muscular movement is permanent and geometrically progressive cellular evolution until perfection is attained and maintained.

15. Physical movement, scientifically applied, again, does not call into play only a certain number of muscles, but practically all the voluntary muscles are brought into action in turn, and moved and developed in balance, whereas agriculture or any physical labour or sports develops some muscles and neglects others, which causes both disturbance of balance not only (1) between muscle-cells and nerve-cells of the voluntary muscles and parts moved and similar cells in unmoved or unequally moved muscles and parts of the voluntary system, but also (2) between the moved and the unmoved or unequally moved cells of the involuntary systems of the body, and, again, (3) between all these respective cells in the internal and involuntary systems and the superficial and voluntary cells. It is this disturbance of balance of some part or parts of the body that diminishes resistant power and leads to disease, and as all parts are inter-dependent and inter-related, all must be equal in balanced strength if a body is to be disease-proof, because what affects one part affects the whole to some extent.

16. Scientific physical movement, on the other hand, by consciously bringing practically each and all of the voluntary muscles of the body in proper order and sequence into balanced movement, with the mind fully concentrated on the muscle or muscles being moved, sets all the involuntary muscles and cells both of body and brain moving to their very maximum of effort and in perfect balance, thus developing all these cells of every system and part of the body to their utmost capacity, vigour and reproductive power, the cells, that is, upon which the performance of function depend. It gives continuous and progressive compensation to these cells in return for movement, whereas games or sports or physical work in which the movement is or becomes sub-conscious, only develop the cells to the point necessary to perform the feat or the work

and then the cells cease to develop further, while some cells again are comparatively neglected altogether.

17. Physical movement scientifically applied not only thus restores external and internal balance and builds the body and brain in symmetrical and harmonious strength everywhere, but it builds up a new and better body in any or every part as desired, by what I have fully described elsewhere as a process of cellular evolution. In other words, the natural movements being scientifically applied and carried out consciously, and not haphazard or sub-consciously, " weed out " weak, old and infirm cells unable to keep pace with the increased demand put upon them, and so are literally worked to death, only the fittest and youngest surviving, through being able to live such a strenuous life of movement. Thus, by scientific movement, we can actually build up an entirely new organ or system, or, in time, an absolutely new and better physical body, including a new and better brain, with healthier and more active and stronger cells in balance, keeping them always youthful and longer youthful, vigorous, and in their highest efficiency, by the physical movement essential to life that maintains them only in their prime, and will not tolerate the existence of weak or unfit cells or cells too old to become diseased, or to combat and conquer disease germs from without.

May I just add, in conclusion, that I shall always be pleased to place any medical man in possession of information on any point regarding the employment of physical movements in a remedial or curative sense which is not still clear to them. I have no desire to dogmatise nor to assume an oracular tone, but I am most anxious that every medical man should divert his mind to a study which the medical profession has admittedly paid but slight attention in the past, and which I personally have found a most fascinating one, and one, I believe, of incalculable benefit to suffering humanity. It is, indeed, as Dr Radcliffe and The Lancet agree, too precious to be exploited by quacks and charlatans to the danger of the sick and the suffering.

Life of the Author as told in Photographs.

Series of Photos

showing the Author at different periods of his varied career. These are presented here for the encouragement of the youth of the nation, and to show what can be accomplished by anyone who patiently and conscientiously follows out the methods described in this book.

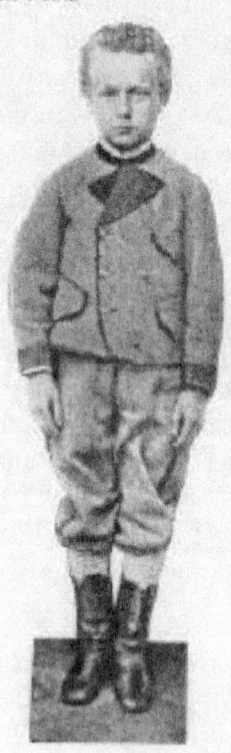

(1)
The Author at the age of 10. Delicate as a boy, he became enthused with a fervour for physical development, after seeing the statues and pictures of ancient and classical heroes in the art galleries of Europe, and lived afterwards with one ambition only, to become as well-developed and strong as they were.

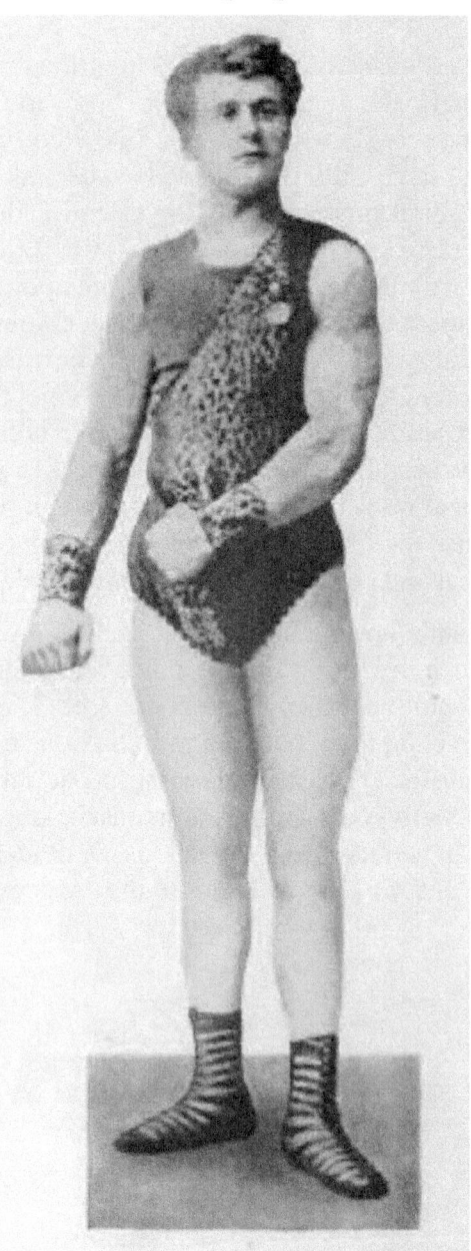

(2)
Photo taken at the age of 18, showing the remarkable increase of development in the intervening eight years.

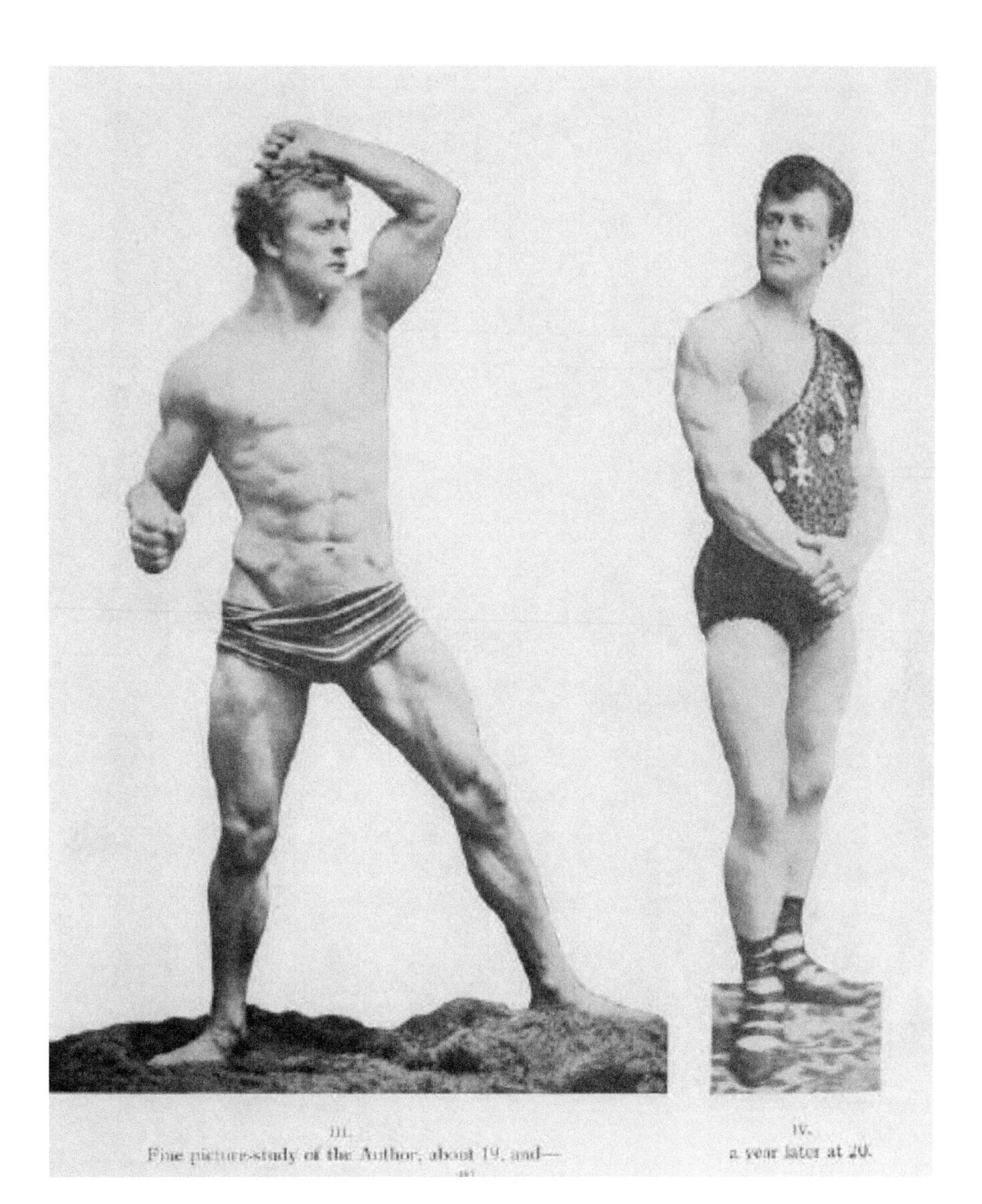

III.
Fine picture-study of the Author, about 19, and—

IV.
a year later at 20.

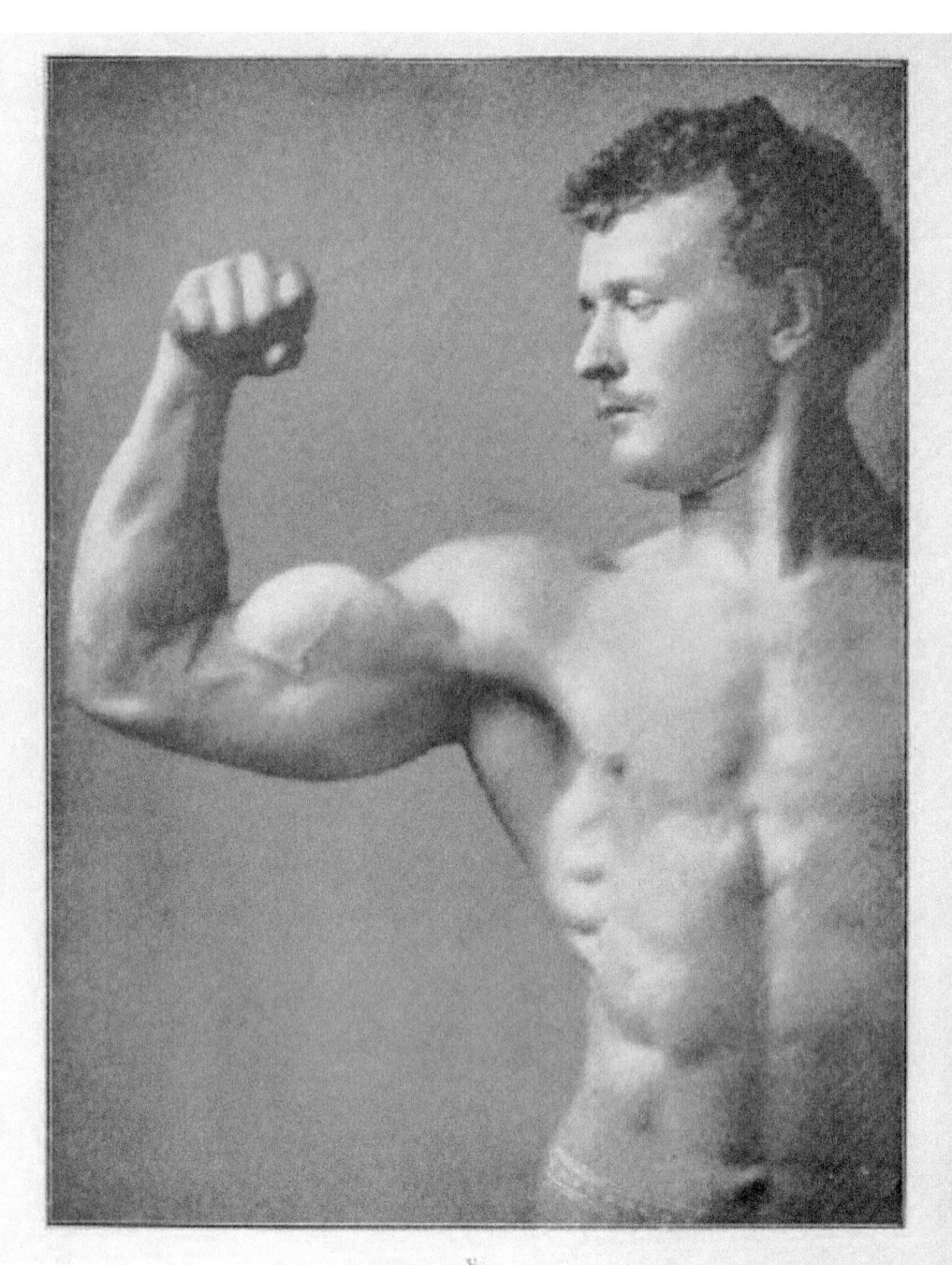

v.
Photo taken at 21, showing great biceps and triceps development of arm. It was about this period that the Author first appeared in London at the Royal Aquarium, accepting Samson's challenge to the world, and defeating the famous pupil of Samson—Cyclops, and subsequently Samson himself, for wagers of £100 and £1,000 respectively.

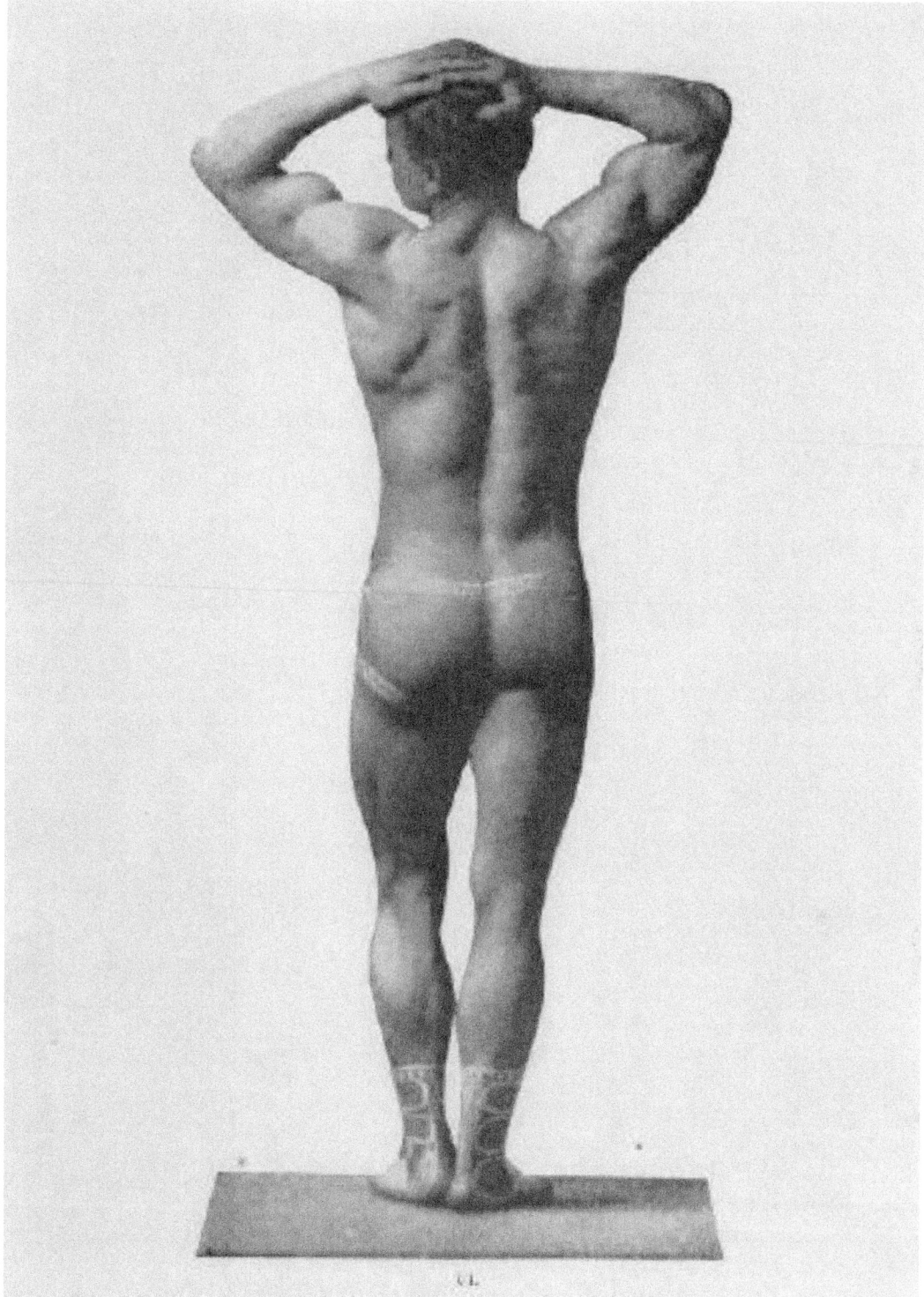

Author at about the same age, showing symmetrical development and balanced physique of back, shoulders and limbs.

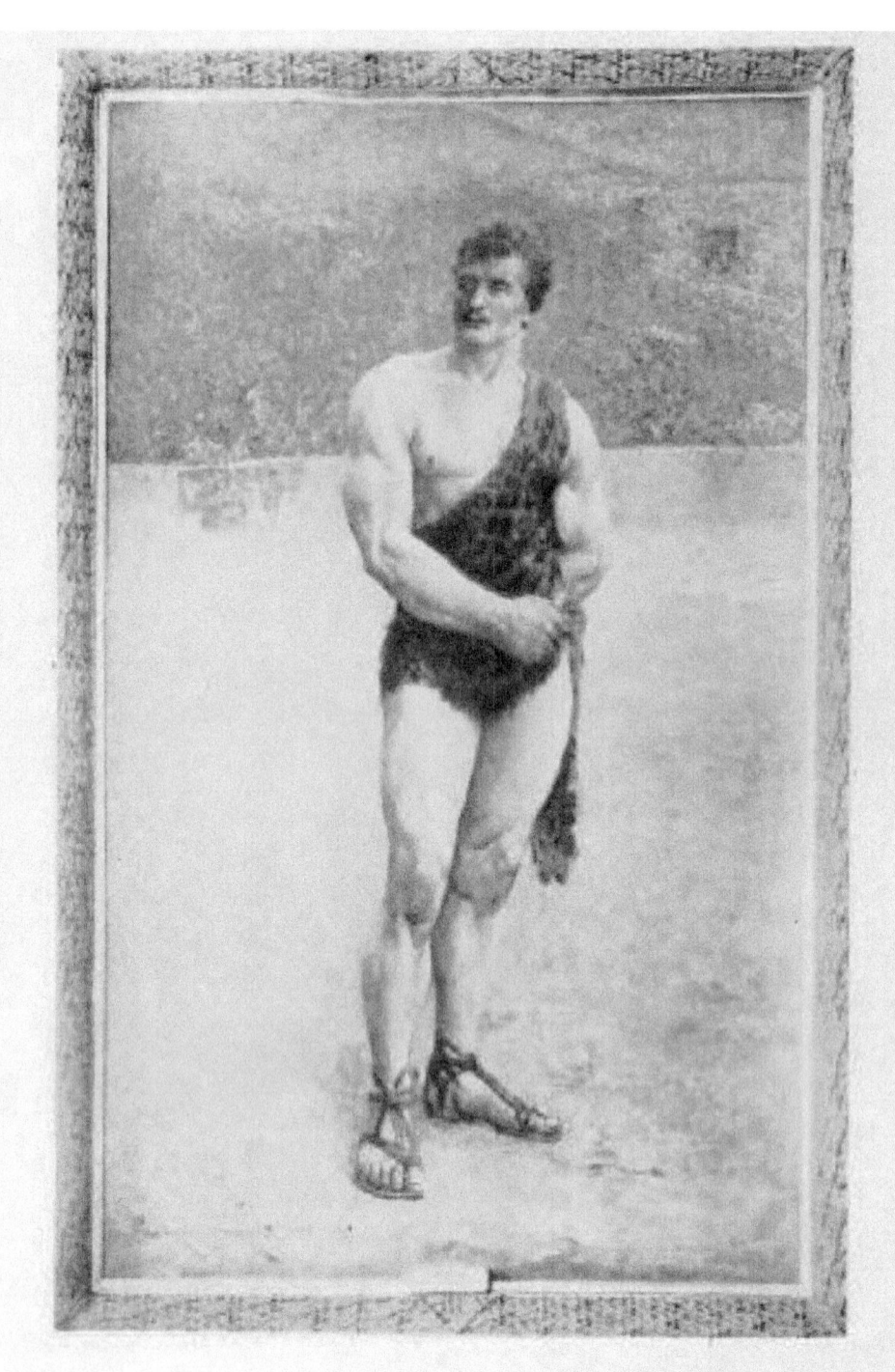

VII.
SANDOW AS GLADIATOR.

Aged 23. Reproduced from the painting made of him by the famous artist, Mr. Aubrey Hunt, who first met Sandow near Genoa, and was struck by his remarkable physique. It was Mr. Hunt who mentioned Samson's challenge to Sandow, and the latter left for London on the same evening to accept it.

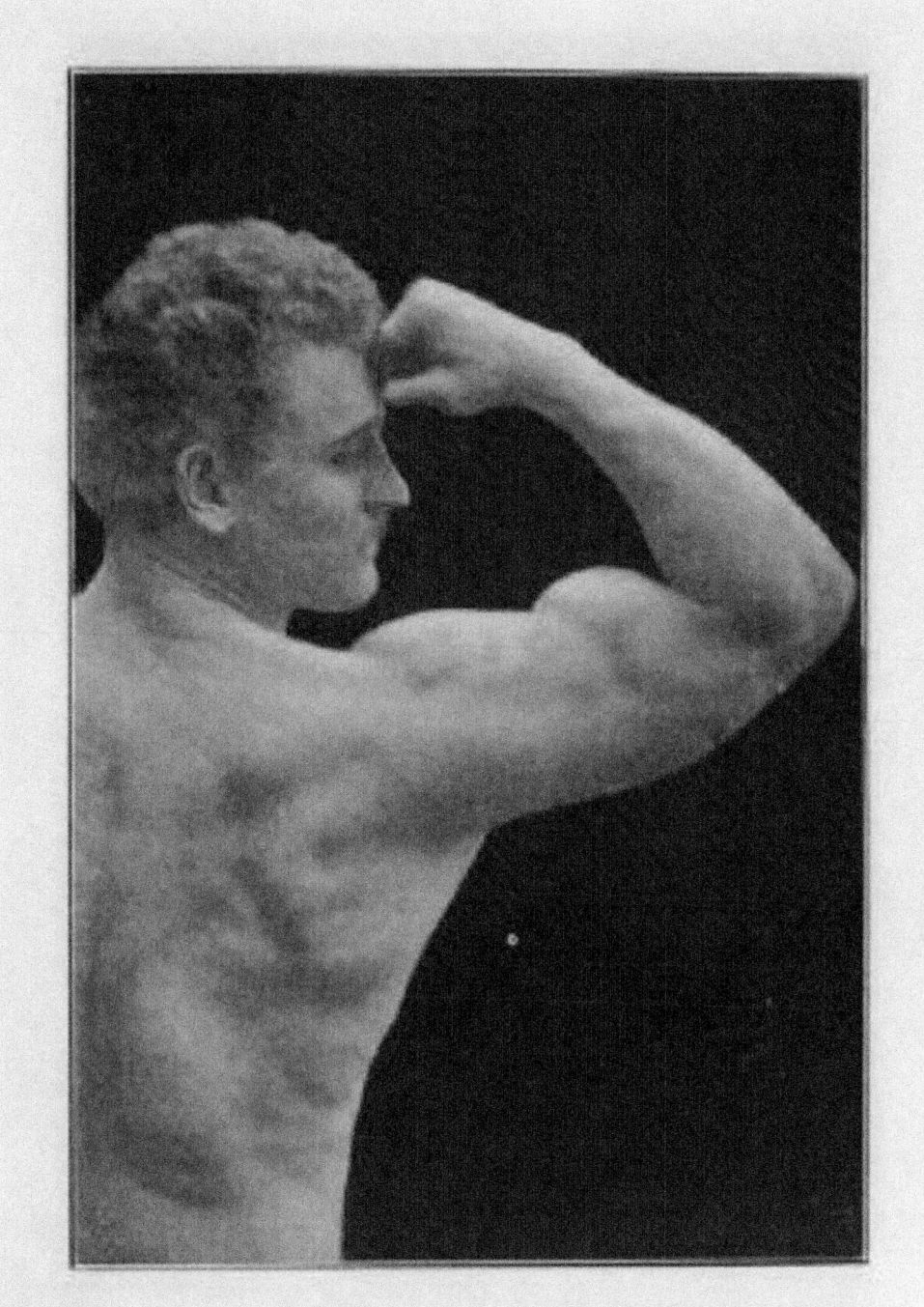

VIII.

Another photo taken at about the same age.

IX.

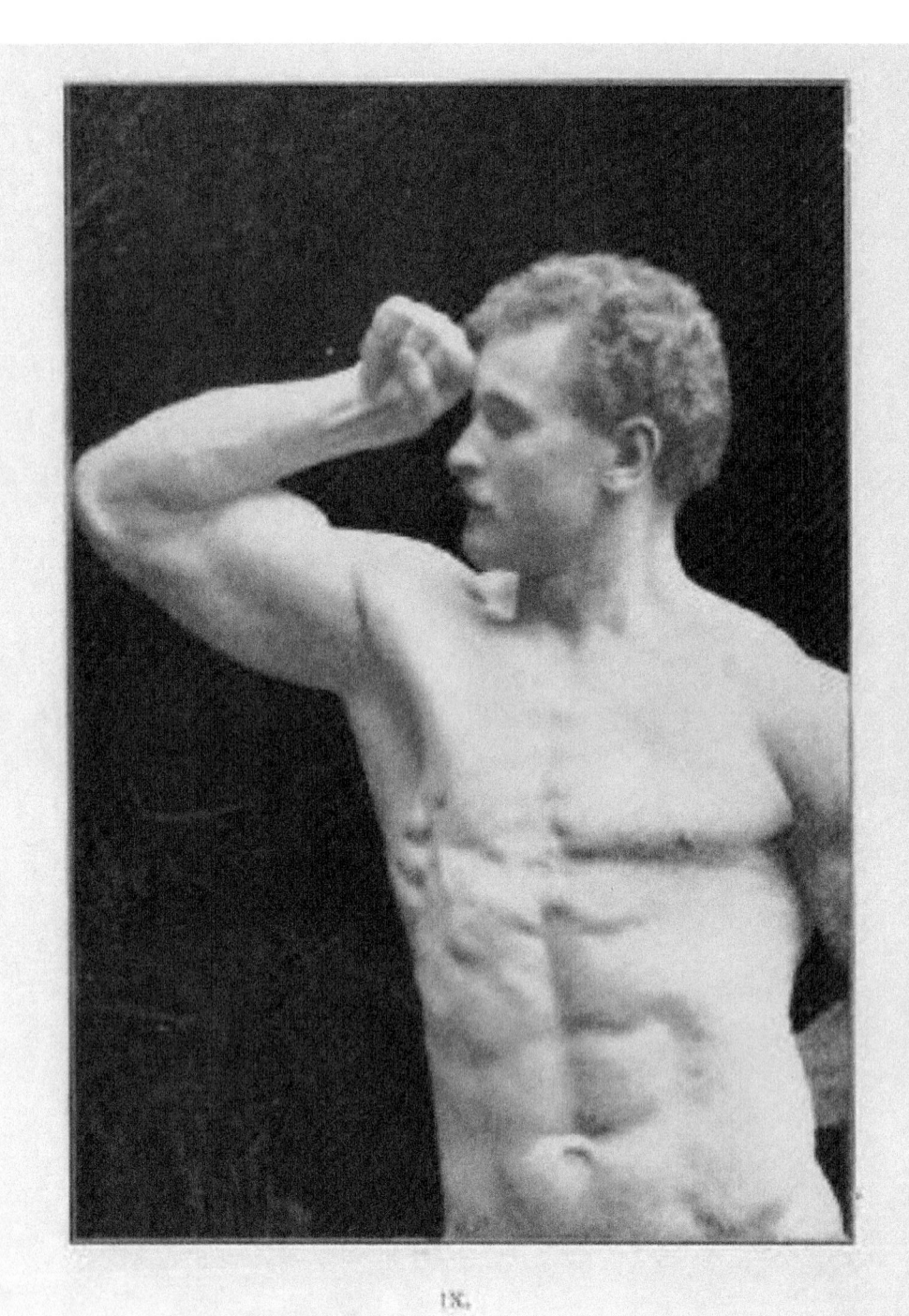

The Author about a year later. A study showing contraction of biceps and flexors of forearm.

Photo-study of the Author at 25.

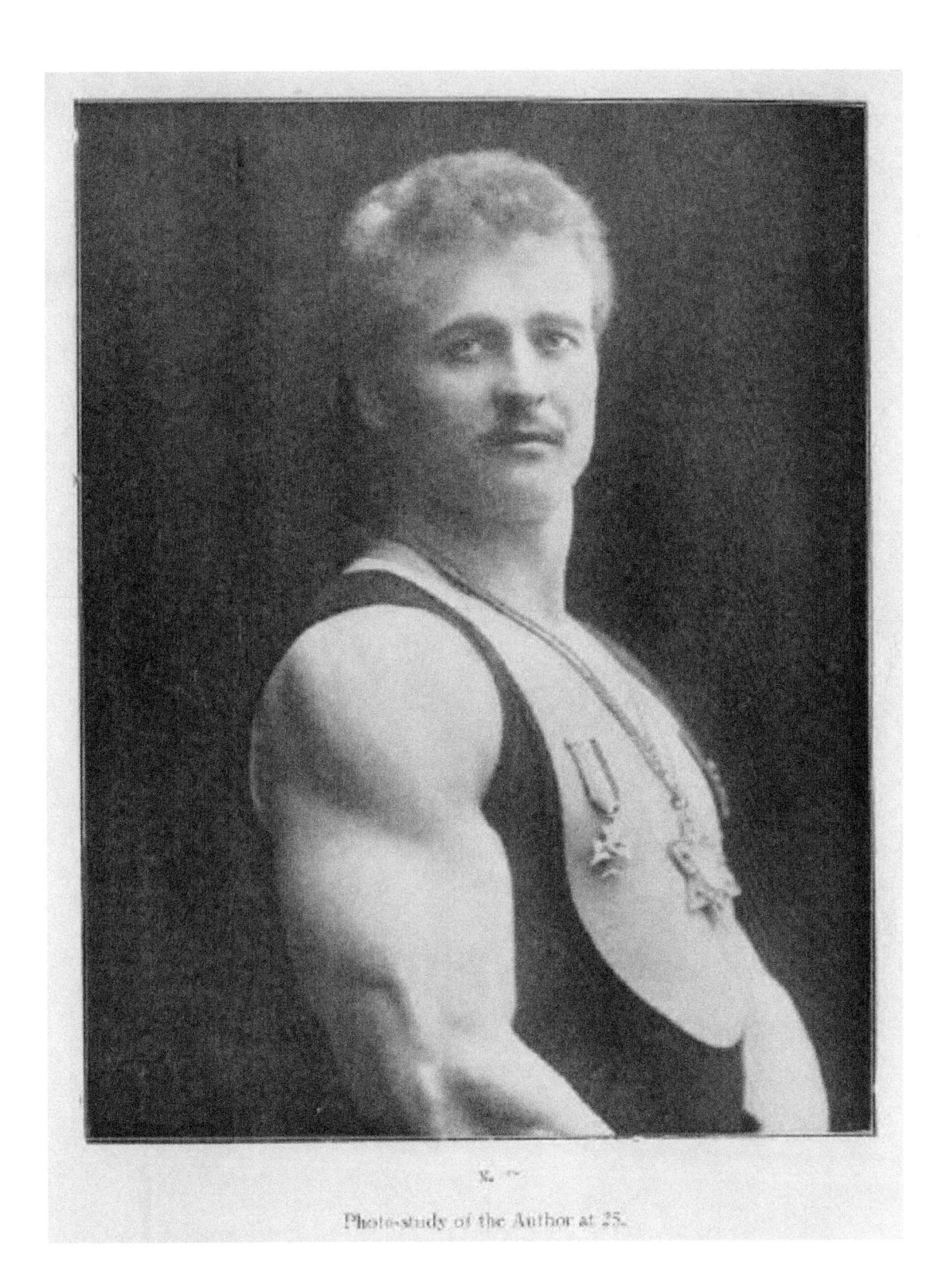

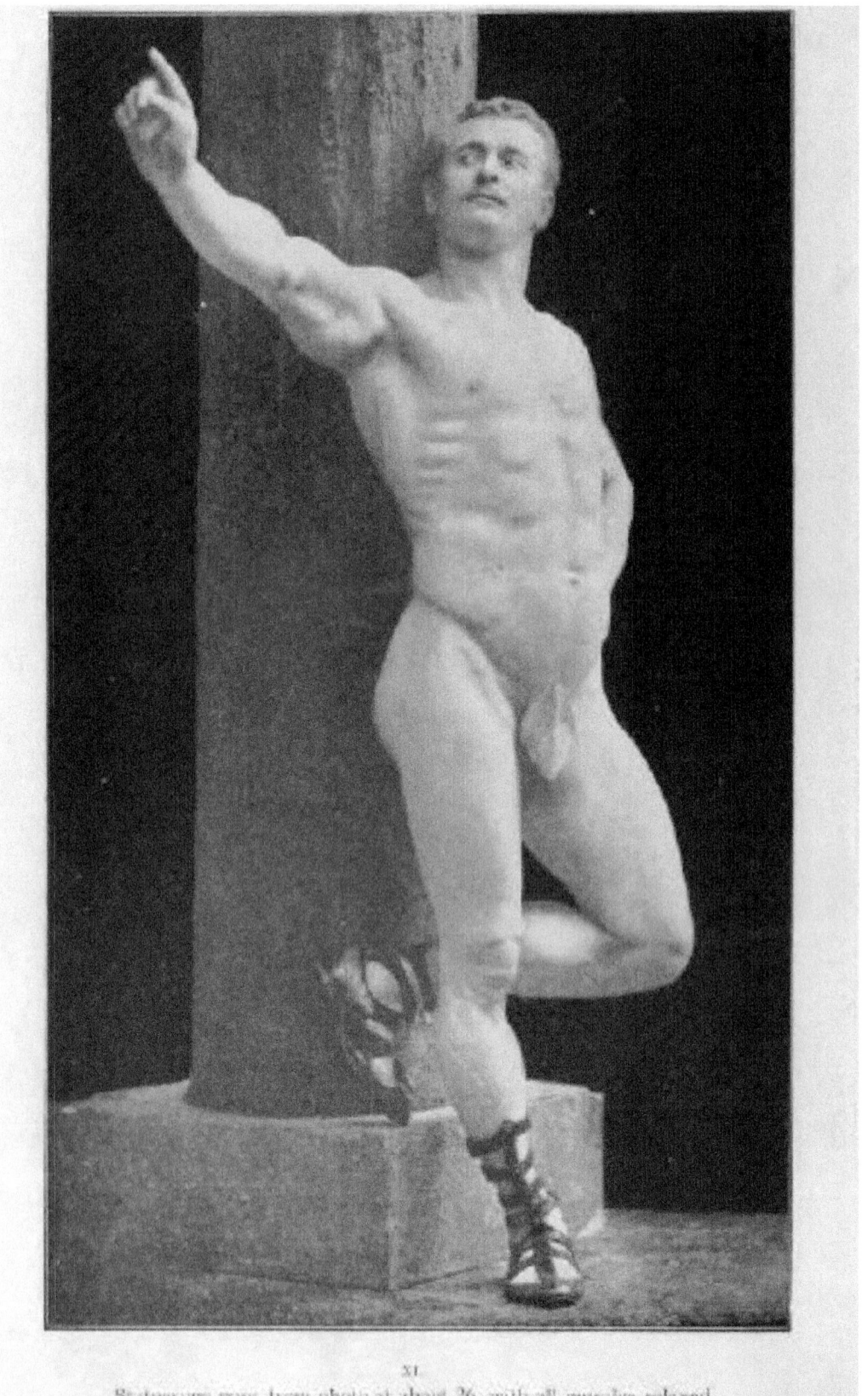

XI.
Statuesque pose, from photo at about 26, with all muscles relaxed.

XII.
The Author at 27.

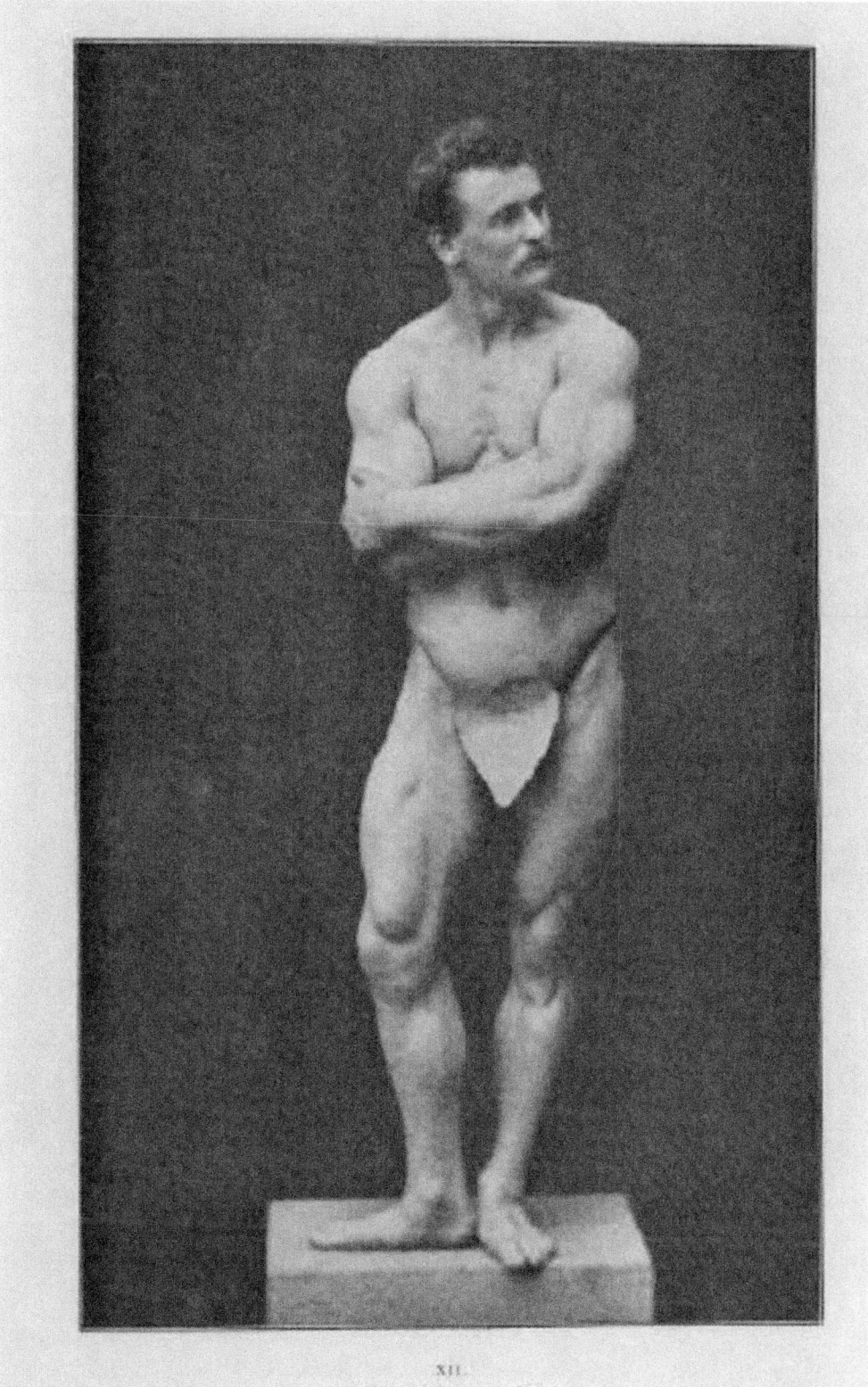

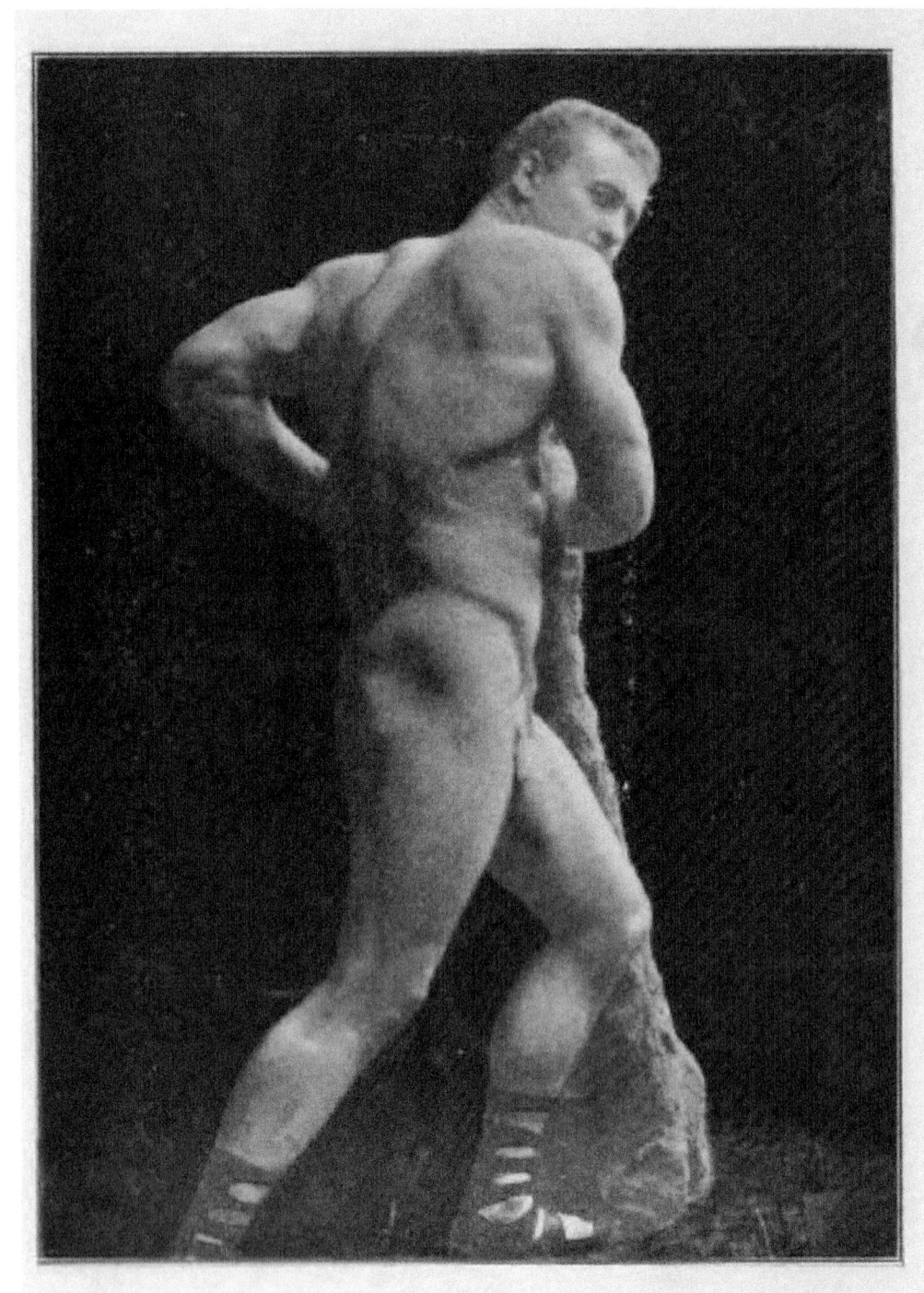

XIII.
At 30, with muscles in contraction.

XIV.
Artistic pose, showing Author at 35.

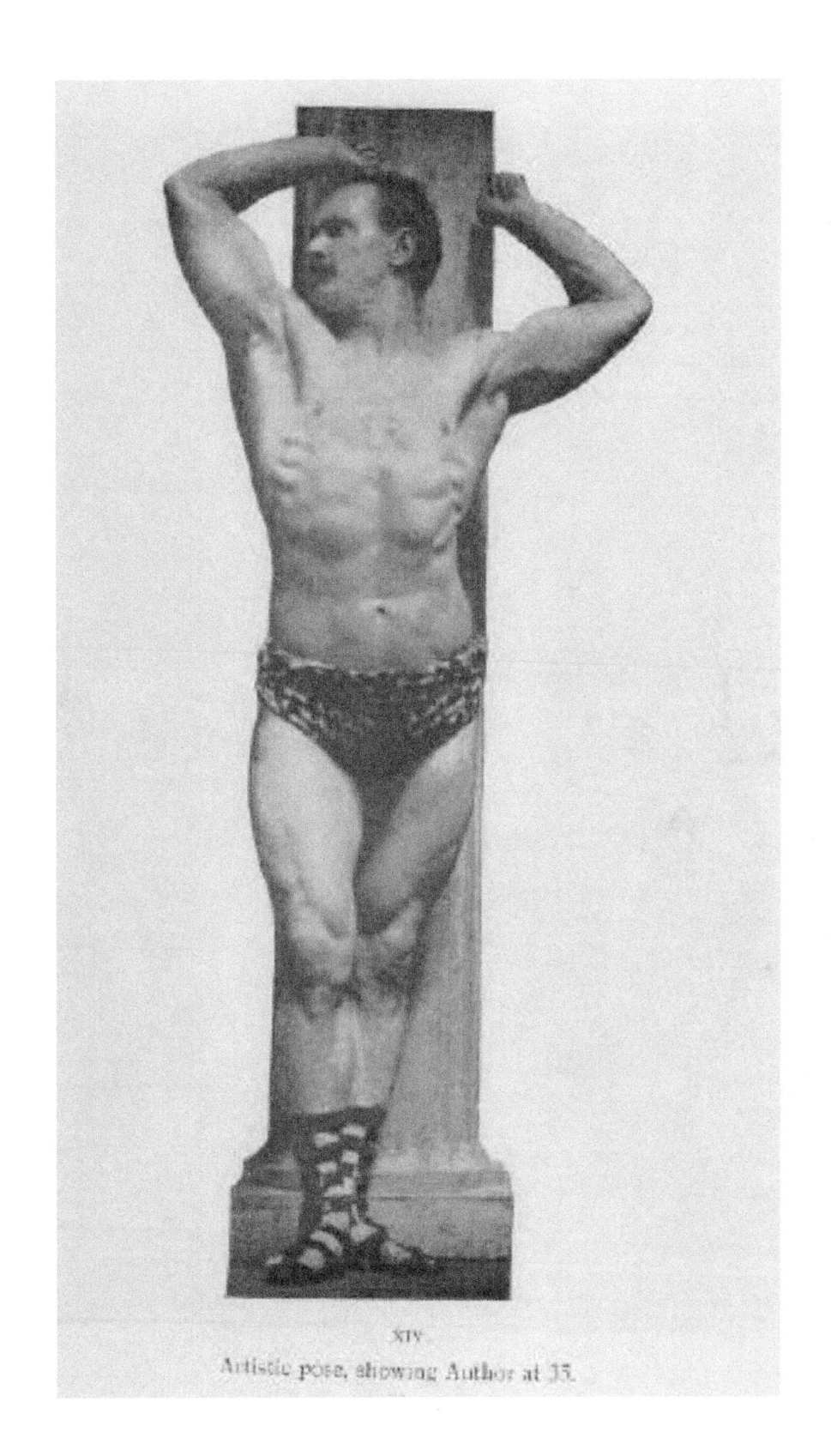

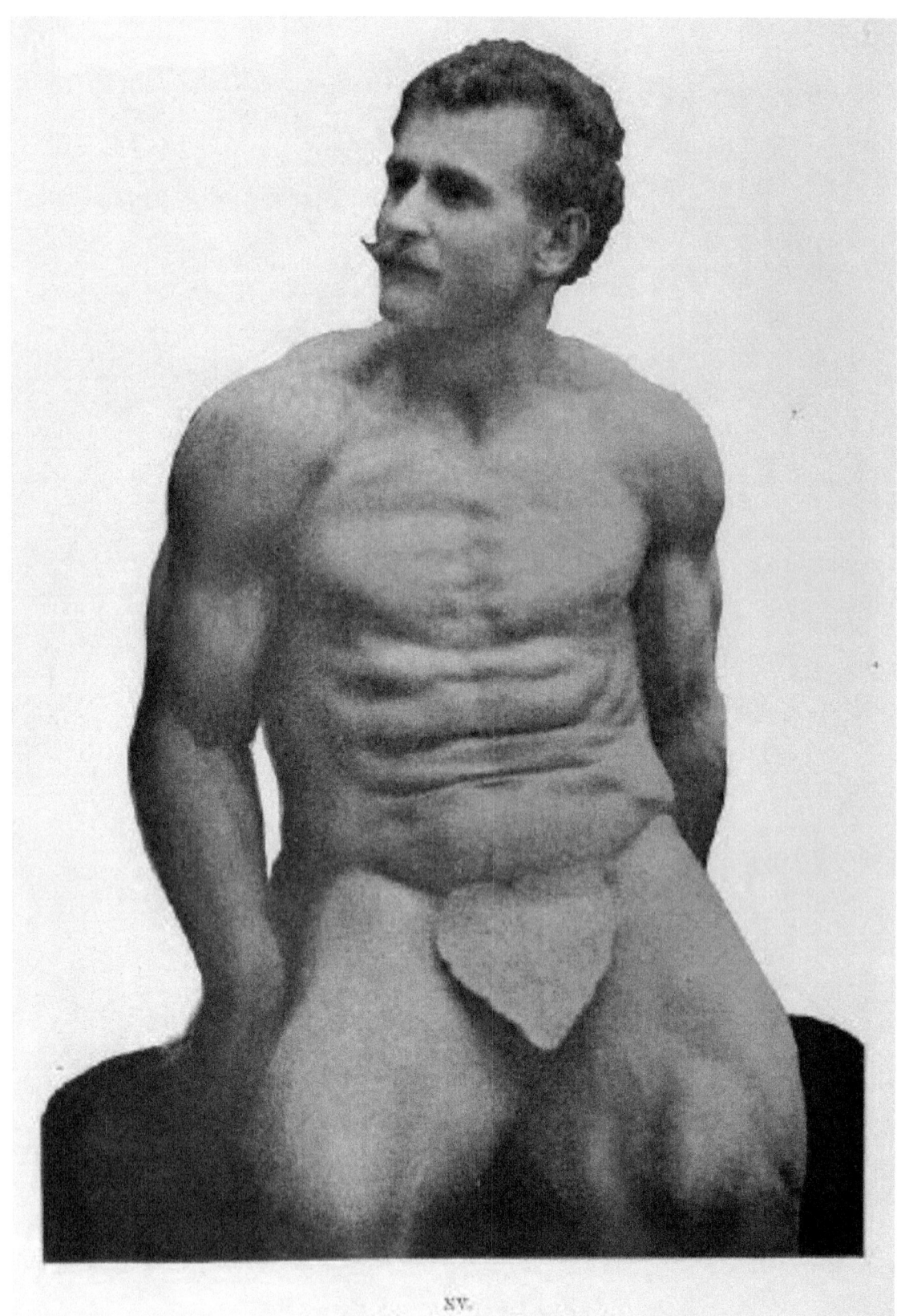

XV.
Photo at 37, with muscles relaxed.

XVI.
Two years later, at 39.

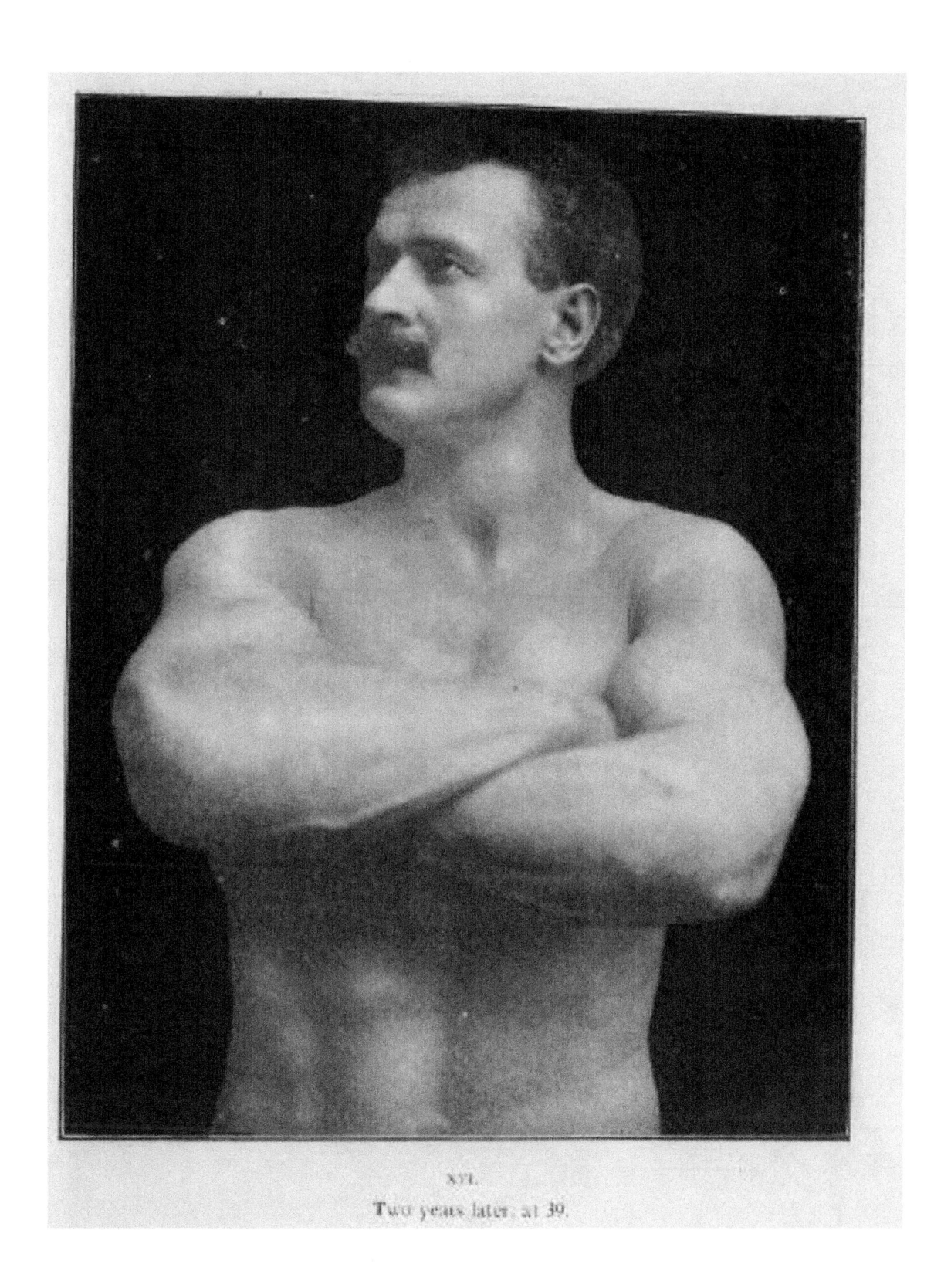

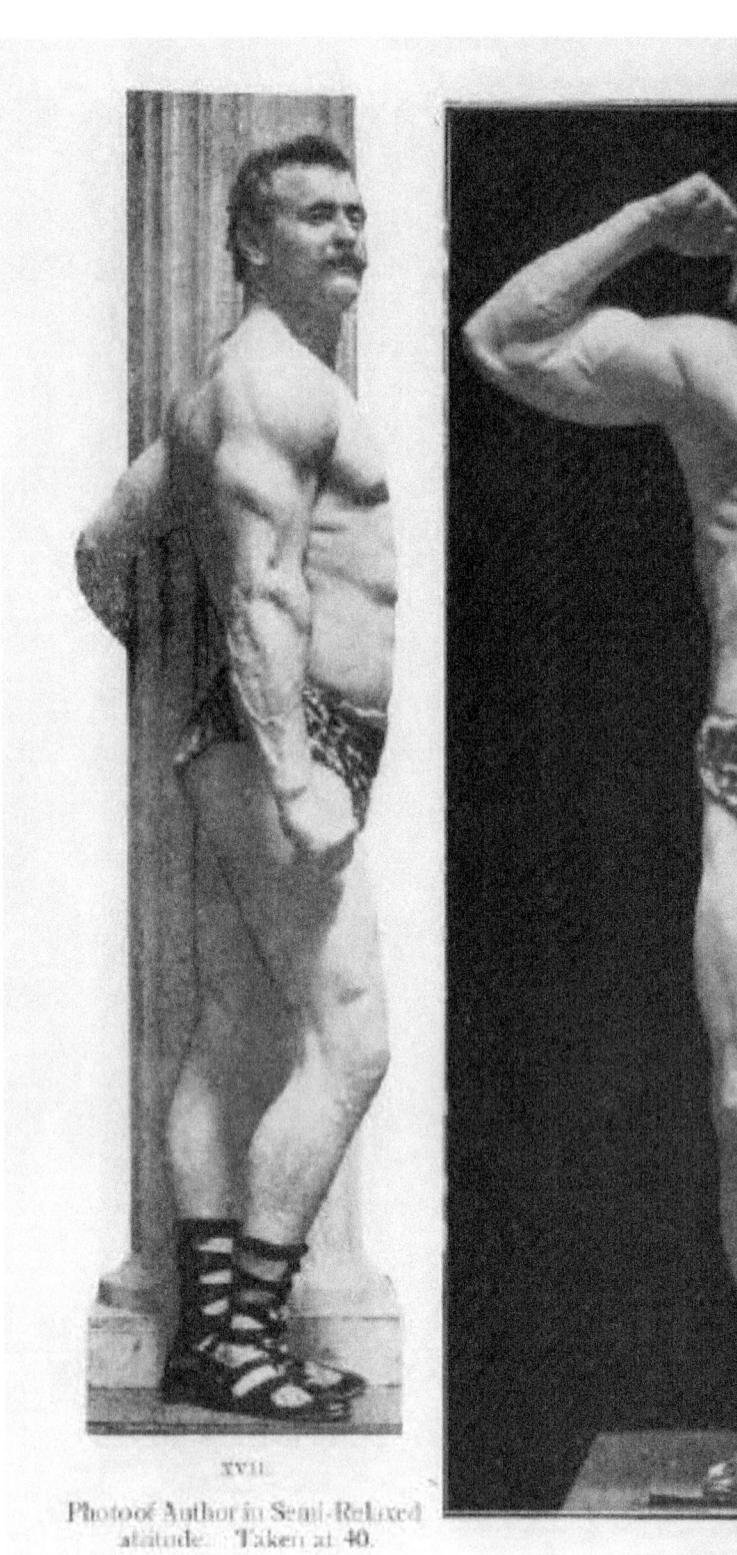

XVII.
Photo of Author in Semi-Relaxed attitude. Taken at 40.

XVIII.
Another study at 40, with muscles contracted.

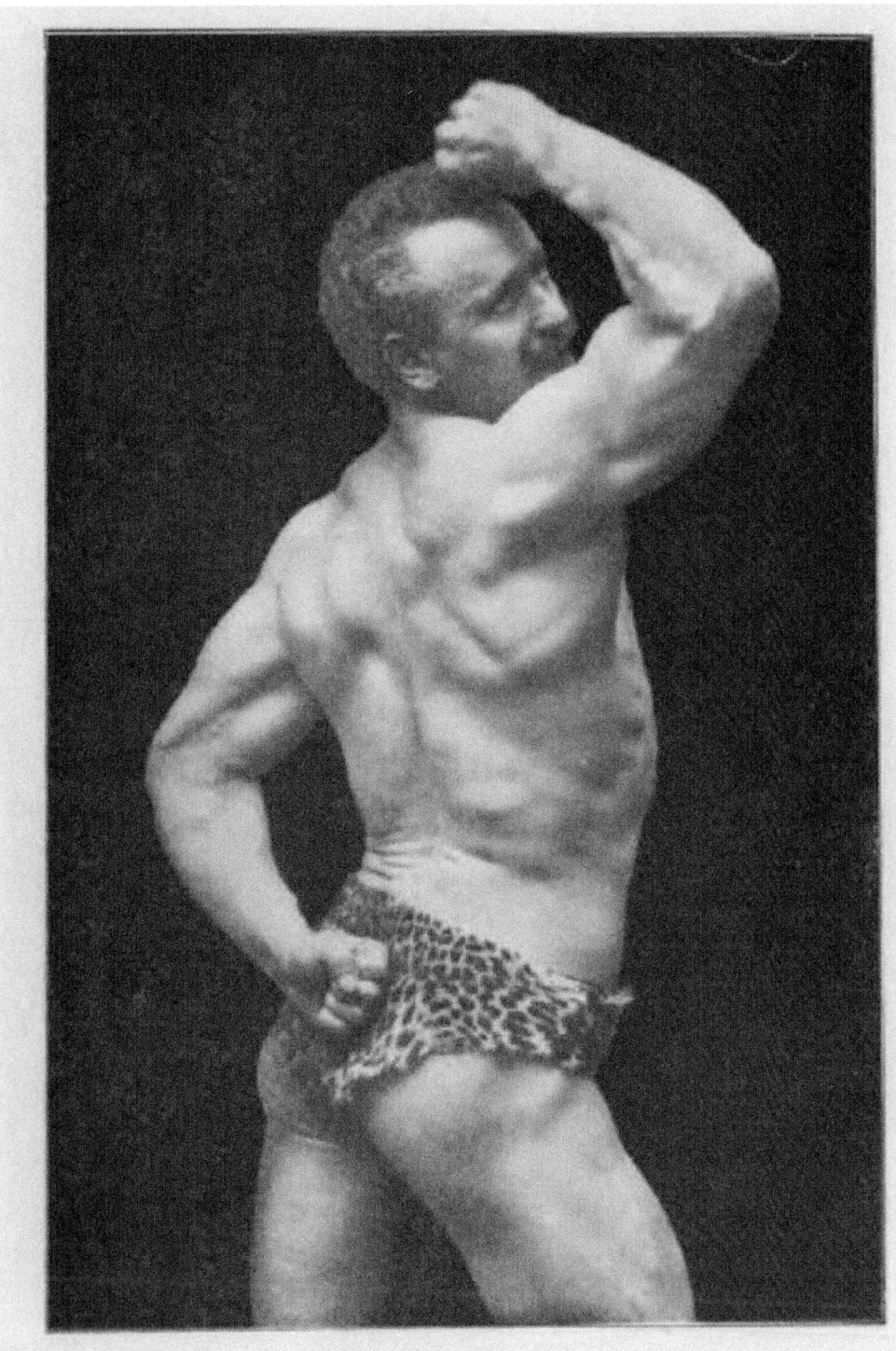

XIX.
The Author as he appeared about 42, showing back muscles contracted.

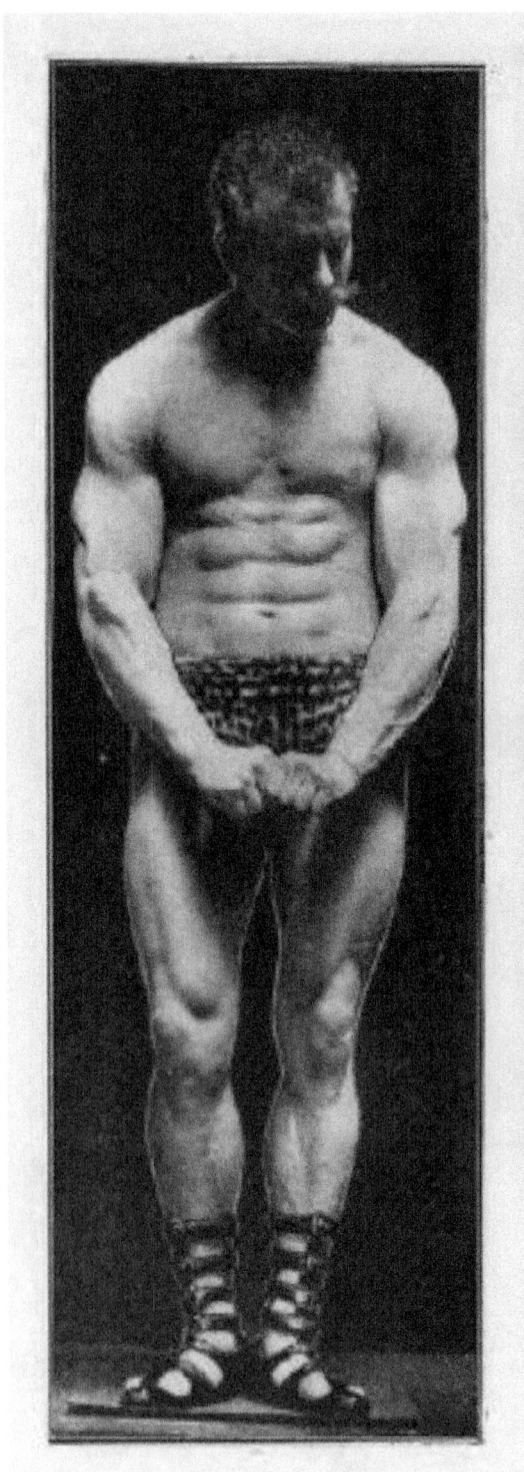

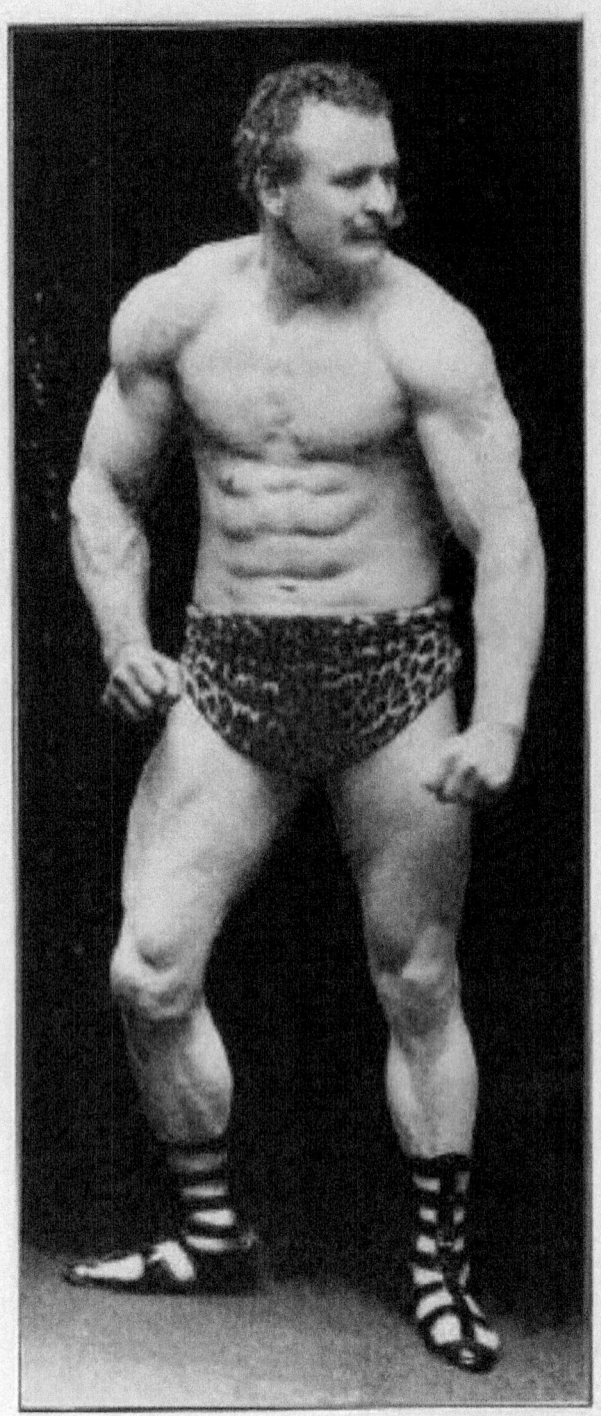

Two studies of the Author at 43. Note development of abdominal muscles in photo on left and triceps development of arms.

XXI.

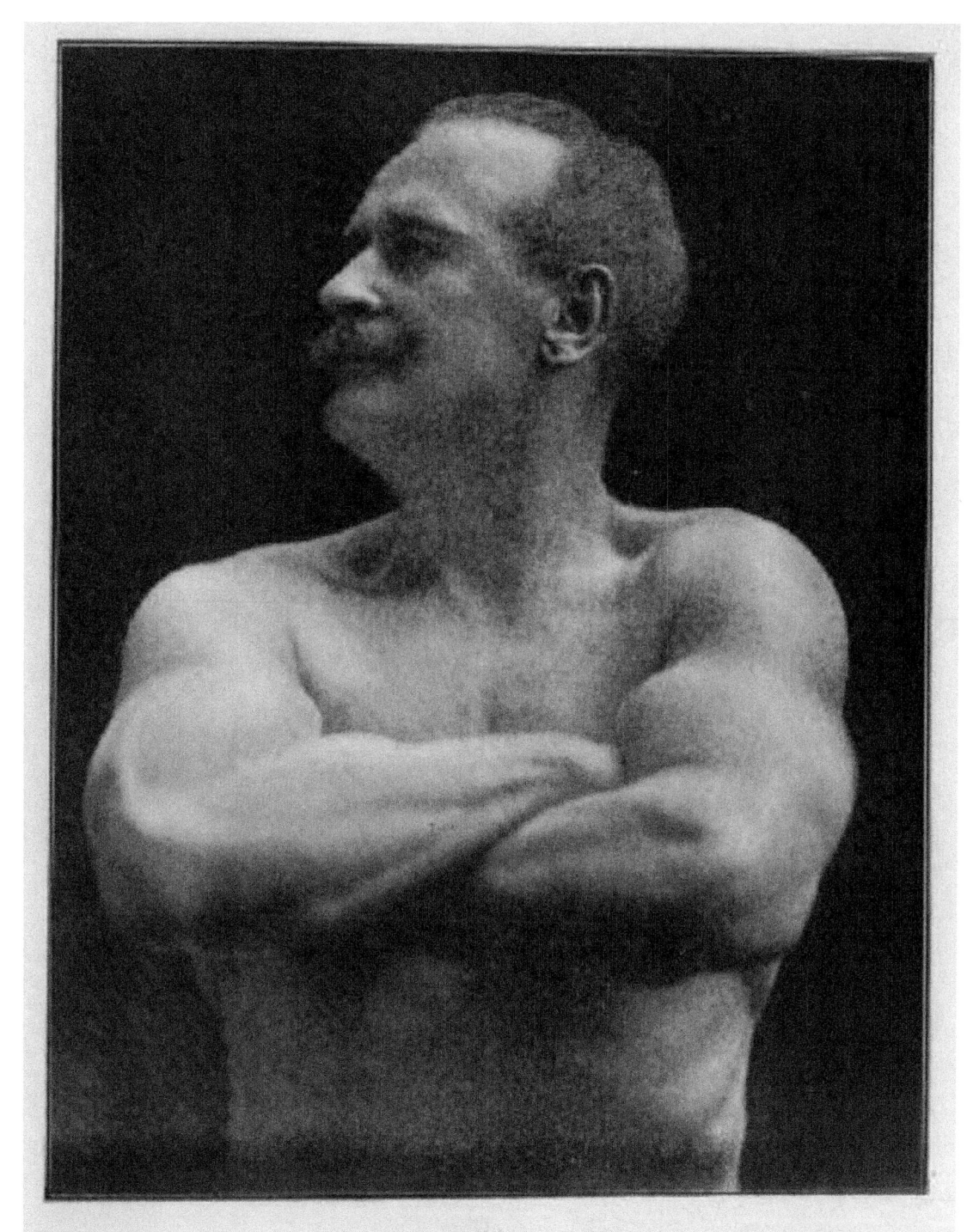

AS HE IS TO-DAY.

Striking photo of the Author at 52, confirming his statement in this book that muscle, once built up, remains, to a great extent, always, provided the body is only given a few minutes daily exercise to maintain balance when once it is established.

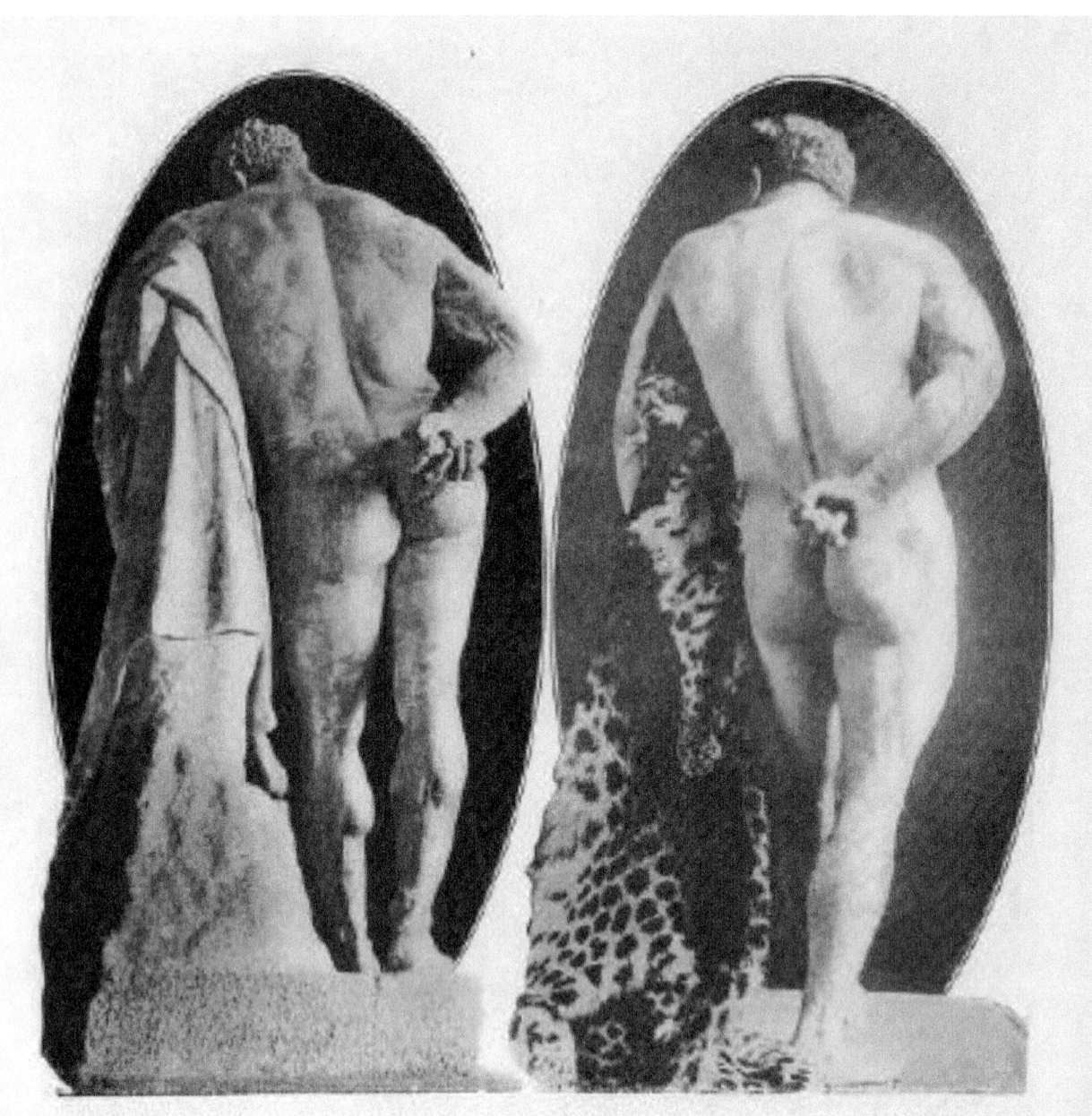

The original Farnese Hercules, to whom the Author has been compared. The accompanying photo shows—

The Author in a similar pose. Many say that the Author's proportions are the more symmetrical of the two.

CHAPTER XXV.

Hints for the Prevention of Disease and Exercises that will help.

THE exercises given here are only for normal men and women who are organically sound and suffering from no disease or weakness tending towards disease. To make certain of this it is always best to consult your own medical man at the beginning, lest there be some latent or inherited weakness entirely unsuspected, as was the case with the million and more rejected, after medical examination, for military service, most of whom were entirely unsuspicious of any physical weakness whatever. These exercises are only meant to be used as a preventive against disease or weakness tending to disease.

Those who are not organically sound, or who are suffering from any actual illness or disease or weakness towards disease, should not use these exercises, but should have exercises specially selected, prescribed and graduated to suit their particular illness, disease or weakness, and this either by a medical man who is familiar with curative exercise treatment or on the advice of an expert in curative physical culture to suit their individual condition and requirements.

The number of movements given here in each exercise, with the increase suggested at the end of every three months, apply only in normal conditions of life, but where there is excessive mental work, great anxiety, grief, loss of sleep, or any other abnormal condition causing great expenditure of nervous energy, which sometimes happens, the number of movements may be curtailed so as to preserve balance between physical and mental expenditure. My chapter on " Neurasthenia " deals with this matter very thoroughly.

Before commencing these exercises, every reader will find it a good plan to take a set of measurements and mark same on chart which is given at the close of this chapter. By keeping this chart posted up to date at the end of each period, the reader will thus have a record of his progress. This is to be recommended in every case, as it will give the reader greater interest in noting increase of measurements every three months, and improving development of physique as the exercises are continued. A photographic record with photos taken in the nude or wearing loin-cloth only or ordinary bathing pants of this progress will show the astonishing improvement made in twelve months, and, again, at the end of every succeeding year.

  1. Study Anatomical Chart herewith and learn the names of all the superficial muscles indicated on it. Repeat the name of the principal muscles used as you carry out each movement.

  2. Perform each movement as if against great resistance, so as to increase force of contraction and with full mental concentration on the muscle or muscles being moved, and keep the mind from wandering. Contraction should be maintained during each movement and the whole number of movements to be made in any exercise. Relax the muscles only between exercises (not between movements in exercise) except in the one relaxation exercise specified where all the muscles are relaxed.

  3. Remember that it is not so much the number of movements made, but the amount of contraction put into each movement that counts. This enhances the benefit of each contraction by assisting in the elimination of the waste caused by the contraction and the bringing up of greater supplies of nutriment by the blood circulation.

4.   By concentrating the mind fully upon the muscle or muscles moved, the cells in the motor areas of the brain associated are also developed. This helps to develop also will power, and to give you control over the voluntary muscles and through them over the nervous system also.

5.   Do the movements exactly as explained, and for the exact number of times given for at least the first three months you may, if you feel very weak, do less, but never do more. After three months they may be increased by five each and similarly every subsequent three months until they can be carried out not more than 50 times.

6.   It is best to use only one arm or leg at a time, except where otherwise advised, as this enables you to concentrate more fully and put more effort into the contraction. This means quicker and better results and tends to develop and strengthen the heart gradually.

7.   Don't be in too great a hurry or grow impatient- It took me years of concentration and conscious effort to build up my own body, and you must not expect to build up a disease- free body in a few weeks or even months.

8.   Do not feel alarmed if after the movements at first you feel stiffness or pain. This is usually only muscular pain through weakness and disuse of certain muscles, and it will pass away as you grow stronger.

9.   Do not introduce " substitutes " for any of the movements here given, as they are all selected after long experience and observation.

10.   The best time to carry out the exercises is in the morning immediately on rising and before breakfast. Those who feel too faint or weak for this might have a cup of tea or coffee or hot milk first with a biscuit, but on no account should exercise be undertaken for at least two hours after a full meal.

11.   Where, however, this is not convenient or against personal inclination, the evening may be chosen and the exercises performed before retiring to bed, unless that interferes with sleep.

12.   The bath should follow the exercises, cold or tepid in the morning and warm in the evening. As far as possible the movements should be carried out at the same time daily, Sundays excepted, for regularity and continuity add to their value.

13.   If possible, the exercises should be carried out stripped to the waist, but a singlet may be worn that allows plenty of room for the free play of the muscles around the shoulder. If convenient, it is a good plan to perform the exercises in front of a mirror, as it is helpful to watch the actual working of the muscles and to see them develop.

14.   At first, the exercises may be divided into two lots, and carried out on alternate days; half being done one day and half the next, the only exception being the breathing exercises, which should be done every day. Exercises should be either divided equally and can be selected at discretion of reader.

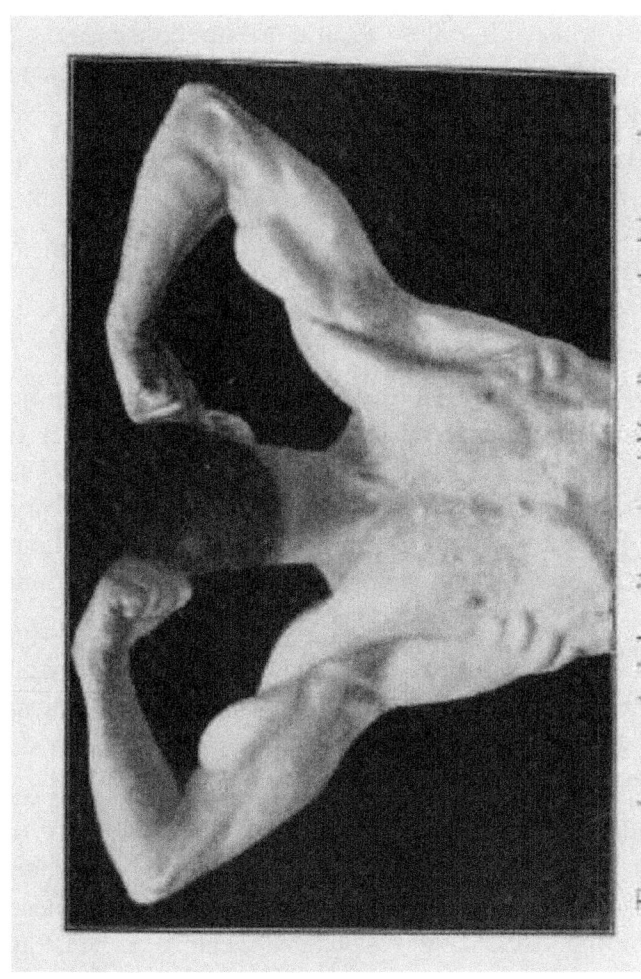

The power latent in such a body as this to resist and defeat disease must be obvious at a glance. Although starting as an adult, this development is the result of the method here described, and shows what we could expect if children were physically educated in the same way from schooldays.

Exercise 1. Stand erect, heels together, toes outwards, chest forward. Upper arm pressed to side and remaining stationary in this position while the lower arm is carrying out the movements. Arm slightly forward, fist closed, knuckles behind. Place right hand on left biceps. Then contract left arm, raising dumb-bell to shoulder, but keeping upper arm close to side and unmoved. Return to first position and repeat movement 10 times, keeping mind concentrated solely on biceps of left arm during the series of movements. Return to original position and repeat with right arm, feeling contraction with left hand. Perform 10 times. Principal muscle brought into play and to be concentrated on, biceps of arm.

Exercise 2. The same movement with forearm reverse knuckles of fist to front. Bring arm, being moved a little forward of body this time, to enable you to catch hold of the triceps of the other arm with free hand to feel and note its contraction. Raise fist to shoulder as before, without moving upper arm, keeping knuckles in front, straighten out again and repeat with each arm 10 times, first feeling contraction of triceps; study contraction in mirror. This movement develops the triceps of the arm as shown in chart. Principal muscle brought into play and to be concentrated upon, triceps of arm.

Exercise 3. Stand as in previous exercise, with arm bent at elbow, palm in front, and fist raised level with shoulder. Feel flexors of left forearm (see chart) with right hand to note muscles contracted. Bend first forward and downward from wrist only, keeping forearm rigid. Raise fist again to former position and repeat 10 times. Return to first position as before and repeat movement with right arm 10 times, feeling contraction with left hand. Principal muscles brought into and to be concentrated upon, flexors of forearm.

Exercise 4. Stand erect as before, both arms hanging by side, knuckles in front. Place right hand on muscle of front forearm, marked in chart, to note contraction. Bend left fist upwards from wrist only, keeping left arm fully stretched out at side of body, and then return fist to original position. Repeat 10 times. Same movement with right arm,, feeling contraction with left hand also 10 times. Principal muscle brought into play and to be concentrated upon, extensors of forearm.

Exercise 5. Stand erect as before, but with left arm bent at elbow, knuckles out, fist at shoulder. Place right hand on left shoulder at muscle marked Anterior and Posterior Deltoid. Now push arm straight upwards over head to full extent as if pushing up heavy weight with all your strength. Bring arm back to original position as if pulling against great resistance whilst doing so. Repeat movement 10 times. Same movement 10 times for right arm, feeling shoulder muscles with left hand. Principal muscles brought into play and to be concentrated upon, Deltoids.

Exercise 6. Erect position as before. Arm hanging loosely at side. Place right hand on top of large muscle marked Trapezius in chart between shoulder and neck just above collar bone. Push shoulder forward and downward without moving body or arm except at shoulder. Repeat 10 times and also same with right shoulder feeling contraction with left hand. Principal muscle brought into play and to be concentrated upon, Trapezius.

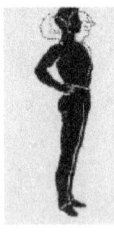

Exercise 7. Stand erect, heels together, toes pointing outwards, and hands on hips. Elbows back, chest raised. Eyes front and head well back. Then tense muscles of neck and press chin downward slowly on to chest. Then press head backwards as far as possible as if against strong resistance. Take one hand from hip and feel contraction of muscles at nape of neck or watch in mirror. Movement to be performed 10 times.

Exercise 8. Position as in last. Press the head slowly to the extreme right and downwards towards right shoulder as if against strong resistant power, and then bring head slowly over to extreme left side in the same way as per diagram. Release right hand and feel contraction of muscles at side of neck with it, and then repeat with left alternately. Keep muscles of neck (marked Sterno-Cleido-Mastoid in chart) thoroughly tensed right through each movement, and carry out each 10 times. Principal muscles brought into play and to be concentrated upon, Sterno-Cleido-Mastoid.

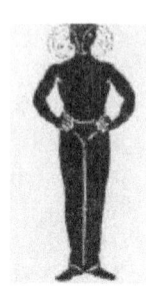

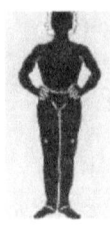

Exercise 9. Stand as in Exercise 8. Without moving the shoulders, turn head as far to the right as possible, and then to the left in the same way, as per diagram, keeping muscles tensed all the time as if moving against great resistance. Hands may be released from hips to feel contraction of Sterno-Cleido-Mastoid muscles as shown in chart, or watch in mirror. Principal muscles engaged and' to be concentrated upon, the Sterno-Cleido-Mastoid.

Exercise 10. Stand with feet apart, left foot slightly in advance of right, and left arm fully extended horizontally, as per diagram, marked Pectoralis Major on chart. Bring left hand slowly down across front of body, slightly bending elbow, as if pulling down heavy weight. Then let hand travel back to level of shoulder again. Repeat 10 times and do same with right. Feel large chest muscle market Pectoralis Major on chart with free hand or keep free hand on hips and watch in mirror. Principal muscle brought into play and to be concentrated upon, Pectoralis Major.

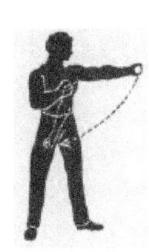

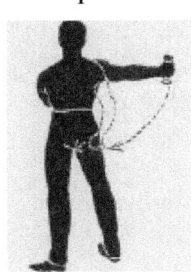

Exercise 11. Stand feet apart, as in movement No. 10, with right hand on hip. Press left arm slowly (1) backwards behind back, (2) downwards, and (3) upwards towards right hip and slightly bending elbow when raising behind back to hip as per diagram. Return to position and repeat 10 times. Same with right arm afterwards. Note contraction of Latissimus Dorsi muscles, as shown in chart, or watch in mirror. Principal muscles used and to be concentrated upon, Latissimus Dorsi as shown in anatomical chart.

Exercise 12. Stand erect, heels together, chest advanced, knuckles downwards, and arms extended, sideways in line with shoulders as per diagram 1. Raise shoulders to dotted line in diagram 1, then bend arms at elbow as in diagram 2, letting shoulder drop again during the bending of the arms. Then, while stretching arms to original position, raise shoulders to dotted line as in diagram once more. Before beginning to bend arms again relax muscles of the shoulder, and allow shoulder to drop as in first position. In other words, raise and lower shoulders alternately as arms are being bent and straightened. Repeat movement 10 times, watching contraction in mirror. Principal muscles used and to be concentrated upon, the Biceps, Triceps, Deltoids and Trapezius, as marked on anatomical chart.

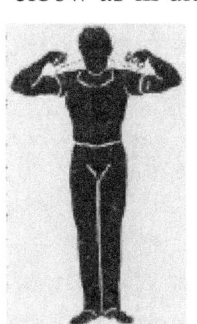

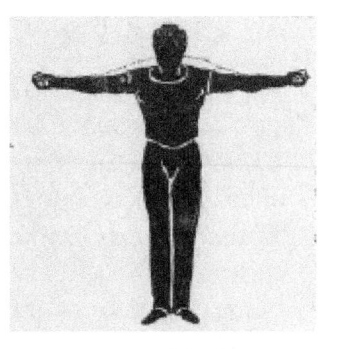

Exercise 13. Stand quite easy, toes at an angle of 45 degrees, arms hanging by sides. Draw in abdomen and raise chest, at the same time pressing out the muscles marked Latissimus Dorsi and Serratus Magnus on chart, the former running from above the waist at back behind the arms and below the armpit, so that the muscles force the arms outwards as if a wedge had been driven between each arm and the side of the body, or, in other words, these back and side muscles are brought under the armpits and show clearly from the front. See photo of author showing chest expansion in chapter on "The Machinery of National Physical Training" (opposite page 241). Repeat 10 times. This is muscular chest expansion, and the breathing must be natural and normal. Principal muscles: Latissimus Dorsi and Serratus Magnus.

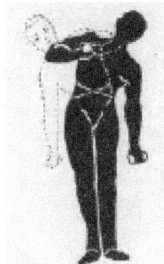

Exercise 14. Stand straight, arms hanging by sides, knees braced. Bend over to left side from hips only as far as possible, at the same time bringing right hand well up under armpit, stretching left arm down as far as possible. Then bend over sideways from hips only on the right side, trying to touch side of leg as far down as possible, and bringing left fist to armpit. Repeat movement 10 times. The principal muscle here employed is the Obliquus Abdominis (see chart) upon which the mind should be fully concentrated. The biceps, triceps and deltoid muscles are also brought into

play.

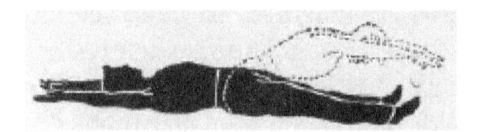

Exercise 15. Lie flat on back, legs close together and straight, toes pointed forward, arms stretched full length behind the head. Inhale deeply through the nostrils and raise the upper part of the body into a sitting position. Do not stop, but continue bending forward till the finger tips reach beyond the toes, as per diagram, then exhale. Return to previous position, inhaling. Keep head between arms throughout the movement. If you cannot do this movement at first, place toes beneath weight so as to get leverage. The principal muscles used and to be concentrated upon are the Rectus Abdominis and the Erector Spinae (see chart). Repeat 10 times.

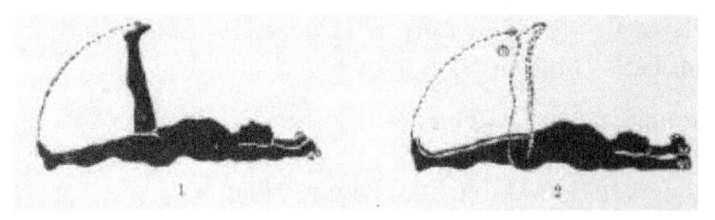

Exercise 16. Lie flat on back, arms fully stretched out behind and with hands underneath head. Heels and head both raised slightly from the ground. Raise the right leg until it is at right angles to the body as per diagram 1. Then lower right leg without touching floor, at the same time raising left. The exercise should be done slowly and not with any jerking movement, the one leg being lowered as the other is raised. Repeat 10 times. Then perform the same movements simultaneously with both legs as per diagram 2, and repeat 10 times. The principal muscles used are the Rectus Abdominis (see chart), upon which concentrate the mind.

Exercise 17. Stand in erect position, chest raised, heels together, toes pointing out. Place both hands on Gluteus Maximus muscle as shown in chart, and push middle part of the body forward, returning to original position, keeping upper part of body and legs quite still and only moving middle part of body forwards and backwards. Repeat 10 times. Concentrate mind on principal muscle brought into play, the Gluteus Maximus.

Exercise 18. Stand easy, and then tense large muscles in front of thigh of left leg by bracing or stiffening knee backwards and feeling muscle in front of thigh contracting with left hand. Repeat same movement with right thigh and right hand, and then with both thighs feeling contraction with one hand on each thigh. Principal muscles brought into play, the Quadriceps Extensor as shown on chart, and mind should be kept fixed on it during movement. Repeat each of these movements 10 times.

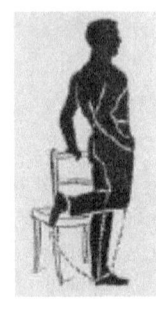

Exercise 19. Stand beside a chair, grasping top rail of chair with left hand. Place right hand on hip or at back of right thigh so that you can feel the contraction of the biceps or flexors muscles of thigh as marked on chart. Press the right leg up behind the body as per diagram, as if trying to raise heavy weight attached to ankle. Recover and repeat. This movement should be performed with each leg alternately 10 times. Principal muscle used, the Biceps of thighs, upon which mind should be centred.

Exercise 20. Again stand at side of chair left hand on hip, other grasping chair as in diagram. Raise left leg as high as possible sideways and outwards as if forcing it upwards against great force and recover position. Repeat 10 times and follow in same way with right leg. Principal muscles brought into play and upon which to concentrate are the Abductor muscles of the thigh as shown in chart.

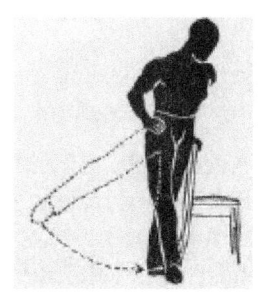

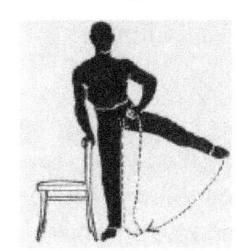

Exercise 21. Same exercise reversed, only stand as in diagram, with right leg raised outwards and sideways before commencing the movement. Bring right leg slowly downwards to ground as if pulling heavy weight down, and then recover original position. Perform exercise with each leg 10 times, alternately. Muscles brought into play, and upon which to concentrate are the Adductor muscles of thigh as marked on the chart.

Exercise 22. Stand easy, and bending down clasp calf of left leg with both hands. Then raise heels from ground, and feel muscles of the back of calf marked Gastrocnemius and Soleus on chart contracting quite hard. Lower heel again to ground and repeat this movement 10 times, first with the left leg and then with the right, using full pressure. Concentrate thoughts on muscles of calf being used.

Exercise 23. Stand as before, with feet firmly on the ground. Stoop and clasp front of lower left leg where muscle Tibialis Anticus is marked on chart. Raise toes of left foot from the ground and note contraction. Lower toes to original position and repeat 10 times, afterwards doing the same with the right leg, using full pressure in both. Principal muscle used and to be concentrated upon, the Tibialis Anticus.

Exercise 24. Stand with feet about 12 inches apart, heels on floor arms, by side, knees pressed back. Sit down slowly, without touching floor, knees apart, as per diagram. Return to original position. Heels should be kept on floor during movement, and leg stiffened when rising up. To increase power of contraction, imagine a heavy weight to be resting on shoulders during the movement. Muscles brought into play and concentrated on, the Quadriceps and Biceps of the thigh as per chart. Other muscles used, the Gluteus Maximus. Repeat 5 times only.

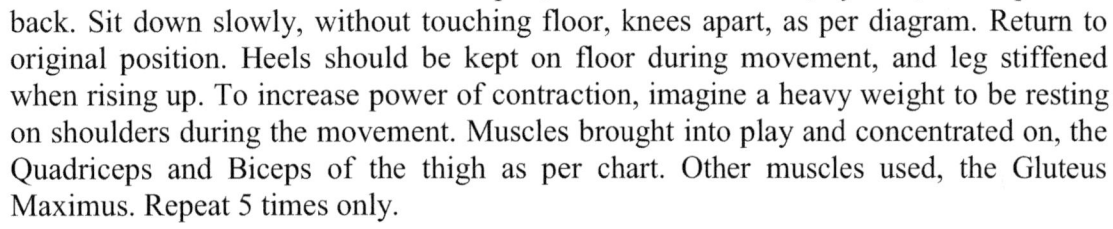

Exercise 25. Same as previous exercise, only before commencing movement, raise heels and stand on tip toes as per diagram. Sit down as in No. 24 and rise slowly up. Again, the pupil should imagine he is raising a heavy weight on back from the ground. Repeat 1 times only.

Exercise 26. Stand with hands at shoulders, elbows bent as per diagram. Body and head well back, face looking upwards. Now bring the body smartly forward, stretching arms above head as you bend forward, keeping head and arms in one line, and without bending the knees, endeavouring to touch the ground about 12 inches in front of the toes, exhaling. Return smartly to first position, inhaling. Repeat 5 times.

Exercise 27. Breathing exercise. Upper chest breathing. Stand erect with heels together, knees braced, hips pressed back, hands crossed over the abdomen. Fully inflate the lungs, raising chest as high as possible, as per diagram, pressing abdomen with hands.

Exhale, relaxing pressure of hands. Keep shoulders down during this movement. Don't hold breath between inhalation and exhalation. Repeat 10 times.

Exercise 28. Breathing exercise (abdominal breathing). Stand erect with neck pressed back, chest relaxed and hands clasped over abdomen as per diagram. Inhale slowly through the nostrils and inflate lungs to the fullest extent allowing the abdomen instead of chest to swell fully and force hands forwards. Expel all air from lungs, drawing in abdomen, and raising the chest. Place hands of abdomen to feel inhalation and exhalation. Don't hold breath. Repeat 10 times.

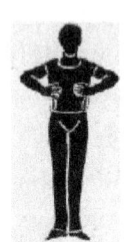

Exercise 29. Breathing exercise (costal breathing). Stand erect, placing hands flatly on ribs, fingers forward, as per diagram. Inhale deeply and slowly, and feel ribs expanding and chest widening as you inhale. Do not raise chest or abdomen. Exhale fastly and fully by mouth. Repeat 10 times. (N.B.—On no account should the breath be held between inspiration and exhalation. This applies equally to all these exercises, apart from breathing exercises, except Exercise 15.)

Exercise 30. Stand erect, feet forming a right angle, left toe pointing in front. Strike out quickly with right hand in front carrying left foot forward, knee bent and right leg braced behind as per diagram 1. Do same movement with left arm, and repeat each movement 10 times. Perform this movement swiftly both in lunging and retreating.

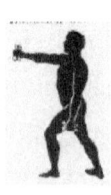

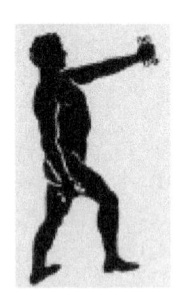

Exercise 31. Stand with right toe pointing forward and left foot at right angles. Strike forward sharply with left hand, at the same time carrying forward right leg, knee bent and left braced as support behind as per diagram. Repeat same movement with right arm carrying forward right leg as before as in diagram. Repeat each 10 times. N.B.—These last two are relaxation movements and should be done with relaxed muscles swiftly, smartly and lightly. Only meant to develop speed and suppleness of muscle. In carrying foot forward let toe touch ground only lightly and almost noiselessly. Repeat 10 times, as before.

Exercise 32. Stand erect, toes at an angle of 45 degrees, arms extended sideways, and level with the shoulders. Knuckles downwards. Bend arms at elbow, without moving upper arm, and bring fists slowly to side of head above ears. Put full effort as if intending to squeeze or crush head. Return to position and repeat 10 times. Principal muscles brought into play and to fix mind upon are the Biceps, Triceps, Deltoids, Trapezius, and Erector Spinae also should be contracted. See chart. Reverse, starting with fists against side of head above ears, bringing arms level with shoulders, putting great power as if striving to stretch to your utmost or attempting to reach with each hand the furthest point possible sideways from each shoulder. Repeat this also 10 times.

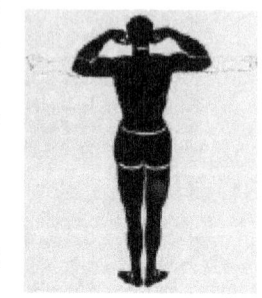

N.B.—The exercises here given are equally suitable and beneficial for people of both sexes, as the voluntary muscular system is the same in both. In a man, however, the muscles developed will always show more prominently than in a woman, because there is greater destruction of fatty tissue between muscle and skin in his case. On the other hand, physical exercise will never cause a woman to develop a masculine and muscular appearance, because Nature in some way preserves from destruction the fatty tissue between muscle and skin in her case. For this reason, the limbs and figure take more beautiful curves when physical exercises are carried out, and the flesh becomes firmer and healthier. These exercises will increase grace and beauty of outline, improve carriage and gait and poise, and benefit health from a preventive point of view, as they have already done for the healthy and well- formed women whose photographs are reproduced in this book.

RELAXATION MOVEMENTS.—It may be well to make quite clear here exactly what I mean by relaxation movements. Strictly speaking, of course, there is no such thing as a relaxation movement, for the complete relaxation of a muscle means absence of all movement. This is a term I have invented to describe any movement when the movement of a muscle or muscles is not performed with full power of contraction but with muscles relaxed instead. In other words, the muscles are held lightly and not braced, so that they are always ready for quick action in response to a command from the will. Such movements are of special value to develop speed and agility. The more relaxed the condition the swifter the execution of the movement. In relaxed movements the contraction takes place quickly at the end of the movement, whereas in contraction movements the muscle is flexed slowly from the very beginning. In other words, the mind must be concentrated on relaxation and not on contraction.

To carry out the exercises may not always be easy or pleasant. Indeed, it will require an effort of will to stick to them under all circumstances. But the reward, though not immediate or visible at once, is great, for the body is not only more healthy and strong, but the mind and will are disciplined and brought into subjection, so that your prospect of success in life will be greater.

MEASUREMENT CHART FOR MEN.

For the benefit of those who would like to note and keep a record of their physical progress, this chart is given. It will be interesting for one who carries out the exercises here given to keep such a record, and to be able to contrast his condition on commencement and at later periods.

THE MEASUREMENTS MUST BE TAKEN ROUND THE BODY AND LIMBS.

DETAILS.	PRESENT DAY.	AFTER 3 MTHS.	AFTER 6 MTHS.	AFTER 1 YEAR	AFTER 18 MTS.	AFTER 2 YRS.
Height						
Weight						
Neck						
Waist						
Chest (contracted)						
Chest (expanded)						
Thigh (left)						
Thigh (right)						
Upper arm (right)						
Upper arm (left)						
Forearm (right)						
Forearm (left)						
Calf (right)						
Calf (left)						

MEASUREMENT CHART FOR WOMEN

Those who wish to keep a record of their progress and improvement will find this chart convenient, and it will be a pleasing experience for them afterwards to contrast their measurements, weight and height then with their original condition. This chart can be used for two years.

THE MEASUREMENTS MUST BE TAKEN ROUND THE BODY AND LIMBS.

DETAILS.	PRESENT DAY	AFTER 3 MTHS.	AFTER 6 MTHS.	AFTER 9 MTHS.	AFTER 18 MTHS.	AFTER 2 YEARS.
Height						
Weight						
Neck						
Waist						
Chest (contracted)						
Chest (expanded)						
Upper arm (right)						
Upper arm (left)						
Forearm (right)						
Forearm (left)						
Thigh (left)						
Thigh (right)						
Calf (right)						
Calf (left)						

CHAPTER XXVI.

My Appeal to the People for a Real League of Nations against Disease.

AN ALL-FOR-HEALTH LEAGUE.

LIKE some stout Cortes of modern times, Mr Lloyd George sees, in his hour of triumph, a new world swimming into his ken. It is as yet an inchoate and shapeless mass, enshrouded in mist and rain, and hung over with many clouds, but through and over all these the sun of hope breaks, to give revealing glimpses of its staggering immensity, its amazing potentialities, its incalculable and immeasurable possibilities, immediate and remote.

MAKING THE NEW WORLD.

The old world, charred, scarred, blackened and half-consumed by the angry flames of war, is already becoming but a blurred and sinking object far away in our wake on the dim and distant horizon. Soon, let us hope, it will sink to be seen no more. We are leaving it fast behind—have left it, let us hope, forever. Let us be quite certain that our compass is true, that our charts are all in order, and that no new siren-voices lure us from our true sea-path to be shattered on rocks or sucked down in maelstroms not less deadly than those from which we have escaped.

To destroy that which is already more than half-destroyed is easy if we are so determined. To reconstruct the new may be more difficult, and to make the new world a better world still will be even harder. Construction and reconstruction demand an architect and a builder, an incendiary can destroy.

One thing is already apparent. In the new world, human life will have a new and added value. Human bodies and brains will be appraised at a higher rate than ever before. But better and stronger bodies and brains will be required in return, and there will be scant mercy for the culpably inefficient, physically or mentally. Old systems and standards of education must give place to new, for the education of the individual is the first step in the upbuilding of a new .and better world. We must begin by building better men, women and children; in other words, by building the builders who are to rebuild and reconstruct a new and better world. Otherwise the new world will prove but little less pleasant to live in than the old.

BETTER BODIES AND BETTER BRAINS.

When, then, is to be the standard by which we shall be judged? It will be a high standard and a severe one—not set by decadent man but by stern and immutable Nature. Man must again become a dual being, with both a higher type of body and a higher type of brain. The old educational shibboleths will be discarded. A better type of brain will be looked for than the mental money-box which modern education gives people to-day in place of that organ.

A better type of body, too, will be necessary to the upbuilding and maintenance of a real thinking-machine that will be asked to create, initiate, produce and put into execution plans, methods and campaigns for something greater and bigger than ever mind of man has yet conceived. The body must be as a strong tower above which flashes the illuminating mind to make safe the new world against the risks and dangers that brought about the destruction of the old.

This is the type of human being of which it may truly be said he was made in the image of his Creator, man, as the Creator intended him to be, as he was, indeed, Divinely created and constructed to be. In attaining to such an ideal all can contribute something, from Premier to peasant, from aristocrat to artisan. Here is work and reward for all, and all will be equally needed.

I have myself spent thousands of pounds of my own money to help mankind to a truer perspective of life. I have—at a great, expense in war time—prepared and written this book and collected these photographs from all parts of the world with the same object, and prepared it for publication at a time when I knew the microscopic searchings of Mars were certain to bring to view the ghastly revelation with which we are all now familiar. My own work does not, cannot, end here, nor will my efforts in this direction end until' the hour of my departing.

To-day, however, I appeal to all sane-thinking men and women, to every father and mother, and to the young men and the young women who will be the fathers and mothers of the future, to add their labour in what I declare to be the first and most necessary step in the restoration, upbuilding, establishment and maintenance of a people truly great, viz., the physical reconstruction of the individual human body and the establishment and sustenance of the human mind on a deep and strong physical foundation. Even the children are invited to put their little hands and brains to this splendid task. No effort can be spared if we are to enter into a new world, that will really-also be a better world, without unnecessary qualms and forebodings as to the future.

OBJECTS OF THE ALL-FOR-HEALTH LEAGUE.

" What can I do?" is the question that I can hear the reader ask. I have thought of a way that will enable every reader to help at a trifling expenditure in the way of labour or time. It is my intention to organise an international All-for-Health League, in this country at first, but I hope increasing and spreading very soon to the uttermost ends of the earth. This will be then a very real League of Nations against man's most treacherous, most relentless and most mischievous enemy, Disease.

The objects of the League will be to enforce Government action for the suppression and prevention of disease, to promote and foster habits of health and strength among the people, to form clubs and organisations everywhere for the diffusion of health knowledge and to popularise the physical culture of the body; above all, to use every possible effort to save the children from educational methods that imperil their physical health and happiness, and, indeed, their whole future life and well-being.

A perusal of this book is sufficient to convey to my readers the principles and objects of the All-for-Health League, because they are all pretty well enunciated in these pages. But I may say, by way of encouragement, that I am confident of enlisting distinguished and powerful patronage from men and women whose names are " familiar in our mouth as household words," and I am hoping also to enlist the gracious services of Royalty to honour us at Patron and President.

EVERY SHOULDER TO THE WHEEL.

The readers of this book will, I hope, form a nucleus around which this real League of Nations against Physical Deterioration and Disease will be upbuilt, for without organisation and united effort we cannot report progress. There will be many obstacles to overcome and many difficulties to be surmounted. Conservatism and tradition may oppose us, but with a clear conscience and a firm faith in what we preach and practise, nothing can daunt or dismay us. On the other hand, we will rally round our banner all those sane- minded men and women who have high ideals and a lofty ambition, who are anxious to give children the physical outfit for life that the strenuous life before them will demand, who seek to help me in the prevention, cure and overthrow of the enemy Disease, and to give us in the new world into which we are about to enter men and women of a physical and mental supremacy and grandeur, besides which the inhabitants of the old will seem but as Liliputians and with but Liliputian ideas and ideals.

As I say elsewhere in this book, no one lives unto himself alone, and no one, however humble his or her position in life, is without influence for good or ill both by precept and conduct. The smallest lever can raise and move a weight many times greater than its own, and a very small wedge in the tiniest crevice is sufficient to remove mountains.' I say this for the encouragement of those whose modesty may paralyse effort, and who may deem their own services too cheaply to enlist them in this great crusade against humanity's most deadly foe. By whole-hearted co-operation now, such a League as I suggest may yet prevent such dread possibilities as the last awful influenza epidemic with its 6,000,000 dead, to say nothing of the millions of others whose innate vitality and resistant power alone pulled them rapidly through. Had all these people been physically fit with bodies charged with vitality and strongly resistant to disease they would not have died, and might never have even succumbed to the disease.

It is good to know at such a time as this that we will have behind us the momentum and impetus of the world's greatest statesmen, and the world's mightiest power, the Press. War and its lessons are too fresh in our minds yet for any statesman or public journal not to profit from them, and to avail themselves of the experience gleaned for the good of the people. But memory is apt to be a treacherous thing at times, especially when new interests will arise and new problems have to be solved. So let us take the present tide at the full, and seize the power and opportunity that patriotism and enthusiasm just now place at our disposal for the physical uplift of the people.

THE HOUR AND THE MAN.

History has again repeated itself in presenting us simultaneously with that ancient and ever-acceptable combination in this country, the hour and the man. The time could not possibly be better suited to the situation than the man, for Mr Lloyd George's great speech at Manchester shows that the head of the Government in this country, at least, sees things clearly and sees them whole, while his war-work shows him the man of action as well as the man of thought and speech. And what Britain does to-day the world will do to-morrow.

But behind the Premier again must be the irresistible sweep of public opinion to support and sustain him, and as he himself has declared, in work of such magnitude everyone can do 'his or her share. It is to provide a channel through which much of this individual effort can flow that I am forming the All-for-Health League. Every reader of this book should join this League and persuade others to join. It will cost nothing, and I am confident the reward will be great, for duty well done and service rendered in any good cause in itself brings reward exceeding great.

The All-for-Health League will aim chiefly at all the chief objects that a perusal of this book would suggest to the reader, viz.:—

    1.   To build up by cellular reconstruction and evolution a stronger, finer, healthier and disease-proof race of men, women and children;

    2.   To agitate for physical education in our schools in precedence of mental education, and by the scientific methods here enunciated and explained;

3. To arouse the intelligent interest of the State in all matters pertaining to individual and national health and physical well-being of the people;

4. To promote legislation that will safeguard the health- rights of the people and enforce them, and to organise public opinion politically;

5. To advocate for the people equal opportunities from childhood for health and hygienic conditions of life;

6. To form social clubs and physical culture organisations throughout the country for the spreading of health knowledge and the culture of the body as described later.

7. To print and distribute helpful literature for the purpose of giving the people higher and better ideals;

8. To take as our League motto, " Life is Movement," and to spread the doctrine of scientific physical movement as the first essential of a healthy and happy life;

9. To assist every movement of a similar kind, and especially to lend our aid to all auxiliary reform movements that are for the hygienic advancement of the people;

10. To agitate for the addition of this subject to the cur-riculum of every medical college, school and 'Varsity, and to advocate the establishment of special colleges for the training of students in scientific and curative physical movement by Nature's methods;

11. To save and rescue this country from that state of physical decline into which it had fallen previous to the war, and to build up a better race of men, women and children, physically, mentally and morally.

12. Last, but not least, will be the foundation of social clubs throughout the country, in every city, town and village, all to be federated in one great international organisation with its headquarters in London, and to be called:

THE BLUE-BLOOD CLUB,

the most exclusive club in the world, but exclusive only in the sense that none but the healthiest, fittest and cleanest living men and women will be permitted to enter its portals or participate in its councils. I have already begun the preliminary negotiations for the establishment of the mother-club in the metropolis, and expect confidently to enlist the co-operation of the greatest in the land in establishing what I really believe will be one of the most uplifting movements for the physical salvation of the people ever undertaken in any country.

The Blue-Blood Club will represent, but on a far greater scale, something like Vincent's, of Oxford, the club reserved only for men who have won their " blue," and by far the hardest of all the 'Varsity clubs to join. But in the case of the Blue- Blood Club, membership will not be restricted to those who have won success or honours in cricket, football, rowing, or any other form of sport.

But success in sports, games and athletics even will not suffice in itself to qualify for membership in the Blue-Blood Club, because, as I have already shown, it is no uncommon thing for even a very successful athlete to possess physical defects and shortcomings that would disqualify him from belonging to a fraternity in which physical and organic fitness in the highest degree is the essential passport to membership. On the other hand, one who possessed a symmetrical and well-formed physical body in perfect balance everywhere, with an organism perfectly sound and disease-free but with no pretensions whatever to athletic supremacy or prowess, will only be assured of a place among these kings among men and queens among women.

In fact, for such a brotherhood only those without physical or organic blemish, and a perfectly balanced physical body, will be able to qualify. Such a club as I propose here will be a body to the membership of which Royalty may well aspire, if only as an example and a pattern to the nation. Membership, indeed, will be something to be prized for more than the entree into the most exclusive circles in Society. It will be a club unique in its kind, and, in time, I hope to see it represented in every city, town and village throughout the world, with an esprit de corps and a spirit of camaraderie among its members unrivalled even to-day by that of the masonic craft.

The highest physical and medical standard will have to be reached by all who aspire to membership, however highly they are placed in the social sphere. Caste, lineage, connections, influence, money, or even fame in any particular sphere of life will not of itself throw open the doors of the Blue-blood Club to anyone, however distinguished. Its members will constitute a real aristocracy of physique, constitution and health, and the essentials of qualification for membership will alone ensure its being truly the most select club in the world.

Only those who can pass the most severe medical tests, whose every system and organ is sound as it was in our original progenitor in the Garden of Eden, whose muscles, nerves, skin, heart, lungs, liver, kidneys and intestines are without flaw or defect, whose bodies are strong, symmetrical, and balanced in their beauty and strength, who are without taint of disease, through heredity or acquired, whose whole character is guaranteed not by others but by the physical condition of bodies that themselves bear evidence of clean thinking, clean living and clean conduct in every affair of life, can hope to belong to this real aristocracy and nobility of an age that has grown iconoclastic towards ancient idols and refuses to bow the knee even before those who boast " the pure blood of an illustrious race " or a man degenerate even though " hung o'er with titles and strung round with strings."

Think with what pride a man or woman will claim membership to such an elite—the real elite—of humanity. Membership of such a club will be an open sesame to every door, a breaker down of every social barrier, a real distinction of " class " that will appeal to a democratic age, and the only and desirable line of cleavage between the millions in the new age that is just about to dawn. Such men and women will be entitled rightly to assess themselves at a higher value to any nation than the men and women who neglect and ignore the cult of the physical body, who shirk their responsibilities to unborn generations, and who violate, either through ignorance or expediency, almost every hygienic law.

In time, and especially with such physical education and " health conscription " as I propose from childhood, I can see branches of this mother-chib springing up in every corner of the globe, and even every man and woman fully qualified to be worthy members of such an organisation. The chief value of the club, in fact, would be that it would constitute and present an ideal to the people, especially to the children, and inspire them to live lives in consonance with Natural and Divine laws, intended to give man from the beginning of the world a body so perfectly balanced in its physical strength as to be successfully resistant to disease in any and every form. In other words, every child would look with admiration and envy towards those whose perfect health and physique enabled them to claim membership of the Blue-Blood Club, and would be inspired to hope and strive one day to join its exclusive ranks.

But, in the meantime, the practical example of the few will be infinitely better than precept and theory. There is no reason to-day why any man or woman should have a 50 per cent, physical body when he or she can have a 100 per cent. one. Look at the splendid types of men, women and children photographically depicted in this book. Most of these are types of normal men and women who have taken the trouble to make their bodies symmetrical and strong in such perfect balance as to be disease-free. Everyone can do the same and should do so, notwithstanding our present abridged and amputated educational methods by which our educational authorities hope, in some way, to develop. Brobdignagian brains on Liliputian bodies.

In fact, to encourage the thousands who will fit themselves to join such a body as the Blue-Blood Club, it is my intention to create also the rank of Associates, so that even those in humble circumstances can stand in equal rank with the fully-qualified members of this most exclusive club, as Associates, provided they can qualify physically. For, in both cases, the qualifying tests will be the same, and Members and Associates will alike occupy a unique position in the eyes of the world as men of impeccable physique and constitution, and pre-eminent above their fellow-men in every physical sense.

This is what every man and woman should strive to be, and this is an especial reason why every reader of this book should, in the first place, become a member of the All-for-Health League, and induce his or her friends, relations and acquaintances to do so also. The objects of the League are such that they will insensibly fit men and women to take their proper place in this true nobility based on the primitive physical grandeur of man, smoothed, embellished and adorned by all the mental refinements and moral improvements that humanity has admittedly gained through civilisation, but too often at the price of those mighty muscles and the sinews of steel with which men once waged unceasing war against his savage enemies in primitive jungle and forest. To-day, I say it is possible for every man and woman to once more regain that muscular grandeur and inviolable health, superadded to the mental and moral glories of modern civilised life.

The high physical standard essential to qualify for membership or association at first may naturally limit the number of those able to join so exclusive an organisation, but membership of or association with such an organisation will mean so much, setting, as it were, the seal and crown on a man's or a woman's health and physical ambition and attainments, that thousands of Leagueites will, I am confident, soon fit themselves in every way to qualify for admission into the magic circle, the innermost temple into which only those who have attained to the highest possible standard of physical worth and excellence can ever hope to obtain admission. However, no matter how many or how few are able to qualify at the outset, the Blue-Blood Club will be formed, and will certainly take rank as the ideal club to which every right-thinking man and woman should belong, or, at least, strive to belong to.

It is intended, as soon as the Roll of Membership justifies it, to provide members with a club-house that will transcend everything of its kind in any part of the world, a real Temple of Health, externally and internally, a worthy habitation for the men and women who shall make it their place of rendezvous. It has long been a dream of mine to see such an establishment and institution erected in this great metropolis of the world, and with the encouragement and support I have so far received, there is every prospect of my dream coming true.

Architecturally, the intention is to have it modelled on the most classic lines, a worthy rival to the architectural and artistic glories of Rome, Florence and Venice. Wide, capacious corridors, galleries and rooms shall be turned into veritable art galleries, with statues and pictures of ancient heroes and heroines, and the mural decorations will be in harmony with the motives and ideals animating the members of such an organisation. Capacious exercising halls with all the most modern devices and apparata to keep the body in its highest state of physical excellence, swimming baths vying with those of Rome in its historic days, hygienic baths of every kind, and every convenience and comfort that can appeal to those who wish to maintain the body in an almost regal dignity as it should and ought always be maintained are to be provided, and the club will be one in every way of which even the most perfect type of men and women may well be proud to claim membership. The intention is at present to provide every modern accommodation and convenience for those who worship at the shrine of Hygeia.

My conception of the All-for-Health League is a world-organisation on as big lines and as powerful in its own way as the Masonic institution, the Blue-Blood Club occupying a position akin to the Grand Lodge of Freemasonry. In the League itself, clubs or branches of the Blue-Blood Club will be formed, in which members and associates unfit, in the high physical sense necessary to qualify for a Club representing the Grand Lodge of the new Order of Health, will be able to prepare and fit themselves for that position. These clubs will, to all intents and purposes, be forerunners and miniatures of the Blue-Blood Club itself, and will be known as All- for-Health Clubs, which I hope and confidently expect to see springing up in every city, town, and village of the United Kingdom, and, indeed, throughout the world Men and women physically unfit to pass the Blue-Blood standards of health and fitness would be initiated into these clubs just as men are initiated into Masonic Lodges, and would then be enabled to pass through various " degrees," or stages, until finally physically fitted to enter the Blue- Blood Club itself as Members or Associates. With such a lever as this we could, to use a famous expression, move the world.

Our purpose as our ideals will be high, to elevate the physical standard of the people, to safeguard and assist the children to enforce that intelligent and active interest of the State in all matters pertaining to health, physical training, housing, the feeding of the children, etc., and to lead mankind at last to a diseaseless world by living lives in strict conformity with the natural law of life, the law of movement.

It is, of course, only possible at present to give the barest outline of what we will be able to achieve when once this great Freemasonry of Health is organised and established. We can safely reckon on the support of that mighty agent of publicity, the Press, which already shows its eagerness to give its potent aid to every movement that makes for the health and efficiency of the people. But individual effort will also count for much, and I want everyone who is interested, no matter in what part of the world they may live, to enlist for service in this great work, and to use his or her influence in every way to help the good cause. In such a work everyone can bring something to the common good, and the humblest can stand side-by side with the wealthiest in this truly democratic army that will wage relentless war against disease, and everything that tends to be productive of disease or arises from the presence in our midst of this common enemy of mankind.

Those who are anxious to serve should communicate, in the first place, with the Secretary of the All-for-Health League, when they will receive a programme of our ideals, plans and arrangements and' a card of membership, as soon as organisation is completed. Those who join will not only derive health benefit themselves but will also be expected to preach and practise the gospel of health, physical fitness and freedom from disease, at every opportunity, to set an example to others of hygienic and cleanly living, and to inspire in all, but especially in the rising generation, the same ardent enthusiasm for whatsoever is noble, whatsoever is good and whatsoever is right for that body which is, or ought to be, the temple of the [human soul. This is a Gospel that the world is much in need of to-day, and I look to our future members or helpers, in however humble a capacity, to do their best to spread it broadcast whenever and wherever they can.

If we can only implant in the children the stimulating ideal of physical beauty and its inseparable companion, health, and arouse the spirit of emulation that now fills them when they seek victory in some form of sport or in some mental examination, a needed impetus will begin to a phase of education and culture that has not yet been approached in the right way. I want to fire the youthful mind with the keen zest for physical well-being with which a boy strives to become a good football player or a girl to excel at tennis. These sports, after all, can never give a boy or girl the perfectly balanced strength that will give him or her a body beautiful and strong, a body, too, able by its very strength to resist and defeat disease.

If the children themselves are given an intelligent interest in their own wonderful bodies they will enter into their physical education with vim, enthusiasm and determination. It is no use to sow seed on soil completely unprepared for it. The children must be taught to admire, covet and strive for a body as perfect as that of an Apollo or an Adonis, and to feel ashamed to remain otherwise. This is what I mean when I speak of giving the children a new ideal. Physical education and bodily reconstruction must not be allowed to be regarded as a task like mastering the Pons Asinorum or conjugating the verbs of a dead language. The subject should be vivified by splendid pictures, sculpture and stories of the great men of bye- gone days, and the children should be so educated that they will- come to regard weakness and disease as things of which they must- feel ashamed. Physical strength and beauty are things that will iriake a powerful appeal to children so long as the lessons are not permitted to become a bore, and the breath of life is breathed into the dry bones of anatomy and physiology. The child should have its natural spirit of emulation turned into a healthy and desirable channel instead of too often being frittered away on useless and even undesirable achievements.

A modification of the training of Spartan children, omitting its ugly and repellent features, might be adopted. Every boy should be- taught to aim and strive only for that which is manly, to shrink from physical weakness and cowardice, to regard disease almost as a sin against his Creator. Each girl, too, should be inspired by the heroic women of the past with a healthy ambition to become I a perfect woman nobly planned." If we do this, and persist along these lines, the seed sown will assuredly fall on fruitful ground.

In the meantime all who can will, I hope, send their names along for membership of the All-for-Health League, or, if they feel that they already possess a sufficiently high organic and physical standard, should apply to become members or associates of the Blue- Blood Club. The Blue-Blood Club, and its contributory clubs, will all be affiliated to the All-for-Health League in one great masonic brotherhood throughout the world, modelled on much similar lines to that other world-famous organisation, and to belong to any of these organisations will be a passport to friendship everywhere throughout the world, and in itself a guarantee that will ensure a welcome from all who admire and respect high thinking and clean living. It will constitute a real brotherhood and freemasonry based on self- respect, physical as well as mental, which alone can ensure life on that grand plane which is essential before we can enter into the new and promised land where disease shall cease from troubling and men and women be at rest from such unnecessary pain and suffering.

Much depends, as I have said, on my readers in beginning, carrying on and helping forward in this splendid work. Many of them will have done the State some service already during the tempestuous days through which we have just passed. Those that have volunteered and risked life and limb to defeat one enemy of the nation will, I am sure, be only too ready to volunteer for service in a less dangerous but quite as necessary a war against a far more malignant and treacherous foe, physical deterioration and disease.

Some of them may have been left scarred and wounded and bruised after fighting for home and kith and kin. They have suffered them-selves, and, alas, too often the children that come after them will also have to bear their cross also.

But, in the new crusade against weakness and disease they will be benefiting themselves and their children, !and their children's children will also reap a harvest of health. Those who join these All-for-Health Clubs, and strive, even if they never succeed, to qualify for membership of the Blue-Blood Club, will, at least, have their reward in the possession of a better and healthier body, of a far higher type in every physical sense, and will be able to offer and bequeath to their children an estate that the money of a million millionaires could never buy.

Let all who can come forward now, and, as a famous martyr once said, " we will light a candle that will never be extinguished." All they are asked to do, in the first place, is to send along their names and address to The Secretary, The All-for-Health League, 67, Jermyn Street, London, S.W. 1., and full particulars, with card of membership, will be sent to them as soon as organisation is completed.

Only by these methods here advocated may we, in accordance with the natural law of evolution, hope to raise mankind from the low estate of physical deterioration into which so great a mass of it has fallen or been driven by cruel circumstance. Fortunately, there are already in our midst many who have either attained and maintained a high degree of physical, organic and constitutional excellence that will enable them to qualify for membership in the world's pioneer Blue-Blood Club, or become Associates, and all who desire to do so should send along their names and addresses to The Secretary, who will be very pleased to send them all further particulars, as soon as arrangements at present in hand are completed. Application to join as Members or Associates should, in the first instance, be addressed to The Secretary, The Blue-Blood Club, 67, Jermyn Street, London, S.W. 1.

In this way, it is hoped that we will set a new fashion and standard for all, so that out of our present decadent state " a loftier race than e'er the world has known may yet arise." It is to that end that all my efforts aim, and I look with every confidence to the people themselves to rally round and accord this movement their hearty support at a time when the physical reconstruction and regeneration of the people is, above all things else, the first and most important step in national and, indeed, international reconstruction.

Printed in Great
Britain
by Amazon